Proceedings of the International Symposium on Medroxyprogesterone Acetate

Geneva, Switzerland, February 24–26, 1982

Editors:
F. Cavalli
W.L. McGuire
F. Pannuti
A. Pellegrini
G. Robustelli Della Cuna

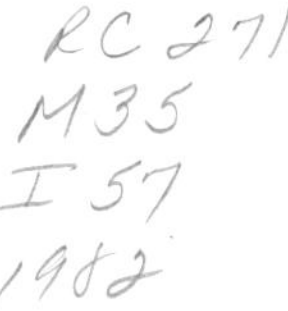

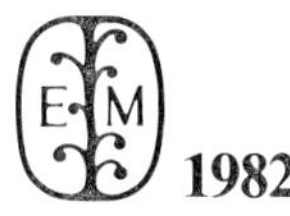

1982
Excerpta Medica
Amsterdam-Oxford-Princeton

International Congress Series No. 611
ISBN Excerpta Medica 90 219 9560 3
ISBN Elsevier Science Publishing Co., Inc. 0 444 90297 X

Publisher:
Excerpta Medica
305 Keizersgracht
1000 BC Amsterdam
P.O. Box 1126

Sole Distributors for the USA and Canada:
Elsevier Science Publishing Co., Inc.
52 Vanderbilt Avenue
New York, NY 10017

Printed in The Netherlands by Casparie, Amsterdam.

Contents

Opening remarks

As a local oncologist, it is my particular pleasure to open this meeting and to welcome you all – participants, organizers and sponsors – to Geneva for this international conference on medroxyprogesterone acetate. I know that your time will be much taken up with the meeting, but I do hope that you will find a few minutes, or perhaps a few hours, for a short walk along the lake or in the streets of the old town, so that your short stay in Geneva will not only be useful but also pleasant.

Geneva has always been – and I believe still is – a place where leading people of the world like to live and to spend as much time as they can; Calvin, Voltaire, Einstein and Lenin all spent a major part of their active life in Geneva. I hope that this particular spirit of Geneva will pervade the next few days and allow us to have a rich, pleasant and useful meeting.

Medroxyprogesterone acetate is an old drug and was probably one of the first agents used in the treatment of cancer. However, despite its long use, its place and usefulness in the treatment of breast cancer is still not completely understood. A major contribution to oncology was made when Professor Pannuti, of Bologna, showed and explained that medroxyprogesterone acetate used at high dose has a particular place in the treatment of different malignancies, and especially in the treatment of breast cancer. Although this problem is not completely solved, I hope we will find a few more answers during this meeting.

I wish you all a pleasant stay in Geneva, and a great success to the Congress.

Professor P. Alberto,
Division d'Onco-Hématologie,
Hôpital Cantonal,
Genève,
Switzerland

It is a great pleasure for me to attend this symposium, representing the UICC. Meetings such as this, to discuss, in depth the different aspects of a limited subject, are a real need in order to facilitate, among specialists in a given field, the exchange of ideas and discussions of details that are so frequently fundamental to the progress of science. This need is a natural consequence of the tremendous input of new information which is continually being added by research workers all over the world.

On the one hand, we need large meetings with a broad coverage of several fields of specialization, such as the international cancer congresses held every 4 years under the auspices of the UICC, for many important reasons, among which may be mentioned:

1. Education in all its aspects.
2. Promotion of the fight against cancer.
3. Feasibility.
4. Social and scientific contact among participants from several specialties.
5. International collaboration and friendship.
6. A multidisciplinary approach to many problems.

On the other hand, such enormous meetings are no longer sufficient to satisfy the needs of the sophisticated specialist who wants to develop as much as possible in his own limited field and to find the answers to his problems.

As a world organization with continuously growing activities, and a privileged international position, the UICC is expanding its activities in many directions. One of these is collaboration with international and regional organizations in order to co-ordinate activities, to join efforts, in order to get greater efficiency and avoid duplication and overlapping in some fields. Along these lines, the UICC is also promoting, supporting and participating in international meetings such as this.

Hormones play an important, complex and, in many aspects, until now, unclear role in human biology. These facts are reflected in their use in the treatment of cancer. Results (in some cases, very favourable ones with complete response in a proportion of cases) are seen frequently by those who use these drugs, attesting to their importance even if many aspects of why, when and how they produce results, remain obscure. However, progress is being made continuously, clarifying little by little these obscurities and, what may be of more significance, expanding the field of tumours susceptible to hormonal manipulation. A typical way of this may be found in the progestogens, and more than justifies the efforts of Farmitalia Carlo Erba in organizing and holding this symposium.

Medroxyprogesterone acetate is a very interesting substance whose antineoplastic action in endometrial and breast cancer has been known for many years. Numerous studies recently conducted in the fields of experimental and clinical pharmacology, pharmacokinetics, mechanism of action, immune and hormone modulation, influence of receptors as well as schedules of treatment and combination with cytotoxic agents have shown a great potential which is already being explored, with good results in some instances.

Interesting studies already demonstrate possible responses in tumors of the prostate, ovary and kidney.

The presentation and discussion of the most recent findings in these fields by a select group of outstanding specialists is the purpose of this meeting. The careful planning, the list of invited speakers and topics to be discussed during the meeting serve as a guarantee of success.

On behalf of the UICC, it is with great pleasure that I congratulate the organizers of this symposium and extend a warm welcome to all the invited speakers and participants.

Professor A.C. Junqueira,
Hospital Santa Cruz,
São Paulo,
Brasil

I am very pleased to add a few words to the opening remarks of Professors Alberto and Junqueira during this opening session. I am here in the double role of scientific secretary of the symposium and also as a representative of Farmitalia Carlo Erba which has been pleased to sponsor this meeting.

As the scientific secretary, I have tried, with the help and collaboration of the Advisory Board, to build up a programme which would provide us with a really up-to-date description of the experimental and clinical profile of this drug. On Friday, at the end of the symposium, we will be able to see whether that target has been reached. Tonight, I am very optimistic, for several reasons. First, the number of speakers who accepted our invitation has been very high, and it includes almost all the investigators who have a direct and large experience with this drug at both the experimental and the clinical levels.

Secondly, the attitude of all the contributors was positive, so that it has been possible to obtain and print in advance before the symposium the abstracts of all the papers, some of which will be presented as posters.

Finally, it has been possible to integrate the presentation of the most recent results of various investigators in round table discussions on specific topics, which will certainly favour an interesting discussion among the experts and the audience.

As a representative of Farmitalia Carlo Erba, first of all I would like to thank everyone who has contributed to the organization of the symposium. I would also like to express our deep gratitude to Professor Alberto who has agreed to be with us and to open the symposium. Professor Junqueira is not only an old friend but he is here also as the official representative of the UICC. The sponsorship of the UICC has been greatly appreciated, and certainly this sponsorship underlines the scientific importance of the meeting.

As both Professor Alberto and Professor Junqueira have said earlier, chronologically speaking, medroxyprogesterone acetate may be considered as an old drug; it was synthesized in the Farmitalia laboratories in 1958. More recently, however, through active clinical research on new dosage schedules – research carried out first in Italy and then in many other countries – it has been possible to identify a new role for medroxyprogesterone acetate in the modern treatment modalities.

As you know, Farmitalia Carlo Erba has been – and still is – involved mainly in anthracycline research, but the increasing interest in medroxyprogesterone acetate (and, in a broader sense, in hormonal therapy) testifies to our intention and to our willingness to follow a multidisciplinary approach (also at the level of industrial research) in line with progress in the oncological field. Thus, I hope that in the next two days this symposium may allow us not only to update the present knowledge of medroxyprogesterone acetate but also give us an opportunity to discuss, in a friendly and relaxed atmosphere, the more general problems concerning the management of hormone-dependent tumours.

Professor C. Praga,
International Division,
Medical Department,
Farmitalia Carlo Erba,
Milano,
Italy

High-dose medroxyprogesterone acetate in oncology. History, clinical use and pharmacokinetics

F. Pannuti[1], A. Martoni[1], C.M. Camaggi[2], E. Strocchi[1], A.R. Di Marco[1], A.P. Rossi[1], L. Tomasi[1], M. Giovannini[1], A. Cricca[1], F. Fruet[1], G. Lelli[1], M.E. Giambiasi[1] and N. Canova[1]

[1]*Divisione di Oncologia, Ospedale M. Malpighi, Bologna; and* [2]*Istituto di Chimica Organica, Università degli Studi, Bologna, Italy*

Introduction

Medroxyprogesterone acetate (MPA) was first synthesized by Babcock et al. [1] and Sala et al. [2], independently (Fig. 1). Its progestogenic activity became evident soon after. In the original papers of Babcock et al. it was, in fact, described as the most active progestational agent so far discovered.

Several published papers support this description, in respect to both animals [3, 4] and man [5].

Macromolecular components of normal human mammary cytosol which bind ^{3}H-labelled MPA in vitro have been largely characterized [6]. These components show a strong affinity for progestins, and are most likely the progesterone receptors of human mammary tissue.

From the clinical point of view, the progestational activity of MPA is clearly shown by delay in menstruation [7, 8], inhibition of ovulation [9], changes in cervical secretion [10], changes in the vaginal karyopyknotic index, and endometrial deposition of glycogen [5]. The active progestogenic dose is well below the doses found useful in the treatment of breast cancer.

At the beginning of 1972, we in Bologna started administering MPA intramuscularly (i.m.) at higher doses than the 100 mg/day traditionally used, to determine the maximum tolerated dose [11].

The results obtained suggested that the increase of dosages given to patients with hormone-sensitive tumours had resulted in significant antitumour activity, and a noticeable improvement in their general condition, especially as regards pain [12].

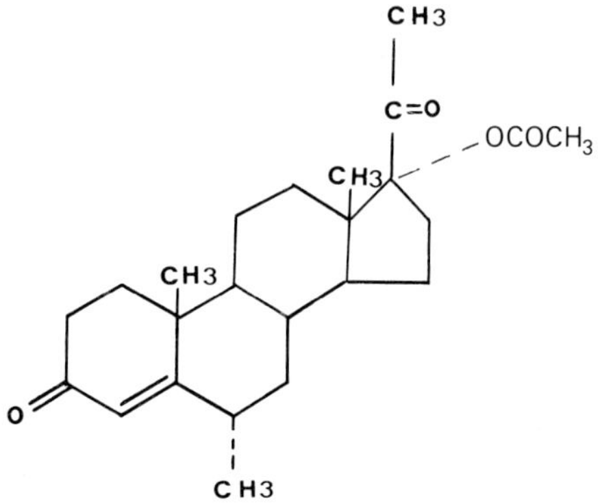

Fig. 1. *6α-Methyl-17α-acetoxyprogesterone (medroxyprogesterone acetate, MPA).*

The effects were particularly apparent in patients with metastatic breast cancer. Further work with high-dose MPA in such patients confirmed that at doses of ≥ 500 mg/day the highest remission rates possible with endocrine treatment could be achieved. These rates could not be obtained using lower doses [13]. Subsequently, we demonstrated that high doses could also be given orally (p.o.), and that tolerance was excellent [14].

In Pavia, Robustelli Della Cuna et al. carried out a very well-designed study on high-dose MPA, which confirmed our results [15].

Other Italian investigators such as Pellegrini et al. [16], Amadori et al. [17], De Lena et al. [18] and Mussa et al. [19] obtained similar results, leaving aside a few differences resulting from different circumstances.

Mattsson, in 1978, was the first non-Italian investigator to confirm the significant antitumour activity of MPA at high doses [20]. Subsequently, Mendiola et al. [21], Madrigal et al. [22], Izuo et al. [23] and Becher et al. [24], reported results similar to ours, and a prospective controlled study by Cavalli et al. has recently demonstrated convincingly that high doses are more efficacious than low doses [25].

In other malignancies, such as endometrial carcinoma and renal carcinoma, in which progestogenic therapy is indicated, no conclusive data regarding the use of MPA at high doses are yet available. There have been encouraging results in relation to treatment with high-dose MPA in prostatic cancer, and in melanoma.

Hormonal interference

The idea of hormone dependence of tumours is based on the experimental and clinical observations of Huggins et al. showing that the metabolism and proliferation of tumour cells, like those of the normal cells from which they originate, depend on the activity of one or more hormones [26].

Tagnon et al. [27] suggested that the term 'hormone sensitivity' rather than hormone dependence should be used. Breast cancer cells do not, for example, necessarily depend on the effects of a single hormone, but may be sensitive to such a hormone, or to several hormones. We distinguish between absolute hormone sensitivity (sensitivity to all hormones, regardless of dose) and relative sensitivity (sensitivity to one or more hormones, or varying sensitivity to different doses of the same hormone).

The classification of hormone therapy as additive or ablative is a simplification, but on the other hand, is an approximate and too schematic an approach to cancer patients.

Ovariectomy, for instance, results in cessation of ovarian hormone production, but the consequent hyperproduction of the relevant pituitary gonadotropins is unavoidable. It is also known that the adrenal glands can start compensatory production of sex hormones, under such circumstances.

Surgery can therefore result in both the interruption of secretion of hormones which can affect the development and proliferation of uterine tumour cells and new secretion of such hormones.

The administration of hormones such as progestins which, in itself, increases hormone levels, can also inhibit the secretion of hormones (ovarian, pituitary and, possibly, adrenal) thus bringing about effects opposite to their intrinsic effects.

The problem is even more complex, however. Some hormones can exert a pharmacological effect on the host, but can also alter the relationships between the tumour and the organism. These overall effects may result in marked objective and subjective improvement. Such hormones can significantly influence the evolution of neoplastic disease considered not only as the manifestation of a pool of proliferating atypical cells, but also as a clinical situation in which relationships between tumour cells and the host overall play a major role.

It is for this reason that we have introduced the term 'hormonal interference', having the oncological significance indicated above, in addition to the term hormone sensitivity. While the latter emphasizes the possibility of response to hormone therapy independent of problems in relation to the direction of this response, the nature of the hormones or the doses used, the term 'hormone interference' shifts attention from the tumour cell to the pharmacological use of the hormone. The aim of this approach is:

1. To highlight the complexities of hormone therapy.

2. To highlight the possibility that there may be interference in the kinetics of tumour cells, independent of the direction of hormonal action.
3. To emphasize that hormones affect both the course of neoplastic disease, and its wider clinical repercussions, i.e. relationships between tumour and host.

MPA and hormone interference

Figure 2 shows the effects of MPA on human endocrine balance, as recorded in the literature, and in relation to our own findings (Table I). The results obtained by the various investigators are in good agreement, and basically coincide with findings in animal studies [35, 36].

Pituitary gonadotropins appear to be inhibited, 17β-oestradiol, testosterone, ACTH and hydrocortisone levels decrease, triiodothyronine (T_3) and thyroxine (T_4) levels fall, and levels of thyroid-stimulating hormone (TSH) rise. Prolactin levels show no change, growth hormone (GH) levels either remain stationary or increase, and insulin levels increase, in animals.

These effects may be due to the influence of MPA on hormone production, but an effect on hormone metabolism has also been demonstrated.

Circulating oestrogen levels are, in fact, reduced, as a result of both inhibition of follicle-stimulating hormone (FSH) and enzymatic induction of hepatic reductase, resulting in increased clearance of testosterone, and consequent decreased conversion of androgens to oestrogens [37, 38]. In addition, MPA induces synthesis of oestradiol-dehydrogenase in the cytoplasms of

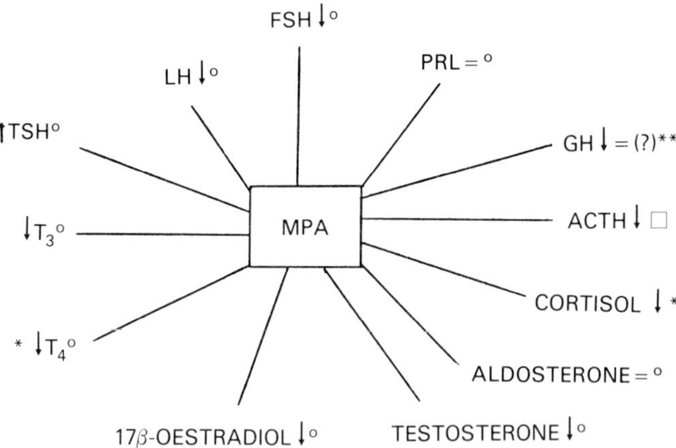

*Fig. 2. MPA: hormonal interference in man (°[33,34], *[30–32], **[28,31], □[29,32].*

Table I. Effect of high doses of MPA on hormone plasma levels in postmenopausal patients.

Hormone	T3	T4	TSH	LH	FSH
Numbers of patients	20	20	20	17	17
Normal values	0.6/1.7 ng	45/110 ng	0.5/4 ng	> 50 mIU	> 50 mIU
Means, before/after	1.3/0.96	83.3/60.3	2.25/3.33	49.17/13.17	47.52/13.58
Standard deviation (mean difference)	−0.47	−28.29	+2.34	−28.85	−32.12
t value	3.15	3.63	2.06	5.14	4.35
P	< 0.01	< 0.01	< 0.05	< 0.01	< 0.01
Hormone	**PRL**	**E_2**	**T**	**ALD I[1]**	**ALD II[2]**
Numbers of patients	15	16	17	12	12
Normal values	5/18 ng	20/60 ng	230/570 pg	30/100 pg	100/300 pg
Means, before/after	18.40/ 19.46	65.15/ 42.11	540.11/ 272.47	147.0/ 129.58	230.16/ 245.9
Standard deviation (mean difference)	−29.37	−32.54	435.57	−72.22	−159.83
t value	0.14	2.83	2.53	0.83	0.34
P	NS[3]	< 0.05	< 0.02	NS[3]	NS[3]

[1]ALD I = aldosterone – patients in orthostatism; [2]ALD II = aldosterone – patients in clinostatism; [3]NS = not significant.

target cells, resulting in increased conversion of oestradiol to oestrone, with a reduction in availability of oestradiol within the cell, as a consequence [39].

MPA also interferes with hormone action on target cells. It has a high affinity for progesterone receptors [5, 6] and, to some extent, also for glucocorticoid receptors [40]. It is also known that MPA reduces 17β-oestradiol binding to its own receptor [41, 42].

Such interference in hormone production and metabolism, and in hormone/hormone receptor interactions, together with a possible nonspecific, direct action, result in target cell damage.

MPA antitumour action

The actual mechanism of the antitumour action of MPA is still under debate. It is accepted that there is interference with both the production and metabolism of hormones. Suppression of the hypothalamic-hypophyseal axis is of course of fundamental relevance.

The cellular basis of the activity of MPA is probably the result of inhibition of mitosis, via a receptor-mediated mechanism. In-vitro studies on experimental mammary tumours of different hormonal sensitivities have shown the role played by specific cytoplasmic receptors in the tumour cells.

MPA is not active against C3H mammary carcinoma, a hormone-independent tumour, and it does not improve the activity of doxorubicin. With the hormone-responsive 13–762 mammary adenocarcinoma, MPA delays tumour onset, and improves doxorubicin activity when the 2 drugs are given together [43]. MPA inhibits ^{3}H-thymidine incorporation, mitotic index and progesterone and oestradiol binding in MCF-7 cells [44].

Iacobelli had recently obtained a variant MCF-7 cell line, designated CG-5, which is highly oestrogen-responsive [45]. The addition of MPA produces a dose-related inhibition of CG-5 proliferation, beginning at hormone concentrations as low as 10^{-10} M.

On the other hand, MPA effects (at doses of 24 or 120 mg/day, i.m.) on dimethylbenzanthracene (DMBA)-induced mammary cancer in rats, have recently been claimed to be similar, regardless of the presence or absence of cytoplasmic oestrogen receptors in the tumours [46]. There would seem to be another endocrinological tumour-suppressing mechanism, apart from the mechanism involving the oestrogen receptor system, in the case of high-dose MPA administration.

MPA toxicity: preclinical studies

The acute toxicity of MPA has proved to be very low. In rats and mice, the LD50 exceeded 10 g/kg, when MPA was administered subcutaneously [47].

Chronic daily doses of up to 15 mg/kg, administered parenterally, do not produce toxic effects in rats. Daily doses of 100–400 mg/kg for 30 days induce severe local reactions, as a result of the accumulation of unabsorbed material [47], together with rapid deterioration in general condition, probably because of resorption of necrotic products.

All animal species exhibit more or less marked signs of liver toxicity (fatty infiltration, cloudy vacuolar infiltration, periportal lesions, cytoplasmic clarification, cloudy hepatosis and glycogen infiltration). These signs are more apparent at high dose levels.

We should like to draw attention to some effects seen following MPA administration which will also be reviewed in the clinical section, namely leukopenia (mainly lymphocytic) and increase in haemoglobin levels in females (both dose-related), increase in body weight in all females treated, and the increase in food intake in all females (not dose-related).

MPA toxicity: clinical studies

Since the early 1960's, MPA has been administered clinically, both p.o. and i.m., at various dosages, but it was only in the 1970's that a dosage of 500 mg/day was exceeded. This is now considered as the boundary between low- and high-dose MPA therapy. The dose limitation had no toxicological justification (see below).

Low-dose MPA showed no side-effects. Between 1972 and 1974, we demonstrated that higher doses could be used. The highest tolerable i.m. dose was 1,500 mg [11]. The occurrence of gluteal abscesses limited the possibility of increasing the i.m. dosage. In our first group of 52 patients with advanced breast cancer, we used 1,500 mg of MPA/day for 30 days at a concentration of 50 mg/ml. Gluteal abscesses were seen in 17 patients (33%) [13].

At our suggestion, Farmitalia supplied us with MPA at a concentration of 200 mg/ml. Using this preparation, we treated 25 patients at a dosage of 2,000 mg/day and recorded 2 cases of gluteal abscess (8%), and 4 cases of infiltration (17%) [48].

More recently, the incidence of gluteal abscess has been further reduced (Table II) through the use of MPA at higher concentrations, and greater accuracy in administration. The incidence of gluteal abscess is now very low.

An interesting, and potentially useful, side-effect of MPA is an increase

Table II. Incidences of gluteal abscess in advanced cancer patients treated with high doses of MPA, 1972 to 1981 (numbers of cases/numbers of patients treated (%)).

Dose (mg)	1972–1975*	1976–1978**	1980–1981**
500	—	1/46 (2.2)	0/10 (—)
1,000	—	—	0/18 (—)
1,500	17/54 (31.5)	7/46 (15.2)	0/5 (—)
2,000	—	2/25 (8)	1/9 (11)
Total	17/54 (31.5)	10/117 (8.5)	1/42 (2.4)

* MPA 50 mg/ml.
**MPA 200 mg/ml.

Table III. High-dose MPA therapy. Statistically significant variations in haemato-chemical parameters after one month of treatment.

	Intramuscular administration (mg)			Oral administration (mg)	
	500	1,500	2,000	2,000	3,000–5,000
White blood cell count	↑	↑	↑	↑	↑
Lymphocytes		=		=	
Neutrophils		↑		↑	
Red blood cell count	=	=	=	=	=
Platelets	=	↑	↑	=	=
Alkaline phosphatase	=	=	↓	=	=
Serum glutamic oxalo-acetic transaminase	=	=	=	=	
Bilirubin	=	=	=	=	=
Blood urea nitrogen	↓	=	=	=	↑
Creatinine	=	=	=	=	=
Uric acid	=	↓	=	=	=
Glucose	=	=	=	↓	=
Cholesterol	=	=	=	=	=
Total protein	↑	=	=	=	=
Albumin		↓	↓		
α_2 Globulin		↑	↑		
(α_1, β γ Globulin)		=	=		
Ca	=	=	=	=	=
P	=	=	=	=	=
K	=	↑	↑		
Na	=	=	=		

↑: Mean increase within normal values; ↓: Mean decrease within normal values; =: No change.

(mean 1,480/mm^3) in white blood cell count (Table III), observed during both i.m. and p.o. treatment, which corresponds with the myeloprotective effect demonstrated by Robustelli della Cuna and ourselves.

During recent pharmacokinetic work, we have observed that the increase in white blood cell count is related to MPA bioavailability rather than to the route of administration. In cases where bioavailability of MPA is high, a higher, statistically significant, increase ($P < 0.01$) in white blood cell count (mean 2,120/mm^3) has been observed.

Table III records the behaviour of some haematochemical parameters following a 30-day course of various p.o. and i.m. dosages of MPA. As pointed out before, an increase in white blood cells which seems to favour neutrophils were recorded at all dosages and by both routes of administration.

Table IV. High-dose MPA. Side-effects in percentages (excluding gluteal abscess (see Table II).

	Intramuscular administration (186 patients)	Oral administration (110 patients)
Sweating	11	14
Vaginal spotting	11	9
Moon face	11	3
Fine tremors	10	16
Cramps	8	6
Insomnia	1	3
Constipation	0.5	4
Itching	0.5	2
Thrombophlebitis	0.5	—
Gastric intolerance	—	4
Anorexia	—	2

In addition, platelet counts, and plasma potassium and α-globulin levels increased with the highest i.m. doses used. Kidney and liver functions were unaffected, except that total protein rose in the case of the 500-mg dosage.

Table IV records clinical side-effects (not gluteal abscess, which has been already discussed) during high-dose i.m. and p.o. MPA in our studies.

In a pilot study, we treated 30 patients with massive daily doses of MPA (3,000, 4,000 or 5,000 mg) orally. Side-effects occurred with the same frequency and to the same degree as after doses of 2,000 mg.

On the basis of our experience, and that of other investigators, it can be assumed that MPA is very well tolerated, and that, with the doses so far used, no clear-cut toxicological profile emerges.

Among the side-effects of MPA, the increase in body weight and in white blood cell counts, far from being detrimental, might form the object of treatment with MPA at high doses, in some cases of cancer.

Effect of MPA therapy on pain

Ever since hormone therapy was first used, it has been recognized that, in some cases of hormone-sensitive tumours, remission of pain can result from treatment.

In advanced breast cancer, MPA at a mean dose of 100 mg/day, p.o. or i.m., has been found to relieve pain in about 21% of cases, on average [51, 52].

When we began using high-dose MPA, we noticed that, even before objective remission became apparent, treatment could induce rapid, subjective remission, and strong analgesic effects.

MPA at a dosage of 1,500 mg/day i.m., for 30 days, in 54 patients with advanced breast cancer, resulted in distinct relief of pain, even after one week, and the relief became more evident as treatment continued [48].

The analgesic effect was particularly marked in patients with well-advanced disease and bone metastases, bedridden, and considered no longer susceptible to chemotherapy.

In connection with the analgesic effect we recorded improvement of walking impairment in 63% of cases. Walking impairment was considered as a symptom related to the presence of neoplastic bone involvement.

We still remember with enthusiasm, those early 1970's when, for the first time, we saw patients who had been bedridden for months, who were in pain, and who were considered incurable, resume walking, free of pain.

The first group treated by us had a 43% objective remission rate (complete response (CR) or partial response (PR)) lasting for 7 months, on average. The mean duration of pain remission was 6 months. Significant pain subsequently tended to recur.

When this happened, 23 patients from this group were again treated with MPA, at higher dosages (2,000 mg/day, i.m., for 30 days). This treatment resulted in pain remission in 21 cases (91%). The objective response rate was 18% [12].

Overall, our breast cancer patients treated with MPA at high doses showed a 65% incidence of pain relief. Pain was relieved in 78% of cases when MPA was administered i.m., and in 49% of cases when MPA was administered p.o. ($P < 0.001$).

A 78% analgesic response is similar to that attained with hypophysectomy, but MPA treatment is less traumatic, and has different side-effects.

Our findings on the analgesic effect of MPA in breast cancer have been confirmed by other investigators [15, 17, 53].

Our experience with other hormone-sensitive tumours is more limited. In advanced prostatic cancer, the use of MPA at high doses gave pain remission in 10/10 cases [54]. We obtained 5 remissions in 12 cases of clear cell renal carcinoma [55].

The above-mentioned findings raise the question of whether the analgesic effect of MPA is closely related to its antitumour effect, or whether a mechanism of action which is at least partially unrelated should be supposed.

This question was studied in a trial in which patients with far advanced, hormone sensitive tumours (HST) or hormone insensitive tumours (HIT) were treated orally with 2,000 mg/day for 30 days. Pain relief occurred in 65% (17/26) of cases of HST and in 43% (16/37) of cases of HIT [56]. This result is highly interesting and suggests new ways of using MPA.

Anabolic effect of MPA

Ever since starting work with MPA at high doses in the treatment of breast cancer, we have noticed a side-effect useful in neoplastic patients, namely, increase in body weight, associated with better appetite and improved performance status.

In patients with advanced breast cancer treated with high doses of MPA, increase in body weight occurred in 50% of cases, improvement of appetite in 71%, and reduction of asthenia in 57%. The objective response rate was 41%.

Two questions arise from these observations:

1. Is the increase in body weight related to the antitumour activity of the drug, or independent of it?
2. Is the increase in body weight the result of either anabolic activity, or a steroid-like effect?

The first question was analysed in a study in which a 30-day course of MPA at a dose of 2,000 mg/day orally, was administered to patients with very advanced HST or HIT. Improvement in anorexia occurred in 49% (37/76) of HST cases and in 62% (40/65) of HIT cases. Improvement in body weight (increase $\geq$ 0.5 kg) occurred in 57% (37/65) of HST cases and 63% (36/57) of HIT cases. Improvement in performance status occurred in 25% (17/67) of HST cases, and in 46% (24/52) of HIT cases [56]. In both groups of patients, therefore, we recorded improvement in the parameters studied. This indicates that the influence of MPA on these parameters is not related to its direct effect on the tumour.

In order to answer the second question, experiments were carried out in both animals (A) and man (B).

Hershberger's method was used to evaluate the increase of weight of the levator ani muscle in castrated rats [57]. Three to four-week-old Sprague-Dawley rats were randomly subdivided, after castration, into 7 groups of 5 animals each. The control group was given saline solution, and the others received various doses of MPA for 7 days. The animals were killed on the eighth day and the levator ani muscle weighed. Two different routes of administration were tested, p.o. and intraperitoneal (i.p.) (Fig. 3).

Increasing doses of i.p. MPA induced a progressive increase in the weight of the levator ani muscle, as compared to weights in the control group. The increase became significant (Duncan's test) at a dose of 20 mg/kg of MPA,

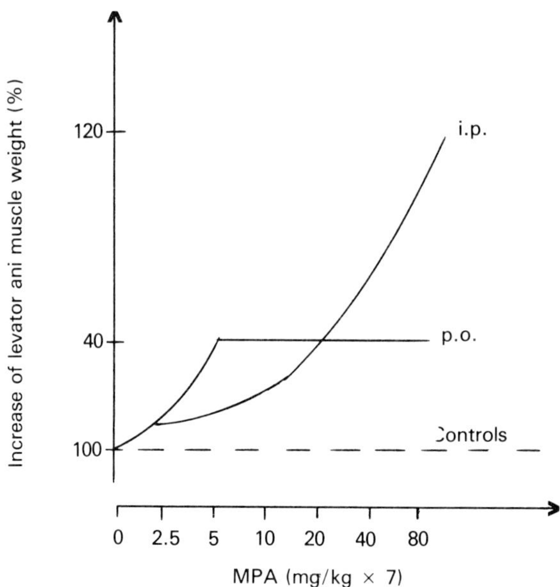

Fig. 3. Anabolic effect of MPA: Hershberger test in rats. Duncan's test: 5 mg → P = 0.05; 20 mg → P = 0.05).

which corresponds to approximately 1,200 mg/day in man. With p.o. MPA, a significant increase in weight was achieved using doses of 5 mg/kg (about 300 mg/day in man). Unlike i.p. MPA, p.o. MPA did not induce increase in weight in proportion to increase in dosage [58].

A trial is at present in progress in which 8 patients with neoplastic cachexia have received high doses of MPA for 30 days.

Before and after treatment, anthropometric parameters (body weight, sum of skin folds, measured using Gershmel's plicometer, lean mass worked out from the sum of the skin folds on the basis of Durnin's tables [59], and elementary strength evaluated using a dynamometer), and metabolic parameters (protein, nitrogen and caloric intakes, determined by means of dietary survey, urinary nitrogen excretion by Kjeldahl's method, and nitrogen balance) were measured. The values for both types of parameter were the averages of data collected 3 days before and 3 days after treatment. The results are shown in Tables V and VI. Elementary strength, protein intake, nitrogen intake and caloric intake all showed significant increases. The increase in nitrogen balance was not significant. If the Steroid Protein Activity Index (SPAI) (Albanese [60]), is positive, an anabolic effect is indicated. MPA gives a SPAI of +28%. Corticosteroids, as is well known, give negative values. For anabolic steroids, the index ranges from +6 to +34%.

Table V. Anabolic effects of high-dose MPA as shown by anthropometric measurements in 8 patients.

	Means		Standard deviation	t value	*P*
	Before	After			
Body weight (kg)	53.45	54.77	2.48	0.94	Not significant
Skinfold thickness (sum) (mm)	27.3	29.5	2.89	2.17	Not significant
Lean body mass (kg)	44.0	44.0	1.94	−0.35	Not significant
Elementary strength (kg)	24.4	22.0	5.43	2.41	0.05

Table VI. Anabolic effect of high-dose MPA as revealed by metabolic parameters in 8 patients.

	Means		Standard deviation	t value	*P*
	Before	After			
Protein intake (g/day)	38.11	60.34	15.56	4.04	< 0.01
Nitrogen intake (I) (g/day)	5.97	9.56	2.50	4.16	< 0.01
Caloric intake (kcal/day)	1,397	2,100	537	3.70	< 0.01
Nitrogen, urinary output (U) (g/day)	5.64	5.38	2.96	1.23	Not significant
Nitrogen balance [B = I − (U + 10%)]	0.67	3.35	3.17	2.35	< 0.05

Advanced endometrial carcinoma

A recent literature review indicates that, on average, advanced endometrial cancer shows a response rate to MPA treatment ranging from 33–44.5% [61]. Well-differentiated tumours are more likely to respond to hormone therapy than poorly-differentiated tumours.

In contrast to breast cancer, endometrial carcinoma seems to respond equally well to either low or high doses of MPA. We are not, however, aware that dosage has ever been investigated systematically, or in controlled studies.

Advanced carcinoma of the prostate

The first use of progestins in prostatic carcinoma dates back to the 1950's, but it was only later that more powerful synthetic compounds, with higher pro-

Table VII. MPA in advanced cancer of the prostate.

	Numbers of investigators	Numbers of patients	Remission rates (%)	
			Objective	Subjective
Low doses (≤ 500 mg/day)	7	224	36	55
High doses (> 500 mg/day)	1	21	19*	95

*More restrictive objective criteria.

gestational activity became available, and led to the wider use of this type of drug.

A review of the literature carried out by us shows that the objective remission rate is, on average, 40–50% [62]. The subjective remission rate is higher.

As to side-effects, the most frequent complaint relating to the injectable preparations is local intolerance. MPA is the most actively studied progestin, as far as mechanisms of action and clinical implications are concerned.

Our experience (Table VII) is similar to that of other investigators, notwithstanding an objective remission slightly lower than those reported elsewhere.

The high subjective response rate (90–100%) observed by us, together with the virtual absence of toxicity, leads us to believe that this drug can also be recommended for use as first-line therapy.

Advanced clear cell renal carcinoma

The rationale for hormonal therapy in clear cell renal carcinoma arises from the observation of Bloom, in 1967, that renal tumours can be induced in male hamsters by oestrogens, and can be made to regress by means of testosterone and progestins [63]. The finding of receptors for oestrogens and progestins in human renal carcinoma has confirmed the supposed hormonal relationships of this malignancy [64]. The earliest studies, between 1968 and 1971, using MPA at low p.o. or i.m. doses, resulted in a 16% objective response rate [47]. Studies between 1971 and 1976 have shown, on average, a 2% objective response rate in 415 patients [65].

Our experience with MPA at high doses (1,500 mg/day i.m. for 30 days) has also been disappointing, with only 2/20 partial remissions [55].

Metastatic melanoma

A number of phenomena indicate some degree of correlation between the behaviour of melanoblastoma and the endocrine situation of the organism (spontaneous regression after childbirth, rapid dissemination during pregnancy, and sporadic partial regressions in connection with hormonal manipulations such as hypophysectomy, oestrogen or androgen therapy).

Fisher, in 1976, was the first to demonstrate the presence of oestrogen receptors in melanoblastoma [66]. Progestin receptors have subsequently been detected.

In 1978, Beretta used MPA to treat melanoblastomas in progression after chemotherapy [67]. A response rate of around 12% in 24 patients was obtained. It is likely that hormone therapy would achieve better results in the 25% of melanoblastoma patients with hormone receptor-positive tumours.

Advanced ovarian carcinoma

For many years, the hormone therapy of ovarian carcinoma has been undertaken empirically, and sporadically, often in association with other drugs. Progestins at doses of 200–600 mg/week have been the hormones most widely used. With these agents, response rates ranging from 9–65% have been reported. From a review of the literature, however, it appears that these response rates include subjective responses (reduction of ascites etc.) [68]. The objective response rate is around 10%. This has also recently been demonstrated by Malkasian, who administered MPA to 19 patients at daily doses of between 100 and 400 mg and obtained an objective response in only one case [69].

Recently, in the light of results obtained in hormone-dependent tumours, ovarian carcinoma has also been treated with high-dose MPA (≥ 500 mg/day) combined with chemotherapy. The median durations of remission seemed to be prolonged by such therapy [70]. A number of studies are in progress, and should provide definitive findings.

Advanced breast cancer

The observation that changing hormone levels can interfere with tumour growth is not new. Ovariectomy, for the palliative treatment of breast cancer, was first successfully performed a century ago [71].

In a review of literature carried out by us, steroids with progestational activity (MPA excepted) were found to result in an average objective remission rate of 23% in advanced breast cancer [72].

Up to 1972, doses of MPA of 500 mg/day or more had never been used. With daily doses of less than 500 mg a 13% objective response rate is obtained on average [72].

In 1972, we demonstrated that higher dosages of MPA could be used, and that 1,500 mg/day for 30 days was the maximum tolerated i.m. dose (MTD) of MPA at a concentration of 50 mg/ml, the concentration available at that time [11]. With this dose, the objective remission rate (complete + partial remissions) was 43% [13]. Subsequently, we compared the MTD with a lower dosage of MPA (500 mg/day, i.m., for 30 days). The objective remission rates and durations of remission were similar (43.5% for 6 or more months in the 500-mg group, and 45.5% for 6 months or more in the 1,500-mg group). However, the higher dosage resulted in longer survival and a better subjective response rate [49]. Believing the response rate to be dose-related, at least within limits, and the i.m. route to be limited by local toxicity, we used MPA at high doses p.o. (2,000 mg/day).

In a controlled study we compared MPA given p.o. with tamoxifen (20 mg/day). The response rates obtained were 37% with MPA and 27% with tamoxifen [14].

We are at present analysing by computer all relevant data on patients treated with MPA in our Institute within the last few years. We are searching a posteriori for factors which might have influenced the various responses to MPA therapy. This can, naturally, only be meaningful with extensive data, for the analysis of which a powerful high-speed computer is needed.

We are using a CDC 730 computer system and the Biomedical Computer Programs-programme package, obtained from the Health Sciences Computing Facility of the University of California at Los Angeles (UCLA) [73]. The complete clinical history of the patients under study is available, allowing every possible kind of uni- and multivariate statistical analysis.

The results that we shall show here were generally obtained by fitting a hierarchical log-linear model to the cell frequencies of a multiway frequency table. The programme tests the validity of models using the 'likelihood G' method, and goodness-of-fit.

Survival distribution was estimated by both the product-limit estimate (based on individual survival times) and by actuarial life tables. Two different, nonparametric rank tests (the Mantel test and the generalized Wilcoxon test) were used to assess the quality of the survival distributions.

The evaluation criteria for objective response have been published before [13]. They are in accordance with indications of the Union Internationale Contre le Cancer [74].

Table VIII gives an outline of patient characteristics. The i.m. daily doses used were 500, 1,500 and 2,000 mg. Treatment lasted for one month. No maintenance therapy was given subsequently. The p.o. daily doses were 2,000, 3,000, 4,000 and 5,000 mg. The duration of therapy was, again, one month,

Table VIII. Treatment of advanced breast cancer with high doses of MPA. Details of patients.

	Intramuscular dosages (mg)			Oral dosage (mg)	
	500	1,500	2,000	2,000	3,000–5,000
Total numbers of patients: 296	50	116	20	80	30
Age (years)					
≤ 50	6	34	5	20	9
51 to 60	19	36	7	30	11
61 to 70	19	36	5	24	8
> 70	6	10	3	6	2
Menopausal status (years since menopause)					
Premenopause/menopause					
< 1 year	6	25	5	14	6
1 to 5	15	30	5	26	6
5 to 10	14	35	5	19	6
> 10	15	26	5	21	12
Disease-free interval (years)					
0	7	13	1	8	3
0 to 2	26	62	10	26	13
> 2	17	41	9	46	14
Performance status (%)					
30 to 50	13	56	15	14	15
60 to 70	24	29	5	36	10
80 to 100	13	31	0	30	5
Dominant metastatic site					
Soft tissue (ST)	10	16	3	15	3
Bone (O)	28	61	11	36	14
Viscera (V)	12	39	6	29	13
C.I.[1] $(\frac{V}{ST + O})$	0.32	0.51	0.43	0.57	0.77
Prior treatment					
Hormone therapy	11	30	8	24	2
Chemotherapy	7	8	4	10	11
Hormone + chemotherapy	8	9	0	5	2
None	24	69	8	41	15

[1]C.I. = Comparative index.

but in this case maintenance therapy was subsequently established at a daily dose of 1,000 mg in the lowest dose level group, and 2,000–3,000 mg in the others. Patients treated with 3, 4 and 5 g/day were evaluated as belonging to a single group, because the number of patients within each dose group was small and many patients had been intensively pretreated. In fact, they had a lower performance status and higher comparative index (see Table VIII).

Table IX shows the response to treatment. The objective remission rate (complete + partial) was 41% overall. Patients with dominant bone and soft-tissue lesions had better remission rates (53.5% and 47%). A lower remission rate (18%) was obtained in patients with mainly visceral lesions.

Patients treated with MPA i.m. had a higher remission rate than those treated p.o. (Table X). The difference is not, however, statistically significant, but there is a significant difference if the patients with visceral lesions are omitted. The objective remission rate did not depend on dose (Table XI) in patients treated by either route of administration. In this connection, it must be borne in mind that the prognoses in patients in the 3,000–5,000 mg group were worse than those in patients in the lower dose groups. Visceral lesions were more common and, on average, performance status was lower. This may account for the lower remission rate in this group. Objective remission rates were not related to the lapse of time since the menopause, length of disease-free interval, or previous treatments.

Table IX. Clinical response to high-dose MPA in cases of advanced breast cancer, according to the predominant site of metastases (number of patients (%)).

Site of metastases	Numbers of patients	Remission		No change	Progression
		Complete	Partial		
Soft tissue	47	4 (9)	18 (38)	11 (23)	14 (30)
Bone	150	1 (0.5)	79 (53)	33 (22)	37 (24.5)
Viscera	99	0 (—)	18 (18)	46 (46.5)	35 (35.5)
Totals	296	5 (2)	115 (39)	90 (30)	86 (29)

Statistical evaluation: Pearson χ^2 test: $P < 0.001$.

Table X. Clinical response to high-dose MPA in cases of advanced breast cancer, according to the route of administration (numbers of patients (%)).

Route of administration	Numbers of patients	Remission		No change	Progression
		Complete	Partial		
I.m.	186	4 (2)	78 (42)	48 (26)	56 (30)
P.o.	110	1 (1)	37 (34)	42 (38)	30 (27)
Total	296	5 (2)	115 (39)	90 (30)	86 (29)

Statistical evaluation (Pearson χ^2 test): i.m. vs. p.o., $P < 0.20$; i.m. vs. p.o., visceral metastases excluded, $P < 0.009$.

The median duration of remission was 7 months (Table XII). Figure 4 shows that the duration of objective remission does not depend upon the predominant site of metastases, but does depend on route of administration; it is longer with i.m. than with p.o. treatment.

Table XIII is an analysis of subjective responses. Remission of pain, a symptom resulting mainly from bone metastases, is significantly higher when the i.m. route is used.

In addition, statistical analysis shows that increase in dose tends to produce improvement in pain relief. Improvement in performance status depends upon the route of administration, and, for each route, tends to improve as the

Table XI. Clinical response to high-dose MPA in cases of advanced breast cancer, according to dosage (numbers of patients (%)).

Dose (mg)	Numbers of patients	Remission		No change	Progression
		Complete	Partial		
500 i.m.	50	1 (2)	21 (42)	8 (16)	20 (40)
1,500 i.m.	116	2 (2)	49 (42)	35 (30)	30 (26)
2,000 i.m.	20	1 (5)	8 (40)	5 (25)	6 (30)
2,000 p.o.	80	0 (—)	28 (35)	32 (40)	20 (25)
3,000 to 5,000 p.o.	30	1 (3)	9 (30)	10 (33.5)	10 (33.5)

No statistically significant difference in remission rates as between i.m. and p.o. administration.

Table XII. Duration of objective remission (complete remission + partial remission) following high-dose MPA treatment in advanced breast cancer.

Route of administration	Dose (mg)	Numbers of patients	Duration of objective remission (months)	
			Median	Range
I.m.		82	7	1 to 95
	500	22	7	2 to 41
	1,500	51	7	1 to 95
	2,000	9	15	5 to 27
P.o.		38	6	1 to 28
	2,000	28	6	1 to 28
	3,000 to 5,000	10	8	3 to 16
Totals		120	7	1 to 95

dose is increased, but not significantly. Asthenia, anorexia and walking impairment tend to improve most when the i.m. route is used, but the improvement is at the limits of significance, and not dose related.

Factors affecting survival are listed in Table XIV.

Survival depends on the dominant metastatic site, performance status, and previous treatment. Patients with visceral metastases, poor performance status, or previous chemotherapy have a shorter life expectancy, independent of the treatment given.

Survival unquestionably depends on the type of objective response to MPA therapy (Fig. 5). The median survival period is 30 months for patients in

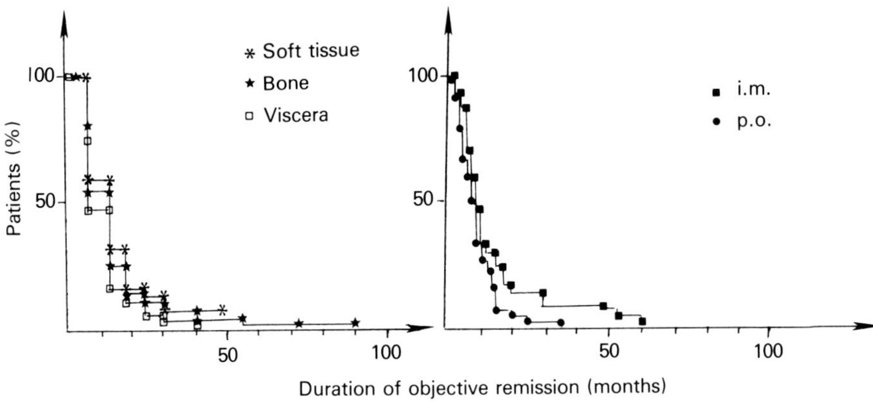

Fig. 4. High-dose MPA in advanced breast cancer. Duration of objective remission (complete remission + partial remission) according to predominant metastatic lesion (Wilcoxon's test, P = 0.24, Mantel-Cox's test P = 1.00), and route of administration (Wilcoxon's test, P = 0.13, Mantel-Cox's test, P = 0.03).

Table XIII. Subjective remission in relation to high-dose MPA treatment in advanced breast cancer (numbers of patients showing improvement indicated/numbers of patients treated (%)).

Symptom	I.m.	P.o.	χ^2
Pain	102/130 (78)	34/79 (43)	$P < 0.0001$
Asthenia	74/123 (60)	23/48 (48)	Not significant
Anorexia	61/83 (73)	22/34 (65)	Not significant
Dyspnoea	28/65 (43)	11/37 (30)	Not significant
Walking impairment	35/77 (45)	11/36 (31)	Not significant
Performance status	93/148 (63)	36/92 (39)	$P < 0.002$

whom there was remission, 19 months for patients whose disease showed no change, and only 6 months for patients whose disease progressed.

This preliminary analysis seems to indicate that survival also depends on the route of administration.

By examining patients participating in a prospective clinical trial comparing i.m. treatment with 500 and 1,500 mg/day, there is some evidence of dependence of duration of survival on dose (Fig. 6). The median survival period was 20 months for patients treated with the lower dose, and 38 months for patients treated with the higher dose.

Table XIV. Treatment of advanced breast cancer with high-dose MPA. Factors affecting survival.

	Numbers of patients	Survival (months)			P	
		75%	50% (Median)	25%	Wilcoxon	Mantel
Predominant metastatic lesion						
Soft tissue	47	17	24	49		
Bone	150	13	22	46	= 0.0001	= 0.0002
Viscera	99	5	12	25		
Performance status						
30 to 50%	113	5	13	25		
60 to 70%	104	11	23	46	= 0.0001	= 0.0001
80 to 100%	79	16	25	47		
Previous treatment						
None	157	12	23	52		
Hormonotherapy	75	10	19	31	= 0.01	= 0.02
Chemotherapy	64	7	13	29		
Response						
Complete remission + partial remission	120	18	30	61		
No change	90	11	19	31	= 0.0001	= 0.0001
Progression	86	3	6	15		
Subsequent treatment						
None	120	4	12	22		
Hormonotherapy	110	14	26	49	= 0.0001	= 0.0001
Chemotherapy	66	13	26	46		

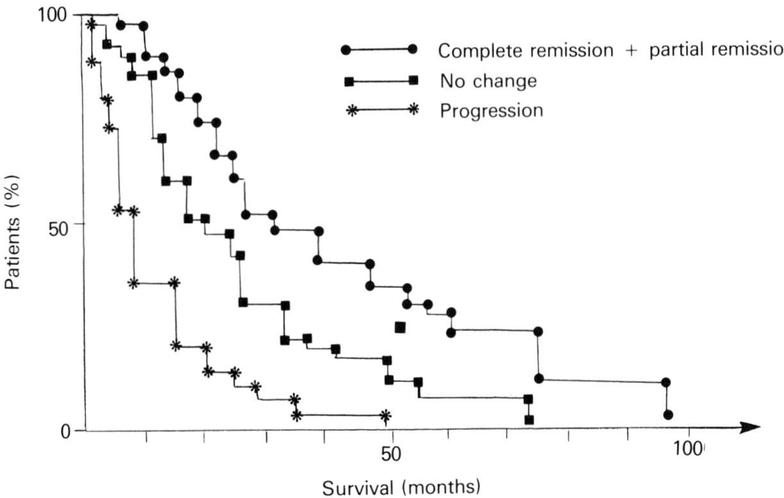

Fig. 5. High-dose MPA in advanced breast cancer. Survival analysis according to objective response (Wilcoxon's test, P = 0.000; Mantel-Cox's test, P = 0.000).

It must be remembered, in this connection, that there is another important, well known, prognostic factor which may influence the outcome of MPA therapy, namely, the receptor content of the tumour cytosol.

Unfortunately, we have no data on this aspect, at present. Most of the patients treated up to now in our Institute had been subjected to mastectomy before receptor analysis was performed. We now perform receptor analyses routinely. Data from these analyses will be used in future studies.

Early breast cancer

In 1975, the Italian Cooperative Chemo-Radio-Surgical Group started a prospective, controlled study on the adjuvant treatment of operable Stage-II breast cancer.

After mastectomy, the patients were randomly allocated to receive either postoperative radiation therapy, or MPA at high doses (1,500 mg/day, i.m., for 30 days, every 6 months, 3 times). At 36 months, there was no statistically significant difference between the 2 groups in relation to either incidence of recurrence or survival [75].

MPA pharmacokinetics

In 1980, we initiated a multidisciplinary study on pharmacokinetics,

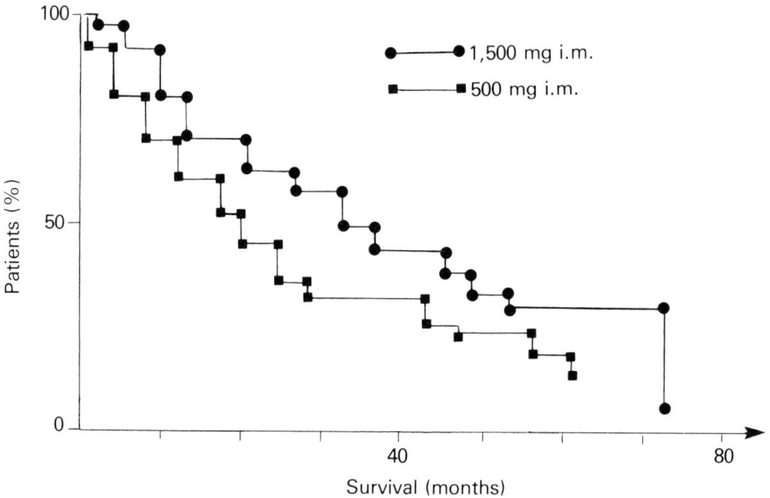

Fig. 6. High-dose MPA in advanced breast cancer. Survival analysis according to i.m. dose level (Wilcoxon's test, P = 0.08; Mantel-Cox's test, P = 0.10).

metabolism and clinical response during MPA treatment, in order to shed some light on the still unresolved problems connected with the clinical use of high doses of MPA.

The subjects entered into this study were hospital in-patients, with histology-proven, far-advanced cancer. All had received prior radiation therapy and/or chemotherapy or hormonotherapy, but oncological treatment had been discontinued at least one month before the study, generally because of lack of response.

All relevant clinical data concerning these patients were recorded in our data system, in a format compatible with the BMDP package of biomedical programmes, obtained from the Health Science Computing Facility of UCLA [73].

Throughout the experiments, the MPA was administered p.o., using commercially available MPA vials, the contents of which were suspended in fruit juice.

MPA plasma levels in each patient were monitored in our laboratory using an automated gas chromatographic procedure characterized by a complete absence of interference from MPA metabolites, an 8% run-to-run coefficient of variation, and a very high linear range.

Although the intrinsic cross-reactivity problem associated with the radioimmunoassay of MPA can now partially be overcome by using a selective extraction technique, we think our chromatographic method is much better suited to routine use, especially because of the very high linear range, which overcomes problems connected with the high interindividual variability in MPA plasma concentrations.

Single dose administration

Figure 7 shows the behaviour of the MPA absorption-decay curve after a single p.o. administration. The MPA plasma profile is easily fitted using a triexponential equation, consistent with a 2-compartment open pharmacokinetic model, and first order absorption. The first decay phase can be attributed to distribution to peripheral tissues, and is characterized by a half-life of about 1.4 hours. The subsequent biological half-life is considerably longer (about 58.8 hours).

Five different dosage levels (250, 500, 1,000, 2,000 and 3,000 mg) were examined in this study. For each level, the mean curve was derived from data from 10 cancer patients. For clarity, we have reported here only data concerning the 2,000 and 3,000 mg dosage levels, using a semilog scale.

The half-lives do not depend on the dosage employed. Dosage contributes instead to the relative bioavailability of the drug, as shown in Figure 8, which

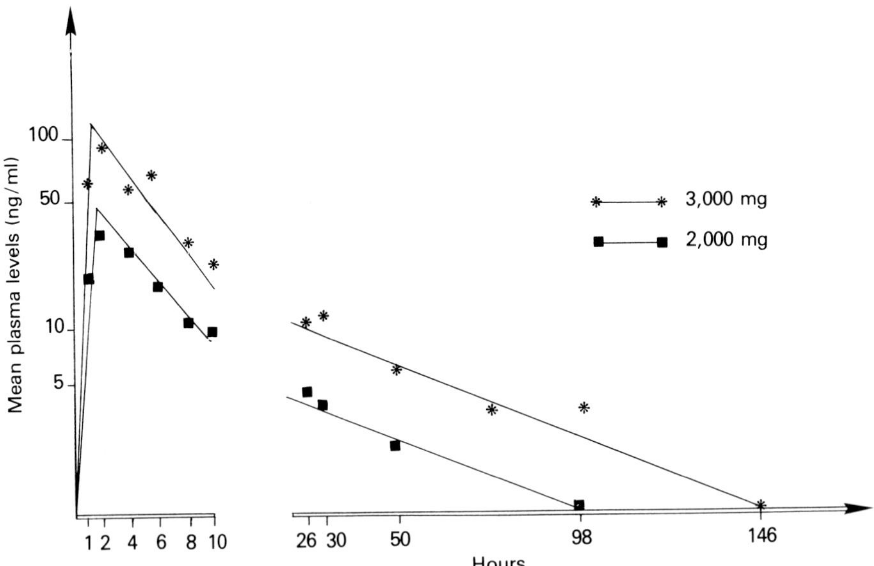

Fig. 7. Mean plasma levels after single p.o. administration of high-dose MPA in advanced cancer patients.

is a scattergram showing the relationship between the dose administered and the area under the absorption/decay curve (AUC), a good index of relative MPA bioavailability.

The wide interindividual variation is very pronounced, as are the relatively low AUC values obtained, even with the highest doses employed. These data are an indication that the extent of absorption of MPA following p.o. administration is relatively small, unless an abnormally high volume of distribution is involved.

Plasma MPA levels obtained after doses given i.m., p.o. and i.m. + p.o., on one occasion in each case, are shown in Figure 9.

Here again, each curve was the mean of determinations involving 10 cancer patients. For clarity, only the profile relative to 2,000-mg doses is shown. It is of particular interest to note the different behaviour of the MPA plasma levels following p.o. and i.m. administration.

Peak levels are higher after p.o. treatment, but appreciably better long-term bioavailability is obtained using i.m. administration.

In this case, the decay phases are obscured by the prolonged absorption phase, and a steady-state concentration is maintained.

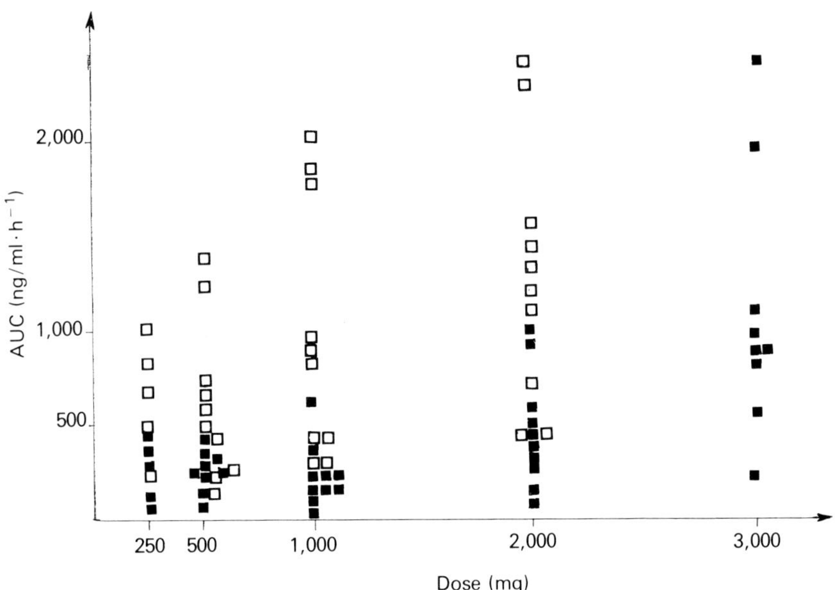

Fig. 8. High-dose MPA. AUC (0 to 146 hours) after single administration in advanced cancer patients (□ = i.m.; ■ = p.o.).

A similar depot effect is observed following intraperitoneal administration. In this case, the steady state level is considerably higher. Simultaneous i.m. + p.o. administration results in the superimposing of the absorption/decay profiles obtained after administration of single doses i.m. and p.o.

The simultaneous administration of MPA by the i.m. and p.o. routes may, in fact, be effective in overcoming the drawbacks of both routes, namely, the local intolerance sometimes observed with high-dose i.m. treatment, and the low percentage of drug absorbed, characteristic of p.o. administration.

I.p. administration guarantees higher MPA plasma levels (Table XV), and may be of value in patients with peritoneal metastases and ascitic effusion.

The most important data obtained from these single dose pharmacokinetic studies are:

1. the relative low plasma MPA levels obtained, even after the administration of very high doses,
2. the significant dose/bioavailability relationship, observed after both p.o. and i.m. administration, and
3. the wide interindividual variation in plasma MPA concentrations.

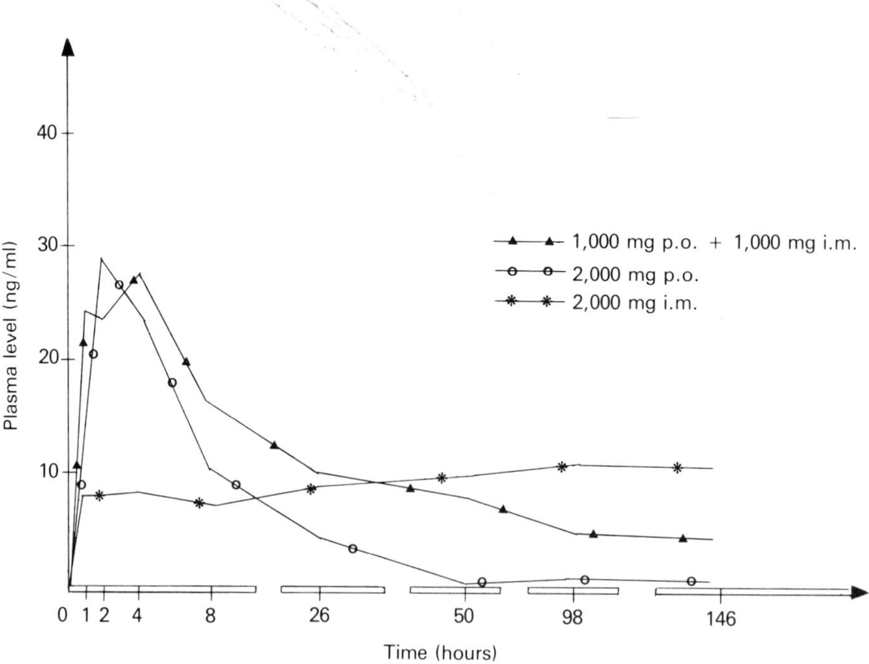

Fig. 9. High-dose MPA in advanced cancer patients. Effects of route of administration on plasma levels after a single 2,000-mg dose.

Table XV. Plasma levels (ng/ml) after single intraperitoneal administration of 2,000 mg of MPA to patients with advanced cancer.

Time (hours)	Patient						
	C.S.	B.A.	B.L.	B.M.	C.T.	P.A.	Z.A.
1	83.0	34.3	76.9	18.3	10.0	48.3	64.7
2	158.0	68.5	133.9	37.0	48.8	95.3	76.7
4	201.0	89.8	176.0	50.1	61.1	65.8	88.6
8	209.0	122.0	266.6	43.2	65.3	215.0	98.2
26	158.5	72.0	156.0	77.1	72.7	240.0	106.4
50	138.7	69.0	94.0	75.5	49.0	106.3	70.1
98	130.6	50.0	40.0	124.0	39.5	59.1	34.4
146	93.7	48.0	14.0	67.0	35.9	30.5	21.1

Repeated administration

In Table XVI, MPA plasma levels after repeated administration, namely, treatment involving MPA daily, p.o. or i.m. for 30 days, are reported.
After p.o. treatment, a relatively steady plasma concentration of MPA is reached in 4–12 days. Even with the extremely high dose of 5 g of MPA, per day, this level did not exceed 350 ng/ml. After discontinuing administration, MPA plasma levels decreased, with a half-life of about 2.5 days. It is of interest that, in a very similar regime, daily administration of 20 mg of tamoxifen (TMX) gives TMX plasma levels at least twice as high over the same time interval.

After i.m. administration, a steady-state is reached only after discontinuing treatment. Plasma levels are dose-dependent, and did not exceed 300 ng/ml, even at the highest dose employed.

The most important differences between the 2 routes of administration are the slower increase in MPA levels following i.m. treatment, and the absence of a depot effect after p.o. administration.

Two clinically relevant phenomena are particularly evident, namely, the logarithmic decay in MPA plasma levels after the last p.o. administration, in contrast to the steady-state levels arising from the depot effect following i.m. treatment, and the higher MPA levels obtained with 30 days of i.m. treatment. In order to attain the ultimate MPA levels found after 1,000 mg of MPA, i.m., about 4,000 mg are necessary, p.o. These data can easily explain the results obtained in previous clinical evaluations, if a bioavailability/response relationship exists.

The wide interindividual variation observed in MPA bioavailability follow-

Table XVI. Mean plasma MPA levels (ng/ml) after repeated administration (for 30 days) to patients with advanced cancer.

Days	Oral administration (mg)						Intramuscular administration (mg)		
	500	1,000	2,000	3,000	4,000	5,000	500	1,000	2,000
4	19.7	88.6	69.9	115.3	138.8	159.8	9.7	28.0	42.9
8	18.5	143.0	115.1	198.3	167.3	295.4	23.8	76.6	102.0
12	15.5	121.4	102.5	261.6	202.6	356.5	44.4	82.7	129.0
15	30.2	117.5	87.5	267.9	209.9	349.3	47.2	103.2	149.6
21	16.0	137.3	117.6	209.6	230.0	384.4	43.2	124.6	201.4
28	14.0	130.7	88.3	203.2	229.2	334.4	53.6	138.3	242.4
30	7.9	82.0	97.5	238.4	182.9	295.6	64.0	142.6	287.2
31	4.2	66.8	60.3	125.1	113.2	164.0	58.1	156.0	248.2
33	3.8	23.2	44.5	65.9	69.1	127.8	44.5	134.3	271.8
35	1.9	10.6	27.8	44.2	39.8	67.6	43.7	142.5	196.6
37	0.0	6.0	17.5	32.5	24.9	34.1	49.6	132.6	225.3
Numbers of patients	5	10	10	8	12	18	6	11	6

ing single p.o. or i.m. administration is also present after repeated administration, as shown in Figure 10.

It should be noted that the AUC values reported relate to the 0 to 37th day interval. In the longer term, the depot effect of i.m. administration will render the bioavailability by this route even more favourable.

Preliminary trials of rectal administration have also been carried out. Using the preparations currently available, this route does not seem to guarantee adequate absorption.

The interindividual variability observed in MPA levels does not seem to be directly related to impaired MPA metabolism induced by the different kinds of tumours or metastases.

Normalized MPA absorption curves for patients, classified according to the primary tumour, are shown in Figure 11. No significant differences are evident.

The relevance of biliary excretion to MPA metabolism can be seen from Figure 12.

A patient (M.E.), previously subjected to cholecystectomy and choledochal drainage was treated in our Institute with 1,000 mg of MPA/day, i.m. Plasma and bile samples were collected simultaneously, and analysed in the usual way for their MPA content. After the initial induction period, there was a marked

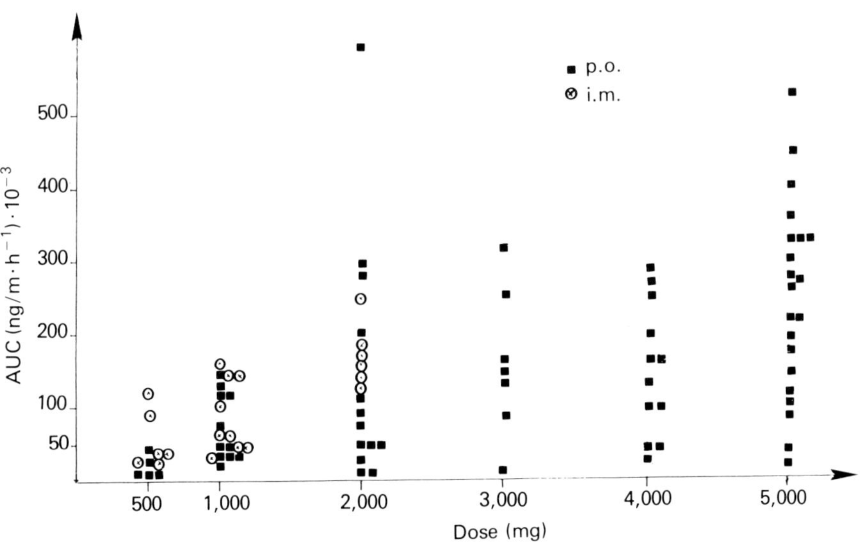

Fig. 10. AUC (0 to 37 day interval) after repeated administration of high-dose MPA to advanced cancer patients.

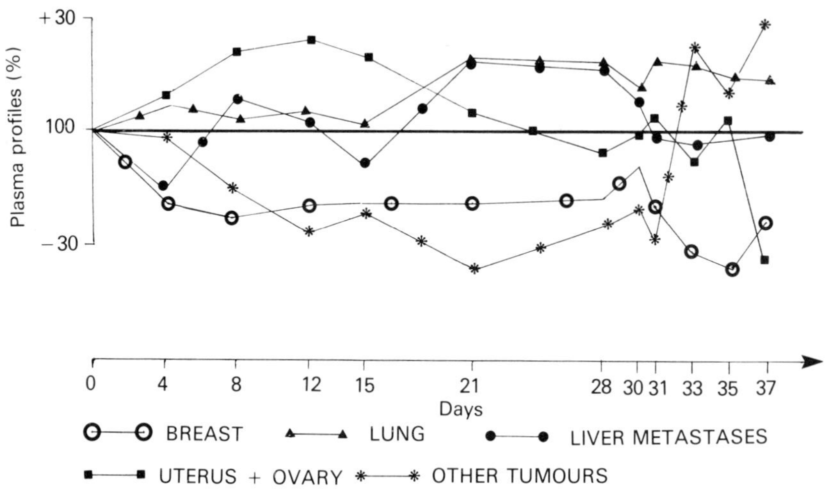

Fig. 11. High-dose MPA administered repeatedly, p.o. and i.m., to advanced cancer patients. Normalized plasma profiles according to site of tumour lesions.

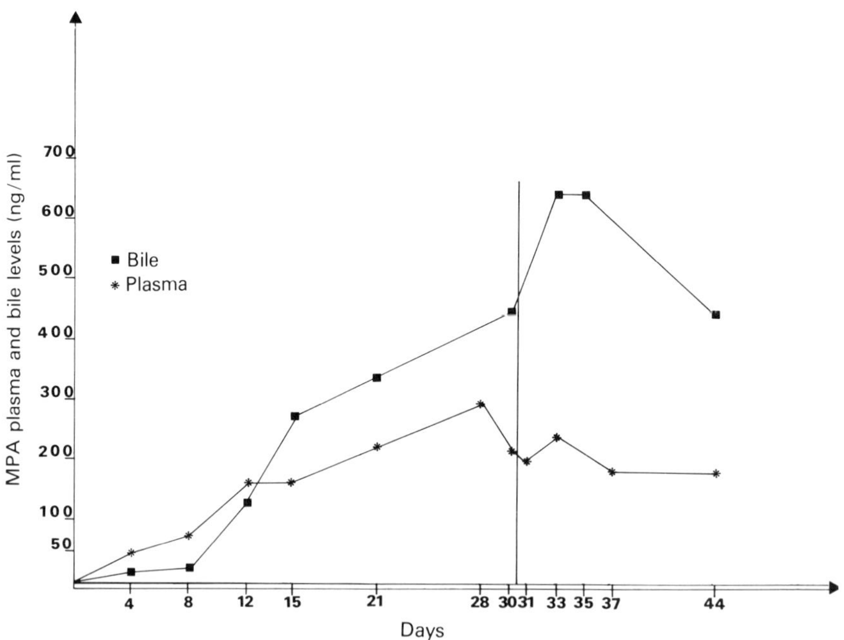

Fig. 12. MPA plasma and bile levels after administration of 1,000 mg/day, i.m., for 30 days to one advanced cancer patient.

Table XVII. MPA levels in cellular cytosol. (Cells from tissues of Sprague-Dawley rats.)

Tissue	Intramuscular adminis-tration (ng/g) (10 mg × 7 days)	Oral adminis-tration (ng/g) (20 mg × 7 days)	Blank
Brain	37.0	—	0.0
Cerebellum	—	0.0	—
Heart	28.9	—	—
Large intestine	—	37.7	2.0
Small intestine	—	—	1.8
Liver	154.7	—	—
Rectum	—	27.4	0.0
Spleen	74.4	20.6	—
Lung	58.1	—	8.2
Stomach	35.6	15.6	3.5
Plasma	—	16.1 ng/ml	—

increase in biliary MPA level. Concentrations of about 2–3 times the corresponding plasma levels were attained.

These results are in accordance with an active transport process across both sides of the hepatocytes. Hepatic functions were found to be normal in this patient, both before and after MPA treatment, using standard clinical tests.

On the basis of these findings, it can be concluded that the use of very high doses of MPA is totally justified from a metabolic point of view.

MPA plasma levels of about 300 ng/ml are cleared in about 10 days, even by patients with impaired hepatic or renal function.

Finally, we should like to present some very recent data concerning MPA distribution in the tissues. Table XVII shows the results of assays carried out on a cellular cytosol obtained from rats of the Sprague-Dawley strain, treated p.o. or i.m. with high MPA doses. Blank analyses are fairly good for almost all samples. The data seem to indicate that MPA tissue distribution is extensive.

At present, we have only one set of data relating to MPA tissue distribution in man. A patient was under treatment with MPA before ovariectomy for ovarian cancer. Samples of the tumour were analysed for MPA. High MPA concentrations were found in the tumour cytosol.

MPA bioavailability/response relationship

Very high MPA doses are necessary consistently to achieve MPA plasma levels of about 100–300 ng/ml, but are these levels clinically useful?

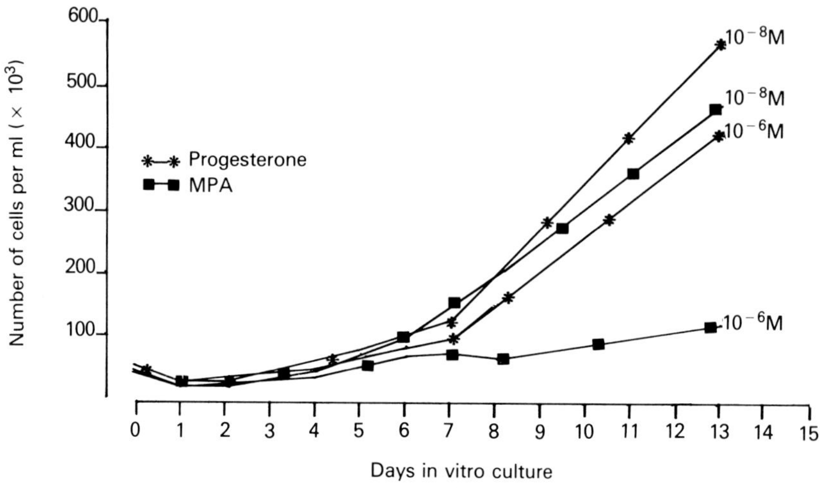

Fig. 13. Effect on growth of the MCF-7 human breast tumour cell line of different molar concentrations of MPA. Reproduced with permission of the Editor from [76].

Figure 13 reports the results of well known, in-vitro studies concerning the growth of MCF-7 cell lines under different conditions. It is evident that MPA added to the culture at a concentration of about 400 ng/ml (10^{-6}M) completely inhibits cellular growth. At the 4 ng/ml (10^{-8}M) level, MPA stimulates cellular division [76].

In order to test whether a similar effect might exist in vivo, we tried to correlate MPA plasma level determinations with clinical responses. This approach is, in our view, more valuable than a simple dose-response correlation, because of the wide interindividual variation in MPA plasma levels.

Unfortunately, at present we can report only preliminary data. Patients are too few in number (only 38 patients with breast cancer), and not sufficiently homogeneous.

There is, notwithstanding, a definite trend towards a better response in patients with high MPA bioavailability (Table XVIII).

Subjects with a MPA AUC of less than 50.10^3 ng/ml$\cdot$h^{-1} showed objective remission in 20% of cases, and 34% of cases have shown progression. With high MPA bioavailability (AUC more than 50.10^3 ng/ml$\cdot$h^{-1}), objective remissions increased to 35% of cases, and progression was seen in 15% of cases.

These patients all had very advanced cancer before treatment, and almost all had been fairly intensively pretreated. This may explain the low overall objective response rate.

Table XVIII. High-dose MPA in advanced breast cancer. Relationship between objective response and bioavailability (numbers of patients (%)).

AUC ($ng/ml \cdot h^{-1}$)	Complete remission + partial remission	No change	Progression	Numbers of patients
$\leq 50 \times 10^3$	2 (22)	4 (45)	3 (33)	9
$> 50 \times 10^3$	11 (38)	13 (45)	5 (17)	29

Pearson χ^2 test: no statistically significant difference ($P < 0.51$).

The trend toward better response with high MPA plasma levels is significant in the case of subjective responses to therapy. In relation to pain, we observed remission in over 50% of cases with high MPA bioavailability but in only 15% of cases with low AUC values (< 50). We found an improvement in performance status (better than 10%) in 37% of cases with high AUC values, and in only 5% of patients in whom bioavailability was low.

Conclusion

We believe that our pharmacokinetic data are in good agreement with findings in the computerized analysis of our clinical experience.

The consistently better results obtained with i.m. treatment schedules are probably related to the good long-term bioavailability generally attained using this route of administration. The absence of a statistically significant dose-response relationship (at high dosages, ≥ 500 mg/day) is probably a result of the high interindividual variation in plasma MPA levels, which results from slow absorption in the case of i.m. administration, and low absorption in the case of p.o. treatment.

There are, of course, several questions still open for discussion in relation to the clinical use of MPA:

1. Does a clear-cut dose/response or bioavailability/response relationship exist?

Our experience seems to indicate that it may. In our opinion, in mammary carcinoma, at least, a minimum plasma MPA concentration exists below which the percentage of objective and subjective remissions is low. Determination of the p.o. MTD is of critical importance in this connection.

2. How can the optimum MPA plasma level be reached?

The same doses of MPA given p.o. or i.m. result in substantially different effects as indicated both by clinical results and pharmacokinetic investigations. The problems of the more rational use of the 2 routes of administration in individual patients, and the evolution of standard maintenance therapies still remain unresolved. We would emphasize again that p.o. treatment requires extremely high doses in order consistently to reach plasma levels equivalent to those attained following i.m. administration of 1,000 or 2,000 mg/day. In addition, after discontinuing p.o. therapy, MPA levels drop to zero in a few days, whereas i.m. therapy results in long-term constant levels of MPA, because of the depot effect. The interindividual variability in MPA absorption also requires routine monitoring of MPA plasma levels.

3. What is the mechanism of action of high-dose MPA?

More sophisticated knowledge regarding the mechanism of action of MPA at the molecular level and its metabolic pathway would be extremely useful, especially in determining the more general strategic role of therapeutic MPA in therapy.

MPA therapy combined with hormonal therapy or chemotherapy, or given sequentially, needs to be studied on a rational basis, rather than empirically, as heretofore was the case.

Ultimately we feel that the use of high-speed computer systems for the analysis of clinical data will come to be more generally accepted.

The importance of critical and accurate statistical analysis in epidemiology is commonly acknowledged. A similar approach to the examination of clinical findings should shed new light on prognostic factors useful for optimizing treatment.

In our hospital we hope eventually to establish a multinational data bank (Fig. 14) relating to hormonotherapy of mammary carcinoma, and are at present working towards this end.

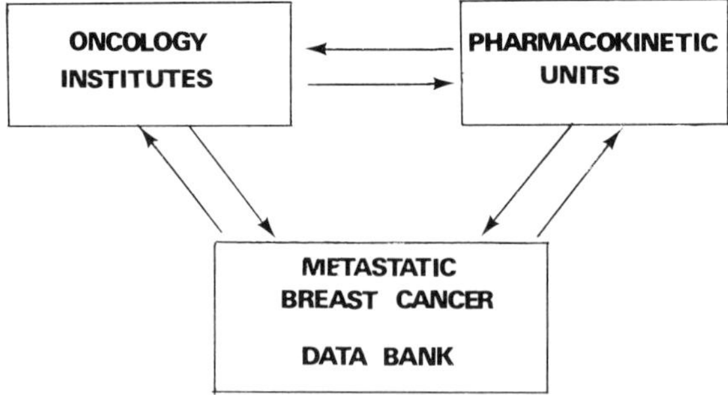

Fig. 14. Proposal for an International Breast Cancer Study Group.

References

1. Babcock, J.C., Gutsell, E.S., Herr, M.E. et al. (1958): 6α-methyl-17α-hydroxyprogesterone 17-acylates, a new class of potent progestins. *J. Am. Chem. Soc. 80,* ,2904.
2. Sala, G., Camerino, B. and Cavallero, C. (1958): Progestational activity of 6α-methyl-17α-hydroxyprogesterone acetate. *Acta Endocrinol. 29,* 508.
3. Briggs, M.H., Caldwell, A.D.S. and Pitchford, A.G. (1962): The treatment of cancer by progestogens. *Lancet II,* 63.
4. Brotherton, J. (1976): *Sex Hormone Pharmacology,* pp. 51–58. Academic Press, New York.
5. Shapiro, S.S., Dyer, R.D. and Colas, A.E. (1978): Synthetic progestins: *in vitro* potency on human endometrium and specific binding to cytosol receptor. *Am. J. Obstet. Gynecol. 132,* 549.
6. Young, P.C.M., Keen, F.K., Einhorn, L.H. et al. (1980): Binding of medroxy-progesterone acetate in human breast cancer. *Am. J. Obstet. Gynecol. 137,* 284.
7. Greenblatt, R.B. (1958): A new clinical test for the efficacy of progesterone compounds. *Am. J. Obstet. Gynecol. 76,* 626.
8. Dickey, R. and Stone, S. (1976): Progestational potency of oral contraceptives. *Obstet. Gynecol. 47,* 106.
9. Powell, L.C. and Seymour, R.J. (1971): Effects of depomedroxyprogesterone acetate as a contraceptive agent. *Am. J. Obstet. Gynecol. 110,* 36.
10. Stoll, B.A. (1967): Progestin therapy of breast cancer: comparison of agents. *Br. Med. J. 3,* 338.
11. Pannuti, F., Martoni, A., Pollutri, E. et al. (1976): Massive dose progestational therapy in oncology (medroxyprogesterone). Preliminary results. *Pan. Minerva Med. 18,* 129.
12. Pannuti, F., Martoni, A., Rossi, A.P. et al. (1979): The role of endocrine therapy for relief of pain due to advanced cancer. In: *Advances in Pain Research and Therapy,* Vol. II, pp. 145–165. Eds: J.J. Bonica and V. Ventafridda. Raven Press, New York.
13. Pannuti, F., Martoni, A., Lenaz, G.R. et al. (1978): A possible new approach to the treatment of metastatic breast cancer: massive doses of medroxyprogesterone acetate. *Cancer Treat. Rep. 62,* 449.
14. Pannuti, F., Martoni, A., Fruet, F. et al. (1982): Oral high dose medroxy-progesterone acetate (MAP) vs. tamoxifen (TMX) in postmenopausal patients with advanced breast cancer. In: *The Role of Tamoxifen in Breast Cancer.* Raven Press, New York. (In press.)
15. Robustelli Della Cuna, G., Calciati, A., Bernardo Strada, M.R. et al. (1978): High dose medroxyprogesterone acetate (MPA) treatment in metastatic carcinoma of the breast: a dose-response evaluation. *Tumori 64,* 143.
16. Pellegrini, A., Massidda, B., Mascia, V. et al. (1978): Advanced breast cancer treatment with chemotherapy and medroxyprogesterone acetate. In: *Proceedings of the XIIth International Cancer Congress, Buenos Aires, 1978,* Vol. 3, p. 48.
17. Amadori, D., Ravaioli, A., Ridolfi, R. et al. (1979): Il MAP ad alte dosi nella terapia del carcinoma della mammella in fase avanzata. *Chemioter. Oncol. 1,* 44.
18. De Lena, M., Brambilla, C., Valagussa, P. et al. (1979): High dose medroxy-

progesterone acetate in breast cancer resistant to endocrine and cytotoxic therapy. *Cancer Chemother. Pharmacol. 2,* 175.
19. Mussa, A., Dogliotti, L. and Di Carlo, F. (1980): Valutazione globale dei risultati ottenuti nel trattamento dei carcinomi metastatici della mammella con terapia combinata MAP-alte dosi e bromocriptina. *Minerva Med. 71,* 391.
20. Mattsson, W. (1978): High dose medroxyprogesterone acetato treatment in advanced mammary carcinoma (a phase II investigation). *Acta Radiol. Oncol. 17,* 387.
21. Mendiola, C., Manas, A., Ramos, A. et al. (1979): High dose medroxyprogesterone acetate (MAP) for the treatment of advanced resistant breast cancer. In: *Proceedings of the 6th Annual Meeting of the Medical Oncology Society, Nice, 1979,* p. 33.
22. Madrigal, P.L., Alonso, A., Manga, G.P. et al. (1980): High doses of medroxyprogesterone acetate (MPA) in the treatment of metastatic breast cancer. In: *Role of Medroxyprogesterone in Endocrine-related Tumors,* pp. 93–96. Eds: S. Iacobelli and A. Di Marco. Raven Press, New York.
23. Izuo, M., Yuichi, I. and Keiichi, E. (1981): Oral high-dose medroxyprogesterone acetate (MAP) in treatment of advanced breast cancer. *Breast Cancer Res. Treat. 1,* 125.
24. Becher, R., Firusian, N., Hoffken, K. et al. (1981): High dose medroxyprogesterone acetate (MAP) in advanced breast cancer. *Abstract from Conference Book, 7th Annual Meeting of the European Society for Medical Oncology, 28–31 October, Lausanne, Switzerland,* pp. 33.
25. Cavalli, F., Goldhirsch, A., Kaplan, E. et al. (1981): High (H) versus low (L) dose medroxyprogesterone Acetate (MPA) in advanced breast cancer. *Abstract from Conference Book, 7th Annual Meeting of the European Society for Medical Oncology, 28–31 October, Lausanne, Switzerland,* p. 32.
26. Huggins, C., Stevens, R. and Hodges, C.V. (1941): Studies on prostatic cancer. II. The effect of castration on advanced carcinoma of the prostate gland. *Arch. Surg. 43,* 209.
27. Tagnon, H.J., Coune, A., Heuson, J.C. et al. (1967): Problems in the treatment of disseminated cancer of the breast: selection of patients for hormone treatment. In: *New Trends in the Treatment of Cancer,* pp. 126–133. Eds: L. Manuila, S. Moles and P. Rentchnick. Springer-Verlag, Berlin–Heidelberg–New York.
28. Lawrence, A.M. and Kirstein, L. (1970): Progestins in the medical management of active acromegaly. *J. Clin. Endocrinol. Metab. 30,* 646.
29. Mathews, J.H., Abrams, C.A.L. and Morishima, A. (1970): Pituitary adrenal function in few patients receiving MAP for true precocious puberty. *J. Clin. Endocrinol. Metab., 30,* 653.
30. Sadoff, L. and Lusk, W. (1974): The effect of large doses of medroxyprogesterone acetate (MAP) on urinary levels and serum levels of cortisol, T4, LH and testosterone in patients with advanced cancer. *Obstet. Gynecol. 43,* 262.
31. Meyer, W.J., Walker, P.A., Wiedeking, C. et al. (1977): Pituitary function in adult males receiving medroxyprogesterone acetate. *Fertil. Steril. 28,* 1072.
32. Novak, E. (1977): Effects of medroxyprogesterone acetate on some endocrine functions in healthy male volunteers. *Curr. Ther. Res. 21,* 320.
33. Sala, G., Castegnaro, E., Lenaz, G.R. et al. (1978): Hormone interference in metastatic breast cancer patients treated with medroxyprogesterone acetate at

massive doses. Preliminary results. *IRCS Med. Sci. 6,* 129.
34. Pannuti, F., Giovannini, M., Martoni, A. et al. (1980): Effects of high dose oral medroxyprogesterone acetate (MAP) on plasma levels of T3, T4, TSH, LH, FSH, PRL, 17β-estradiol, testosterone and aldosterone. *IRCS Med. Sci. 8,* 764.
35. Frank, D.W., Kirton, K.T., Murchison, T.E. et al. (1979): Mammary tumors and serum hormones in the bitch treated with medroxyprogesterone acetate or progesterone for four years. *Fertil. Steril. 31,* 340.
36. Concannon, P., Altszuler, N., Hampshire, J. et al. (1980): Growth hormone, prolactin, and cortisol in dogs developing mammary nodules and an acromegaly-like appearance treatment with medroxyprogesterone acetate. *Endocrinology 106,* 1173.
37. Gordon, G.G., Southren, A.L., Tochimoto, S. et al. (1970): Effect of medroxyprogesterone acetate (Provera) on the metabolism and biological activity of testosterone. *J. Clin. Endocrinol. 30,* 449.
38. Gurpide, E. (1976): Hormones and gynecologic cancer. *Cancer 38,* 503.
39. Tseng, L. and Gurpide, E. (1975): Induction of human endometrial estradiol dehydrogenase by progestins. *Endocrinology 97,* 825.
40. Bojar, H., Maar, K. and Staib, W. (1979): The endocrine background of human renal cell carcinoma. *Urol. Int. 34,* 330.
41. Taylor, C.W., Brush, M.G., King, R.J.B. et al. (1971): The uptake of oestrogen by endometrial carcinoma. *Proc. R. Soc. Med. 64,* 407.
42. Di Carlo, F., Conti, G., Marsanich, P. et al. (1979): Effetti dei progestinici sui recettori per gli estrogeni. *Boll. Soc. Piem. Chir. 49,* 261.
43. Formelli, F., Zaccheo, T., Casazza, A.M. et al. (1981): Effect of medroxyprogesterone acetate and doxorubicin on sublines of 13762 mammary adenocarcinoma in rats. *Eur. J. Cancer Clin. Oncol. 17,* 1211.
44. Di Marco, A. (1980): The antitumor activity of 6α methyl-17α acetoxyprogesterone (MPA) in experimental mammary cancer. In: *Role of Medroxyprogesterone in Endocrine-Related Tumors,* pp. 1–20. Eds: S. Iacobelli and A. Di Marco. Raven Press, New York.
45. Iacobelli, S., Natoli, C. and Sica, G. (1982): Inhibitory effects of medroxyprogesterone acetate on the proliferation of human breast cancer cells. In: *Role of Medroxyprogesterone acetate (MPA) in Endocrine-Related Tumors II.* Raven Press, New York. (In press.)
46. Tominaga, T., Kitamura M., Saito T. et al. (1981): Effects of hexestrol, medroxyprogesterone acetate and chlormadinone acetate on 7-12-dimethylbenz[a]-anthracene-induced rat mammary cancer in relation to estrogen receptor. *Gann 72,* 604.
47. *Farmitalia monograph, Brochure 311276,* 1980.
48. Pannuti, F., Martoni, A., Lenaz, G.R. et al. P. (1976): Management of advanced breast cancer with medroxyprogesterone acetate (MAP, F.I., 5837, F.I. 7401, NSC-26386) in high doses. In: *Functional Exploration in Senology,* pp. 253–265. Eds: C. Colin, P. Franchimont, W. Gordenne, P. Juret, R. Lambotte, J. Lavigne, G.F. Leroux, B.A. Stoll and R. Vokaer. European Press, Ghent.
49. Pannuti, F., Martoni, A., Di Marco, A.R. et al. (1979): Prospective, randomized clinical trial of two different high dosages of medroxyprogesterone acetate (MAP) in the treatment of metastatic breast cancer. *Eur. J. Cancer 15,* 593.
50. Pannuti, F., Fruet, F., Piana, E. et al. (1978): The anabolic effect induced by high

doses of medroxyprogesterone acetate (MAP) orally in cancer patients. *IRCS Med. Sci. 6,* 118.
51. Bucalossi, P., Di Pietro, S. and Gennari, L. (1963): Trattamento ormonico del carcinoma mammario diffuso con un progestativo sintetico: il 6α-methyl-17α-acetossiprogesterone. *Minerva Chir. 9,* 358.
52. Klaassen, D.J., Rapp, E.F. and Hirte, W.E. (1976): Response to medroxyprogesterone acetate (NSC 26386) as secondary hormone therapy for metastatic breast cancer in postmenopausal women. *Cancer Treat. Rep. 60,* 251.
53. Martino, G. and Ventafridda, V. (1976): Effetto antalgico dell'alcoolizzazione ipofisaria, del Medrossiprogesterone acetato ad alte dosi e della loro associazione nel carcinoma mammario in fase avanzata. *Tumori 62,* 93.
54. Pannuti, F., Rossi, A.P. and Piana, E. (1977): Massive doses of medroxyprogesterone acetate (MAP): pilot study in the treatment of advanced prostate cancer. *IRCS Med. Sci. 5,* 375.
55. Pannuti, F., Martoni, A. and Cricca, A. (1978): Treatment of renal clear cell carcinoma by high doses of medroxyprogesterone acetate (MAP): pilot study. *IRCS Med. Sci. 6,* 177.
56. Pannuti, F., Burroni, P., Fruet, F. et al. (1980): Anabolizing and antipain effect of the short-term treatment with medroxyprogesterone acetate (MAP) at high oral doses in oncology. *Pan. Minerva Med. 22,* 149.
57. Hershberger, L.G., Shipley, E.G. and Meyer, R.K. (1953): Myotrophic activity of 19-nortestosterone and other steroids determined by modified *levator ani* muscle method. *Proc. Soc. Exp. Biol. Med. 83,* 175.
58. Pannuti, F., Gaggi, R., Murari-Colalongo, G. et al. (1981): Experimental study on the anabolic and androgenic/antiandrogenic activity of different dose levels of medroxyprogesterone acetate (MAP) in rats. *Oncology 38,* 307.
59. Durnin, J.V.G.A. and Womersley, J. (1974): Body fat assessed from total body density and its estimation from skinfold thickness: measurements on 481 men and women aged from 16 to 72 years. *Br. J. Nutr. 32,* 77.
60. Albanese, A.A. (1967): Clinical techniques for evaluating anabolic agents, II. *In: Animal and Clinical Pharmacologic Techniques in Drug Evaluation,* pp. 763–778. Eds: P.E. Siegler and J.H. Moyer III. Year Book Medical Publishers, Chicago.
61. Marzi, M.M., Bianchi, U., Pecorelli, S. et al. (1980): Progestins in advanced endometrial cancer. In: *Role of medroxyprogesterone in Endocrine-Related Tumors,* pp. 137–143. Eds: S. Iacobelli and A. Di Marco. Raven Press, New York.
62. Lelli, G., Giovannini, M., Gentili, M.R.A. et al. (1982): Carcinoma della prostata. Ormonoterapia: fase precoce, fase avanzata. In: *Trattato di Clinica Oncologica,* Ed: F. Pannuti. Piccin, Padua. [In press].
63. Bloom, H.J.C., Roe, F.J.C. and Mitchley, B.C.V. (1967): Sex hormones and renal neoplasia. *Cancer 20,* 2118.
64. Concolino, G., Marocchi, A., Conti, C. et al. (1978): Human renal cell carcinoma as a hormone-dependent tumor. *Cancer Res. 38,* 4340.
65. Holland, J.M. (1973): Cancer of the kidney. Natural history and staging. *Cancer 32,* 1030.
66. Fisher, R.I., Neifeld, J.P. and Lippman, M.E. (1976): Oestrogen receptors in human malignant melanoma. *Lancet II,* 337.
67. Beretta, G. (1978): High dose medroxyprogesterone acetate (MAP) as secondary

treatment for advanced melanoma. In: *Proceedings of the XIIth International Cancer Congress. Buenos Aires,* Vol. 3, p. 187.
68. Pannuti, F., Pollutri, E. and Giovannini, M. (1982): Il trattamento medico dei tumori ovarici. In: *Trattato di Clinica Oncologica.* Ed: F. Pannuti. Piccin, Padua. [In press].
69. Malkasian, G.D., Decker, D.G., Jorgensen, E.O. et al. (1977): Medroxyprogesterone acetate for the treatment of metastatic and recurrent ovarian carcinoma. *Cancer Treat. Rep. 61,* 913.
70. Gallo Curcio, C., Casali, A., Gianciotta, A. et al. (1979): Trattamento chemioormonoterapico in venti casi dell'ovaio metastatizzato. *Clin. Ter. 90,* 137.
71. Beatson, G.T. (1896): On the treatment of inoperable cases of carcinoma of the mamma: suggestion for a new method of treatment, with illustrative cases. *Lancet 2,* 104.
72. Pannuti, F., Martoni, A., Fruet, F. et al. (1979): Il tumore della mammella: il trattamento della fase avanzata. In: *Chemioterapia dei Tumori Solidi,* pp. 439–509. Ed: F. Pannuti. Patron, Bologna.
73. Dixon, W.J. and Brown, M.B. (1979): *BMDP-79 Biomedical Computer Programs, P-Series.* University of California Press, Berkeley.
74. Hayward, J.L., Carbone, P.P., Heuson, J.C. et al. (1977): Assessment of response to therapy in advanced breast cancer. *Eur. J. Cancer 13,* 89.
75. Pannuti, F., Martoni, A., Fruet, F. et al. (1982): Surgical adjuvant hormonal therapy with high dose medroxyprogesterone acetate (MAP) in breast cancer: results 36 months after mastectomy. *Pan. Minerva Med.* [in press].
76. Bodgen, A.E. (1978): Personal communication.

Session I: Experimental pharmacology and mechanism of antitumour activity

Chairmen: A. Di Marco – Milan, Italy
J.C. Heuson – Brussels, Belgium

Antitumour activity and pharmacokinetics of medroxyprogesterone acetate in experimental tumour systems*

F. Formelli[1], T. Zaccheo[2], A. Mazzoni[1], A.M. Isetta[2], A.M. Casazza[2] and A. Di Marco[2]
[1]National Tumour Institute; and [2]Farmitalia Carlo Erba, Milan, Italy

Introduction

Medroxyprogesterone acetate (MPA) is a synthetic steroid with progestational activity which has been employed in the treatment of a wide range of hormone-dependent tumours such as advanced breast cancer [1], endometrial adenocarcinoma [2], prostatic carcinoma [3], hypernephroma [4], testicular teratoma [5], bladder carcinoma [6] and ovarian carcinoma [7].

In an endeavour to understand the mechanism of the antitumour activity of MPA better, we investigated its effects on the growth of experimental tumours of different hormone sensitivities in mice and rats, and the pharmacokinetics of the compound in the same 2 species. The activity of a combination of MPA and doxorubicin (DX) was also examined.

Materials and methods

Tumour systems

Rat tumours Mammary tumours were induced in 50-day-old inbred Fischer 344 female rats by feeding 15 mg of 7,12-dimethylbenzanthracene (DMBA) per rat. Primary tumours were excised and transplanted subcutaneously (s.c.) into syngeneic intact and ovariectomized (OVX) female rats. Tumours growing only in intact animals were used as second generation transplants for ex-

* This work was supported in part by Grant No. 80.02371.96 of the Consiglio Nazionale delle Ricerche project 'Control of Tumour Growth'.

periments. OVX host animals were used in each experiment to check the hormone dependence of tumours. Three sublines, obtained in our laboratory from the hormone-responsive 13762 adenocarcinoma, were transplanted into syngeneic Fischer 344 female rats. These sublines were obtained following transplantation, freezing and in-vitro cultivation of the 13762 adenocarcinoma [8] and were shown to have different histological and oncogenic patterns. The Walker carcinosarcoma 256 was transplanted s.c. as tumour fragments into female Sprague-Dawley rats.

Mouse tumours MS-2 sarcoma [9] and colon 26 were transplanted s.c. into BALB/c mice. MXT adenocarcinoma, colon 38 and melanoma B16 were passed s.c. into BALB/c x/DBA/2 (BDF_1) mice. The third generation transplant of a spontaneous mammary carcinoma, inoculated s.c. into C3H/He female mice, was also used.

Tumour diameters were measured by means of calipers twice weekly, and tumour weights were estimated according to Geran et al. [10]. All animals used were supplied by the Charles River Laboratories (Calco, Como, Italy) and maintained under standard laboratory conditions.

Drugs MPA (Farmitalia Carlo Erba, Milan, Italy) and 17β-oestradiol (E_2) (Sigma Chemical Co., St. Louis, MO., U.S.A.) were suspended in sesame oil and administered s.c. in a volume of 2 ml/kg to rats and 5 ml/kg to mice, 5 days a week, for 4–7 weeks. DX (supplied as hydrochloride by Farmitalia Carlo Erba, Milan, Italy) was dissolved in distilled water immediately before use, and injected intravenously (i.v.) in a volume of 5 ml/kg once a week for 4–5 weeks. In combined treatment, MPA and DX were each administered in accordance with their respective treatment schedules, at the same doses as those used in treatment with each drug alone.

MPA serum levels in rats and mice were evaluated by radio-immunoassay (RIA) [11] after extraction with diethylether [12]. Animals were treated 5 times a week for 2 and 3 weeks, and, on days 1, 12 and 19, 3 animals per group were killed at various times following the final treatment, and their sera analysed to determine MPA levels.

Results

Effect of MPA on transplanted DMBA-induced mammary tumours

The sensitivity of second generation transplants of DMBA-induced tumours to high doses of E_2 and MPA, as well as to ovariectomy, was studied. Ovariectomy was performed 3 days before tumour transplantation. Oestradiol and MPA were administered from 3 days after tumour implant, 5 days a week, for 7 weeks. Results are shown in Figure 1. MPA at a dose of 100 mg/kg, was

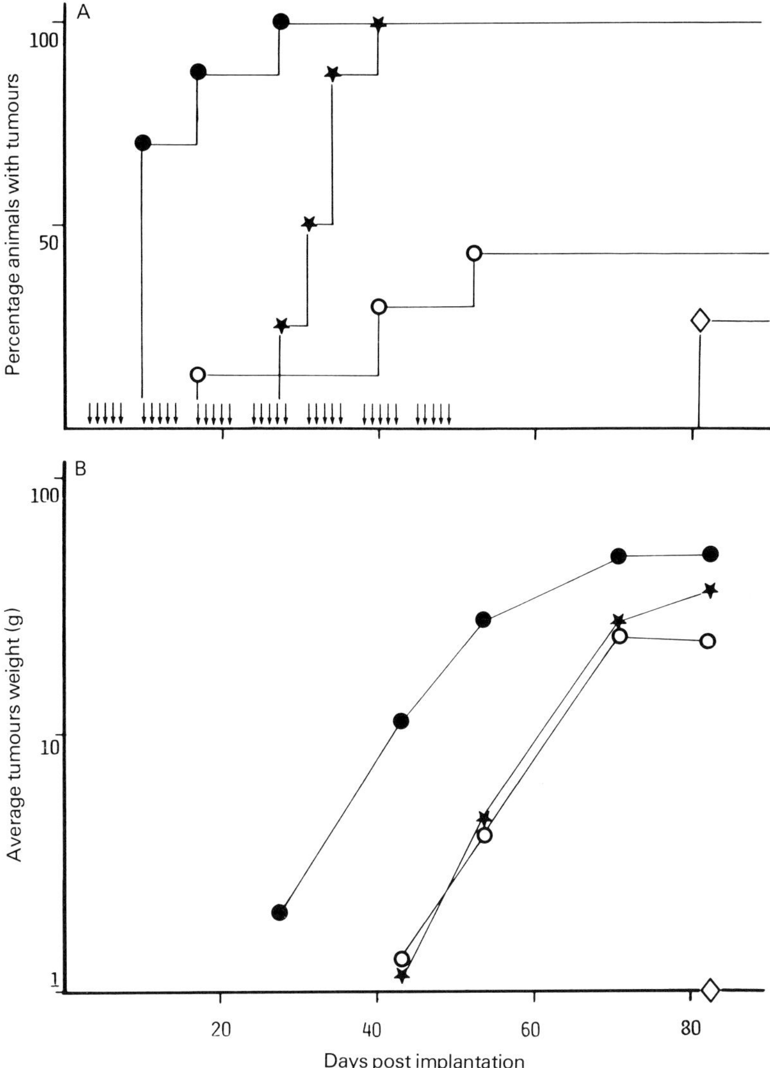

Fig. 1. Effects of MPA, 100 mg/kg s.c. (○), E_2, 0.1 mg/kg s.c. (●) and OVX (◇) on second generation transplants of DMBA-induced mammary tumours. Controls were treated with sesame oil (★). Animals were treated starting 3 days after tumour implantation, 5 days a week for 7 weeks. Ovariectomy was performed 3 days before implantation.

highly effective in delaying tumour onset. Eighty days after tumour implant, tumours were present in less than 50% of MPA-treated animals, though evident in 100% of the controls (Fig. 1A). The average tumour weight in MPA-treated, tumour-bearing animals was similar to that in controls (Fig. 1B). As expected, ovariectomy almost completely inhibited tumour growth. The opposite effect was obtained in rats treated with 0.1 mg/kg of E_2. This substance enhanced the speed of onset (Fig. 1A) and growth (Fig. 1B) of tumours.

Late tumours grown in MPA-treated and OVX rats (Fig. 1) were transplanted into both intact and OVX rats, to check the hormonal

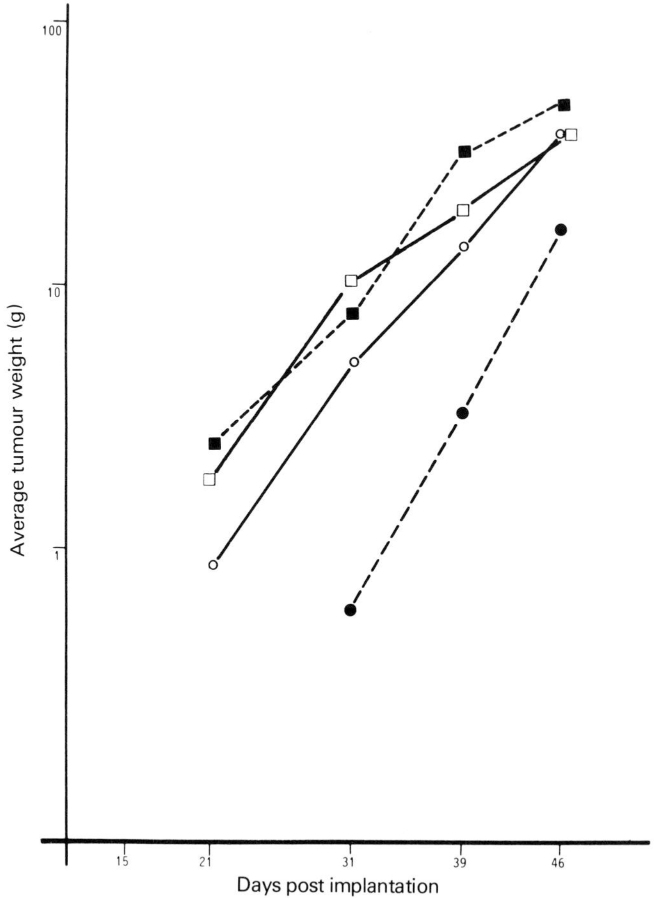

Fig. 2. Growth of transplanted DMBA-induced mammary tumours from OVX rats in intact (□) and OVX rats (■), and from MPA-treated rats in intact (○) and OVX rats (●).

dependence of the tumour cells predominating after the 2 hormonal manipulations. The results, recorded in Figure 2, show that tumours growing after ovariectomy were hormone-independent, since they grew in both intact and OVX animals. Tumours growing in MPA-treated rats were still hormone-dependent, as indicated by their retarded growth in OVX animals.

The activity of MPA on established DMBA-induced transplanted tumours was also tested (Fig. 3). In rats treated with MPA at a dose of 100 mg/kg, tumours were significantly smaller than in controls. The onset of growth of the tumour was delayed in animals ovariectomized at the beginning of the experiment and used to check hormone dependence.

Effects of MPA on sublines of 13762 mammary tumour

The 3 sublines obtained in our laboratory from the 13762 mammary tumour have different histological characteristics. Subline 2A maintained the

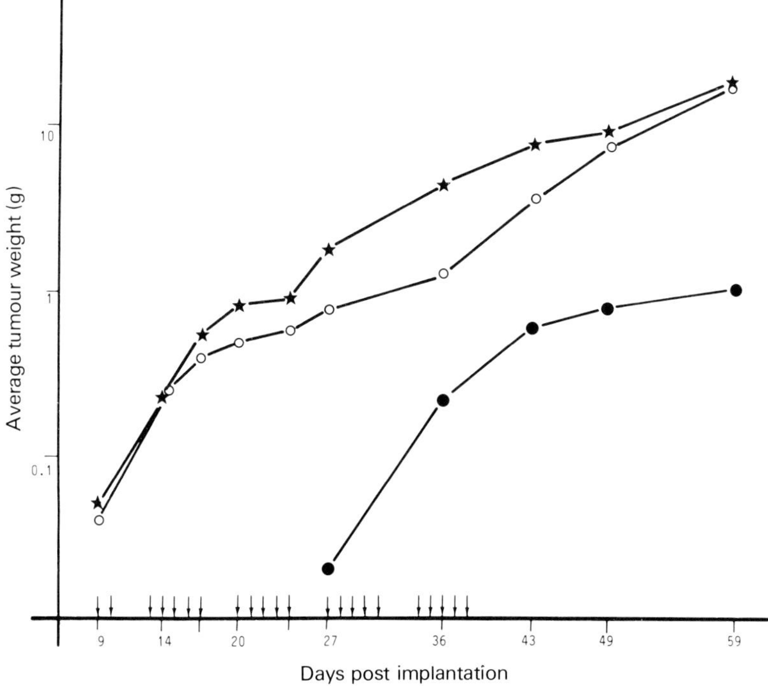

Fig. 3. Effects of MPA, 100 mg/kg s.c. (○) on established transplanted DMBA-induced tumours. Ovariectomy (●) was performed 3 days before implantation. Controls (★) were treated with sesame oil.

histological features of a mammary adenocarcinoma like those of the original 13762 tumour. Subline 2B was a poorly-differentiated mammary adenocarcinoma with small areas of fibrosarcomatous-like cells. Subline 2BV was composed mainly of spindle-shaped tumour cells, typical of a fibrosarcoma [8]. The oestrogen receptor contents of subline 2A (14th passage) and subline 2B (31st passage) were, respectively, 4.03 and 3.6 femtomoles/mg protein. Progesterone receptors were not detectable in either of the 2 sublines [13].

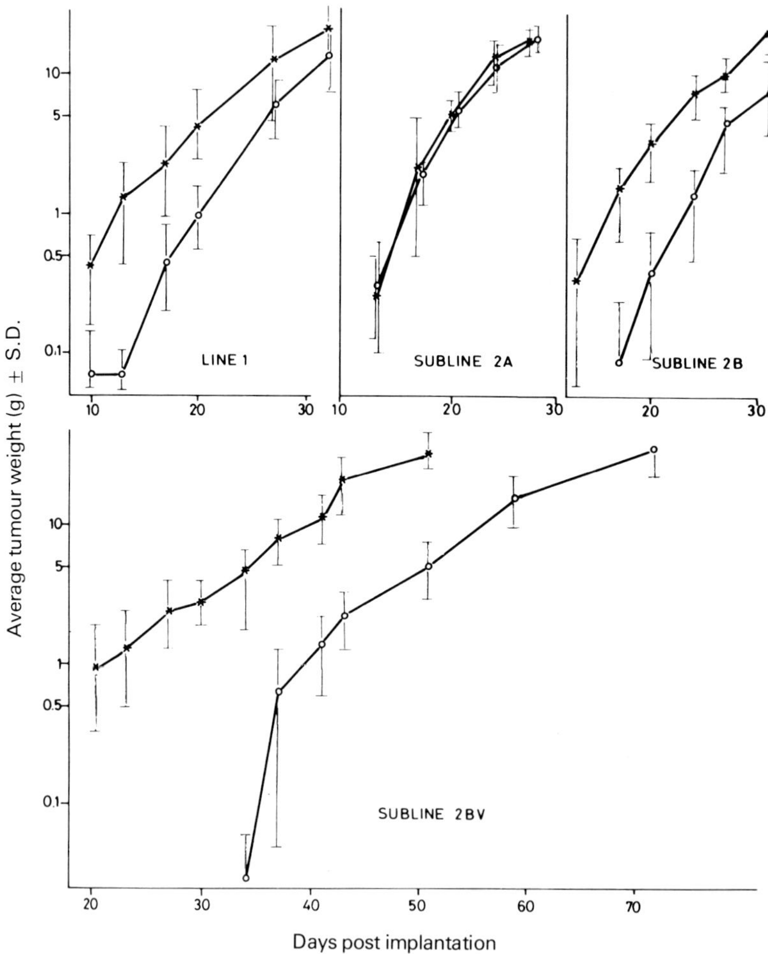

Fig. 4. Effects of MPA (○) on 13762 sublines. MPA was suspended in sesame oil and given s.c. at a dose of 100 mg/kg. Controls were treated with sesame oil (★). Animals were treated 5 days a week for 4–5 weeks.

The activity of MPA on the 3 sublines described was studied. The results are shown in Figure 4. MPA, given s.c. at a dose of 100 mg/kg 5 times a week for 4 weeks, was highly effective in delaying tumour onset in the case of the original tumour (line 1), subline 2B and subline 2BV, but had no activity on subline 2A. With subline 2B, sensitivity to MPA was lost with increase in the number of tumour passages (Table I).

The activity of MPA administered at different doses, and the dependence of the effect on the time of starting treatment is recorded in Figure 5. When treatment started 3 days after tumour implant, a good correlation was found between delay in onset of tumour growth and MPA dosage. MPA was also active when given to animals with already established tumours, but its activity was less than that observed when MPA was given immediately after tumour inoculation.

The effects of combined hormonal therapy and chemotherapy were investigated using MPA and DX against subline 2A, which was MPA-insensitive at the 14th passage, and on subline 2B, which was MPA-sensitive at the 34th passage. MPA was given s.c. at a dose of 100 mg/kg 5 times a week for 4 weeks. DX was given i.v. at the maximum tolerated dose (3.6 mg/kg, i.v.) once a week for 4 weeks. Results are shown in Figure 6. As previously shown, MPA delayed the growth of 13762 subline 2B, but was not active on subline 2A. DX produced a significant inhibition of tumour growth of sublines 2A and 2B, but its activity was higher against subline 2B than against subline 2A, with tumour growth inhibition of 81.8% and 40.6%, respectively, at the end of treatment. Figure 6 also shows that combined treatment with these agents resulted in higher growth inhibition than with either MPA or DX

Table I. MPA sensitivity of 13762 tumour, subline 2B. Relationship to number of serial passages. Subline 2B of 13762 tumour was implanted s.c. as fragments into female rats (8/group).

Number of passages	Control rats		MPA-treated rats	
	Mean days to tumour weight equivalent to:		Mean delay (days) in growth of tumour to weight equivalent to:	
	1 g	10 g	1 g	10 g
32	16	26	6.0	6.0
33	15	25	9.0	10.0
34	11	20	4.3	7.0
43	11	18	3.0	2.0
	13	19	3.8	3.6
45	13	21	0.5	0.0

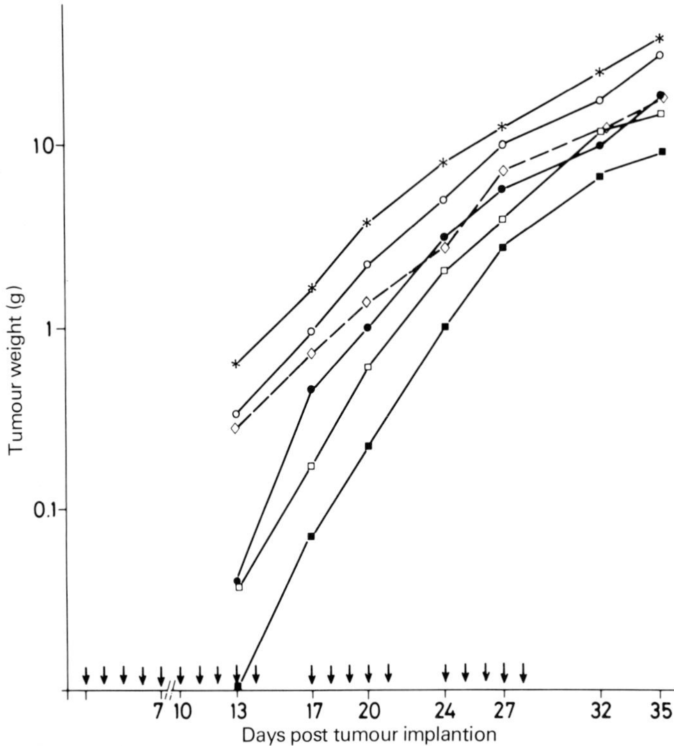

Fig. 5. Effects of various doses of MPA on 13762 mammary carcinoma (line 1). MPA was given s.c. at the doses of 12.5 mg/kg (○), 25 mg/kg (●), 50 mg/kg (□) and 100 mg/kg (■), 5 days a week for 4 weeks, starting 3 days after tumour implant. Treatment with MPA 100 mg/kg was also started when tumours were established (◇). Controls were treated with sesame oil (★).

given alone, for both sublines. However, the difference was not statistically significant.

Effect of MPA on Walker 256 carcinosarcoma

MPA, given s.c. at a dose of 100 mg/kg 5 times a week for 2 weeks, had no activity on the Walker 256 carcinosarcoma transplanted into female Sprague-Dawley rats.

Effect of MPA on experimental tumour systems in mice

The activity of MPA administered s.c. 5 times a week for 4 weeks against a

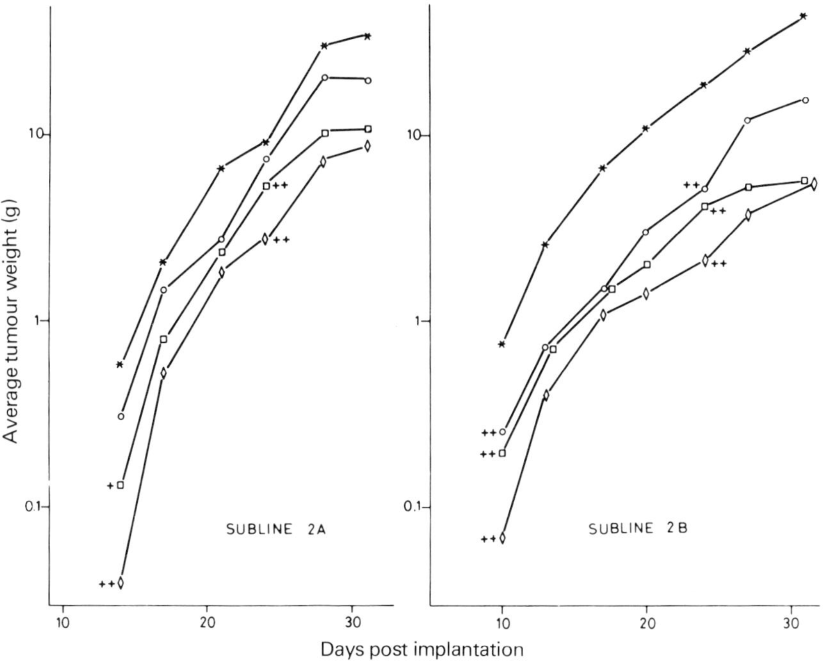

Fig. 6. Effect of MPA (○) and DX (□) as single agents and in combination (◇) on growth of sublines 2A and 2B of 13762 mammary carcinoma. Animals were treated s.c. with MPA 100 mg/kg 5 days a week for 4 weeks, and i.v. with DX 3.6 mg/kg once a week. In combined treatments each drug was given according to its treatment schedule. Controls were treated with sesame oil (★). + = $P \leq 0.05$, + + = $P \leq 0.01$ (Student's t-test) as compared to controls at tumour onset and at end of treatment.

panel of tumours transplanted into mice was tested. The results are reported in Table II.

In female mice, MPA at high doses (150–300 mg/kg/day) had no activity on MS-2 sarcoma, slightly increased the growth of C3H mammary carcinoma and melanoma B16, and significantly enhanced the growth of MXT adenocarcinoma and colon 38.

In mice bearing colon 26, an undifferentiated colon carcinoma which induces rapid cachexia and weight loss in the host animals, MPA significantly increased the life span but had no effect on tumour growth. In female mice, MPA also caused an increase in body weight. In male mice, MPA had no effect on either body weight or the growth of colon 38 and melanoma B16.

Table II. Effect of MPA on experimental tumour systems in mice.

Tumour	Sex	Dose (mg/kg)	Percentage differences between tumour weights in treated animals as compared with tumour weights in controls at end of experiment				Percentage increases in life spans in comparison with controls				Percentage differences in body weights in treated animals as compared with controls			
MS2-sarcoma	♀	150	−9				−18				+5			
C3H mammary	♀	150	+70				0				+14			
carcinoma		300	+72				0				+10			
MXT adeno-	♀	3	+94*				−7				+13			
carcinoma		300	+67*				−3				+9			
Colon 26	♀	3		−6				+21				+8		
		150	+3	+39			+35**	+93**			+11,	+11		
Colon 38	♀	3		−16				+4				+1		
		30		+4				+9				+9		
		150	+193**	+28	+373*		−40	−6	ND		+14,	+4,	+12	
		300	+144*	+43		+268*	−16	−16		ND	+10,	+6,		+12
	♂	3	−8				ND				0			
		300	−7				ND				−8			
Melanoma B16	♀	3			+3				−21				+11	
		30		−18				ND				+10		
		150	+17	+3			+2	ND			+7	+12		
		300		+57	+45			ND	−2			+12,	+12	
	♂	3	−10				−6				−2			
		300	−20				+23				−3			

$*P \leq 0.05$; $**P \leq 0.01$ (Student's *t*-test).
ND = not determined.

Pharmacokinetics of MPA in rats and mice

MPA serum levels in rats

MPA serum levels were measured in rats bearing 13762 tumours which were treated s.c. with 50 and 200 mg/kg MPA 5 times a week for 3 weeks.

The results, recorded in Table III, show that peak levels after the first treatment with 200 mg/kg MPA were higher than those found on days 12 and 19 of treatment. Plasma clearance was fairly slow: drug levels at 24 hours were about half the 7 hour levels. In addition, high drug levels were constantly found before each administration. A slight increase in drug levels was found between treatments on days 12 and 19 at both dose levels, suggesting that a steady state had not been reached by day 19 of treatment.

MPA serum levels in mice

MPA serum levels were also investigated in mice. C3H mice were treated with 300 mg/kg MPA, s.c. (500 mg/m^2, equivalent to 200 mg/kg in rats) and with 1,000 mg/kg MPA, s.c., 5 times a week for 2 weeks. Results are shown in Table IV.

On day 1, peak levels were similar to those found in rats. The rate of elimination 24 hours after the first treatment was higher than that found in

Table III. MPA serum levels in rats bearing 13762 tumour (ng/ml ± standard deviation).

Time of serum level determination		Dose (mg/kg)	
Day	Hours	50	200
1	2		206 ± 342
	7		2360 ± 994
	24		1070 ± 592
12	0	272 ± 14	358 ± 46
	2	316 ± 23	471 ± 52
	7	367 ± 21	465 ± 20
19	0	303 ± 19	516 ± 29
	2	411 ± 28	707 ± 61
	7	439 ± 206	524 ± 20

MPA equivalent levels in untreated rats were 13.9 ± 8.8 ng/ml.

Table IV. MPA serum levels in C3H mice (ng/ml ± standard deviation).

Time of serum level determination		Dose (mg/kg)	
Day	Hours	300	1000
1	2	1890 ± 229	2102 ± 540
	6	2086 ± 322	1389 ± 465
	24	149 ± 36	204 ± 32
12	0	699 ± 70	930 ± 61
	2	1660 ± 357	3150 ± 711

MPA equivalent levels in untreated mice were 10.5 ± 1 ng/ml.

rats. No difference was found in peak levels after administration of the 2 doses. On day 12, peak levels were higher than those found in rats, and there was a relationship between the dose administered and serum drug levels.

Discussion

The data reported in the present study show that MPA can have different effects, depending on the hormone sensitivity of the tumour and the species and sex of the host animal, and that the effects are related to constant high serum levels of the drug.

In rats, MPA at high dosage was very effective against a hormone-dependent tumour such as the transplanted DMBA-induced mammary carcinoma, and against hormone-sensitive tumours such as the 13762 adenocarcinoma, but had no activity against a hormone-independent tumour such as the Walker 256 carcinosarcoma.

Other authors have found that MPA at high dosage was highly active against the primary DMBA-induced mammary carcinoma, which is also a hormone-dependent tumour [14, 15], and that it was effective regardless of whether cytoplasmic oestrogen receptors were present in the tumour or not [15]. The original 13762 adenocarcinoma, and one of the selected sublines, both sensitive to MPA, had low contents of oestrogen receptors [13, 16] and no detectable progesterone receptors [13]. These findings suggest that, in rats, MPA at high doses may act as a 'chemical ovariectomizing' agent, by inhibiting the hypothalamo-hypophyseal axis, but that other endocrine-inhibiting mechanisms apart from the mechanism involving the oestrogen receptor system may also contribute to antitumour activity of MPA. In addition, a direct effect of MPA at high doses on hormone-sensitive tumour cells is suggested by in-vitro data [17, 18].

The results obtained in the study of the activity of MPA and DX administration against the 13762 adenocarcinoma confirm both laboratory [19] and clinical data [20], and suggest that combinations of endocrine treatment and chemotherapy may be more effective than either treatment alone, against both hormone-sensitive and apparently hormone-insensitive tumours. In fact, potentiation of the antitumour activity of DX by MPA against the 13762 subline which was not sensitive to MPA, was also observed, suggesting that the selection of cell clones following transplantation, freezing and thawing was not complete, and that tumour cells responsive to hormonal treatment may also have been present in the insensitive tumour.

In the transplanted DMBA-induced mammary tumour, we have shown that treatment with MPA, in contrast to ovariectomy, did not result in the selection of exclusively hormone-independent cells, since the onset of growth of transplanted MPA-treated tumours was delayed in OVX rats as compared to intact animals. This suggests that therapy with different hormones might be advantageous in the case of hormone-dependent tumours, a possibility which deserves further investigation in the hope of improving the utility of hormone therapy.

The lack of antitumour activity of MPA against mouse tumours and its stimulant effect on some tumours at high doses are intriguing, and difficult to explain. The hormone sensitivity of mouse tumours has not been so widely investigated as that of mammary tumours in rats. Serial passages of these tumours may have resulted in selection of lines with different hormone sensitivities. The C3H/He mammary carcinoma was chosen by us as a hormone-independent tumour, but has been reported to have oestrogen [21] and glucocorticoid receptors [22]. B16 melanoma, according to some authors, has a different growth rate in male and female mice [23], and it has been reported that oestrogens hinder its growth [24]. MXT adenocarcinoma has oestrogen and progesterone receptors, and is ovarian-dependent [25]. As for colon 38, we have found it to be oestrogen receptor-positive (manuscript in preparation). These data suggest that several tumours transplanted into mice remain hormone-sensitive, a conclusion supported by the fact that their growth is influenced by high doses of MPA. Similar growth-stimulating properties of MPA have been reported in 2 patients with renal cell carcinoma [26], and in rats with a transplanted uterine adenocarcinoma [27] and with DMBA-induced mammary tumours [14]. In both the experimental tumour systems mentioned, the stimulant effect was seen at low MPA doses. In the case of the DMBA-induced rat mammary tumour, while MPA stimulated tumour growth at a low dose (1 mg/kg), a high dose (100 mg/kg) was strongly inhibitory towards the same tumour [14]. The low dose also caused an increase in body weight, while the high dose did not. In female mice, we observed a similar correlation between increase in body weight and tumour-stimulating effect, but in males MPA had no effect on either body weight or tumour growth. This suggests that MPA has an endocrine-inhibitory activity in mice, which may be responsible for its stimulant effect on the tumour systems mentioned. Further studies on the hormone sensitivity of the experimental systems used, might help towards understanding of the mechanism of action of MPA and might reveal, in particular, if MPA has a different endocrine activity in mice and in rats. From the data reported by other authors on the DMBA-induced rat mammary tumour [14], it seems that, in the rat, MPA may vary in activity according to dose. It is interesting to note that MPA, without affecting tumour growth, significantly increased the life span of mice bearing colon 26, a tumour which grows very quickly, and which induces rapid cachexia in host animals. This may be due to an anabolic effect of MPA in mice as previously reported in man [28] and rats [29].

The pharmacokinetic studies on MPA show that, on giving the drug repeatedly, s.c., constant high drug levels are attained in the blood of both rats and mice. Analogous constant high drug levels have been found in man after i.m. administration [30] and may result from both slow release from the site of injection and slow elimination of MPA.

References

1. Ganzina, F. (1979): High dose medroxyprogesterone acetate (MPA) treatment in advanced breast cancer. *Tumori 65*, 563.
2. Bonte, J., Decoster, J.M., Ide, P. and Billiet, G. (1978): Hormonoprophylaxis and hormonotherapy in the treatment of endometrial adenocarcinoma by means of medroxyprogesterone acetate. *Gynecol. Oncol. 6*, 60.
3. Rafla, S. and Johnson, R. (1974): The treatment of advanced prostatic carcinoma with medroxyprogesterone. *Curr. Ther. Res. 16*, 261.
4. Concolino, G., Marocchi, A., Conti, C. et al. (1978): Human renal cell carcinoma as a hormonedependent tumor. *Cancer Res. 38*, 4340.
5. Klepp, O., Klepp, R., Host, H. et al. (1977): Combination chemotherapy of germ cell tumors of the testis with vincristine, adriamycin, cyclophosphamide, actinomycin D and medroxyprogesterone acetate. *Cancer 40*, 638.
6. Francone, E. (1974): Medroxyprogesterone acetate and bladder tumors. *Minerva Urol. 26*, 32.
7. Malkasian, G.D., Decker, D.G., Jorgenstens, E.O. and Edmondon, J.H. (1977): Medroxyprogesterone acetate for the treatment of metastatic and recurrent ovarian carcinoma. *Cancer Treat. Rep. 61*, 913.
8. Formelli, F., Zaccheo, T., Casazza, A.M. et al. (1981): Effect of medroxyprogesterone acetate and doxorubicin on sublines of 13762 mammary adenocarcinoma in rats. *Eur. J. Cancer Clin. Oncol. 17*, 1211.

9. Giuliani, F., Bellini, O., Casazza, A.M. et al. (1978): Biologic characterization and chemotherapeutic response of MS-2 tumor: a non-regressive mouse sarcoma derived from MSV-M induced sarcoma. *Eur. J. Cancer 14*, 555.
10. Geran, R.I., Greenberg, N.H., McDonald, M.M. et al. (1972): Protocols for screening chemical agents and natural products against animal tumors and other biological systems. *Cancer Chemother. Reports 3*, 1.
11. Shrimanker, K., Sakena, B.N. and Fotherby, K. (1978): A radioimmunoassay for serum medroxyprogesterone acetate. *J. Steroid Biochem. 9*, 359.
12. Zaccheo, T., Formelli, F., Casazza, A.M. and Isetta, A.M. (1981): Antitumor activity and pharmacokinetics of medroxyprogesterone acetate (MPA) in experimental tumor systems. *Proceedings of 12th International Congress of Chemotherapy, Florence, Italy*. (In press.)
13. Ronchi, E., Zaccheo, T., Di Fronzo, G. and Formelli, F. (1981): Estrogen and progesterone receptors in sublines of 13762 mammary adenocarcinoma in rats. *IRCS Med. Sci. 9*, 960.
14. Danguy, A., Legros, N., Devleeschouwer, N. et al. (1980): Effects of medroxyprogesterone acetate (MPA) on growth of DMBA-induced rat mammary tumors: histopathological and endocrine studies. In: *Role of Medroxyprogesterone in Endocrine-Related Tumors*, pp. 21–28. Eds: S. Iacobelli and A. Di Marco. Raven Press, New York.
15. Tominaga, T., Kitamura, M., Saito, T. and Itoh, I. (1981): Effects of hexestrol, medroxyprogesterone acetate and chlormadinone acetate on 7,12-dimethylbenz(a)anthracene-induced rat mammary cancer in relation to estrogen receptor. *Gann 72*, 604.
16. Bodwin, J.S., Clair, T. and Cho Chung, Y.S. (1980): Relationship of hormone dependency to estrogen receptor and adenosine 3', 5'-cyclic monophosphate-binding proteins in rat mammary tumors. *J. Nat. Cancer Inst. 64*, 395.
17. Di Marco, A. (1980): The antitumor activity of 6α-methyl-17α-acetoxy progesterone (MPA) in experimental mammary cancer. In: *Role of Medroxyprogesterone in Endocrine-Related Tumors*, pp. 1–20. Eds: S. Iacobelli and A. Di Marco, Raven Press, New York.
18. Natoli, C., Sica, G. and Iacobelli, S. (1981): Effects of medroxyprogesterone acetate on cell cultures of carcinoma of the human breast. *Tumori 67 (2 Suppl. A)*, 185.
19. Sluyser, M., Degoeij, C.C.J. and Evers, S.G. (1981): Combined endocrine therapy and chemotherapy of mouse mammary tumors. *Eur. J. Cancer 17*, 155.
20. Robustelli Della Cuna, G. and Bernardo-Strada, M.R. (1980): High dose medroxyprogesterone acetate (HD-MPA) combined with chemotherapy for metastatic breast carcinoma. In: *Role of Medroxyprogesterone in Endocrine-Related Tumors*, pp. 53–64, Eds: S. Iacobelli and A. Di Marco. Raven Press, New York.
21. Richards, J.E., Shymala, G. and Nandi, S. (1974): Estrogen receptor in normal and neoplastic mouse mammary tissues, *Cancer Res. 34*, 2764.
22. Braunschweiger, P.G. and Schiffer, L.M. (1981): Antiproliferative effects of corticosteroids in C3H/HEJ mammary tumors and implications for sequential combination chemotherapy. *Cancer Res. 41*, 3324.
23. Proctor, J.W., Auclair, B.G. and Stokowski, L. (1976): Endocrine factors and the growth and spread of B16 melanoma. *J. Nat. Cancer Inst. 57*, 1197.

24. Proctor, J.W., Yamamura, Y., Gaydos, D. and Mastromatteo, W. (1981): Further studies of endocrine factors and growth and spread of B16 melanoma. *Oncology 38*, 102.
25. Watson, C.S., Medina, D. and Clark, J.H. (1979): Characterization and estrogen stimulation of cytoplasmic progesterone receptor in the ovarian-dependent MXT-3590 mammary tumor line. *Cancer Res. 39*, 4098.
26. Tchaod, R., Easty, G.C., Ambrose, E.J. et al. (1968): Effect of the chemotherapeutic agents and hormones on organ cultures of human tumors. *Eur. J. Cancer 4*, 39.
27. Sekiya, S., Yano, A. and Takamizawa, H. (1974): Enhancement of tumor growth and metastases by medroxyprogesterone acetate in transplanted uterine adenocarcinoma cells of the rat. *J. Nat. Cancer Inst. 52*, 297.
28. Pannuti, F., Fruet, F., Piana, E. et al. (1978): The anabolic effect induced by high doses of medroxyprogesterone acetate (MPA) orally in cancer patients. *IRCS Med. Sci. 6*, 118.
29. Pannuti, G., Gaggi, R., Murari-Colalongo, G. et al. (1981): Experimental study on the anabolic and androgenic/antiandrogenic activity of different dose levels of medroxyprogesterone acetate (MPA) in rats. *Oncology 38*, 307.
30. Cornette, J.C., Kirton, K.T. and Duncan, G.W. (1971): Measurement of medroxyprogesterone acetate (Provera) by radioimmunoassay. *J. Clin. Endocrinol. Metab. 33*, 459.

Effects of medroxyprogesterone acetate on the development of dimethylbenzanthracene-induced mammary tumours: possible modes of action*

A. Danguy[1], N. Legros[2], G. Leclercq[2] and J.C. Heuson[2]
[1]Histological Laboratory, Faculty of Medicine, University of Brussels; and [2]Department of Medicine and Laboratory of Clinical Investigation H.J. Tagnon, Clinic and Laboratory of Mammary Oncology, Institute J. Bordet, Brussels, Belgium

Introduction

The semisynthetic steroid 6α-methyl-17α-acetoxypregn-4-ene-3,2-dione (medroxyprogesterone acetate, MPA) has an intense progestational activity in animals [1]. The compound was first synthesized in 1958 [2]. MPA has been used for a number of years with some success in the treatment of endometrial adenocarcinoma [3], prostatic carcinoma [4], testicular teratoma [5, 6], ovarian carcinoma [7] and breast cancer [8–12].

The present investigation was undertaken in the hope of achieving a better understanding of the antitumour activity of MPA. The effect of the drug on the growth of 7,12-dimethylbenz(a)anthracene-(DMBA)-induced mammary tumours in the rat was studied. This model is extensively used in the study of dependence of breast cancer on hormones. Histological modifications in elements of the pituitary-gonadal and adrenal axes and endocrinological alterations which occurred after administration of the drug are also described.

* This study was supported by the Fonds Cancérologique de la Caisse Générale d'Epargne et de Retraite, Belgium. Thanks are also due to Farmitalia Carlo Erba, who provided progestagen and financial support.

Material and methods

Animals and carcinogen

Mammary tumours were induced in 50-day-old female Sprague-Dawley rats, bred in our laboratory, by means of a single, intravenous injection of 5 mg of DMBA (Eastman, Rochester, NY, U.S.A.) dissolved in sesame oil. The first tumours appeared 2 months after administration of DMBA.

The study was made up of experiments on intact and ovariectomized (OVX) animals. The studies in OVX rats were designed on the basis of results in the experiment using intact animals.

In the latter experiment, the animals were divided at random into 4 groups. There were equal numbers of tumours, of equal sizes in each of the 4 groups. A control group received sesame oil only. The 3 other groups, A, B and C, received subcutaneous (s.c.) injections of 1 mg/kg, 10 mg/kg and 100 mg/kg of MPA, respectively, dissolved in the vehicle.

In the experiment involving OVX animals, 6 groups were formed. These consisted of 3 groups of nonovariectomized animals and 3 groups of OVX animals. One group of intact animals received no MPA, but only sesame oil. The other 2 groups, A and C, received 1 and 100 mg/kg MPA, respectively, s.c., as in the experiment involving only intact animals. In the OVX animals, group F received no MPA, only sesame oil, and groups D and E, 1 and 100 mg/kg of MPA, respectively, s.c. The animals were ovariectomized before drug administration.

In both studies, MPA was administered for 6 weeks, 6 days a week. Body weight and tumour surface area were recorded at the beginning and end of the experiments. Tumour size was measured by means of calipers, and expressed as a surface area by multiplying 2 diameters at right angles to each other. Total tumour surface per rat is the sum of the surface areas of all tumours.

At the end of treatment the animals were killed by decapitation (Guillotine, Harvard apparatus Co., Dover, Ma., U.S.A.). Blood was collected and allowed to clot at room temperature. After centrifugation the serum was collected and stored at $-20\,^{\circ}C$ until assay for hormone levels [13].

Histological procedures

Pituitaries, mammary gland tumours, adrenals and ovaries were collected quickly after decapitation and fixed in Bouin-Hollande fluid for at least one week. Mammary glands, tumours, ovaries and adrenals were stained using haematoxylin, eosin and saffron. The adenohypophyses were studied using the unlabelled antibody peroxidase-antiperoxidase (PAP) method [14] for the detection of adrenocorticotropic hormone (ACTH) and prolactin (PRL). Antiserum to rat prolactin was kindly supplied by Dr A.F. Parlow of the National Institute of Arthritis and Metabolic Diseases (NIAMD), Rat Pituitary Hormone Program. An antiserum to synthetic 17–39 ACTH prepared in our laboratory, and of known specificity was used [15]. The same pituitaries were analysed using an immunofluorescence method, to detect luteinizing hormone (LH) cells, using an antiserum to ovine LH [16].

Radioimmunoassays (RIA)

Plasma LH and PRL levels were measured using double antibody radioimmunoassays (RIA kits supplied by NIAMD, Bethesda, MD, U.S.A.). The results were expressed in ng NIAMD-Rat-LH-RP1 and ng NIAMD-Rat-PRL-RP1 standards/ml. The results were subjected to analysis of variance [17].

Results

Effects of MPA and/or ovariectomy on DMBA-induced mammary tumours

The effects of MPA are summarized in Table I. In intact animals, 1 mg/kg of the drug significantly enhanced tumour growth. Tumour growth was significantly inhibited by 100 mg/kg of MPA. Ovariectomy alone resulted in tumour regression, as expected. Administration of MPA at 1 mg/kg and 100 mg/kg to OVX animals did not affect the course of tumour regression brought about by ovariectomy.

Effects of MPA on body weight

The results are summarized in Table II. In intact animals, the administration of 1 mg/kg or 10 mg/kg of MPA significantly increased body weight. Ovariectomy also produced an increase in body weight. Administration of 1 mg/kg of MPA to OVX animals resulted in no greater increase than ovariectomy alone. A dose of 100 mg/kg significantly inhibited the increase in body weight resulting from ovariectomy.

Effects of MPA on plasma LH and PRL levels

Plasma concentrations of PRL and LH are shown in Figures 1 and 2, respectively.

Table I. Effect of MPA and/or ovariectomy on DMBA-induced mammary tumours (adenocarcinomas). Data analysed statistically using Wilcoxon test for paired differences.

Group	MPA dose (mg/kg)	Mean total tumour area per rat (mm^2)			Group	MPA dose (mg/kg)/ OVX status	Mean total tumour area per rat (mm^2)		
		Before MPA	After MPA	Difference			Before MPA	After MPA or OVX	Difference
Control		184	376	+ 192	Control		267	334	+ 67
A	1	173	725	+ 552*	A	1	331	1234	+ 904*
B	10	199	359	+ 160^{+}	C	100	301	135	− 166***
C	100	165	31	− 134***	D	1 + OVX	362	159	− 203**
					E	100 + OVX	225	291	+ $66^{+‡}$
					F	OVX only	328	146	− 182^{**++}

* Significantly different from control, $P<0.01$.
** Significantly different from control, $P<0.02$.
*** Significantly different from control, $P=0.02$.
$^{+}$ No significant difference from control.
‡ No significant difference from group F result.
$^{++}$ No significant difference from group D result.

Table II. Effects of MPA and/or ovariectomy on rat body weight.

Group	MPA dose (mg/kg)	Mean weight of rats (g)			Group	MPA dose (mg/kg)/ OVX status	Mean weight of rats (g)		
		Before MPA	After MPA	Difference			Before MPA	After MPA or OVX	Difference
Controls		288	298	+ 10	Controls		254	265	+ 11
A	1	285	316	+ 31*	A	1	274	329	+ 55**‡
B	10	305	329	+ 24*	C	100	264	266	+ 2+
C	100	280	290	+ 19+	D	1 + OVX	258	312	+ 54**‡
					E	100 + OVX	273	272	– 1+‡‡
					F	OVX only	260	310	+ 50**

* Significantly different from control, $P<0.05$.
** Significantly different from control, $P<0.02$.
+ Not significantly different from control.
‡ Not significantly different from group F value.
‡‡ Significantly different from group D value, $P<0.05$.
‡‡‡ Significantly different from group E value, $P<0.05$.

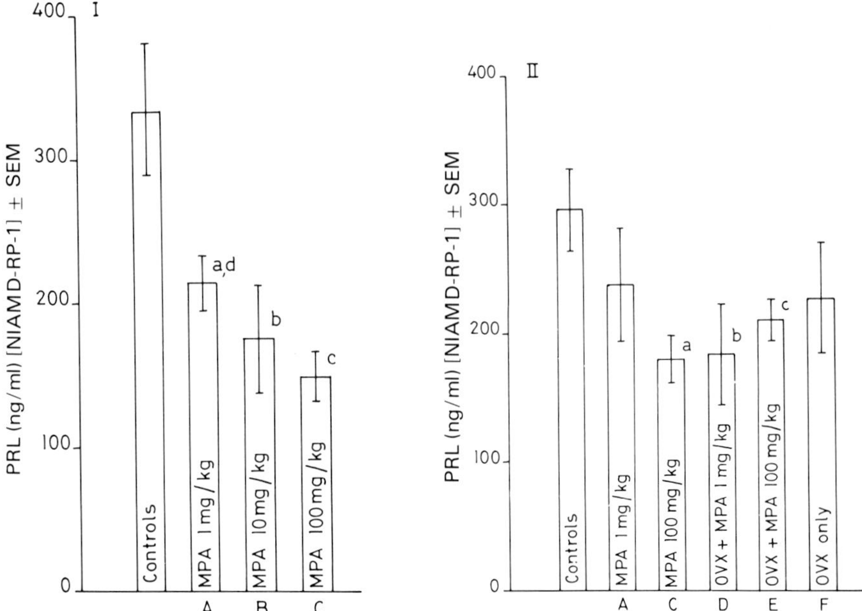

Fig. 1. Serum levels of PRL in tumour-bearing rats at the end of the 6-week experimental period. I. MPA alone. Fisher F test: a. A vs controls: NS; b. B vs controls $P<0.05$; c. C vs controls $P<0.001$; d. A vs C $P<0.05$. II. MPA with or without OVX. Fisher F test: a. C vs controls $P<0.001$; b. D vs controls $P<0.05$; c. E vs controls $P<0.05$.

PRL concentrations Neither 1 mg/kg of MPA alone nor ovariectomy modified plasma concentrations of PRL significantly. (Controls 337 ± 46 ng/ml, 1 mg/kg MPA 214 ± 19 ng/ml, ovariectomy 225 ± 41 ng/ml.) In intact animals, the level of PRL following a dose of 10 mg/kg MPA, was 175 ± 37 ng/ml. The lowest level, 148 ± 16 ng/ml, was measured in animals treated with 100 mg/kg MPA. Ovariectomy did not lower PRL levels further in animals receiving 100 mg/kg MPA.

LH concentrations MPA at doses of 10 and 100 mg/kg resulted in a significant decrease in LH concentrations (21 ± 3 ng/ml and 15 ± 3 ng/ml, respectively) as compared to controls (31 ± 5 ng/ml). Ovariectomy alone resulted in a marked increase in LH level (840 ± 45 ng/ml) as expected. MPA, 1 mg and 100 mg/kg, reduced the effects of ovariectomy significantly (215 ± 34 ng/ml and 113 ± 31 ng/ml, respectively).

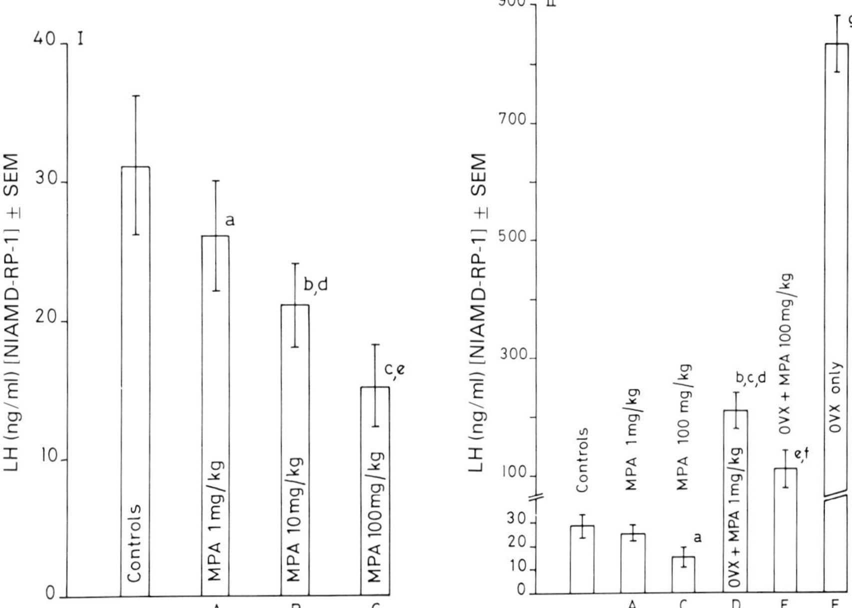

Fig. 2. Serum levels of LH in tumour-bearing rats at the end of the 6-week experimental period. I. MPA alone. Fisher F test: a. A vs controls: NS; b. B vs controls P<0.05; c. C vs controls P<0.01; d. A vs B NS; e. A vs C P<0.05. II. MPA with or without OVX. Fisher F test: a. C vs controls: NS; b. D vs controls P<0.001; d. D vs E P<0.05; e. E vs controls P<0.001; f. E vs F P<0.001; g. F vs controls P<0.001.

Morphological data

The ovaries after administration of 1 mg/kg of MPA were normal. In animals treated with 10 and 100 mg/kg of MPA, the ovaries were atrophic, and contained very small, often atretic, follicles, with no corpora lutea. In both intact and ovariectomized animals, the adrenals were notably small at the higher doses, with atrophy of the cortical components and thickening of the connective capsule. Necrosis and adenomas of the adrenocortical tissue were also observed.

In the mammary glands, secretion was evident, with patency of alveoli and presence of casein and lipid materials in the excretory ducts of all except the control group and OVX group of animals.

Ovariectomy produced no detectable histological modifications in the adrenal or mammary glands.

The vaginal epithelia were atrophic in all animals except intact animals

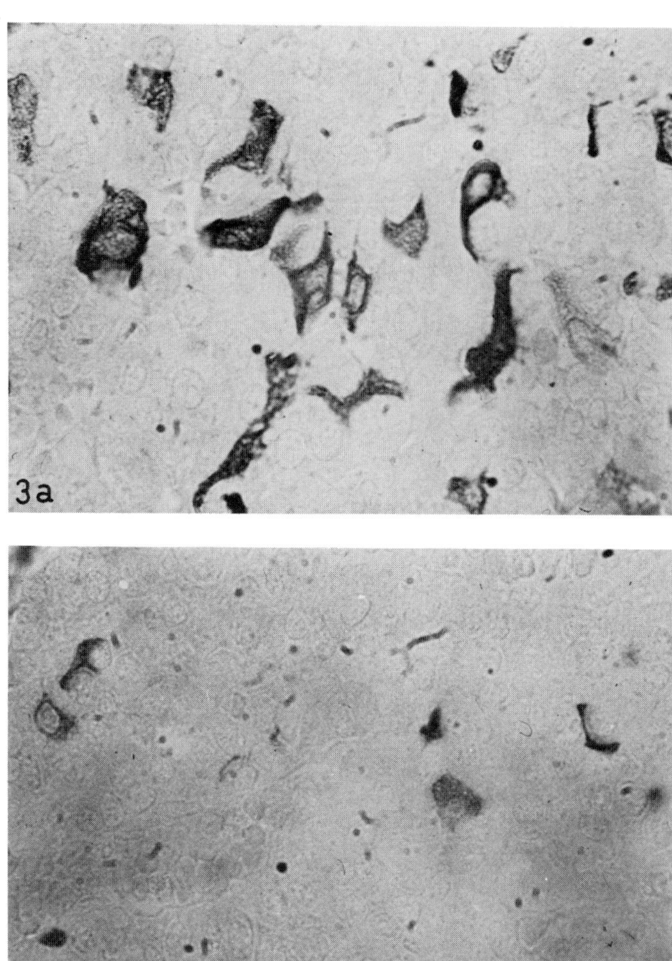

Fig. 3. 5-μm Paraffin sections of rat pituitaries stained by the unlabelled PAP method with antiserum to rat ACTH. a. Pars distalis of a control animal. Immunoreactive ACTH cells are more numerous as compared to b. b. Pars distalis of a MPA 100 mg/kg treated animal. ACTH cells are scarce as compared to a. 1 cm = 5 μm.

receiving 1 mg and 10 mg/kg of MPA, in which pseudogestational changes were seen.

Using PAP unlabelled antibody preparation, PRL and ACTH cells in all pituitaries were found to be as well developed after treatment with 1 mg/kg of MPA as in controls. In contrast, after 10 mg/kg of MPA, and, more especial-

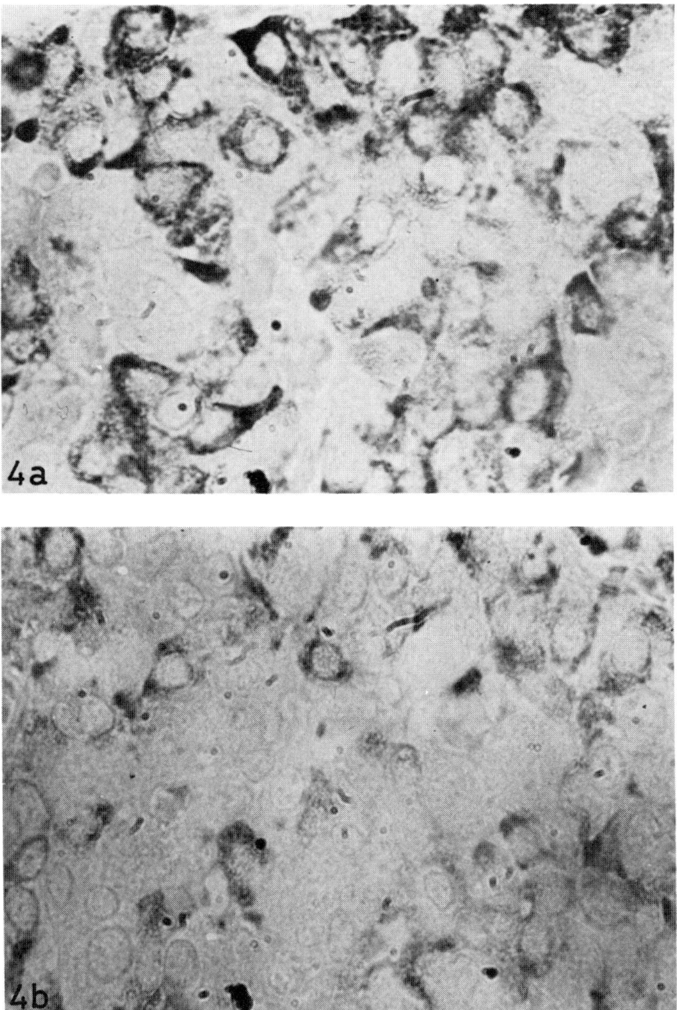

Fig. 4. 5-μm Paraffin sections of rat pituitaries stained by the unlabelled PAP method with antiserum to rat PRL. a. Pars distalis of a control animal. Cells containing PRL are more numerous than in b. b. Immunoreactive PRL cells in the pars distalis of a MPA 100 mg/kg treated rat. 1 cm = 5 μm.

ly, after 100 mg/kg of MPA, mammotrophs and adrenocorticotrophs were few and atrophic (Figs. 3 and 4).

Using the immunofluorescence technique, the gonadotrophs in animals treated with 100 mg/kg of MPA were also found to be fewer in number than in control animals or those treated with 1 mg/kg of MPA (Fig. 5).

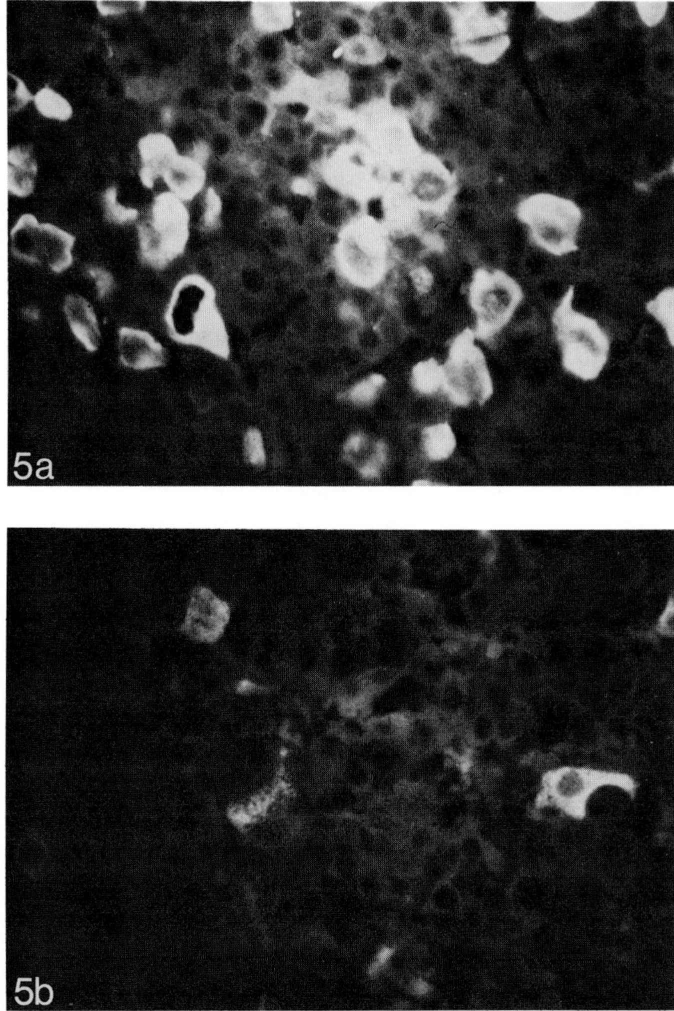

Fig. 5. 5-μm Paraffin sections of rat pituitaries stained using immunofluorescence and antiserum to ovine LH. a. Pars distalis of a control animal. The gonadotrophs are fairly well developed. b. Pars distalis of a MPA 100 mg/kg treated rat. The gonadotrophs are developed to a much lesser extent than in (a). 1 cm = 5 μm.

Discussion

Under the conditions in the study described here, 1 mg/kg of MPA was found to stimulate the growth of DMBA-induced rat mammary tumours. Growth of these tumours was strongly inhibited by 100 mg/kg of MPA.

Table III. Effects of treatments on tumour growth, body weight and histological and endocrine parameters (comparisons with control results).

Dose of MPA (mg/kg)	Tumour growth	Body weight	ACTH cells	PRL		LH	
				Cells	Blood concentration	Cells	Blood concentration
1	↑	↑	0	0	0	0	0
10	0	↑	↓	↓	↓	↓	↓
100	↑	↓	↓↓	↓↓	↓↓	↓	↓↓

0 = no significant effect, ↑ = increase, ↓ = decrease, ↓↓ = marked decrease.

Using modern immunohistochemical methods, such as the PAP technique and immunofluorescence, we were able to assess the modifications produced by MPA in the adenohypophysis. Atrophy of adrenocorticotrophs (ACTH cells), gonadotrophs (LH cells) and mammotrophs (PRL cells) was observed following 100 mg/kg of MPA. Atrophy of the adrenals and ovaries was also found in these animals. The histological changes relating to PRL and LH cells were consistent with results of RIA for these hormones in plasma.

The histological and endocrinological changes could be responsible for atrophy of the adrenals and ovaries. The observations complement those first reported by Logothetopoulos et al. in the normal rat [18]. The occurrence of adrenal adenomas in our experimental animals confirms results already reported [19, 20].

The effects of MPA on the adrenal glands has also been demonstrated in man by Hellman et al., who showed that MPA decreases plasma ACTH values, and suggested that it acts through negative feedback on the hypothalamus or adenohypophysis [21]. More recently, MPA has been shown to have androgenic and glucocorticoid activities [22, 23], which may explain the suppression or diminution of adrenal function, via the hypothalamo-hypophyseal axis. In this connection, some years ago in our laboratory Ectors et al., using stereotactic implantation, were able to locate the hypothalamic areas sensitive to MPA [24, 25]. In man, MPA decreases serum gonadotropin and plasma testosterone concentrations [26].

The effect of MPA on body weight is worthy of comment. As shown in Table II, ovariectomy produced the expected increase in body weight and administration of 1 mg or 10 mg/kg of MPA had a similar effect. From this, it is clear that MPA acts as a 'chemical ovariectomizing' agent. The absence of significant change in body weight following a dose of 100 mg/kg is probably a result of drug toxicity.

The observations, summarized in Table III, can be explained as a partial 'pharmacological hypophysectomy'. However, alternative hypotheses cannot be ruled out. Other investigators have, in fact, shown that the antitumour activity of MPA may be exerted via steroid hormone receptors in the cancer cells. MPA has a high affinity and specificity for progesterone receptors [27]. A direct cytotoxic effect of the drug, suggested by preliminary findings [28] also needs to be taken into consideration.

References

1. Glenn, E.M., Richardson, S.L. and Bowman, B.G. (1959): Biologic activity of 6-alphamethyl compounds corresponding to progesterone, 17-alpha-

hydroxyprogesterone acetate and compounds. *Metabolism 8*, 265.
2. Sala, G., Camerino, B. and Cavallero, C. (1958): Progestational activity of 6 alpha-methyl-17-alpha-hydroxyprogesterone acetate. *Acta Endocrinol. 29*, 508.
3. Bonte, J., Decoster, J.M., Ide, P. and Billiet, G. (1978): Hormonoprophylaxis and hormonotherapy in the treatment of endometrial adenocarcinoma by means of medroxyprogesterone acetate. *Gynecol. Oncol. 6*, 60.
4. Rafla, S. and Johnson, R. (1974): The treatment of advanced prostatic carcinoma with medroxyprogesterone. *Curr. Therapy Res. 16*, 261.
5. Bloom, H.J.G. and Hendry, W.F. (1973): Possible role of hormones in treatment of metastatic testicular teratoma tumor regression with medroxyprogesterone acetate. *Br. Med. J. 3*, 563.
6. Kleep, O., Kleep, R., Host, H. et al. (1977): Combination chemotherapy of germ cell tumors of the testis with vincristine, adriamycin, cyclophosphamide, actinomycin D and medroxyprogesterone acetate. *Cancer 40*, 638.
7. Malkasian, G.D., Decker, D.G., Jorgensen, E.O. and Edmonson, J.H. (1977): Medroxyprogesterone acetate for the treatment of metastatic and recurrent ovarian carcinoma. *Cancer Treat. Rep. 61*, 913.
8. Cooperative Breast Cancer Group (1961): Progress report: Results of studies by the Cooperative Breast Cancer Group. *Cancer Chemother. Rep. 11,* 109.
9. Cooperative Breast Cancer Group (1964): Results of studies of the Cooperative Breast Cancer Group, 1961–1963. *Cancer Chemother. Rep. (Suppl. 1) 41*, 1.
10. De Lena, M., Branbilla, C., Valagussa, P. and Bonadonna, G. (1979): High-dose medroxyprogesterone acetate in breast cancer resistant to endocrine and cytotoxic therapy. *Cancer Chemother. Pharmacol. 2*, 175.
11. Della Cuna, G.R., Calciati, A., Srada, M.R.B. et al. (1978): High dose medroxyprogesterone acetate (MPA) treatment in metastatic carcinoma of the breast: a dose-response evaluation. *Tumori 64*, 143.
12. Pannuti, F., Martoni, A., Lenaz, G.R. et al. (1978): A possible new approach to the treatment of metastatic breast cancer: massive doses of medroxyprogesterone acetate. *Cancer Treat. Rep. 62*, 499.
13. Danguy, A., Legros, N., Heuson-Stiennon, J.A. et al. (1977): Effects of a gonadotropin-releasing hormone (GnRH) analogue (A-43818) on 7,12-dimethylbenz(a)anthracene-induced rat mammary tumors. Histological and endocrine studies. *Eur. J. Cancer 13*, 1089.
14. Sternberger, L.A. (1979): *Immunocytochemistry*, 2nd Ed., John Wiley & Sons, New York.
15. Toubeau, G., Desclin, J., Parmentier, M. and Pasteels, J.L. (1979): Compared localizations of prolactin-like and adrenocorticotropin immunoreactivities within the brain of the rat. *Neuroendocrinology 29*, 374.
16. Pasteels, J.L., Gausset, P., Danguy, A. and Ectors, F. (1974): Gonadotropin secretion by human foetal and infant pituitaries. In: *Sexual Endocrinology of the Perinatal Period,* pp. 13–36. Ed: M.G. Forest and J. Bertrand. INSERM, Paris.
17. Cochran, W.G. and Cox, G.M. (1960): *Experimental Designs.* John Wiley & Sons, New York.
18. Logothetopoulos, J., Sharma, B.B. and Kraicer, J. (1961): Effects produced in rat by the administration of 6-α-methyl-17-hydroxyprogesterone acetate from birth to maturity. *Endocrinology 68,* 417.
19. Danguy, A., Heuson-Stiennon, J.A., Toubeau, G. and Pasteels, J.L. (1978):

Long term action of 7,12-dimethylbenz(a)anthracene (DMBA) on pituitary and adrenals in the rat. *IRCS Med. Sci. 6,* 79.

20. Danguy, A. (1981): Altérations histologiques de quelques glandes endocrines chez la rate après l'administration d'un carcinogène chimique. *Arch. Biol. 92*, 219.
21. Hellman, L., Yoshida, K., Zumoff, B. et al. (1976): The effect of medroxyprogesterone acetate on the pituitary-adrenal axis. *J. Clin. Endocrinol. Metab. 42,* 912.
22. Bullock, L.P., Bardin, C.W. and Sherman, M.R. (1978): Androgenic, antiandrogenic and synandrogenic actions of progestins: role of stearic and allostearic interactions with androgen receptors. *Endocrinology 103*, 1768.
23. Winneker, R.C. and Parsons, J.A. (1981): Glucocorticoid-like actions of medroxyprogesterone acetate upon Mt TW 15 rat mammosomatotropic pituitary tumors. *Endocrinology 109*, 99.
24. Ectors, F. and Pasteels, J.L. (1967): Action antiovulatoire de la medroxyprogestérone, implantée en quantités minimes dans l'hypothalamus antérieur de la ratte. *Comptes Rendus des séances de l'Acádémie des Sciences (Paris), 265*, 758.
25. Ectors, F., Pasteels, J.L. and Herlant, M. (1966): Action de la medroxyprogestérone (Provera) sur l'hypophyse, les glandes mammaires et les ovaires chez la ratte. *Comptes Rendus des séances de l'Académie des Sciences (Paris) 263*, 1988.
26. Meyer, W.J., Walker, P.A., Wiedeking, C. et al. (1977): Pituitary function in adult males receiving medroxyprogesterone acetate. *Fertil. Steril. 28*, 1072.
27. Young, P.C.M., Keen, F.K., Einhorn, L.H. et al. (1980): Binding of medroxyprogesterone acetate in human breast cancer. *Am. J. Obstet. Gynecol. 137*, 284.
28. Blossey, H.C. and Koebberling, J. (1981): The mechanism of the antitumor activity of medroxyprogesterone acetate in breast cancer. *Acta Endocrinol. 97 (Suppl. 243),* abstract no. 208.

Discussion

R. Bianco (Naples, Italy): If line 2B is treated with, for example, anti-oestrogens, is there any response on tumour growth?

F. Formelli: That was not tried. The hormone sensitivity of this tumour line is lost very quickly, and we proved that MPA sensitivity was lost with an increasing number of tumour passages – so perhaps that should have been investigated in the beginning before the hormone sensitivity was lost.

S. Iacobelli (Rome, Italy): I was worried by the high dosage of MPA with which the rats were treated by Dr Formelli; if I understood correctly, this was up to 300 mg/kg. With such a high dosage there may be many other effects in addition to those on the tumour itself, in that the drug may interact with many other systems including, possibly, the immune system. Is there any way of monitoring the immune system in these animals to find out whether some of Dr Formelli's results can be explained by modulation of the immune response?

F. Formelli: Perhaps our doses were misunderstood. In fact, in rats the highest dose used was 200 mg/kg, which corresponds to a dose of 1,000 mg/kg in man if expressed in mg/m, but most of the trials were done with 100 mg/kg. In mice, we went up to 300 mg/kg, and that is equivalent to 200 mg/kg in the rat and 1,000 mg/kg in man.

Dr Iacobelli may be right, and these high doses may have some effect on the immunological response – but that has not been investigated.

A. Di Marco: I think that Dr Spreafico will present data on the immunological effects of MPA – so this question could be postponed.

What about the stimulatory effect of low-dosage MPA, Dr Danguy? It is well-known from earlier experiments (Pearson and others, 1969) that progesterone has a stimulatory effect on 7,12-dimethylbenz(a)anthracene (DMBA)-induced tumours in Sprague-Dawley rats. It is not surprising, therefore, that with low-dosage MPA a stimulatory effect is also observed in almost every hormone-dependent tumour in Dr Danguy's system, and in Dr

Formelli's model. But what about the change in the dose-response curve when moving to the high dosage? In this case there is a qualitative change of hormone activity or of the synthetic hormone analogue.

How may this change in dose-response be explained?

A. Danguy: That is a difficult question to answer. Perhaps at high dosage there is a toxic effect at the hypothalamus-pituitary level.

A. Di Marco: You do not think that the direct effect on tumour cells may help to explain the effect? (Dr Danguy: 'Certainly...') The in-vitro antitumour effects are observed with dosages of some hundreds of nanograms – effects which would be difficult to observe with the low dosage but which are achieved with the high dosage. At the high dosage, in addition to the effect on the hypothalamus-pituitary axis, there may be free MPA which acts directly.

J.C. Heuson (Brussels, Belgium): I am not sure that there is any need to invoke this mechanism because there is very strong inhibition of the hypothalamic-hypophyseal axis in these rats that are treated with very high doses of MPA. This may be a direct cause of tumour regression. This is especially likely because these rat tumours are highly prolactin-dependent, so that when the prolactin secretion is suppressed with MPA in high doses, tumour regression would be expected.

A. Di Marco: In that case, an inhibitory effect of antiprolactin drugs would be expected.

J.C. Heuson: That has been clearly demonstrated in these animals. For example, ergocryptine very effectively inhibits tumour growth in these animals.

A. Di Marco: This is partially confirmed by the observations of Dr T. Zaccheo presented in the Poster Session.

A. Fuchs (Freiburg, Federal Republic of Germany): I still do not understand how, according to Professor Heuson, the antiprolactin effect may cause tumour reduction. In the papers that have been presented it was stated that there is tumour growth with low MPA dosage. On the other hand, an attempt is made to correlate tumour growth or tumour reduction to hormone sensitivity, which would explain a local effect. So how can there be a general explanation for those contradictory phenomena? On the one hand, prolactin is being reduced, so the tumour would be expected to become smaller. On the other hand, we want to discover the local effect on the cell, and this would require receptors. However, we do not have progesterone receptors in these tumours. Is there some way to explain these phenomena?

Editor's note added in proof: The inhibitory effect of MPA on prolactin secretion was observed by Danguy and Heuson (pp. 63–76), but only with the high MPA dosage and not with the low stimulatory dosage. In vitro, a specific inhibitory effect of MPA was observed on deoxyribonucleic acid synthesis and mitotic activity in the human mammary cancer line MCF-7 cells which in fact have oestrogen as well as progesterone receptors (Di Marco, 1981). In vivo, the antitumour effect is of more concern in tumours such as DMBA-induced adenocarcinoma in rats which have oestrogen receptors and are susceptible to ovariectomy (Di Marco et al. 1981, Danguy and Heuson 1981, Spreafico see pp. 103–113).

In conclusion, to answer this question it may be said that the presence of oestrogen and possible progesterone receptors is a requisite for the specific activity of MPA in vitro and in vivo, and that in vivo the inhibitory effect on prolactin secretion as well as other inhibitory effects on the pituitary hormone secretion may also play a role.

F. Formelli: As to the results obtained in mice, it should be said that the hormone sensitivity of these experimental tumours is not well known and may be quite different from that of DMBA-induced tumours in rats. In fact, I am studying the growth of these tumours (MXT adenocarcinoma and Colon 38) in ovariectomized animals and, so far, it seems that the growth of these tumours is also stimulated in ovariectomized mice. It is therefore possible that MPA at high doses in mice has a prominent anti-gonadotropic effect.

In rats, I think that the activity of MPA might depend on the presence of hormone receptors in hormone-dependent tumours, like the DMBA-induced tumour presented by Dr Danguy and the hormone-dependent tumour model I used, *i.e.,* the second-generation transplant of DMBA-induced tumours in syngeneic Fisher rats.

In the 13762 mammary tumour, which is hormone-responsive, the activity of MPA at high doses was mostly on early growth and this tumour had a very low level of oestrogen- and non-progesterone receptors. It is therefore hard to relate the effect of MPA on this tumour with the presence of these receptors.

Common and distinctive features in the growth-inhibitory activity of medroxyprogesterone acetate and tamoxifen on oestrogen-sensitive human breast cancer cells

S. Iacobelli[1], C. Natoli[1], G. Sica[2] and P. Marchetti[1]
[1]Molecular Endocrinology Laboratory and [2]Institute of Histology and General Embryology, Catholic University of the Sacred Heart, Rome, Italy

Introduction

The 2 main forms of treatment in the medical management of advanced breast cancer are chemotherapy and hormonotherapy. At present, the response rates to these 2 types of therapy average approximately 60% and 35%, respectively, and have not improved despite the introduction of new drugs and new combinations.

As far as hormonotherapy is concerned, greater success in predicting response can be achieved through the use of steroid-receptor assays. Approximately 50% of patients whose tumours are oestrogen-receptor positive (ER+) (more than 10 femtomoles ($=10^{-15}$ moles) (fmol)/mg protein) derive some benefit from hormonal treatment [1]. The majority of these ER+ cancers also contain progesterone receptors (PR), which are end points of oestrogen action [2], and a large percentage of such patients (80%) are responsive to hormonotherapy [3]. However, hormone receptors are not absolute indicators of tumour responsiveness to endocrine therapy, since approximately 20% of ER+ and some PR+ cancers do not respond. Conversely, similar percentages of ER− and PR− tumours are responsive to hormonal therapy.

We have recently shown that medroxyprogesterone acetate (MPA), a potent semisynthetic progestational agent, is able to inhibit macromolecular synthesis in cultured human endometrial carcinoma explants, and that this effect is presumably mediated by a mechanism involving progesterone receptors [4]. In this paper, we report inhibition of human breast cancer cell proliferation by MPA, and an increase in this effect in cells which have been previously exposed to either oestrogens or anti-oestrogens. Evidence is also presented that, during long-term in vitro incubation, MPA is metabolized to only a minimal extent, suggesting that an active metabolite is not necessarily implicated in the action of MPA.

Materials and methods

CG-5 cells, a new oestrogen-supersensitive variant of the MCF-7 human breast cancer cell line, recently established in our laboratory [5], were grown in Dulbecco's modified Eagle's Medium (DMEM) supplemented with 10% foetal calf serum (FCS) and antibiotics. Cells from stock cultures were trypsinized weekly, and incubated at 37° C under a high humidity, 5% CO_2/95% atmosphere.

Cell growth experiments

Fifty thousand cells/ml were plated in DMEM, supplemented with 5% charcoal-treated serum [6] and antibiotics, in 4 ml plastic culture dishes. After 24 hours the culture medium was changed, and hormones were added. Cell cultures were fed with fresh medium every 3 days. Quadruplicate counts of triplicate culture dishes were carried out at the intervals specified below.

Steroid metabolism

(^{3}H)-MPA (1×10^6 counts per minute) (specific activity 60 Ci/mmol; New England Nuclear Cooperation, Boston, MA, U.S.A.) was added to subconfluent cultures growing in DMEM supplemented with 10% FCS and antibiotics in 10 ml plastic culture dishes. The same amount of radioactive steroid was added to dishes containing medium alone, without cells. After 24, 48 and 72 hours, the culture media, from either dishes containing cells, or from controls, were collected, centrifuged at 1,400 revolutions per minute for 10 minutes, and stored at −20° C. Cells were washed twice with 0.9% NaCl, and stored at −20° C. Cells were thawed, resuspended in 1 ml of 0.9% NaCl and disrupted by sonication. Disrupted cells, or aliquots of the culture medium, were extracted with 10 volumes of diethylether over a period of 30 minutes, and the ether extracts evaporated at 40° C. The residues were redissolved in 20–30 μl of benzene:ethanol (9:1, volume/volume (v/v)) and applied to silica gel plates. Plates were developed using a mobile phase consisting of ethyl acetate:hexane (1:1, v/v). After drying at room temperature, the plates were cut into one-centimetre segments. Radioactivity was measured after extraction with 6 ml of toluene-based scintillation fluid for 6 hours. The identity of radioactive MPA was established by running pure, unlabelled MPA simultaneously.

Results

Effects of MPA alone

Table I indicates that the addition of physiological doses of oestradiol (1 nM) to CG-5 cells increases the number of cells about 3-fold, as compared to control cultures. Under the same conditions, MPA in concentrations ranging from 0.1 nM up to 1 μM inhibits cell proliferation by approximately 40%. The inhibition produced by MPA appears 3 days after the addition of hormone, and remains at the same level up to day 9.

Effects of MPA on oestrogen-stimulated cell proliferation

Approximately half of all patients with breast cancer are premenopausal, and have high levels of circulating oestrogens. It was therefore felt to be important to evaluate whether or not MPA could counteract oestrogen-stimulated proliferation in this category of patients. Cells were simultaneously exposed from the start of culture to fixed concentrations of oestradiol (1 nM) and varying doses of MPA, and the numbers of cells were evaluated after 6 days. The results of this experiment are shown in Table II. Cells exposed to oestradiol alone tripled in number, as compared to control cultures without addition of hormone. In the presence of both oestradiol and MPA, the proliferation rate

Table I. Proliferative effects of oestradiol and MPA added separately to CG-5 cell cultures. Cell counts were performed at varying intervals after hormone addition. Standard deviations were less than 5%.

Steroid	Concentration (M)	Cell numbers (% of control numbers)		
		Day 3	Day 6	Day 9
Control		100	100	100
Oestradiol	10^{-9}	160	305	320
MPA	10^{-10}	77	70	72
MPA	10^{-9}	74	62	59
MPA	10^{-8}	60	58	64
MPA	10^{-7}	65	57	54
MPA	10^{-6}	62	55	64

Table II. Proliferative effects of oestradiol (10^{-9}M) and varying concentrations of MPA added simultaneously to CG-5 cell cultures. Cell counts were performed 6 days after hormone addition. Standard deviations were less than 5%.

Steroids and concentrations	Cell numbers (% of control numbers)
Control	100
Oestradiol 10^{-9}M	286
Oestradiol 10^{-9}M + MPA 10^{-10}M	230
Oestradiol 10^{-9}M + MPA 10^{-9} M	211
Oestradiol 10^{-9}M + MPA 10^{-8} M	210
Oestradiol 10^{-9}M + MPA 10^{-7} M	196
Oestradiol 10^{-9}M + MPA 10^{-6} M	205

was only moderately inhibited, as compared with oestrogen-treated cultures. The mean inhibition was about 35%. The effect was dose-dependent, and started at low, physiological doses (0.1–1 nM) of MPA. The absolute number of cells was double that found in untreated control cultures, which suggests that MPA only partially antagonizes oestrogen-dependent cell proliferation. This may have important clinical implications for the preferential use of MPA in postmenopausal women with low levels of circulating oestrogens. Alternatively, its use might be recommended following ovariectomy, or in association with an anti-oestrogenic compound, to reduce the degree of oestrogenic effect at the cellular level.

Combined effects of MPA, oestradiol and tamoxifen

Recent evidence from different laboratories shows that the anti-oestrogen tamoxifen, a compound widely used for the management of advanced breast cancer, especially in ER+ cases, has the oestrogen-like property of stimulating the synthesis of specific proteins, in particular that of progesterone receptor, in oestrogen-sensitive cells [7]. A hormonal challenge test, consisting of measuring PR in tumour samples before and after the administration of tamoxifen, has, in fact, recently been introduced, with promising results [8].

Tamoxifen and MPA share the common property of being tumoricidal towards breast neoplasms. However, it can be assumed that the mechanisms of action of these 2 drugs are different, and fairly complex.

Tamoxifen binds to oestrogen receptors [9], or perhaps, as has recently been suggested, to specific anti-oestrogenic receptors [10]. The anti-oestrogen receptor complex does not promote progesterone-induced effects on target cells [11]. In vivo, tamoxifen is converted to its hydroxylated and demethylated metabolites. Both tamoxifen and its metabolites have minimal effects on the pituitary-gonadal axis [12].

In contrast, the effects of MPA are mediated by specific progesterone receptors, and possibly also by androgen and glucocorticoid receptors, as far as the anabolic activity of this steroid is concerned [4, 13, 14]. In addition, MPA profoundly alters pituitary function, and ultimately brings about chemical ovaro-adrenalectomy [15–17].

Study of the interactions between MPA and tamoxifen in the control of breast cancer cell proliferation, with the twin aim of verifying whether these 2 compounds have an additive inhibitory effect, and whether tamoxifen or oestradiol increase cell responsiveness to MPA by increasing the progesterone receptor was therefore of interest.

In the first experiment, cells were exposed for 6 days to a fixed concentration of tamoxifen (100 nM), and varying doses of MPA were added simultaneously, from the start of culture. As shown in Table III, inhibition, as compared with untreated cultures, was about 60% under these conditions. The effect was dose-dependent, and became evident at a hormone concentration of 10 nM. In the second series of experiments, CG-5 cells were pretreated for 7 days with either oestradiol (1 nM) or tamoxifen (100 nM) in order to increase progesterone receptor synthesis. The cells were then trypsinized, and tested for responsiveness to MPA alone. As reported in Table IV, cell sensitivity to MPA was greatly increased, and about 60–70% inhibition of growth was achieved under these conditions.

Steroid metabolism

Table V shows that MPA added to CG-5 cell cultures is only minimally

Table III. Proliferative effects of tamoxifen and MPA added simultaneously to CG-5 cell cultures. Cell counts were performed 6 days after hormone addition. Standard deviations were less than 5%.

Compounds and concentrations	Cell numbers (% of control numbers)
Control	100
Tamoxifen 10^{-7}M	74
Tamoxifen 10^{-7}M + MPA 10^{-10}M	66
Tamoxifen 10^{-7}M + MPA 10^{-9} M	60
Tamoxifen 10^{-7}M + MPA 10^{-8} M	48
Tamoxifen 10^{-7}M + MPA 10^{-7} M	42
Tamoxifen 10^{-7}M + MPA 10^{-6} M	40

Table IV. Proliferative effects of MPA added to CG-5 cell cultures pretreated for 7 days with either oestradiol (10^{-9}M) or tamoxifen (10^{-7}M). Cell counts were performed 6 days after hormone addition. Standard deviations were less than 5%.

MPA-concentrations (M)	Cell numbers (% of control numbers)	
	Oestradiol-pretreated	Tamoxifen-pretreated
Control	100	100
10^{-10}	51	47
10^{-9}	44	42
10^{-8}	38	46
10^{-7}	31	41
10^{-6}	19	40

Table V. Metabolism of ^{3}H-MPA by CG-5 cells.

	Radioactivity in MPA area after times shown (%)		
	24 hours	48 hours	72 hours
Cells	87.4	91	82
Medium	94	94	92.5
Control medium	94.5	93.5	92.3

metabolized (less than 10% at 72 hours). The radioactivity appearing is currently under evaluation, to identify the metabolite into which MPA is converted. It should be noted that, in cell growth experiments, the culture medium is changed every 3 days. Each time, new steroid solutions are added. The minimal extent of MPA metabolism we observed is, therefore, not at all relevant to the action of MPA. The results suggest that the MPA molecule itself is the compound having an effect on CG-5 cell proliferation.

Discussion

In the present study, we evaluated the antiproliferative activity of MPA on CG-5 cells, an oestrogen-supersensitive variant of the MCF-7 human breast cancer cell line [5]. CG-5 cells were established in the Molecular Endocrinology Laboratory in February 1981, and are characterized by a very high sensitivity to oestrogen-induced cell proliferation and high levels of steroid and thyroid hormone receptors [unpublished data].

MPA has a direct inhibitory effect on CG-5 cell proliferation. The effect occurs 3 days after addition of hormone. The degree of inhibition is 40%, and this remains constant on subsequent days. MPA metabolism was assessed during the experimental growth period, and it was found that the molecule is metabolized to only a minimal extent within the cells (less than 10% in 72 hours), and not at all in the culture medium, suggesting that the intact MPA molecule itself is the agent affecting cell proliferation.

When CG-5 cells are exposed to oestradiol and MPA simultaneously, the latter is unable to completely inhibit the 3-fold increase in cell proliferation induced by oestradiol. This weak anti-oestrogenic activity of MPA needs to be taken into account from the clinical point of view. MPA should be used preferentially in postmenopausal women with low levels of circulating oestrogens, or in premenopausal women after ovariectomy, or in combination with anti-oestrogenic drugs in order to decrease the proliferative effects of oestrogens.

Interesting results were obtained on testing the antiproliferative effects of MPA in the presence of the anti-oestrogen tamoxifen. The combined use of these 2 drugs resulted in an additive inhibition of cell proliferation (about 60%). This can be explained on the basis of the different, noninteracting mechanisms of action of the different, noninteracting mechanisms of action of the 2 drugs. At least as far as growth inhibitory effects are concerned, MPA presumably interacts with progesterone receptors, while tamoxifen interacts with oestrogen or anti-oestrogen receptors, as has recently been suggested [10]. It is also known, from in vitro [2, 6, 7] and in vivo [8] studies, that both oestradiol and tamoxifen can increase progesterone receptor synthesis in breast cancer cells. On the basis of these observations, we pretreated CG-5 cells for 7 days with oestradiol and tamoxifen, and then tested the cells for their responsiveness to MPA alone. Under these conditions, MPA alone, when added to pretreated CG-5 cultures was able to inhibit cell proliferation by 60 to 70% as compared with controls.

Our findings, overall, suggest that clinical trials based on the combined or sequential use of MPA and anti-oestrogens, to maximize the tumoricidal activity of these drugs in hormone-dependent neoplasms, would be of interest, especially since the drugs have nonadditive side-effects in breast cancer patients.

References

1. McGuire, W.L., Zava, D.T., Horwitz, K.B. and Chamnes, G.C. (1978): Steroid receptors in breast tumors. Current status. In: *Current Topics in Experimental Endocrinology,* pp. 93–129. Eds: L. Martini and V.H.T. Janes. Academic Press, New York.
2. McGuire, W.L. and Horwitz, K.B. (1978): Progesterone receptors in breast

cancer. In: *Hormones, Receptors and Breast Cancer,* pp. 31–42. Eds: W.L. McGuire. Raven Press, New York.
3. McGuire, W.L. (1980): An update on estrogen receptors in prognosis of primary and advanced breast cancer. In: *Hormones and Cancer,* pp. 337–343. Eds: S. Iacobelli, R.J.B. King, H.R. Lindner and M.E. Lippman. Raven Press, New York.
4. Iacobelli, S., Longo, P., Scambia, G. et al. (1980): Progesterone receptors and hormone sensitivity of human endometrial carcinoma. In: *Role of Medroxyprogesterone Acetate in Endocrine-Related Tumors,* pp. 97–106. Eds: S. Iacobelli and A. Di Marco. Raven Press, New York.
5. Natoli, C., Sica, G., Natoli, V. et al. (1982): Two new estrogen supersensitive variants of MCF-7 human breast cancer cell line. *Breast Cancer Res. Treat.* (In press.)
6. Horwitz, K.B. and McGuire, W.L. (1978): Estrogen control of progesterone receptors in human breast cancer. Correlation with nuclear processing of estrogen receptor. *J. Biol. Chem. 253,* 2223.
7. Horwitz, K.B. and McGuire, W.L. (1980): Studies on mechanism of estrogen and antiestrogen action in human breast cancer. In: *Endocrine Treatment of Breast Cancer. A New Approach,* pp. 45–48. Eds: B. Henningsen, H.R. Lindner and C. Steichele. Springer Verlag, Berlin, Heidelberg, New York.
8. Namer, M., Lalanne, C. and Baulieu, E.E. (1980): Increase of progesterone receptor by tamoxifen as a hormonal challenge test in breast cancer. *Cancer Res. 40,* 1750.
9. Wakeling, A.E. and Slater, S.R. (1980): Estrogen-receptor binding and biological activity of tamoxifen and its metabolites. *Cancer Treat. Rep. 64,* 741.
10. Sutherland, R.L., Murphy, L.C., Foo, M.S. et al. (1980): High-affinity antioestrogen binding sites distinct from the oestrogen receptor. *Nature 288,* 273.
11. Jordan, V.C., Dix, C.J., Naylor, K.E. et al. (1978): Nonsteroidal antiestrogens: their biological effects and potential mechanisms of action. *J. Toxicol. Environ. Health. 4,* 363.
12. Patterson, J.S. (1981): Clinical aspects and development of antioestrogen therapy: a review of the endocrine effects of tamoxifen in animals and man. *J. Endocrinol. 89,* 67P.
13. Gupta, C., Bullock, L.P. and Bardin, C.W. (1978): Further studies on the androgenic, anti-androgenic and synandrogenic actions of progestins. *Endocrinol. 120,* 736.
14. Feldman, D., Funder, J. and Loose, D. (1978): Is the glucocorticoid receptor identical in various target organs? *J. Steroid Biochem. 9,* 141.
15. Rifkin, A.B., Kulin, H.E., Cargille, C.M. et al. (1977): Suppression of urinary excretion of luteinizing hormone (LH) and follicle stimulating hormone (FSH) by MAP. *J. Clin. Endocrinol. Metab. 29,* 506.
16. Novak, E. (1977): Effects of medroxyprogesterone acetate on some endocrine functions of healthy male volunteers. *Curr. Ther. Res. 21,* 320.
17. Sala, G., Castegnaro, E., Lenaz, G.R. et al. (1975): Hormone interferences in metastatic breast cancer patients treated with medroxyprogesterone acetate at massive doses: preliminary results. *IRCS Med. Sci. 6,* 501.

Comparison of the effects of medroxyprogesterone acetate and tamoxifen on cell growth in a human breast cancer cell line (MCF-7)*

Y. Nomura, K. Matsui, K. Kanda, Y. Hamada and H. Tashiro
Department of Breast Surgery, National Kyushu Cancer Centre Hospital, Fukuoka, Japan

Introduction

It has been reported that a high dose of medroxyprogesterone acetate (MPA), given intramuscularly or orally, had a distinct effect on advanced breast cancer [1, 2]. However, the exact mode of action of MPA on breast or other cancers has yet to be clarified [3]. Studies on rat mammary cancers showed that the therapeutic effect of MPA may be related to inhibition of the pituitary-gonadal axis [4] and to the hormone receptor system [5]. Di Marco et al. studied the effects of MPA on macromolecular synthesis and levels of cytoplasmic oestrogen receptors (ER) and progesterone receptors (PgR) in a hormone-responsive human breast cancer cell line, MCF-7, and pointed out the similarity between these effects and those of progesterone [3]. These workers reported a direct inhibitory effect of the synthetic progestogen on mitotic activity and macromolecular synthesis in the cells.

Following treatment with anticancer agents, which have a variety of mechanisms, the ability of cancer cells to survive can be assessed by monitoring their continuing proliferation. This can be accomplished in vitro using the colony formation method [6].

We have used this method for comparison of the effects of MPA with those of the anti-oestrogen, tamoxifen, and of steroid hormones in MCF-7 cells and 2 other human breast cancer cell lines recently established in our laboratory.

* This study was supported in part by grants in aid of Cancer Research by the Japanese Ministry of Education, Science and Culture (501045) and by the Japanese Ministry of Health and Welfare (54–3).

Materials and methods

Cells and growth medium

The hormone-responsive human breast cancer cell line MCF-7 was provided by the Mason Research Institute (Rockville, MD, U.S.A.). Cells were grown in plastic culture flasks in RPMI 1640 medium (Dainippon Pharmaceutical Co., Osaka, Japan), supplemented with 10% fetal calf serum (Flow Labs Inc., McLean, VA, U.S.A.), insulin (10^{-4} g/ml), and kanamycin (10^{-4} g/ml). Cells were grown at 37 °C in an incubator with a 5% CO_2: 95% humidified air atmosphere.

Two human breast cancer cell lines (Miyajima and Koike) have been established in our laboratory. Both were derived from advanced primary tumours from breast cancer cases, and have been continuously cultured for 3 years and 4 months, and 2 years and 10 months, respectively.

Chemicals

Medroxyprogesterone acetate (FI 7401) was a gift from Farmitalia Carlo Erba, Milan, Italy, and tamoxifen (ICI 46474) was a gift from Imperial Chemical Industries Ltd., London, U.K. The steroids 17β-oestradiol (E_2), progesterone, 5α- and 5β-androstanolone, and dexamethasone were purchased from the Sigma Chemical Co., St. Louis, MO, U.S.A. All other chemicals were of reagent grade, and were purchased from the Sigma Chemical Co. or the Wako Pure Chemical Co., Tokyo, Japan.

Colony formation

Unless otherwise stated, all sera used in the experiment had been deprived of endogenous steroids, including oestradiol, by 2, 30-minute incubations at 45 °C with a pellet of dextran-coated charcoal (DCC, 0.5% activated charcoal and 0.05% dextran, centrifuged). Monolayers of cell lines were detached by means of trypsin, and the resultant cell suspensions plated out on 60-mm plastic petri dishes (Nunc, Roskilde, Denmark) at a concentration of 400 cells per 3 ml of media. After the cells had attached themselves (24 hours), E_2-deprived sera containing concentrations ranging from 10^{-9}M to 10^{-5}M of MPA, tamoxifen, or the other steroid hormones were added. MPA, tamoxifen and steroids were dissolved in ethanol. The final concentration of ethanol in the medium was not more than 0.2%. In addition to culture in the absence of E_2, a parallel series of cultures in the presence of E_2 (10^{-8}M) were also car-

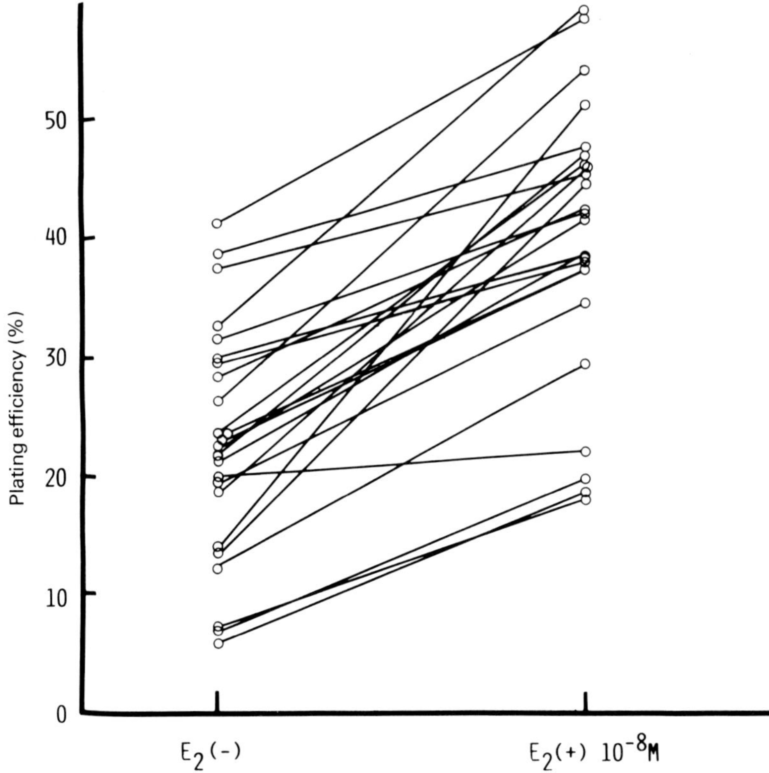

Fig. 1. Effects of oestradiol-17β on MCF-7 cell colony formation. $E_2(-)$: E_2-deprived medium, $E_2(+)10^{-8}M$: E_2-deprived medium with $10^{-8}M$ of E_2 added. Each value represents the mean of 3 experiments.

ried out. Three culture dishes were incubated for each concentration in 5% CO_2: 95% humidified air for a further 18 days. The various drugs under investigation remained present during the entire course of colony formation, i.e. there was no change of medium. On the 19th day, the contents of the dishes were fixed using methanol, and stained with Giemsa stain. The number of colonies per dish was counted and the size of each colony measured.

The plating efficiency (PE) of the cells was calculated from the following formula:

$$PE = \frac{\text{number of colonies per dish}}{\text{number of cells plated}} \times 100.$$

The relative plating efficiency (RPE) was calculated by dividing the PE in the case of cells treated with one of the drugs by the PE for cells not exposed to drugs.

The MCF-7 cells under these conditions showed a PE ranging from 6–41% in cultures in E_2-deprived media. There was a 13–250% increase in colony numbers when 10^{-8}M of E_2 was added (Fig. 1). These variations in PE in the E_2-deprived media and increase in PE through the addition of E_2 were considered to be mainly due to differences between batches of the fetal calf serum used, and the DCC procedures for removing E_2 and other constituents from the serum. The medium was, therefore, discarded if the PE of the cells cultured in the presence of 10^{-8}M E_2 failed to reach a level significantly different ($P<0.05$) from that for cells cultured in an E_2-deprived medium. Throughout this experiment, accordingly, E_2 was considered to be fully active in influencing the PE of MCF-7 cells.

Results

As shown in Figure 2, MPA showed distinct inhibitory effects on the colony-forming activity of MCF-7 cells. This effect was not influenced by the addition of 10^{-8}M of E_2. When cells were treated with tamoxifen in E_2-deprived media, suppression of PE was noted at concentrations greater than 10^{-6}M of tamoxifen, as shown in Figure 3. Unlike MPA, tamoxifen showed no inhibitory effects at a concentration of 10^{-7}M. When cells were cultured in the media to which E_2 had been added, the inhibitory effects of tamoxifen were suppressed, except at a very high concentration (10^{-5}M). The response of MCF-7 cells to these 2 substances was, therefore, different, particularly in the presence of a physiological concentration of E_2.

Figure 4 shows that progesterone had almost no effect on the PE of MCF-7 cells, irrespective of whether E_2 was present or not. The question of whether or not this lack of effect of progesterone was affected by E_2 priming was studied. After the cells were incubated for 3 days in a medium to which E_2 had been added, they were cultured with increasing concentrations of progesterone in the presence of E_2. There was no effect on the PE of the cells, and the relative plating efficiency of the cells with a concentration of 10^{-6}M of progesterone was shown to be 85.7 ± 0.8% (compare with Table). MCF-7 cells therefore failed to respond to progesterone, regardless of whether or not there had been E_2-priming, under these conditions.

As indicated in Figure 5, in the absence of E_2, 5α-androstanolone affected the PE of MCF-7 cells increasingly as concentration increased. The PE did not, however, surpass that obtained in the presence of E_2. In the presence of E_2, 5α-androstanolone had no effect. MCF-7 cells did not respond to increas-

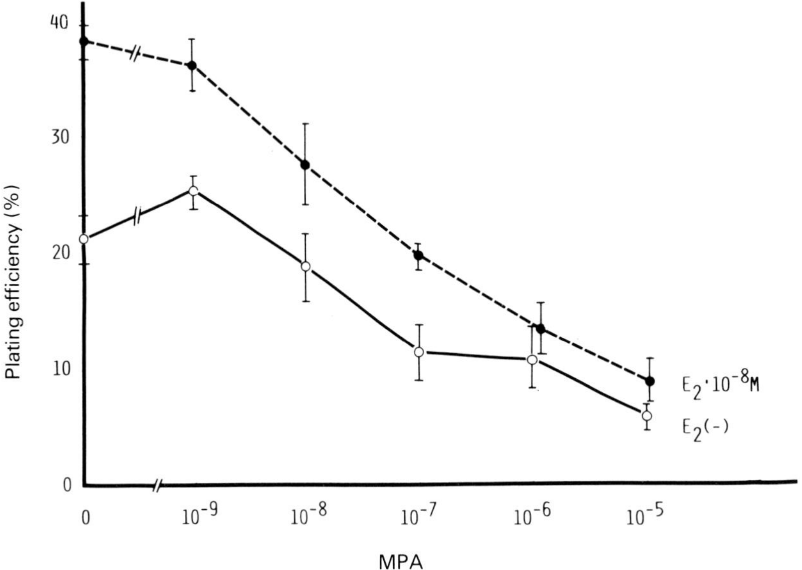

Fig. 2. Effects of MPA on MCF-7 colony formation.

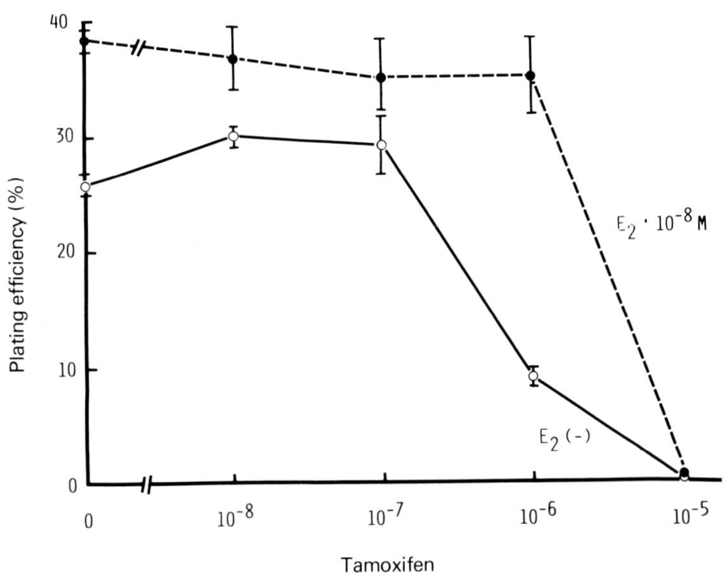

Fig. 3. Effects of tamoxifen on MCF-7 colony formation.

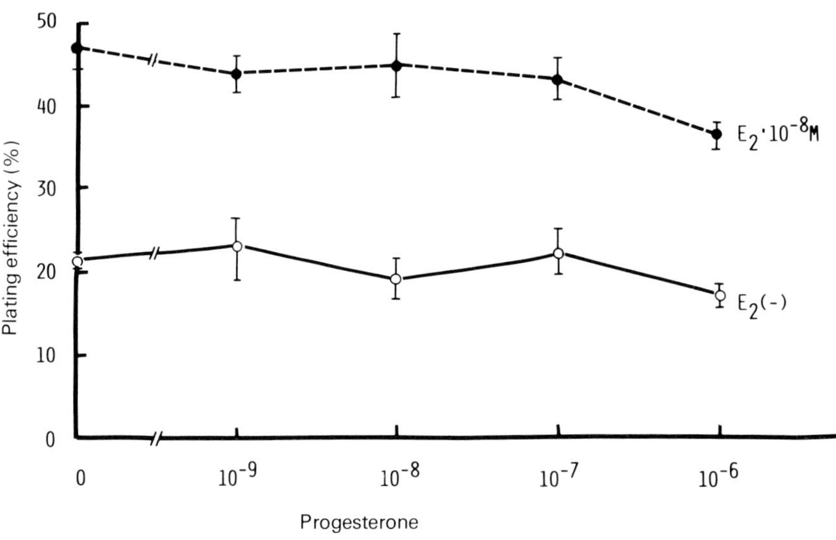

Fig. 4. Effects of progesterone on MCF-7 colony formation.

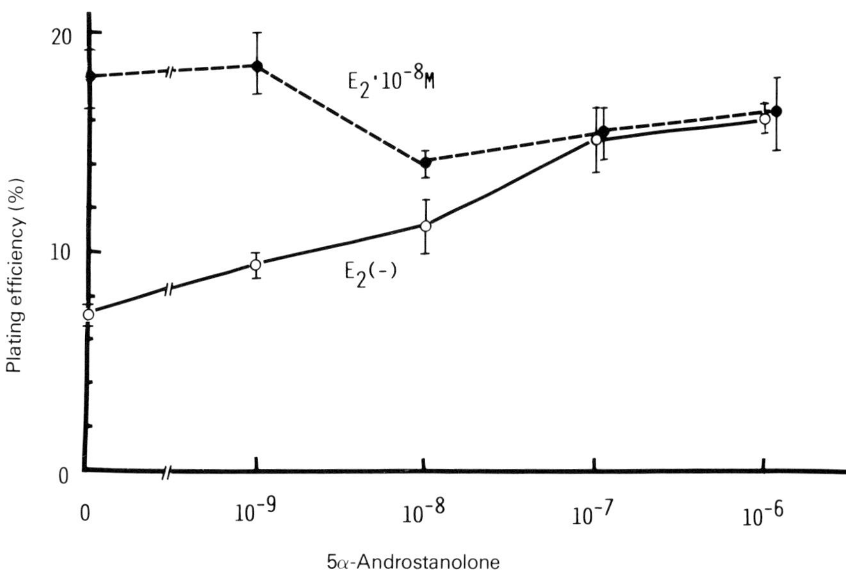

Fig. 5. Effects of 5α-androstanolone on MCF-7 colony formation.

Table. Effects of MPA, tamoxifen and steroid hormones on relative plating efficiency of MCF-7 cells.

Drug (10^{-6}M)	Relative plating efficiency (%)	
	E_2-deprived	E_2-present (10^{-8}M)
Control	100.0	100.0
MPA	44.6 ± 6.8	35.5 ± 5.6
Tamoxifen	42.6 ± 4.6	91.1 ± 8.5
Progesterone	78.8 ± 2.3	77.0 ± 1.4
5α-androstanolone	219.0 ± 7.2	90.7 ± 8.1
5β-androstanolone	86.3 ± 11.1	88.2 ± 5.4
Dexamethasone	30.4 ± 4.6	28.4 ± 7.7

ing concentrations of 5β-androstanolone regardless of whether or not E_2 was present. Dexamethasone had suppressive effects on the PE of MCF-7 cells similar to those of MPA, whether E_2 was present or not (Fig. 6).

The effects of the steroid hormones studied, including MPA and tamoxifen, on the colony-forming activity of MCF-7 cells are shown in the Table in terms of RPE values at concentrations of 10^{-6}M. Under these conditions, the

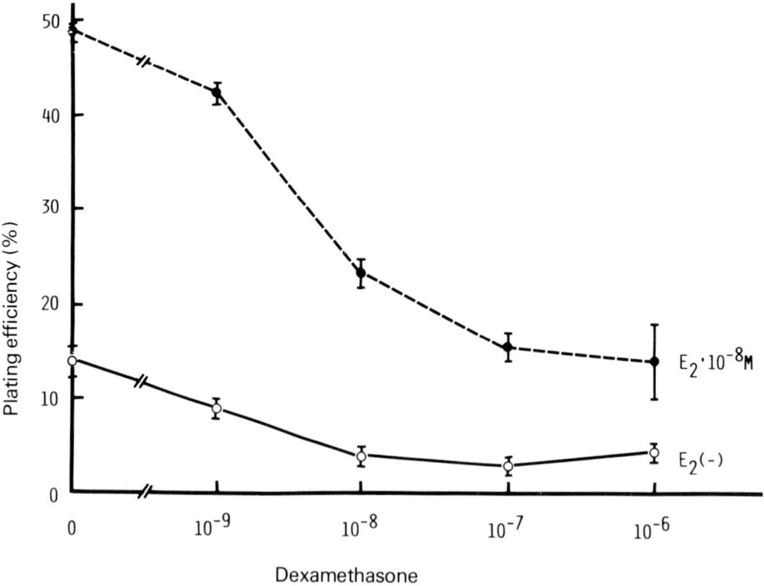

Fig. 6. Effects of dexamethasone on MCF-7 colony formation.

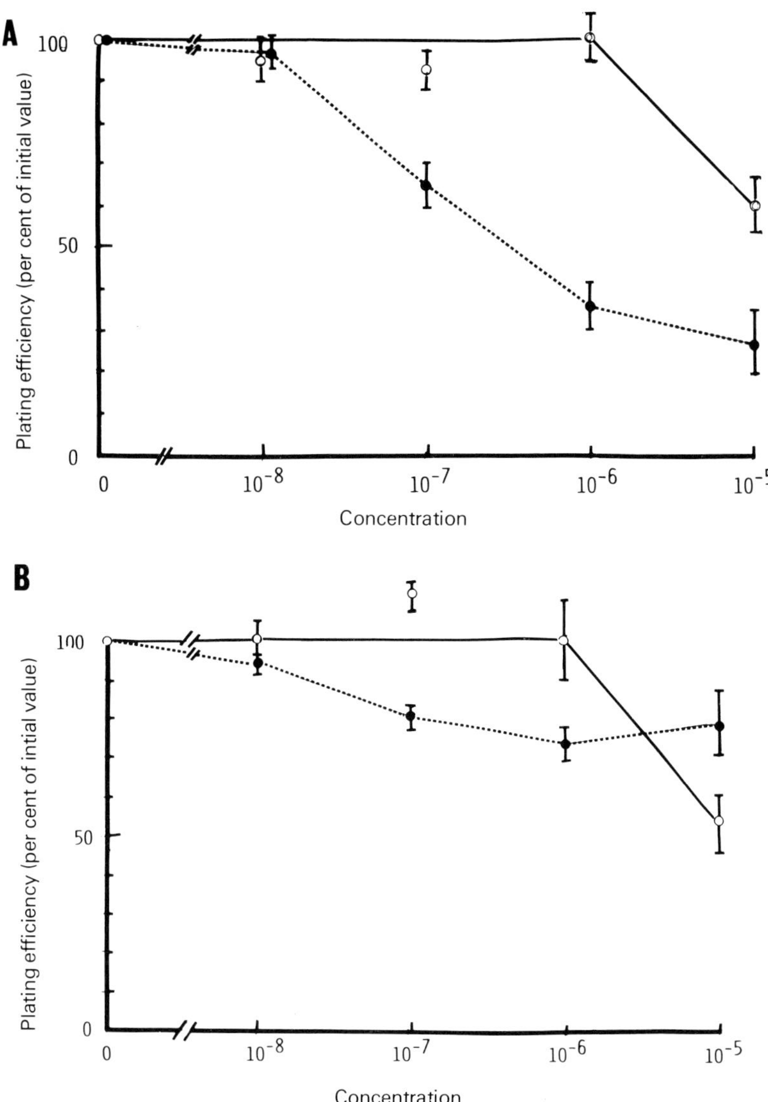

Fig. 7. Effects of MPA and tamoxifen on Miyajima cell (A) colony formation and Koike cell (B) colony formation. ○——○ *tamoxifen;* •···• *MPA.*

effects of MPA appear to be similar to those of dexamethasone, but different from those of tamoxifen, progesterone, or 5α-androstanolone.

The responses of the other 2 cell lines established in our laboratory to MPA or tamoxifen were compared. The Miyajima cells had no oestrogen receptors, and failed to respond to various concentrations of E_2. The colony-forming activity of the cell line was studied in an E_2-deprived medium (Fig. 7A). The PE of the cells was shown to be dose-dependently inhibited by MPA, but there was no effect following the addition of tamoxifen at any except a very high dose. The Koike cells had no oestrogen receptors and did not respond to E_2. The colony-forming activity of the cells was not affected by the addition of MPA or tamoxifen (Fig. 7B). The sensitivities of these 2 cell lines to MPA and tamoxifen were accordingly shown to be different. The sensitivities also differed from those of MCF-7 cells.

Discussion

For comparison of the effects of MPA on the proliferation of MCF-7 cells with those of tamoxifen or steroid hormones, we used the method of colony formation in plastic dishes. Despite some technical limitations, particularly as regards delay in obtaining the results, this method can be one of the most reliable, dose-dependent indices of cell lethality [6].

The hormone-responsive MCF-7 cell line is known to have receptors for oestrogens, progesterone, androgen, glucocorticoids etc. [7], and has been extensively used as a model for hormone-responsive human breast cancer. As Figure 1 shows, however, endogenous oestrogens and other factors in the fetal calf sera used for culture can cause variations in cell proliferation, in spite of DCC adsorption procedures. This phenomenon may partly be attributable to variations between batches of serum [8] and also by the degree of adsorption. It leads to confusing results. We therefore selected only batches of E_2-deprived serum with which there was a significant increase in PE after E_2 treatment.

As Figures 2 and 3 show, the dose-response curve for the effect of MPA on colony formation in the case of MCF-7 cells is different from that for tamoxifen, particularly in the presence of E_2. The inhibitory effect of tamoxifen is suppressed by adding E_2 to the medium. This effect is not observed with MPA. Di Marco et al. showed that MPA inhibits macromolecular synthesis and cell division in MCF-7 cells, but that the inhibitory effect is prevented by treatment with equimolar concentrations of E_2 [3]. The discrepancy between the results of Di Marco et al. and our results may be attributable to differences in methods, and in concentrations of the drugs. In the Miyajima cells (Fig. 7A), where E_2 has no effect on the cell growth, there was a marked difference in inhibitory effects on plating efficiency as between MPA and tamoxifen. These findings may indicate a different mode of action for these 2 agents, and also suggest that MPA may be clinically effective in premenopausal patients.

MPA might also be effective in advanced breast cancer patients who are refractory to tamoxifen.

The inhibition of proliferation of MCF-7 cells caused by a number of steroid hormones was compared with that caused by MPA (Table). Progesterone showed little effect on growth of the cells, whether they had been pretreated with oestrogens or not (Fig. 4). Lippman et al. dit not observe any effect of progesterone on macromolecular synthesis in MCF-7 cells [9]. MPA does not, therefore, appear to act on the cells as a pure progesterone, in vitro at least.

The capacity of the MCF-7 cells to form colonies was stimulated by 5α-androstanolone only in the absence of E_2 (Fig. 5). This seems to be a property specific to this steroid, because there was no effect after treatment with its isomer, 5β-androstanolone (Table). Lippman et al. demonstrated stimulation of thymidine incorporation into DNA in MCF-7 cells following 5α-androstanolone treatment, and its inhibition by antiandrogens such as cyproterone acetate and R 2956 [10]. The androgenic effect of MPA does not, therefore, seem to be predominant in inhibiting proliferation in MCF-7 cells [3]. Teulings et al., however, have drawn attention to the close relationship between the effects of progestogens such as megestrol acetate and MPA and hormone receptors, particularly androgen receptors, in human breast cancer [11].

As shown in Figures 2 and 6, and in the Table, the dose response curve for the inhibitory effects of MPA are very similar to those of dexamethasone, particularly in that the inhibitory effects are not altered by the presence of E_2. A glucocorticoid action for MPA in vivo has been suggested by Sala et al. [12], and by Guthrie and John [13], and for MPA in vitro by Svec et al. [14]. It is, therefore, possible that a glucocorticoid-like activity is exerted by MPA or its metabolites on the proliferation of MCF-7 cells.

This investigation is still in its early stages, and more detailed studies will be necessary to clarify the exact points at which MPA attacks breast cancer cells. Such clarification may be possible by study of the effects of MPA and its metabolites together with antihormones on cell growth in hormone-responsive and hormone-nonresponsive cell lines. It may also be necessary to study the correlation between the response to MPA in advanced breast cancer and the distribution patterns of hormone receptors in the breast cancer concerned. Such a study will have to deal not only with oestrogen and progesterone receptors, but also with others, such as androgen and glucocorticoid receptors.

References

1. Pannuti, F., Di Marco, A.R., Martoni, A. et al. (1980): Medroxyprogesterone acetate in treatment of metastatic breast cancer: seven years of experience. In: *Role of Medroxyprogesterone in Endocrine-Related Tumors,* pp. 73–92. Eds: S. Iacobelli and A. Di Marco. Raven Press, New York.
2. Research Group on FI 7401 (MAP) Treatment for Breast Cancer in Japan (Tominaga, T., Izuo, M., Abe, O., Enomoto, K., Takatani, O., Kubo, K. and Nomura, Y.) (1981): Oral high dose medroxyprogesterone acetate (MPA) in treatment of advanced breast cancer. *12th Internat. Congr. Chemotherapy,* Abstract 102.
3. Di Marco, A. (1980): The antitumor activity of 6α-methyl-17α-acetoxy progesterone (MPA) in experimental mammary cancer. In: *Role of Medroxyprogesterone in Endocrine-Related Tumors*, pp. 1–20. Eds: S. Iacobelli and A. Di Marco. Raven Press, New York.
4. Danguy, A., Legros, N., Devleeschouwer, N. et al. (1980): Effects of medroxyprogesterone acetate (MPA) on growth of DMBA-induced rat mammary tumors: Histopathological and endocrine studies. In: *Role of Medroxyprogesterone in Endocrine-Related Tumors*, pp. 21–28. Eds: S. Iacobelli and A. Di Marco. Raven Press, New York.
5. Di Carlo, F., Conti, G. and Reboani, C. (1978): Interference of gestagens and androgens with rat uterine oestragen receptors. *J. Endocrinol. 77*, 49.
6. Roper, P.R. and Drewinko, B. (1976): Comparison of in vitro methods to determine drug-induced cell lethality. *Cancer Res. 36*, 2182.
7. Horwitz, K.B., Costlow, M.E. and McGuire, W.L. (1975): MCF-7: a human breast cancer cell line with estrogen, androgen, progesterone, and glucocorticoid receptors. *Steroids 26*, 785.
8. Esber, H.J., Payne, I.J. and Bogden, A.E. (1973): Variability of hormone concentrations and ratios in commercial sera used for tissue culture. *J. Nat. Cancer Inst. 50*, 559.
9. Lippman, M., Bolan, G. and Huff, K. (1976): The effects of glucocorticoids and progesterone on hormone-responsive human breast cancer in long-term tissue culture. *Cancer Res. 36*, 4602.
10. Lippman, M., Bolan, G. and Huff, K. (1976): The effects of androgens and antiandrogens on hormone responsive human breast cancer in long-term tissue culture. *Cancer Res. 36*, 4610.
11. Teulings, F.A.G., van Gilse, H.A., Henkelman, M.S., Portengen, H. and Alexieva-Figusch, J. (1980): Estrogen, androgen, glucocorticoid, and progesterone receptors in progestin-induced regression of human breast cancer. *Cancer Res. 40*, 2557.
12. Sala, G., Castegnaro, E., Lenaz, G.R. et al. (1978): Hormone interference in metastatic breast cancer patients treated with medroxyprogesterone acetate at massive doses: preliminary results. *IRCS Med. Sci. 6*, 129.
13. Guthrie, Jr., G.P. and John, W.J. (1980): The in vivo glucocorticoid and antiglucocorticoid actions of medroxyprogesterone acetate. *Endocrinology 107*, 1393.
14. Svec, F., Yeakley, J. and Harrison III, R.W. (1980): Progesterone enhances glucocorticoid dissociation from the AtT-20 cell glucocorticoid receptor. *Endocrinology 107*, 566.

Discussion

R. Bianco: Would the simultaneous presence of tamoxifen and MPA in tissue culture fluid counteract the negative feedback on the progesterone receptor by MPA on these cells? That would be interesting in terms of the therapeutical approaches shown by Dr Iacobelli.

E. Bercovich (Bologna, Italy): In 1975, Horwitz, Costolow and McGuire (*Steroids 26,* 785–795), in a paper on human breast cancer, expressed the opinion that the progesterone receptors are a reflection of the presence and function of the oestrogen receptors. Please would both Dr Iacobelli and Dr Nomura comment on that opinion?

S. Iacobelli: I think that it is true. We carried out the same experiments some time later and found that indeed administration of oestrogen to oestrogen-positive receptor cells increases the progesterone receptor level.

E. Bercovich: As far as I know, it seems from that paper that the progesterone receptor does not have an independent role in the antitumour response, but that it is more or less an indication of the function and role of the oestrogen receptors.

A. Di Marco: If the antitumour effect is bound to the presence of oestrogen as well as to progesterone receptors, it may be thought that the reduction in progesterone receptors may impair the effect of MPA because of a reduced possibility to bind to cellular progesterone receptors.

E. Bercovich: I have no experience with breast cancer, but in our experience with kidney and prostate while using MPA, we observed that the presence of androgenic receptors is of more relevance than that of progesterone receptors (as shown in posters at this meeting). I have some doubts about the central role that has been given to the progesterone receptors. However, it appears from the paper by Horwitz, Costolow and McGuire that progesterone receptors do not have a mechanistic role in the hormonal responsiveness of breast cancer.

W.L. McGuire (San Antonio, U.S.A.): I had not intended to comment on this subject, but perhaps I should say something.

I think the hypothesis, presented several years ago, that the presence of the progesterone receptor was a marker of oestrogen stimulation – oestrogen binding to oestrogen receptor, translocation, protein synthesis and so on – was quite clear. I do not think that it was our intention (or that of others working in this area) to suggest that the progesterone receptor *itself* was intimately involved in tumour growth or regression.

Having said that, there are some new data, actually, some old and some new, indicating that the presence of the progesterone receptor is a very good marker for oestrogen dependence both in advanced disease and in predicting recurrence or disease-free interval, if measured in primary breast cancer. I will show some data to that effect during the Round Table at the end of the meeting.

Furthermore, it can not be assumed that the high doses of progesterone that are used in breast cancer – sometimes more than pharmacological doses – are working through progesterone receptors. In fact, I think that the opposite can be assumed, namely, that they are probably *not* working through progesterone receptors. I would like to think that the effects of high-dose progesterone would be on a cell that contains either an oestrogen receptor or perhaps a progesterone receptor, but that these receptors do not play a role in tumour regression. They are simply markers, just saying that these cells are likely to respond to high-dose oestrogen or high-dose progesterone – even though those biochemical pathways responsible for tumour regression are unknown.

If I understood Dr Iacobelli correctly, he was giving approximately 10^{-7} molar tamoxifen and observed an intermediate growth inhibition of his cells. I do not believe he showed the data, but presumably there was also induction of progesterone receptors. Then, by adding MPA, he was able, synergistically or additively, to increase the amount of growth inhibition. Some time ago we carried out a similar type of experiment in which 10^{-6} molar tamoxifen was given, which does not induce progesterone receptors. In fact, there is inhibition of progesterone receptor synthesis, at least in our hands. However, the growth inhibition is much pronounced.

If Dr Iacobelli tried using higher doses of tamoxifen, 10^{-6} molar, would he still observe a synergistic or additive effect of MPA? I would predict that he would not.

S. Iacobelli: The answer is no. One of our main aims was to try to reduce the dosage to pharmacological levels by combining the 2 drugs. A dose of 10^{-7}

molar tamoxifen, which corresponds to an in-vivo schedule of about 20 or 30 mg, seems to be the reasonable concentration to use. In fact, under these conditions, if MPA is added also at a concentration of 10^{-7} molar, there is about 80% inhibition of cell proliferation.

W.L. McGuire: When Dr Nomura used 5α-dihydrotestosterone (DHT) in cells treated without oestrogen, as the amount of 5α-DHT was increased there seemed to be the same result as in the oestrogen-treated cells. How can that be interpreted?

Y. Nomura: One possibility is that the androgen acts like the oestrogen through some sort of metabolism.

W.L. McGuire: In fact, the explanation is that at the doses used (that is 10^{-6}), 5α-DHT binds to the oestrogen receptor and translocates it, and that is why Dr Nomura obtains the same result as with the oestrogen-treated cells.

E. Milgrom (Paris, France): Dr Iacobelli said that he wants to increase the number of progesterone receptors by giving, first, tamoxifen and, secondly, MPA. By doing so he wants to enhance what could be called a 'progestinic' effect. But, if this kind of mechanism works, I predict that he would find a similar effect using progesterone itself and not the synthetic derivative.

Dr Nomura demonstrated that there was no effect of progesterone. This brings us again to the question whether or not the effect of MPA goes through the progesterone receptor. Could both speakers comment on this, please?

S. Iacobelli: If the cells are exposed to progesterone, the level of the progesterone receptor will decrease.

E. Milgrom (interrupting): If the progesterone receptor is induced with tamoxifen and progesterone is then added, there should be a decrease in the rate of cell proliferation in the same way as if MPA is used, that is, *if* the effect goes through the progesterone receptor. Apparently, from data shown by Dr Nomura, this effect was not observed.

S. Iacobelli: As can be seen from the abscissa scale used, it was possible to observe an inhibitory effect with an MPA concentration as low as 10^{-10} molar. It is therefore highly probable that with this dosage (at least in our continuous in-vitro exposure) the effect is mediated through a receptor mechanism.

E. Milgrom: Was progesterone itself tried?

S. Iacobelli: No.

A. Di Marco: We studied the effect of progesterone in comparison to MPA, measuring the thymidine incorporation, and found that under these conditions progesterone has a similar effect to that of MPA but at concentrations from 10 to 10^2 times higher than MPA.

Another point that may be of interest is the effect of MPA on oestrogen and progesterone receptors. After MPA administration to MCF-7 cells in vitro at concentrations of 10^{-9} or 10^{-8} molar, there is a strong reduction in oestrogen receptors as well as in progesterone receptors measured on whole cells.

I would like to know more about Dr Nomura's experimental conditions. He apparently worked in the presence of oestrogen-deprived serum, but in that serum other hormones, such as glucocorticoid hormones, are present. May there not be interference between glucocorticoid hormones, MPA and oestradiol?

Y. Nomura: That may be possible. However, by giving 2 or even 3 treatments with dextran-coated charcoal to remove oestradiol, it is possible that some other hormones, such as hydrocortisone, may also be removed. We think, therefore, that there are almost no other hormones in that medium.

S. Iacobelli: The problem of serum stripping is quite important in this kind of experimental procedure. Many authors have shown that under the strong conditions required to remove free and loosely bound steroids the cancer cells still grow at a very rapid rate. This is because some conjugated oestrogens remain and are not absorbed by the dextran-coated charcoal procedure. Even with the strong treatment on charcoal, 10% of serum still contains a lot of active steroid (oestrogen) which can stimulate the cells to grow fast.

Y. Nomura: Yes, I know. However, in the near future we should have a conditioned medium without serum, which will be a very important method.

Medroxyprogesterone acetate: experimental studies on its antineoplastic activity and its effect on immunological reactivity*

F. Spreafico, S. Filippeschi, C. Malfiore, M.L. Moras and L. Marmonti
Mario Negri Pharmacological Research Institute, Milan, Italy

Introduction

The studies reported here had, essentially, 2 aims. Our first objective was to obtain information in a well-defined preclinical model which could be of relevance to improving the utility of medroxyprogesterone acetate (MPA) in cancer. Our second objective was to examine as yet unexplored aspects of the biological activity of this drug, which might contribute both to a better understanding of its antitumour activities, and to completion of the assessment of the pharmacotoxicological properties of MPA. More specifically, this paper describes the results seen with MPA, and with the widely employed cytotoxic agent doxorubicin (AM), in the classical animal model of a hormone responsive tumour, the DMBA-induced rat mammary carcinoma. Our immediate aim was thus to obtain results allowing more precise evaluation of the therapeutic potential of MPA vis à vis chemotherapy with AM. Two categories of tumours were chosen for study, analogous to moderately advanced and well advanced human disease. Although the uncertainties connected with the extrapolation of animal data to man are well known it was felt to be of interest to attempt in this way to investigate aspects which were still uncertain at the time these studies were begun, such as whether or not there was a dose-response effect with MPA, and whether it could be used as first-line treatment in some neoplastic conditions, at least. Having regard to the well-known capacity of cancer chemotherapeutic agents to modify immune responses [1, 2], it was felt, in addition, to be of relevance to explore whether MPA

* This work was supported by EURATOM contract BIO-C-355-811 and by a grant in aid from the Italian Association for Cancer Research, Milan, Italy.

could affect the immune defences of the host animals. This might also be of significance in assessing the therapeutic value of MPA.

Material and methods

Two categories of rat mammary carcinoma induced in CD-COBS female rats by a single intravenous (i.v.) injection of 5 mg of 7,12-dimethylbenz(a)anthracene (DMBA), were investigated. In the small tumour category, tumour dimensions on initiation of treatment (day 1) were between 1.0 and 1.5 cm. Since 1 g tumours are believed to involve approximately 10^9 cells, the term small is relative. This category was regarded as analogous to moderately advanced disease. The second category, analogous to advanced disease states in which MPA has, so far, been preferentially employed, comprised rats with primary tumours of between 4.5 and 5.5 cm in diameter on initiation of treatment. The smallest and largest tumour dimensions were determined, using Vernier calipers, by 2 independent observers at 3–4 day intervals in individually marked animals, and the results averaged. Rats with grossly ulcerated tumours were discarded.

It is well known that human neoplasms, even of a specific histological type, grading and stage, can exhibit marked heterogeneity in their responsiveness to treatment. A similar heterogeneity can also be seen in neoplasms, especially solid neoplasms, in animals if the investigations do not involve long-transplanted cancers. It was with the object of more closely approaching the situation in man that MPA activity was tested not on transplanted tumours but in hosts in which the neoplasm had been induced by DMBA. The response criteria used in this study were also chosen to simulate those commonly employed clinically.

Accordingly, in the small tumour category, tumours which grew to 3 cm or over and remained above this size throughout the 120-day observation period were considered as progressive. Tumours the dimensions of which remained between 1 and 3 cm were rated as stable. Decreases in mean tumour dimensions which were either incomplete (i.e. tumour dimensions between 1 and 0.2 cm) and/or not maintained throughout the entire observation period were rated as partial regressions (PR). In cases of tumour regrowth, however, the dimensions had to be 3 cm or less to the rated PR. Complete regressions (CR) were confirmed by autopsy. In the large tumour class, neoplasms growing to 6.5 cm in size or more were considered as progressive, and those remaining between 3.5 and 6.5 cm were rated as stable. Any decrease in tumour size which was either incomplete (i.e. tumour more than 0.2 cm in size) or not maintained throughout the observation period (provided regrowths did not exceed 3.5 cm in size) was considered as PR.

Antitumour activity

Table I presents data from one representative experiment of the series, and clearly shows that MPA treatment was effective when applied to animals with a tumour burden of the order of one billion cells at the start of treatment. MPA activity under these circumstances is revealed not only by the reduced percentage of progressive tumours as compared with that in untreated controls, but also by the finding of a high percentage of tumour regressions, with between 50 and 60% CR when a 100 mg/kg dosage (5 days a week for 4 weeks) was used. Table I shows that when a dosage of 25 mg/kg was used, results were clearly worse than with 50 mg/kg and 100 mg/kg. No significant differences were evident between 50 and 100 mg/kg doses. However, these experiments showed, overall, that a dose-response effect existed within the MPA dose range investigated, in the sense that the 100 mg/kg dose was always slightly more effective than the 50 mg/kg dose, in terms of the percentage of CR + PR, and the time to reach CR.

These experiments do not, however, provide an answer to the clinically relevant question of whether, if dosage had been increased further, there would have been any further increase in effectiveness. As this volume reveals, there is still controversy on the relative therapeutic values of different MPA doses in breast and other cancers.

The results in Table I also show that the effectiveness of MPA, 100 mg/kg (5 days a week for 4 weeks), was similar to that of AM (4 mg/kg i.v. on days 1, 8, 15 and 22). The latter was, however, used as doses which were already toxic, as evidenced by the substantial percentage of early deaths in this ex-

Table I. Effect of MPA on small DMBA-induced mammary carcinomas in primary rat hosts (10 rats per treatment group).

Treatment, dosage and administration	Tumour rating at end of treatment (numbers of animals)				Days of occurrence of	
	CR	PR	Stable	Progressive	CR	Death
Control animals	0	0	4	6	–	81
MPA 100 mg/kg, s.c. 5 d/wk for 4 wk	5	3	2	0	10,16,21,29,37	–
MPA 50 mg/kg, s.c. 5 d/wk for 4 wk	4	4	2	0	25,34,50,70	–
MPA 25 mg/kg, s.c. 5 d/wk for 4 wk	2	2	4	2	17,18	108
AM 4 mg/kg i.v. on days 1,8,15,22	5	2	3	0	7,9,13,28,31,45	28,33,58,79

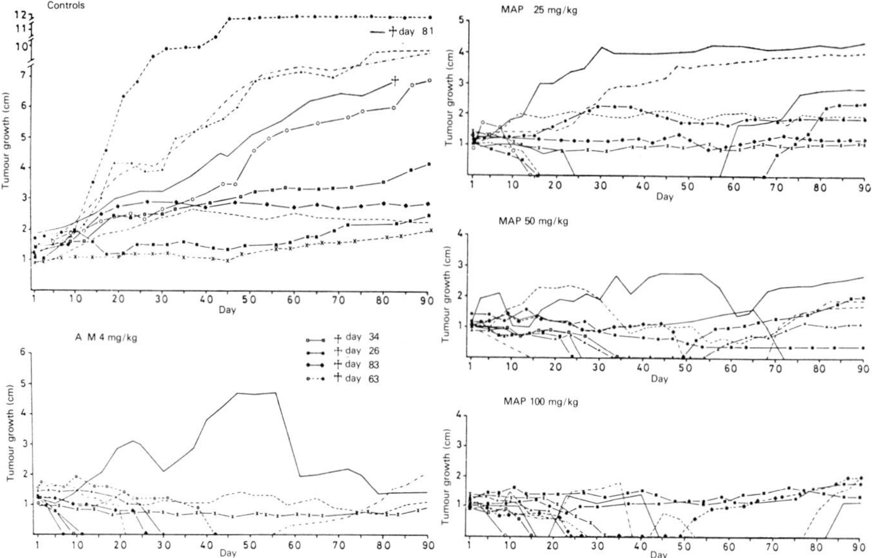

Fig. 1. Effects of various doses of MPA and 4 mg/kg of AM on small tumour growth in rats with DMBA-induced mammary carcinoma.

perimental group. The times to CR were also essentially the same for 100 mg/kg of MPA and AM, as Figure 1, in which the variations in tumour sizes in individual animals are presented, shows clearly. It is evident that, although the times to CR varied, in some animals it could be observed relatively early with both AM and MPA. The same figure shows that, in a few animals, tumours grew again after a variable period of apparent total disappearance (i.e. tumour size less than 0.2 cm). It is impossible on the basis of this study to say whether a further MPA course would have resulted in renewed response of these neoplasms, or whether such regrowth has to be interpreted as an expression of the selection and progressive development of hormone-insensitive cell clones.

Figure 2 shows the results of a representative experiment in which MPA was administered to rats with large tumours at the start of treatment. It is evident that in such animals MPA was effective at both dosages investigated, producing a very distinct shift from progressive disease to arrest of tumour growth and evident regression, even although, as would be expected, the degree of MPA activity was lower than that seen in animals with smaller tumours. In this experiment also, MPA effectiveness was similar to that of a toxic AM regimen, i.e. a course producing a significant percentage of deaths not related to tumours.

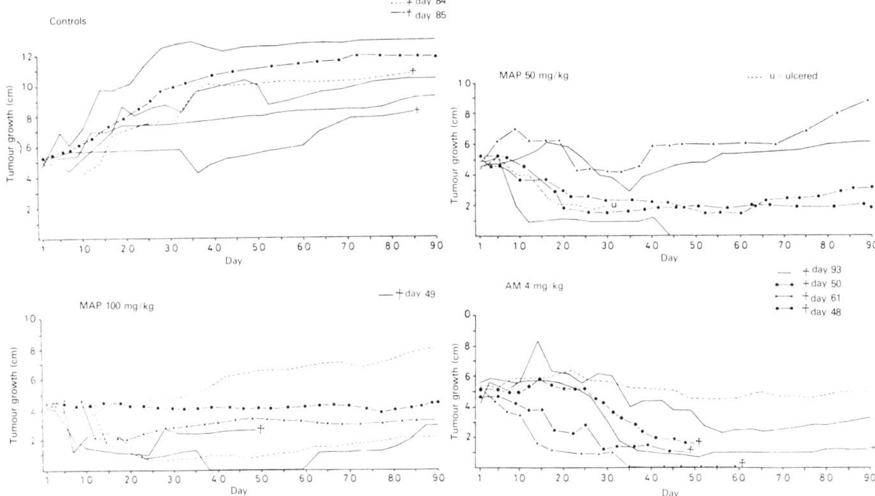

Fig. 2. Effects of various doses of MPA and 4 mg/kg of AM on large tumour growth in rats with DMBA-induced mammary carcinoma.

In a relatively small number of these animals with large tumours, combination therapy with MPA + AM was investigated. Results of representative experiment are presented in Table II. Although the small numbers of animals used prevent any firm conclusion, the findings suggest the possibility, at least, of an additive effect. An extension of work with this type of experiment, with emphasis on the exploration of clinically important, practical aspects of such combination therapy (e.g. sequence of treatments) therefore appears warranted. Such endeavour would also appear justified by the reflection that the remarkable activity of MPA in advanced tumours, described above, may be the experimental counterpart of the clinical findings, discussed by other investigators in this volume, observed in advanced human cancer resistant to other treatments.

Immunological responsiveness

Having confirmed the findings of other groups on the activity of MPA against hormone-responsive tumours in rats (in parallel pilot tests employing a series of murine leukaemias and hormone-independent solid tumours [3–5], no significant activity had been seen), it was felt to be of interest to explore whether MPA administration affected immunological responsiveness. Although such studies were partly directed towards obtaining information on

Table II. Effect of MPA on small DMBA-induced mammary carcinomas in primary rat hosts.

Treatment, dosage and administration	Tumour rating at end of treatment (numbers of animals with rating shown/total number of animals per group)				Days of occurrence of	
	CR	PR	Stable	Progressive	CR	Death
Control animals	0/6	0/6	0/6	6/6	–	84,85
MPA 100 mg/kg, s.c. 5 d/wk for 4 wk	0/6	4/6	1/6	1/6	–	49
MPA 50 mg/kg, s.c. 5 d/wk for 4 wk	1/6	3/6	1/6	1/6	44	–
AM 4 mg/kg i.v. on days 1,8,15,22	1/6	3/6	2/6	0/6	35	48,50,61,93
AM + MPA 100 mg/kg	0/4	4/4	0/4	0/4	–	44,60,93
AM + MPA 50 mg/kg	3/4	1/4	0/4	0/4	23,36,38	41,50,70

whether modification of host defence mechanisms could be contributory to the antineoplastic activity of this agent, the main motive was to learn more about this steroid in relation to an important biological activity, and thus contribute to a better appraisal of the risk-benefit ratio in its therapeutic use. It is, in fact, well known that immunomodulation occurs when standard cancer chemotherapeutic agents are used, and the immunodepression associated with cytoreductive treatment is believed to be an important determinant of a number of acute and long-term complications of such therapies, ranging from infection to increased risk of second malignancies [1]. As reported elsewhere, progestogens and other steroid hormones have also been reported to cause immunodepression in animals [6, 7].

In an attempt to investigate whether MPA treatment could modify host resistance to tumour-associated antigens, we explored whether MPA treatment could modify resistance to challenge with living, syngeneic tumour cells in animals previously immunized with inactivated cells of the same immunogenic tumour. As shown by representative data in Table III, different schedules of MPA treatment given before, concomitantly with, or after immunization did not significantly modify host resistance to subsequent inoculation with neoplastic cells, since the survival of MPA-treated animals was essentially identical with that of the appropriate control animals. It should be noted, in this connection, that our group has previously shown that this model

Table III. Effect of MPA on the survival of pre-immunized, L1210 Ha leukaemia-challenged CD2F$_1$ mice.

10^6 X-rayed L1210 Ha cells, i.p., on day −10	MPA (100 mg/kg s.c.) on days shown	Numbers of L1210 Ha cells, i.p., on day 0	Median survival time (days)
−	−	10^6	7.3
−	−	10^5	9.5
+	−	10^6	12.7*
+	−	10^5	16.8*
+	day 14–5	10^6	12.2
+	day 14–5	10^5	17.4
+	day 19–10	10^6	13.5
+	day 19–10	10^5	16.0
+	day 9–1	10^6	11.9
+	day 9–1	10^5	17.6
+	day 19–1	10^6	13.1
+	day 19–1	10^5	16.4
−	day 19–1	10^6	7.1
−	day 19–1	10^5	9.6

* $P<0.05$ vs untreated controls.

situation is appropriate for revealing the immunomodifying activity of immunodepressive agents, such as nitrosoureas [8], and of immunostimulants, of either natural or synthetic origin [9–11].

In an extension of these experiments, the effect of MPA was investigated in relation to production of antibodies to an antigen such as sheep red blood cells (SRBC). In rodents, the collaboration of macrophages, and T and B lymphocytes is required for optimal response to this antigen. For maximal sensitivity of the evaluation, a technique permitting enumeration of the actual number of antibody-producing cells in the lymphoid organs was used. As shown in Table IV, rodents given a variety of MPA doses and treatments had peak values of antibody-producing cells in the spleen at peak responses not significantly different from controls. It should be emphasized that no significant variations from control values were found when the kinetics of the response were followed in MPA-treated animals. The inclusion of mice in these tests was justified by previous findings of our group indicating this species to be more sensitive than others to immune interference by oestrogens and progestins. It is well known that the sensitivity of primary immune responses to modifying agents is clearly greater than that of secondary responses.

Although our findings did not support the possibility that MPA possesses a strong immunodepressive effect, it was, nevertheless felt to be appropriate to test whether MPA could modify immunodepression induced by a chemotherapeutic agent.

The data in Table V indicate that the immunodepression induced in mice by dimethyltriazenoimidazolecarboxamide (DTIC), was not significantly affected by MPA, which neither reduced nor worsened DTIC-induced reduction of antibody-forming cells. On the basis of not wholly convincing data it has been claimed that MPA can reduce the myelotoxicity of cancer chemotherapeutic agents in man. The findings just described would tend to support the possibility that, if such a protective activity of MPA exists, it does not involve humoral immune capacity, in animals at least.

Table IV. Effect of MPA on primary anti-SRBC response.

Species	Experimental group	Dose (mg/kg)	Number of injections	PFC/spleen
Mouse	Control animals	–	–	46,875
	MPA-treated animals	100	1	44,630
		500	1	45,310
		1,000	1	43,845
		100	5	46,625
		500	5	48,090
Rat	Control animals	–	–	36,470
	MPA-treated animals	100	1	33,905
		100	10	45,260
		100	20	40,125

MPA was stopped 1 d after SRBC in any case; when multiple injections were used MPA was given 5 d/wk for consecutive weeks.

Table V. Effect of MPA on antibody response in DTIC-immunodepressed mice.

Experimental group	Dose (mg/kg)	Number of injections	PFC/spleen
Control animals	–	–	58,270
DTIC-treated animals	75	1	22,480*
DTIC + MPA-treated animals	75 100	1 10	23,265
MPA-treated animals	50	20	63,400
	100	20	61,145

DTIC was injected 4 d before SRBC.
* $P<0.01$.

Table VI. Effect of MPA on splenocyte mitogen responsiveness in mice.

Experimental group	Dosage (mg/kg)	Number of injections	SI* at ConA concentration shown (μg/ml)			SI* at LPS concentration shown (μg/ml)	
			0.2	0.8	1.6	0.5	50
Control animals	–	–	2.18	7.44	5.75	1.57	3.77
MPA-treated animals	100	1	2.01	6.73	4.86	1.83	3.94
	1000	1	2.31	7.26	6.08	1.67	3.65
	100	10	2.47	6.69	5.07	1.87	3.87
	50	20	1.87	7.68	5.35	1.72	4.55
	100	20	2.38	6.58	6.27	1.96	4.38

* = Stimulation index (ratio of mean counts per minute in cultures with and without mitogen). Splenocytes were placed in culture one day after last MPA injection and ^{3}H-thymidine uptake measured after 3 days of culture.

To obtain further information allowing assessment of the possible immunological effects of MPA, it was felt to be of interest to test its effect on cell-mediated imune reactivities. The first parameter investigated in this connection was the *in vitro* responsiveness to polyclonal activators, such as Concanavalin A (ConA), of lymphoid cells obtained from animals treated *in vivo* with MPA. Technical details of the immunological tests have been given elsewhere [6]. Table VI shows that, with regard to this parameter also, MPA administration, in a range of doses and dosage schedules including those shown to be antineoplastically active, was essentially without effect in both rats and mice. A similar lack of effect of MPA was found when the lymphocytes were stimulated using *Escherichia coli* lipopolysaccharide (LPS), which is a preferential stimulant for B cells. ConA is a selective mitogen for T cells.

Finally, it may be worth mentioning that MPA did not significantly modify the expression of Natural Killer (NK) or macrophage-dependent spontaneous cytotoxic activities, both of which are credited with a major role in host resistance, not only as regards neoplastic progression, but also in relation to infectious challenges.

Conclusions

Our experimental observations have confirmed the high activity of MPA in a classic model of a hormone-responsive tumour. The compound exhibited dose related activity, even in animals bearing a very high tumour burden at the start of treatment, under the conditions studied. This activity resulted, in our studies, in a very significant percentage of complete or partial tumour regressions, and was similar to that of a toxic dose of AM. The effects of MPA and AM were additive.

Our immunological findings support 2 general conclusions. Firstly, there was no evidence in favour of the possibility that modification of host antitumour defences plays a role in MPA antitumoral activity. Under our experimental conditions, MPA was essentially immunologically inactive. In addition, no evidence was obtained in our studies for a protective role of MPA, at least as regards immunodepression associated with chemotherapy. Secondly, MPA does not appear to possess any significant immunodepressive activity on either humoral or cell-mediated reactivities when used at dosages exhibiting marked antineoplastic effects. This experimental conclusion appears of direct clinical interest for assessment of the safety and therapeutic potential of MPA, and the evaluation of possibilities of its use in a wider range of neoplastic disease states, alone or in association with other forms of treatment. The fact that, so far, clinical experience with this agent has not been associated with any significant increase in infectious side-effects supports the possibility that our immunological findings in animals might be extrapolated to man.

References

1. Spreafico, F. and Mantovani, A. (1981): Immunomodulation by cancer chemotherapeutic agents and antineoplastic activity. In: *Pathobiology Annual 1981*, pp. 177–195. Ed: H.L. Ioachim. Raven Press, New York.
2. Spreafico, F., Tagliabue, A. and Vecchi, A. (1982): Chemical immunodepressants. In: *Immunopharmacology*. Ed: P. Sirois. Elsevier/North-Holland, Amsterdam. (In press.)
3. Formelli, F., Zaccheo, T., Mazzoni, A. et al. (1982): Antitumour activity and pharmacokinetics of medroxyprogesterone acetate in experimental tumour systems. In: *Proceedings of an International Symposium on Medroxyprogesterone Acetate*, pp. 47–62. Eds: F. Cavalli, W.L. McGuire, F. Pannuti, A. Pellegrini and G. Robustelli Della Cuna. Excerpta Medica, Amsterdam.
4. Di Marco, A. (1980): The antitumor activity of 6α-methyl-17α-acetoxyprogesterone (MPA) in experimental mammary cancer. In: *Progress in Cancer Research and Therapy*, Vol. 15, pp. 1–20. Eds: S. Iacobelli and A. Di Marco. Raven Press, New York.
5. Danguy, A., Negros, N., Devleeschouwer, N. et al. (1980): Effects of medroxyprogesterone acetate (MPA) on growth of DMBA-induced rat mammary tumors: Histopathological and endocrine studies. In: *Progress in Cancer Research and Therapy*, Vol. 15, pp. 21–28. Ed: S. Iacobelli and A. Di Marco. Raven Press, New York.
6. Spreafico, F., Filippeschi, S., Malfiore, C. et al. (1982): Effect of medroxy-

progesterone acetate on DMBA-induced rat mammary carcinoma and on immunological reactivity. *Eur. J. Cancer Clin. Oncol. 18,* 45.

7. Spreafico, F., Vecchi, A., Anaclerio, A. et al. (1977): Experimental analysis of the effects of oral contraceptives on the function of the lymphoid system. In: *Pharmacology of Steroid Contraceptive Drugs*, pp. 267–276. Eds: S. Garattini and H.W. Berendes. Raven Press, New York.
8. Spreafico, F., Filippeschi, S., Falautano, P. et al. (1981): EORTC studies with novel nitrosureas. In: *Nitrosureas. Current Status and New Developments*, pp. 27–42. Eds: A.W. Prestayko, L.H. Baker, S.T. Crooke, S.K. Carter and P.S. Schein. Academic Press, New York.
9. Tagliabue, A., Alessandri, G., Polentarutti, N. et al. (1978): The immunostimulatory activity of 3-(p-chlorophenyl)-2,3-dihydro-3-hydroxytriazolo [3,2-α]-benzimidazole-2-acetic acid (NSC 208828). *Eur. J. Cancer 14,* 393.
10. Vecchi, A., Sironi, M. and Spreafico, F. (1978): Preliminary characterization in mice of the effect of isoprinosine on the immune system. *Cancer Treat. Rep. 62,* 1975.
11. Spreafico, F., Filippeschi, S., Polentarutti, N. and Malfiore, C. (1980): The immunostimulatory capacity of B. subtilis spores. *Chemiotherapia Antimicrob. 3,* 259.

The effects of medroxyprogesterone acetate and tamoxifen on breast cancer in the human tumour cloning assay*

C.K. Osborne and D.D. Von Hoff
Department of Medicine, University of Texas Health Science Centre, San Antonio, Texas

Introduction

Currently, a large variety of cytotoxic drugs and hormones are used in the management of patients with breast cancer. Clinical guidelines have not proven effective in determining which of these therapies is optimal in an individual patient, and the choice of which to use is, therefore, largely empirical. The development of the oestrogen receptor (ER) assay has been a major advance, allowing selection of patients with endocrine-responsive tumours, but the assay is of no value in determining which endocrine therapy should be employed in a given situation, and has not been useful in the selection of appropriate patients for cytotoxic chemotherapy. Furthermore, the ER assay is liable to give a large number of false positive results. Forty per cent of patients with ER-positive tumours fail to respond to hormonal manipulation. Thus there is still a need for an accurate method of determining the best cytotoxic or hormonal agent to use in an individual patient.

The human tumour cloning system developed by Hamburger and Salmon [1, 2] has shown substantial promise as a method for cultivating human tumours in vitro, a task which was largely impossible in the past. More importantly, this system now permits analysis of the effects on human cancers of cytotoxic agents, hormones, growth factors, or other biological response modifiers. Preliminary results using the assay to select drugs which are likely to have in vivo antitumour activity were encouraging [3]. A drug that was inactive in the assay was usually inactive when given to the patient, whereas significant in vitro activity correlated well with in vivo antitumour effects.

*Supported by a grant from Farmitalia Carlo Erba, Milan.

We have considerable experience in growing human breast cancer specimens in the cloning assay [4]. We have now cultured breast cancer specimens from more than 1,000 patients. Overall, about 50% of both primary and metastatic specimens grow sufficiently well to detect drug-induced inhibition of colony formation accurately. Specimens from a variety of metastatic sites, including those from effusions and solid visceral nodules, grow equally well in the assay. Anticancer drugs with known clinical activity against breast cancer show activity in the cloning assay, suggesting that the in vitro activity may reflect activity in patients with the disease. Furthermore, a more recent analysis of results of a prospective trial in patients with breast and other cancers supports the validity of the assay [5]. Cytotoxic drugs showing 50% or greater inhibition of breast tumour colony forming units (TCFU) were found likely to result in tumour regression when given to the patient. Although many problems have been identified, which will be the subject of future work [4], the cloning assay has tremendous potential in helping to individualize the treatment of patients, and to screen new agents.

We have now initiated studies of the effects of hormones and other biological response modifiers on human breast tumour cells in the cloning assay. Our objective has been to identify those hormones or other factors that have direct effects on the clonogenic fraction of the tumour, and to determine whether the assay might be useful in predicting the hormonal dependence of a tumour in individual patients. In this report, we describe our preliminary experience in studying the effects of 2 hormones frequently used in breast cancer patients, medroxyprogesterone acetate (MPA) and tamoxifen (TAM). Both agents inhibit colony growth of certain human breast cancer specimens, as well as growth of the ER-positive breast cancer cell line MCF-7.

Methods

We have recently obtained information on 16 primary or metastatic breast cancer specimens cultured in the human tumour cloning assay in the presence of MPA and/or TAM. The methods used for the collection of cells, the preparation of single cell suspensions, and the cloning assay itself have been described in detail elsewhere [1, 2, 4]. Briefly, the tumour specimens are minced to 2-mm fragments and placed in tissue culture medium. The fragments are then mechanically disrupted and single-cell suspensions obtained. Hormones dissolved in ethanol are then added to the cell suspensions to achieve 1 μM final concentrations and ethanol concentrations of 0.1%. A similar volume of ethanol is added to control cell cultures. The suspensions are then plated in the top layer of agar at a concentration of 500,000 cells per Petri dish. The plates are incubated at 37 °C in a 7% CO_2 humidified atmosphere for 14–21 days. Colonies are then counted by hand, with viewing through a Zeiss inverted phase microscope.

MCF-7 cells are a continuous tissue culture line derived from a malignant effusion from a woman with metastatic breast cancer [6]. The methods used in the cultivation of these cells have been summarized elsewhere [7]. For the cloning assay, MCF-7 cells are harvested in 0.02% EDTA, and single cell suspensions prepared by passage of the cells through progressively smaller gauge needles. After the addition of hormones, the cells are plated in the top layer of agar at a concentration of 2×10^4 cells per ml. Colonies are counted by hand as described above. In addition, colony growth is measured using a Bausch and Lomb FAS-II image analysis system.

Results

The trial is continuing, but we have now accumulated 16 evaluable breast cancer specimens tested with either MPA and/or TAM in the cloning assay. The median number of colonies growing in the control dishes was 94 (range 29–1,216). MPA and TAM on their own significantly inhibited TCFU in several of these specimens. Three out of 16 specimens (19%) had a 50% or greater inhibition of TCFU when incubated with the hormones. Eight out of 16 specimens (50%) had a 20% or greater inhibition of TCFU.

Activity rates for each drug are shown in Table I. Six out of 9 specimens (67%) incubated with MPA showed at least a 20% inhibition of TCFU, and 2 out of 9 (22%) showed a 50% or greater inhibition. Less activity was observed with TAM, but this group included a larger number of metastatic specimens from previously treated patients. Such patients would normally be expected to have inferior response rates to endocrine therapy. However, in the 8 specimens with which both MPA and TAM were assayed, 5 showed at least 20% inhibition with MPA, whereas only one was inhibited by TAM. Obviously, the relative activities of these drugs in the cloning assay can only be determined with greater certainty once more results are available.

Table I. Effect of MPA or TAM on colony growth.

Drug	Number of specimens tested	Number (%) of specimens showing degree of inhibition of TCFU indicated	
		≥50%	≥20%
MPA	9	2 (22)	6 (67)
TAM	14	1 (7)	3 (21)

Assessment of correlations between in vitro activity in the cloning assay, and ER or progesterone receptor (PgR) status, or in vivo response, will also require more results. Thus far, 0/5 ER-negative and 1/3 ER-positive tumours have shown 50% or greater inhibition with either drug. The ER-positive patient whose tumour responded in the cloning assay, had a significant partial tumour regression when treated with another progestational agent, megestrol acetate.

The relatively modest in vitro activity observed with MPA and TAM could have several explanations. One factor could be that endogenous hormones (particularly oestrogens) present in the serum used in the cloning assay stimulate colony growth, thus masking or blocking inhibition by the drugs. The MCF-7 human breast cancer cells, for instance, are not inhibited by TAM when grown in medium containing 10% fetal bovine serum. Cell growth is, however, inhibited when serum which has been treated with dextran-coated charcoal (DCC) to reduce the concentration of endogenous hormones is used. To investigate further the feasibility of using such DCC-treated serum in the clonogenic assay, we used the MCF-7 cells as a model. These cells grow readily in the soft agar cloning assay in the presence of DCC-treated serum. The effects of MPA and TAM on colony growth are shown in Figure 1.

A significant, dose-dependent inhibition of colony growth is evident with TAM in concentrations greater than 10 nM. More than 50% inhibition of TCFU is observed with concentrations of 1 μM. On the other hand, no significant inhibition is seen with MPA at any concentration. These results were obtained from several experiments in which colonies were counted microscopically, by hand. In this method, a colony is defined as a cluster of 50 or more cells. Each colony is usually 50–60 microns in diameter. Quite different results were seen when colonies were counted and analysed using an automated computer-assisted image analysis system, which calculates a size distribution for the colonies (Fig. 2). TAM inhibited the formation of both large and small colonies. Sixty-eight per cent of all colonies greater than 60 microns survived TAM treatment. When a progressively larger diameter was used as criterion for a 'colony', the effect of TAM became more dramatic. Less than 10% of colonies greater than 124 microns survived TAM. No inhibition of colony formation was observed with MPA for colonies greater than 60 microns in diameter, consistent with the results obtained by visual counts (Fig. 1). However, as with TAM, the formation of larger colonies was significantly inhibited by MPA, and only 25% of colonies greater than 124 microns in diameter survived MPA treatment. Thus both TAM and MPA significantly inhibit colony formation by MCF-7 breast cancer cells growing in DCC-treated serum in the soft agar cloning assay.

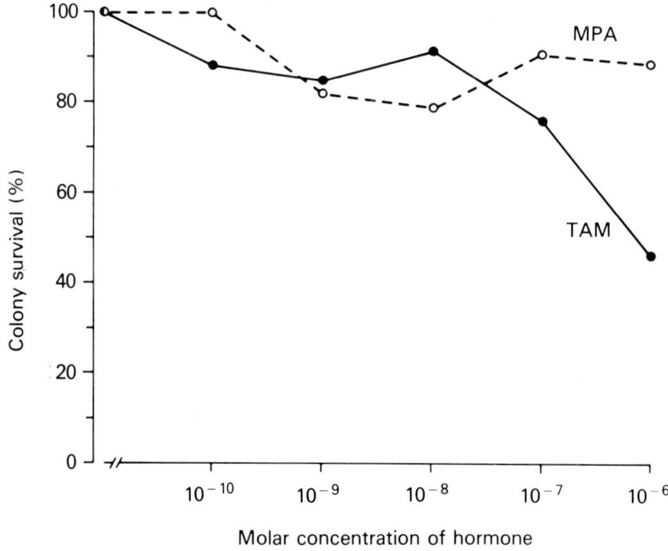

Fig. 1. Effect of MPA and TAM on clonal growth of MCF-7 cells. Averages of 5 experiments, each in triplicate.

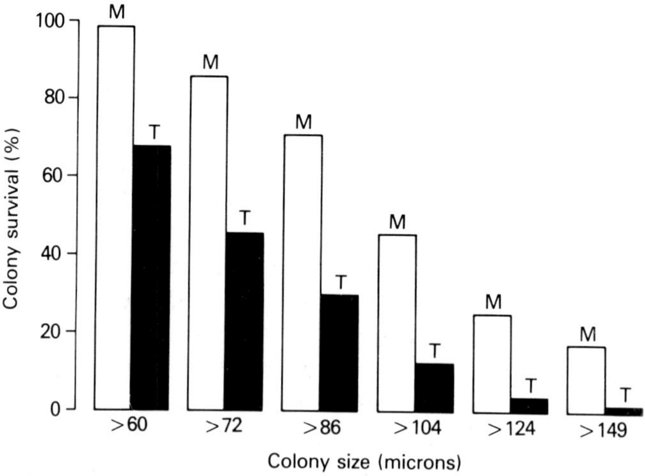

Fig. 2. Effect of MPA and TAM on colony size distribution. Colonies were counted using a Bausch and Lomb image analysis system after continuous exposure to hormones (1 μM). Averages of 2 experiments, each in triplicate.

Discussion

This study, though very preliminary, demonstrates that MPA and TAM have direct inhibitory effects on certain human breast cancer specimens in the cloning assay. In most specimens, the degree of inhibition is not dramatic, and is less than that which we associate with a high predictive index for in vivo response to cytotoxic drugs ($\geq 50\%$ inhibition). However, the mechanism of the antitumour activity of the hormonal agents, although poorly defined, is likely to be quite different from that of cytotoxic drugs, and a different level of in vitro activity for predicting in vivo response may need to be defined. This will require a large prospective study of in vivo response as a function of in vitro activity in the cloning assay.

There are several other potential explanations for the modest activity of these agents in the cloning assay. First, MPA and TAM are not likely to inhibit the growth of hormone receptor-negative cells which may be present in a heterogeneous tumour which is 'ER-positive' by biochemical assay. The development of histochemical assay methods for ER and PgR will permit the quantification of receptors in cells comprising individual colonies growing in soft agar, and will help to clarify this question. Second, as discussed earlier, the endogenous hormones present in the serum used in the assay may mask or minimize the effects of hormones or antihormones added to the system. We are currently attempting to perform the assay with DCC-treated serum, which should minimize the effects of endogenous hormones, and perhaps increase the sensitivity of the assay. Finally, it is known that hormonal inhibition of breast cancer growth requires prolonged exposure to the hormonal agent. Although the assay is performed using a 'continuous' exposure method, it is possible that the duration of incubation is too brief to see a maximal effect. Furthermore, degradation or metabolism of the agents could occur during the assay, and this would also reduce any inhibitory effects. These possibilities are now being investigated.

MPA and TAM also inhibit colony growth of the hormone-responsive MCF-7 breast cancer cell line. It is interesting that the most dramatic effect is a marked reduction in the formation of the larger colonies. A reduction in the larger colonies might indicate a reduction in the most highly proliferative stem cell population. This would correlate best with therapeutic efficacy. The small colonies might be composed of proliferative but nonclonogenic cells of intermediate differentiation, capable of replicating for a finite period of time. Such a compartment has been identified in human cancers [8]. We are currently investigating the effects of MPA and TAM on colony size distributions from actual human breast cancer specimens.

References

1. Hamburger, A. and Salmon, S.E. (1977): Primary bioassay of human myeloma stem cells. *J. Clin. Inv. 60*, 846.
2. Hamburger, A. and Salmon, S.E. (1977): Primary bioassay of human tumor stem cells. *Science 197*, 461.
3. Salmon, S.E., Hamburger, A.W., Soehnien, B.J. et al. (1978): Quantitation of differential sensitivities of human tumor cells to anticancer drugs. *N. Engl. J. Med. 298*, 1321.
4. Von Hoff, D.D., Sandbach, J., Osborne, C.K. et al. (1981): Potential and problems with growth of breast cancer in a human tumor cloning system. *Breast Cancer Research and Treatment 1*, 141.
5. Von Hoff, D.D., Page, C., Harris, G. et al. (1981): Prospective clinical trial of a human tumor cloning system (Abstract). *Proc. Am. Assoc. Cancer Res. 22,* 154.
6. Soule, H.D., Vezquez, J., Lang, A. et al. (1973): A human cell line from a pleural effusion derived from a breast carcinoma. *J. Nat. Cancer Inst. 51*, 1409.
7. Osborne, C.K., Bolan, G., Monaco, M.E. and Lippman, M.E. (1976): Hormone responsive human breast cancer in long-term tissue culture: effect of insulin. *Proc. Natl. Acad. Sci. U.S.A. 73*, 4536.
8. Mackillop, W.J. and Buick, R.N. (1982): Cellular heterogeneity in human ovarian carcinoma studied by density gradient fractionation. *Stem Cells.* (In press.)

Discussion

W. Jonat (Bremen, Federal Republic of Germany): How many breast cancer patients form these large colonies? Dr Osborne said that approximately 50% of patients form 30 colonies, for example, and surely that number will decrease perhaps to 10% if we are considering only those who form a large number of colonies. That means that only about 10% of the patients can be analysed.

C.K. Osborne: That is a good point and it may be true. We do not have data available yet – this is relatively new information about the large colonies and has not yet been published. Our specimens have not yet been analysed with regard to that, but Dr Jonat may be right, and it may further reduce our ability to test significant numbers of patients.

F. Formelli: What were the doses used by Dr Osborne in his studies, in terms of the pharmacological doses of the 2 drugs?

C.K. Osborne: Is the amount of drug in the serum of a patient treated with tamoxifen or MPA correlated in some way? *(Dr. Formelli assented).* I think that they are fairly close. Tamoxifen, at a dose of 0.1–1 μmolar, is fairly close to the levels obtained in vivo. With regard to MPA, I would have to ask one of the experts in that area whether doses of that level are close to those achieved in vivo because I do not know the answer. I might add that when only the large colony formation in the MCF-7 cells is studied, there is a clear dose-response curve. Even doses of 10^{-9} molar MPA have inhibitory activity on the large colonies.

A. Di Marco: Is it possible that Dr Osborne's assay selects for autonomous hormone-independent cells?

C.K. Osborne: At the moment we do not really know about that, except that with regard to oestrogen receptor status, if the oestrogen receptor status of the tumour is determined before it is put into the assay, oestrogen receptor-positive tumours grow just as well as oestrogen receptor-negative tumours. It is not known whether those colonies that are actually forming in the assay are oestrogen receptor-positive or -negative. Histochemical analysis of oestrogen receptor (which is now being worked on) will be required to answer that question.

J.C. Heuson: Has Dr Osborne ever observed a stimulatory effect of either tamoxifen or MPA in this clonogenic assay?

C.K. Osborne: Occasionally minor degrees of stimulation are observed, but I think they are within the standard deviation of the counts. Except in an occasional tumour, where significant stimulation has been observed (which makes one wonder whether there is something wrong with the control dishes in that experiment), nothing consistent has been observed. Dose-response curves have not been possible to do in the human specimens because we do not get sufficient tumour cells.

J.C. Heuson: Jan Bernheim, who is working with us in Brussels, has produced some data. They are completely anecdotal because they come from only one human breast cancer specimen cloning assay. This specimen was taken from a tumour in a patient treated with large doses of MPA, whose tumour was growing. Two weeks after stopping the treatment, a specimen was taken and subjected to the clonogenic assay. As regards the concentration of MPA (abscissa) versus the number of colonies (ordinate), without MPA there were no colonies at all, and with increasing concentrations of MPA the number of colonies can be seen. As I say, this is completely anecdotal and I did not do this assay myself – but I was asked to present the results.

A. Di Marco: In conclusion, perhaps it may be said that there are very nice in-vitro experimental tests showing that there is a direct effect of MPA. There are also in-vivo data demonstrating that there may be effects which are not immediate but are mediated by the endocrinal effects on the other hormones. Perhaps in the future it is important to study which of these factors are relevant for the clinical use of MPA.

Session II: Clinical pharmacology and pharmacokinetics

Chairmen: G. Robustelli Della Cuna – Pavia, Italy
I.R. Hesselius – Uppsala, Sweden

Introduction

Since 1974, MPA has been employed with interesting results in advanced breast cancer at the so-called high doses. The recent evidences coming from controlled clinical trials have confirmed the results of the first-generation trials. Unfortunately, the early clinical experiences did not give enough room to pharmacology and the pharmacokinetic aspects related to the use of this compound, as well as to an exhaustive analysis of the adverse events during the long-term treatments with high-dose MPA. This seems, however, a good time to fill in this gap. This session will be devoted to clinical pharmacology and pharmacokinetic aspects of high-dose MPA as well as to some specific positive side-effects such as the myeloprotective action of this compound observed during cytotoxic treatment.

G. Robustelli Della Cuna

Endocrinological properties of medroxyprogesterone acetate

G. Sala[1], F. Iannotta[1] and A. Facchinetti[2]
[1]Medical Department B, and [2]Nuclear Medicine, Varese Regional Hospital, Varese, Italy

Introduction

Medroxyprogesterone acetate (MPA) is a synthetic progestational agent, active by both the oral (p.o.) and intramuscular (i.m.) routes, which was independently developed by 2 research groups in 1958 [1, 2].

In the 1960's MPA at an average daily dosage of 100 mg gave generally poor clinical results when used against hormone sensitive tumours. The clinical studies carried out during the 1970's by some Italian investigators using much higher daily dosages (1,000–2,000 mg) by the i.m. and p.o. routes of administration, gave far better clinical results. These stimulated renewed interest in establishing the effect of high doses of MPA at the endocrine level, and in correlating biological effects with serum MPA concentrations, in order to understand the mechanism of its antitumour effect.

Material and methods

During the last 20 years, we have studied the endocrinological effects of MPA under various experimental conditions [3–7]. The subjects examined have included adult men and women with normal adrenal function, adrenalectomized men and women, women in a state of natural or surgical menopause, mostly affected by mammary cancer. The endocrinological study was carried out with the methods currently in use in our hospital. A summary of the most pertinent data from these studies will be given in the present report.

MPA was administered at daily dosages of 100, 500, 1,000 or 2,000 mg, i.m., (in aqueous or oily solution), or p.o. (tablets or aqueous suspension) for 5, 8, 10 or 30 days.

Determinations carried out included:
- Serum follicle stimulating hormone (FSH) and luteinizing homone (LH) (radioimmunoassay (RIA), Serono Kits, double antibody method).
- Gonadotropin stimulation with gonadotropin releasing hormone (GnRH) (100 or 200 μg, intravenously (i.v.)).
- Serum prolactin (PRL) (RIA, Serono Kit, double antibody method).
- Prolactin stimulation with thyrotrophin releasing hormone (TRH) (200 μg, i.v.).
- Prolactin stimulation with arginine (0.5 g/kg, i.v., over a 30-minute period).
- Urinary 17-hydroxycorticosteroids (Porter and Silber chromogens (PSC)) [8].
- Urinary tetrahydrocortisol (THF) and tetrahydrocortisone (THE) [9].
- Plasma cortisol (RIA, Sorin Kit, coated tube method).
- Cortisol stimulation with adrenocorticotrophic hormone (ACTH) (0.5 mg of Synacthen®, i.v., in 500 ml of physiological saline over an 8-hour period).
- Cortisol stimulation with insulin (0.1 U/kg by rapid i.v. injection).
- Urinary 17-ketosteroids [10].
- Serum human growth hormone (GH) (RIA, Biodata Kit, double antibody method).
- Human GH stimulated with arginine (0.5 g/kg, i.v., over a 30-minute period).

Serum MPA was determined by RIA after diethylether extraction, using the method of Shrimanker et al. [11]. In these experiments, MPA was administered one hour before blood sampling.

Results

Figure 1 shows the decrease in serum FSH and LH produced by MPA, 0.5 g, i.m., daily, for 10 days, in 6 menopausal women. Figures 2 and 3 show the stronger inhibition of serum FSH and LH obtained with 2 g of MPA, i.m., daily, for 15 and 30 days in 10 menopausal women with breast cancer. While MPA at a daily dosage of 0.5 g, i.m., for 8 days, inhibits the basal levels of gonadotropins in the serum but maintains the hypophyseal reserve of FSH and LH [12], at a daily dose of 0.5 g, i.m. for 30 days (Fig. 4) or 1 g p.o. for 30 days (Fig. 5), MPA reduces gonadotropin reserve, as shown by the reduced absolute release of FSH and LH after GnRH stimulation. △ represents the mean difference in absolute terms between the basal values and GnRH-

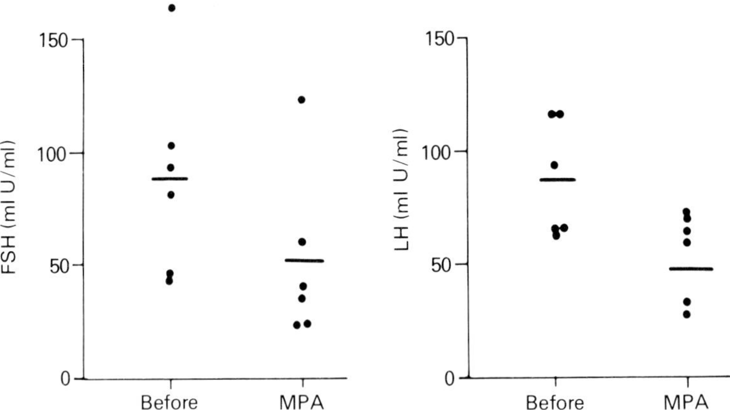

Fig. 1. Effects of 0.5 g of MPA, i.m., per day, for 10 days, on serum FSH and LH.

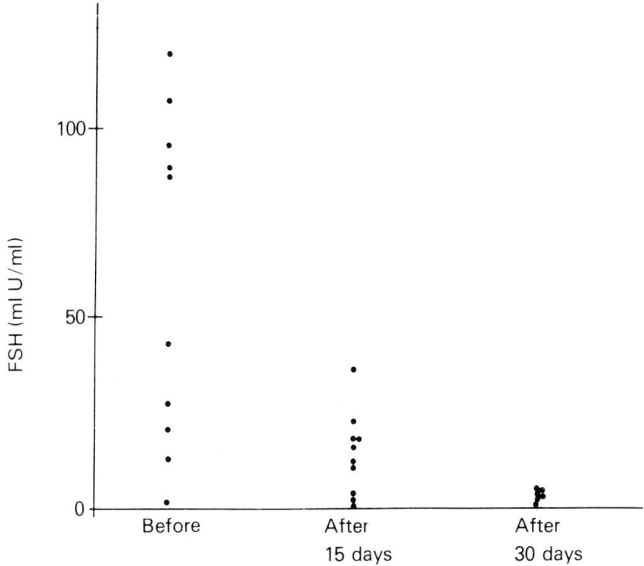

Fig. 2. Effects of 2 g of MPA, i.m., per day, for 10–30 days, on serum FSH.

stimulated values. After both i.m. and p.o. administration, the release of gonadotropins after 30 days of treatment is lower than release before MPA. The effect observed after treatment with 1 g of MPA, p.o., is higher than that observed after 0.5 g of MPA, i.m., reflecting the higher serum concentrations of MPA (197 vs 91 ng/ml).

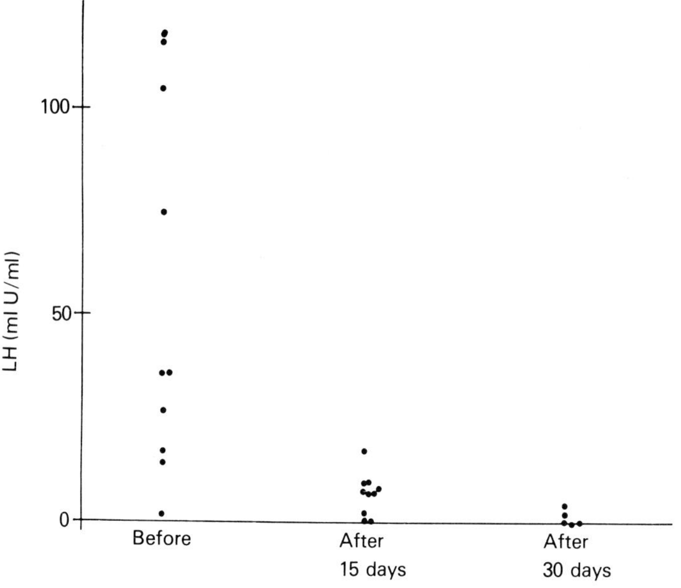

Fig. 3. Effects of 2 g of MPA, i.m., per day, for 10–30 days, on serum LH.

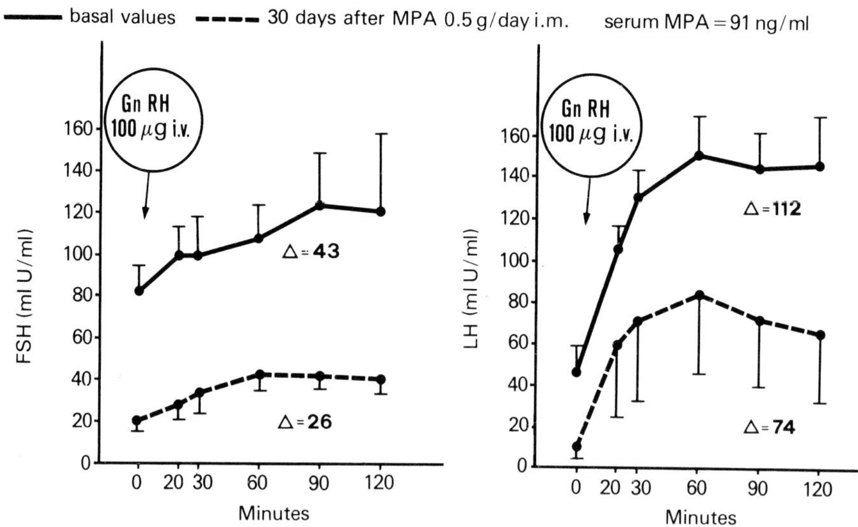

Fig. 4. Effects of 0.5 g of MPA, i.m., per day, for 30 days, on basal and GnRH-stimulated serum gonadotropins.

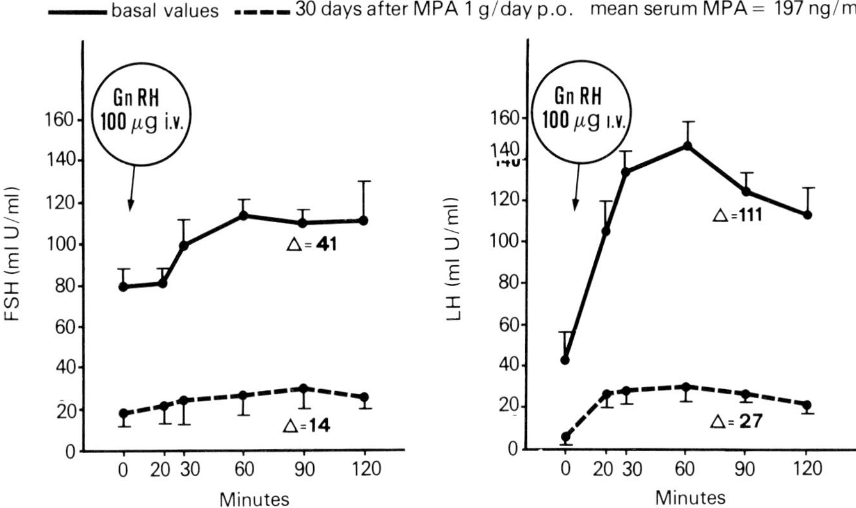

Fig. 5. Effects of 1 g of MPA, p.o., for 30 days, on basal and GnRH-stimulated serum gonadotropins.

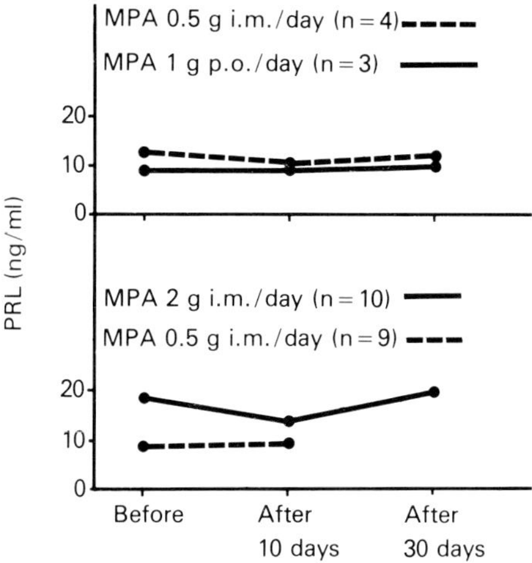

Fig. 6. Effects of MPA under different experimental conditions on serum prolactin levels.

Figure 6 summarizes the behaviour of serum prolactin in 4 different experiments. No change of basal values was apparent. When prolactin is stimulated with thyrotrophin-releasing hormone (TRH) (Fig. 7) or arginine

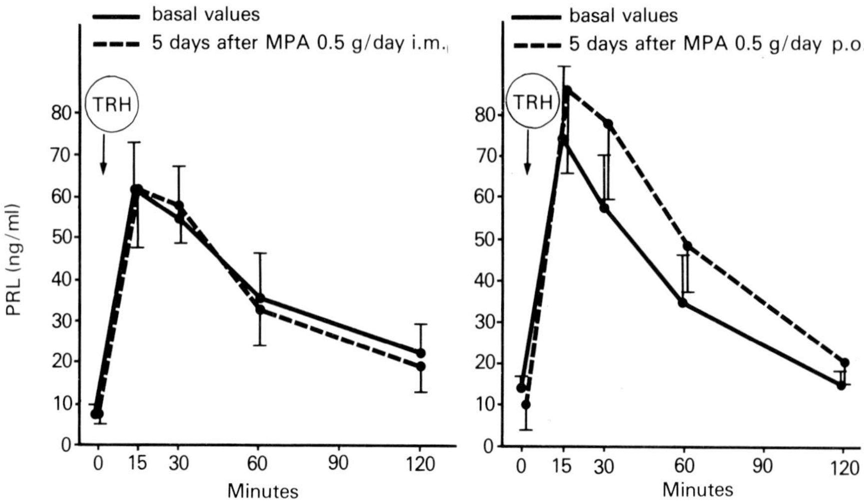

Fig. 7. Effects of MPA (0.5 g per day, for 15 days, i.m. and p.o.) on prolactin stimulated by TRH.

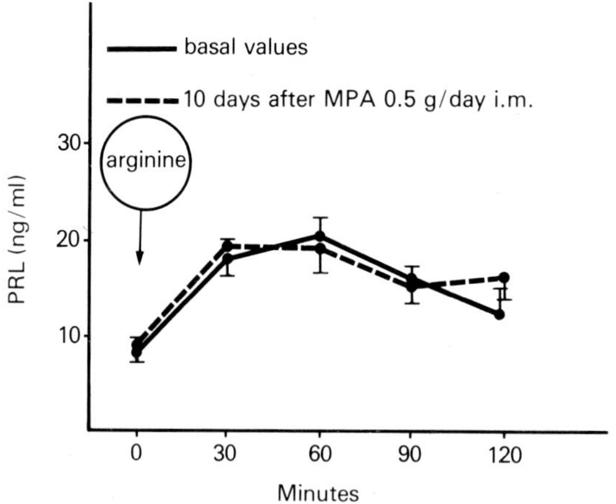

Fig. 8. Effects of MPA (0.5 g per day, for 10 days, i.m.) on prolactin stimulated by arginine.

(Fig. 8), there is no effect of MPA at different doses and by different routes of administration.

Table I shows the urinary excretion of PSCs after the administration of MPA for 10 days under various experimental conditions. A definite increase in urinary corticosteroids is evident after the i.m. administration of 2 g/day of

Table I. Effect of MPA on urinary PSC under various conditions.

Experimental condition	Urinary excretion (mg/day)	
	Before	After 10 days
Subjects with normal adrenal function		
100 mg/day i.m. (N = 5)	6.53	6.02
500 mg/day i.m. (N = 7)	6.09	5.92
2,000 mg/day i.m. (N = 5)	4.45	19.09
100 mg/day p.o. (N = 14)	3.53	10.93
Ovaro-adrenalectomized subjects		
100 mg/day i.m. (N = 5) (oily solution)	0.33	9.80

MPA in aqueous suspension, of 100 mg/day of MPA, p.o., or of 100 mg/day of MPA, i.m., in oily solution. On the other hand, 100–500 mg/day of MPA in aqueous suspension did not produce increases in urinary PSC.

From Table I, it may also be concluded that MPA can be hydroxylated in the C-21 position, even in the absence of the adrenal glands. In fact, PSCs increase remarkably after p.o. administration, even in the adrenalectomized subject.

The effect of high i.m. daily dosages of MPA in aqueous suspension on the urinary excretion of 17-hydroxycorticosteroids and 17-ketosteroids is summarized in Figure 9, which illustrates the progressive increase in urinary PSC caused by the accumulation of MPA administered i.m., with 17-ketosteroids showing a slight, late rise. The increase in urinary PSCs is not correlated with the presence of endogenous adrenal catabolites (Table II), but is correlated with the presence of MPA metabolites, with M1 (6-beta-17-alpha-21-trihydroxy-6-alpha-methyl-Δ^4-pregnene-3,20-dione-21-acetate), isolated by us in 1962 [5], and devoid of corticoid-like properties, prevalent in the urine.

Figure 10 shows the effect of 2 MPA dosages (0.5 g daily, i.m., and 1 g daily, p.o.) on the plasma levels of cortisol in the menopausal woman after 15 and 30 days' treatment. It is evident that the p.o. administration of 1 g daily produces a greater reduction in plasma cortisol, and that this reduction is apparent after only 15 days' treatment. High MPA serum levels are reached sooner after the administration of 1 g daily, p.o., than after 0.5 g daily, i.m., confirming the direct relationship between serum concentrations and endocrine effects of MPA.

Figure 11 summarizes the inhibitory effect produced by 0.5 g of MPA daily, i.m., for 30 days, or 1 g daily, p.o., for 30 days, on the plasma levels of cortisol after stimulation with ACTH or insulin. The response of the adrenals to

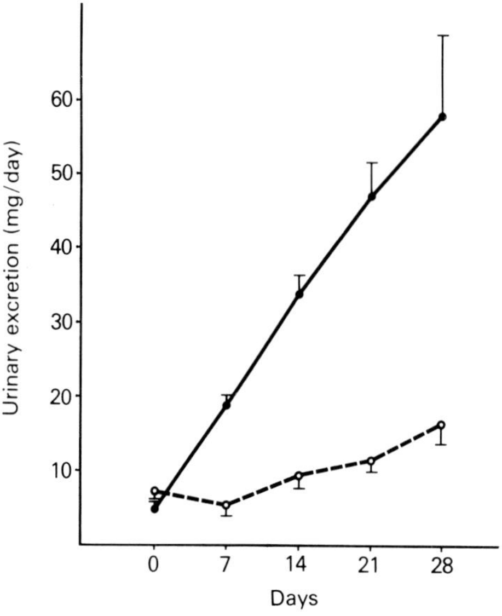

Fig. 9. Effects of repeated MPA administration (2 g per day, for 30 days, i.m.) on urinary 17-hydroxycorticosteroids (•———•) and 17-ketosteroids (○– – –○).

Table II. Effect of MPA on urinary THF under various experimental conditions.

Case number	Experimental condition	THF (mg/day)	THE (mg/day)
4	Before	1.42	1.92
	After 100 mg/day, i.m.	1.18	1.74
2	Before	0.96	1.91
	After 500 mg/day, i.m.	0.56	0.57
3	Before	1.84	2.75
	After 100 mg/day, p.o.	1.96	2.76

the direct or indirect stimulus is strongly inhibited, especially after oral MPA. This stronger inhibition can, again, be correlated with the higher serum concentrations of MPA obtained after oral administration.

Figure 12 shows the effect of MPA (2 g/day, i.m., for 30 days) on serum growth hormone (GH) levels. A trend toward a decrease is apparent, but the difference between basal and 30-day levels is not statistically significant. The number of observations is limited. Similarly, there is no difference between

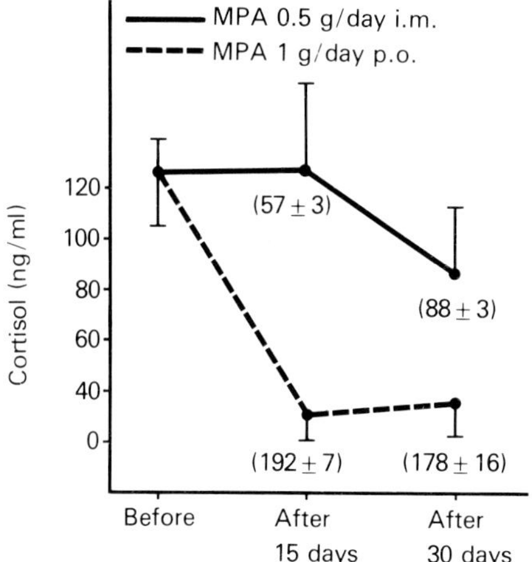

Fig. 10. Effects of 2 dosages of MPA (0.5 g i.m. per day, for 15–30 days, and 1 g, p.o., per day, for 15–30 days) on plasma cortisol. Numbers in parentheses are serum MPA concentrations (ng/ml).

arginine stimulation of GH values before and after treatment with 0.5 g of MPA, i.m., per day, for 10 days (Fig. 13).

Discussion

MPA has been repeatedly shown to be endowed with the progestational activity of natural progesterone. The main differences between the 2 steroids lie in the facts that MPA is effective when administered by the p.o. route, and that MPA is more active [4]. After MPA administration, endometrial tissue undergoes secretory transformation typical of the luteal phase. Cervical mucus decreases in quantity and increases in density, body temperature rises, menstruation is postponed, and premature delivery and threatened abortion are inhibited.

However, in addition to its progestational activity, other endocrine properties of MPA have been demonstrated in the animals and man. MPA is devoid of androgenic and oestrogenic activities, but, on the other hand, has both anti-oestrogenic [13] and anti-androgenic [14] properties.

The anti-oestrogenic activity leads to an anti-ovulatory effect, and reduction of the vaginal kariopyknotic index. The decrease in plasma oestradiol is caused by both the inhibition of ovarian hormonogenesis and increased clearance of androgens induced by MPA. The decrease in intracellular

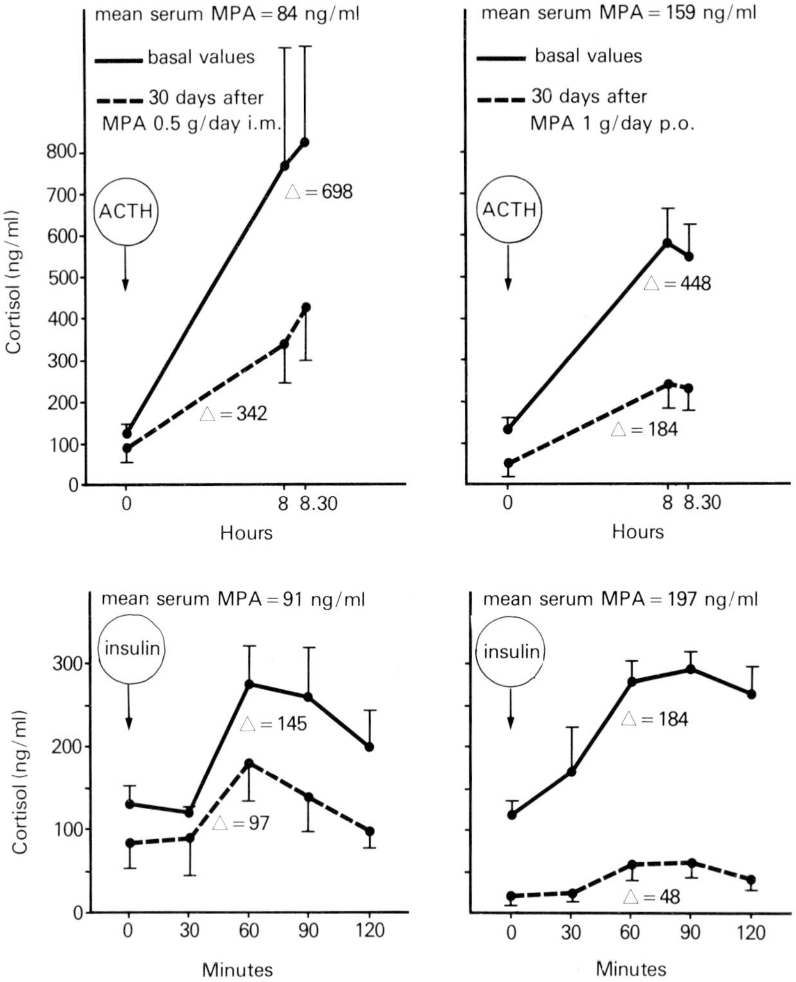

Fig. 11. Effects of 2 dosages of MPA (0.5 g i.m. per day, for 30 days, and 1 g p.o. per day, for 30 days) on plasma cortisol stimulated by ACTH and insulin.

oestradiol is a result of its increased transformation to oestrone by a 17β-dehydrogenase. Finally, MPA is able to block the oestrogen and progesterone receptors in normal and neoplastic mammary and uterine tissues [15].

The anti-androgenic activity of MPA accounts for the inhibition of spermatogenesis and the decrease in libido observed in both healthy subjects and tumour patients. A decrease in plasma testosterone, dehydroepiandrosterone

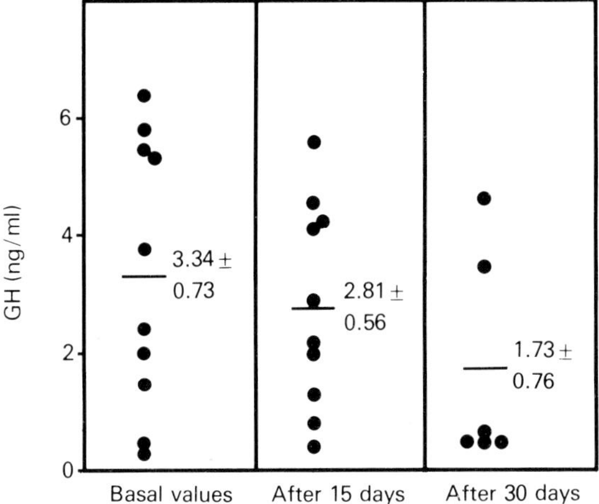

Fig. 12. Effect of MPA (2 g i.m. per day, for 30 days) on serum GH levels.

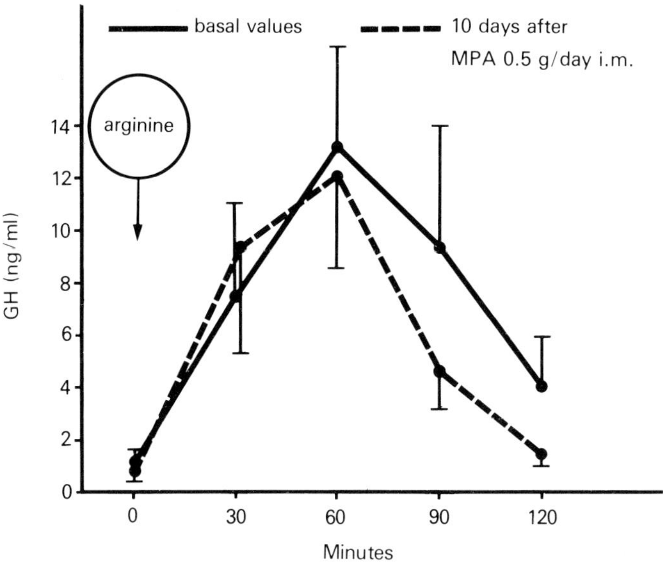

Fig. 13. Response of serum GH values to arginine stimulus before and after MPA 0.5 g i.m. per day, for 10 days.

(DEA), and androstenedione, and reduced production of testosterone and dihydrotestosterone (DHT) can be observed. MPA increases the metabolic clearance of androgens by activating 5α-reductase, alters the stability of the link between testosterone and the carrier protein, and competes with DHT for specific receptors. It has been shown for many years that the anti-gonadotropin effect is responsible for the contraceptive activity of MPA, and affects the basal secretion of FSH and LH, as well as the pre-ovulatory LH peak. Our experiments show clearly that, in menopausal women, high doses of MPA decrease serum FSH and LH levels. The decreases in gonadotropins levels are closely related to serum concentrations of MPA. MPA appears to act at different levels. With low, cumulative dosages (0.5 g daily for 8 days) the decrease in serum gonadotropins is due to a diencephalic block, while for higher, cumulative doses (0.5 g i.m., or 1 g p.o. for 30 days) a hypophyseal block is also present, as demonstrated by the evident reduction in pituitary reserve after GnRH stimulation. Although an increase in prolactin levels has occasionally been observed after MPA administration, our data tend to exclude any effects of the progestational steroid on basal or stimulated serum prolactin values.

The effect of MPA on adrenal function is more difficult to define, inasmuch as the progestational steroid simultaneously has corticoid effects, and inhibits the adrenal glands. In addition, it has recently been shown that MPA behaves both as a corticosteroid agonist and antagonist [16].

Smith et al. reported in 1958 that the urinary excretion of 17-hydroxycorticosteroids and 17-ketosteroids increases after the oral administration of 150 mg of MPA [17]. In 1962, Castegnaro and Sala [5] and Helmreich and Huseby [18] confirmed that urinary PSC levels increased after oral MPA administration; the increase in urinary 17-hydroxycorticoids is attributable to the presence of an MPA metabolite having a dihydroxyacetonic chain at C-17 [5]. The increase in urinary PSC levels (Fig. 9) depends on the degree of bioavailability of MPA, which is governed by pharmacokinetic factors [19], which are now well established through the availability of reliable methods of determination of MPA in the serum [11].

In 1963, Camanni et al. reported the ability of 100 mg of MPA, i.m., daily to replace cortisone acetate 50 mg p.o. daily in adrenalectomized women [20], and it is now well known that women treated with high doses of MPA for long periods of time may present signs of hypercorticoidism, including Cushingoid features, a sense of well being, an increase of appetite, and improvement of coenesthesia [21].

However, the increase in urinary corticosteroids after MPA administration coincides with reduced adrenal function, as shown by inhibition of endogenous cortisol production, reduced urinary excretion of THF and THE, lowered basal concentration of plasma cortisol, and reduced response of plasma cortisol to ACTH and insulin stimulation.

As a plausible explanation of the above-mentioned facts, we postulate the existence of one or more metabolites of MPA having the chemical and biological properties of a glucocorticoid responsible for the adrenal inhibition and for the cortisone-like phenomena caused by the prolonged administration of high doses of MPA.

The isolation, in consistent amounts, of a steroid with a dihydroxy ketonic side chain at C-17 (6-beta, 17-alpha, 21-trihydroxy-6-alpha-methyl-$\triangle_4$-pregnene-3, 20-dione-21-acetate) in the urine of subjects treated with MPA is consistent with this interpretation.

As regards the possible location of the effects of MPA within the hypothalamic-pituitary-adrenal axis, both the adrenal glands and diencephalic-hypophyseal tract appear implicated, as shown by the inhibitory effect of MPA treatment on the cortisol response to ACTH and insulin stimulation.

Literature data do not all agree on the effect of MPA on GH in man [22, 23]. Our data favour stability of serum GH values, both basal and stimulated, although trends towards a decrease in the basal values after 30 days' treatment, and towards a late, reduced response to arginine stimulation are evident.

The recent report by Meyer et al. showing an increase in serum somatomedin C after treatment with 4 g of MPA, i.m., weekly, for 6 months, independent of GH, oestradiol and testosterone variations, is noteworthy [24].

References

1. Sala, G., Camerino, B. and Cavallero, C. (1958): Progestational activity of 6 alpha-methyl-17alpha-hydroxyprogesterone acetate. *Acta Endocrinol. 29,* 508.
2. Babcock, J.C., Gutsell, E.S., Herr, N.H. et al. (1958): 6 alpha-methyl-17 alpha-hydroxyprogesterone-17-acylates: a new class of potent progestins. *J. Am. Chem. Soc. 80,* 2904.
3. Sala, G. and Castegnaro, E. (1962): Biotransformation of 21-methyl into 21-methoxyl steroids. In: *Structure and Metabolism of Corticosteroids,* pp. 95–102. Academic Press, London.
4. Sala, G. (1960): Effetti biologici dei nuovi progestativi – rapporti fra struttura e azione. *Ann. Ostet. Ginecol. 82,* 321.
5. Castegnaro, E. and Sala, G. (1962): Isolation and identification of 6 beta-17 alpha-21-trihydroxy-6 alpha-methyl $\triangle_4$-pregnene-3, 20-dione (21-acetate) from the urine of human subjects treated with 6 alpha-methyl-17 alpha-acetotoxyprogesterone. *J. Endocrinol. 24,*445.
6. Castegnaro, E. and Sala, G. (1971): Pharmacokinetics and metabolism of medroxyprogesterone acetate. Influence of the route of administration and of its physical state. *Steroidol. 2,* 13.

7. Polli, E., Sala, G. and Castegnaro, E. (1963): Effects of a derivative of progesterone (6 alpha-methyl-17 alpha-acetoxyprogesterone) on the adrenal function in man. In: *Research on Steroids,* pp. 167–182. Tipografia Poliglotta Vaticana, Roma.
8. Porter, C. and Silber, R.H. (1954): The determination of 17,21-dihydroxy-20-ketosteroids in urine and plasma. *J. Biol. Chem. 210,* 923.
9. Nowaczynski, W.J., Goldner, M. and Genest, J. (1955): Microdetermination of corticosteroids with tetrazolium derivatives. *J. Lab. Clin. Med. 45*, 818.
10. Medical Research Council Committee on Clinical Endocrinology (1963): A standard method of estimating 17-oxosteroids and total 17-oxogenic steroids. *Lancet I,* 1415.
11. Shrimanker, K., Saxena, B.N. and Fotherby, K. (1977): A radioimmunoassay for serum medroxyprogesterone acetate. *J. Biochem. 9,* 359.
12. Jannotta, F., Pinotti, G. and Pollini, C. (1980): Medroxyprogesterone action on gonadotropins in postmenopausal women. In: *The Menopause: Clinical, Endocrinological and Pathophysiological Aspects.* Eds: Fioretti, Melis. Yen, Viareggio.
13. Tseng, L. and Gurpide, E. (1975): Induction of human endometrial estradiol dehydrogenase by progestins. *Endocrinol. 97,* 825.
14. Nolten, W.E., Sholiton, L.J., Srivastava, L.S. et al. (1976): The effects of diethylstilbestrol and medroxyprogesterone acetate on kinetics and production rate of testosterone and dihydrotestosterone in patients with prostatic carcinoma. *J. Clin. Endocrinol. 22,* 1018.
15. Tseng, L. and Gurpide, E. (1975): Effects of progestins on estradiol receptor levels in human endometrium. *J. Clin. Endocrinol. Metab. 41,* 402.
16. Guthrie, G.P. and John, W.J. (1980): The *in vivo* glucocorticoid and antiglucocorticoid actions of medroxyprogesterone acetate. *Endocrinol. 107*, 1393.
17. Smith, R.W., Mellinger, R.C. and Kline, I.T. (1958): Measurements of adrenocortical function in subjects receiving oral 17-acetoxyprogesterone. *J. Lab. Clin. Med. 52,* 947.
18. Helmreich, M.L. and Huseby, R.A. (1962): Identification of a 6,21-dihydroxylated metabolite of MPA in human urine. *J. Clin. Endocrinol. 22,* 1018.
19. Tamassia, V. (1981): Dose schedules of medroxyprogesterone acetate for breast cancer treatment: a pharmacokinetic approach. Paper read at: Symposium on Progesterone and Progestins, Paris, 7th to 9th May, 1981.
20. Camanni, F., Massara, F. and Molinatti, G.M. (1963): The cortisone-like effect of 6 alpha-methyl-17 alpha-acetoxyprogesterone in the adrenalectomized man. *Acta Endocrinol. 43*, 477.
21. Pannuti, F., Fruet, F., Piaha, E. et al. (1978): The anabolic effect induced by high doses of medroxyprogesterone acetate (MPA) orally in cancer patients. *IRCS Med. Sci. 6*, 118.
22. Simon, S., Schiffer, M., Glick, S.M. and Schwartz, E. (1967): Effect of medroxyprogesterone acetate upon stimulated release of growth hormone in man. *J. Clin. Endocrinol. Metab. 27,* 1633.
23. Lawrence, A.M. and Kirsteins, L. (1970): Progestin in the medical management of active acromegaly. *J. Clin. Endocrinol. Metab. 30,* 646.
24. Meyer, W.J., Furlanetto, R.W. and Walker, P.A. (1980): Medroxyprogesterone acetate (Depo-Provera) increases plasma radioimmunoassayable somatomedin C concentration. *Ped. Res. 14,* 334.

The effects of high parenteral doses of medroxy-progesterone acetate on myelopoiesis in patients with malignant disease*

F. G. Gercovich, E. Morgenfeld, M. Dragosky, H. Murro, M. Sorrentino, A. Presman and R.E. Martinez
Azcuénaga 769 2° 9, 1029 Capital Federal, Argentina

Introduction

Medroxyprogesterone acetate (MPA) (17-alpha-acetoxy-6-alpha-methyl-pregn-4-ene-3,20-dione) is a progesterone derivative which was first synthesized in 1958 [1]. It has proved to be the most powerful and effective progestogen used in hormone treatment to date [2]. It has no toxic effects on myelopoietic tissues and, at certain doses, it blocks pituitary function [2–6]. It has been used on its own for the treatment of carcinoma of the endometrium [7], and hypernephroma [8], and alone or together with chemotherapy for cancer of the prostate [2–6, 9–14], and breast [5, 10, 12, 15].

In the present study, the haematological changes produced by high parenteral doses of MPA in 2 groups of patients with cancer were assessed.

MPA was employed alone or in combination with chemotherapy, and its effects on myelopoiesis were compared with those of similar regimens in which chemotherapy was used alone or together with hormonal therapy or immunotherapy.

Material and methods

Twenty patients with a confirmed diagnosis of advanced cancer (stages III and IV) were divided into 2 groups similar in terms of age (median 57 years) and

*This paper is an English translation published with the editor's permission from *Sangre*.

Table I. Patient characteristics in relation to treatment.

Treatment					
MPA alone			MPA + CT		
Patient no.	Initials	Diagnosis	Patient no.	Initials	Diagnosis
1	AG	Ductal carcinoma of the breast	1	AL	Cancer of the breast
2	AR	Primary unknown	2	CA	Cancer of the breast
3	CA	Cancer of the breast	3	DA	Lymphoma of the breast
4	DA	Cancer of the breast	4	FA	Cancer of the breast
5	GA	Cancer of the oesophagus	5	KL	Cancer of the breast
6	GO	Cancer of the breast	6	LA	Cancer of the ovary and endometrium
7	MU	Cancer of the breast	7	LE	Cancer of the breast
8	PE	Cancer of the breast	8	MA	Cancer of the breast
9	RA	Cancer of the breast	9	TR	Cancer of the breast
10	ZA	Cancer of the lung	10	VA	Cancer of the breast

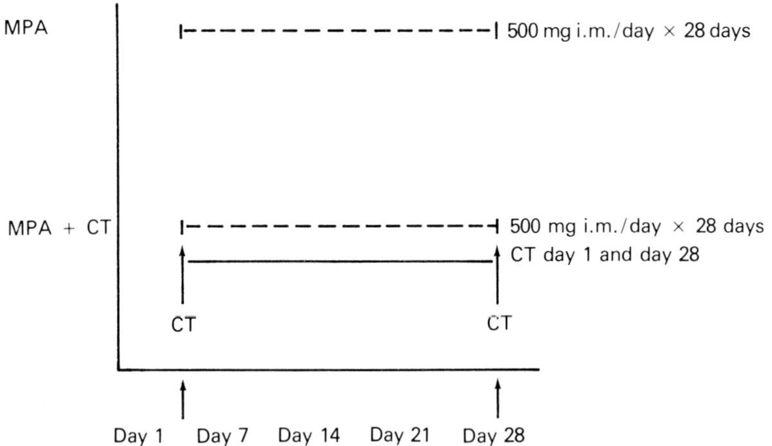

Fig. 1. Treatment schedule.

diagnosis. Ten patients (group A) were given MPA as sole medication, and the other 10 (group B) a combination of MPA and chemotherapy (CT) (Table I, Fig. 1). Both groups were in a position potentially to derive benefit from the treatments mentioned. These groups were compared retrospectively with control patients (group C) who had been given similar CT combinations, (FAC and CMF). The antimitotic drugs used (doxorubicin, cyclophosphamide, fluorouracil and/or methotrexate) produce a predictable pattern of myelodepression, with a leucocyte minimum between the 10th and 14th days of each treatment cycle. To be eligible for enrolment in this study, patients had to be not more than 70 years of age and not undergoing any simultaneous anabolic or steroid therapy. There had to have been an interval of at least 21 days since any previous treatment (irradiation, chemotherapy, steroids or hormones). Patients with gynaecological disorders which precluded the use of MPA, or with thrombo-embolic disorders, liver insufficiency (bilirubin ≥ 2 mg %) and/or hypercalcaemia (Ca ≥ 11 mg %) were excluded. Before, during and after treatment, full clinical history, Karnofsky's performance index and results of laboratory investigations were assessed (Fig. 2). Haematological evaluation comprised full blood count, platelet count, and a marrow cell count, with histological examination of the marrow aspirate (Fig. 2).

MPA was given at a dose of 500 mg intramuscularly, as a 5% solution, for 28 consecutive days. The clinical effects of this regimen were also assessed.

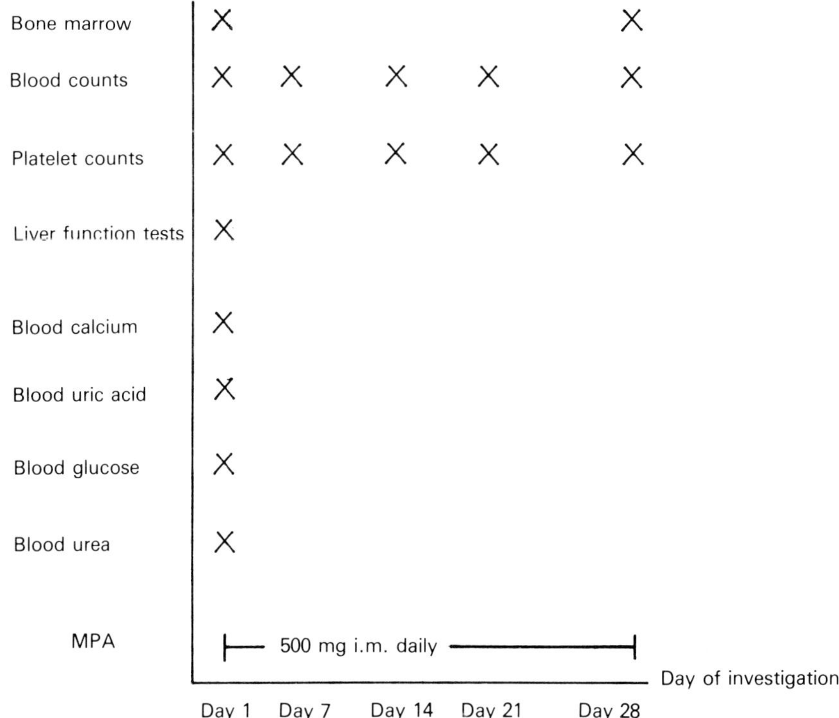

Fig. 2. Laboratory investigations.

Results

There were changes in findings in relation to haemoglobin, haematocrit, platelet count, blood sugar, blood urea, blood calcium, blood uric acid, bilirubin, the transaminases and erythrocyte sedimentation rate (ESR), which were randomly distributed, and would not appear to be of any particular significance.

There were significant changes in the white blood cell counts (Table II) and in the curves designated 'myelostimulation' and 'myeloprotection' in Figure 3, in both MPA and MPA + CT groups.

The median white cell count in group A before treatment was 4,900/mm^3, and rose to 7,900/mm^3 after the 4-week period of investigation had been completed (Table II, Fig. 3). There was a complete absence of myelosuppression in group B, even though it had been expected because of the CT administered. There were 5,300 median white cell count/mm^3 before treatment, 5,500/mm^3 on the 14th day and 6,200/mm^3 on the 28th day of the study (Table II, Fig. 3).

Table II. Changes in white blood cell counts in peripheral blood (all values $\times 10^3$).

Patient no.	Treatment	Day 1	Day 8	Day 15	Day 22	Day 29
1	MPA alone	4.4	5.6	4.3	4.8	5.4
2		6.7	10.7	11.8	11.0	10.2
3		4.0	4.0	5.4	6.8	6.2
4		5.2	4.8	6.0	4.4	6.0
5		17.6	8.6	9.0	5.8	10.0
6		4.7	6.8	4.8	5.4	10.0
7		7.2	8.6	7.0	7.0	11.0
8		4.4	7.6	5.4	4.2	6.0
9		3.6	5.7	5.2	5.4	6.5
10		6.0	7.4	6.4	8.4	9.4
Median value		4.9	7.1	5.7	5.6	7.9
1	MPA + CT	5.8	5.5	7.4	4.8	7.9
2		7.5	2.8	6.4	4.0	9.0
3		5.0	5.6	7.2	6.0	4.7
4		10.0	5.0	4.8	2.4	6.6
5		5.6	5.8	5.6	6.1	6.5
6		3.9	3.1	2.7	2.6	3.8
7		5.1	4.6	4.5	4.4	5.6
8		4.8	5.5	3.5	5.1	5.1
9		6.8	3.8	5.8	4.2	6.0
10		4.8	7.4	5.5	6.7	6.7
Median value		5.3	5.3	5.5	4.6	6.2

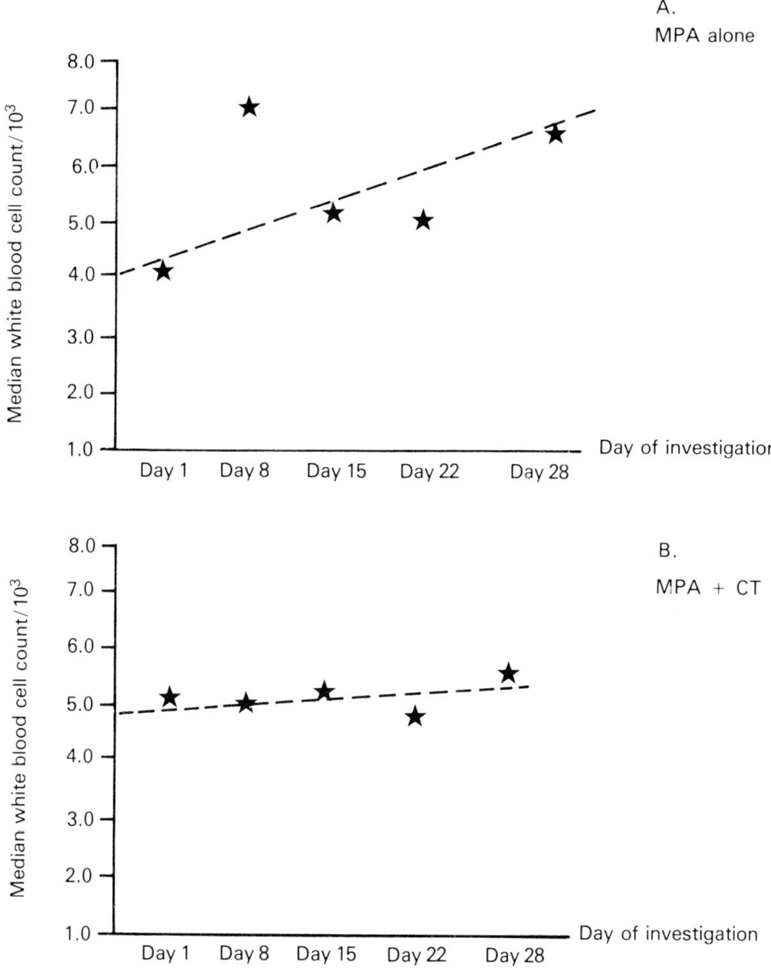

Fig. 3. A. 'Myelostimulation' and B. 'myeloprotection' diagrams.

In patients treated with the FAC regimen, the median lowest white cell count was 2,400/mm^3, on the 14th day. The median lowest count in those treated with CMF, which was found in 50% of these patients [2, 3, 9–11, 16], was 3,000/mm^3.

The median lowest white cell count in those treated with a combination of FAC and testolactone [11] was 2,600/mm^3, and in those treated with a combination of FAC and bacillus of Calmette-Guérin [4] it was 2,400/mm^3. We

Table III. White blood cell counts ($\times 10^3$). Statistical data.

Treatment		1	8	15	22	29
MPA	Median value	4.9	7.1	5.7	5.6	7.9
	Mean value	6.4	7.0	6.5	6.3	8.1
	Standard deviation	3.9	1.9	2.2	2.0	2.1
	Standard error of mean	1.2	0.6	0.7	0.6	0.7
MPA + CT	Median value	5.3	5.3	5.5	4.6	6.2
	Mean value	5.9	4.9	5.3	4.6	6.2
	Standard deviation	1.7	1.3	1.4	1.4	1.4
	Standard error of mean	0.5	0.4	0.4	0.4	0.4

have reported findings in a previous investigation in which a combination of FAC and MPA was given, the latter at a dose of 1,000 mg each week, intramuscularly. The median lowest white count in these patients was 4,200/mm^3 [10].

The white cell counts in group A and B were higher than those in group C. The increase in median white cell count in group A was from 4,900 WBC/ml (day 1) to 7,900/ml (day 28). The white cell count in group B was 4,900 WBC/ml. In group C it was 2,700/ml. Table III shows mean and median values, and corresponding standards deviations and errors. It should be noted that the values for the levels of significance (*P*) are not recorded because of the influence which the sample size has upon them.

The assessment of the bone marrow carried out before and after treatment (Table IV) did not show any changes conclusively attributable to the use of MPA. No variations in cellularity overall before and after treatment were detected for the 2 groups (Table IV). In the posttreatment marrow study in group B (Tables I and IV), none of the progency cell showed diminution of function. In the posttreatment study in the 2 groups of patients, an insignificant number exhibited erythroid hyperplasia, and accentuation of megaloblastic characteristics (Table IV). The clinical results showed a clear improvement in the performance of the patients (increase of 20 points in the Karnofsky Index), in both groups studied. Appetite increased, and pain decreased in patients with bone metastases.

Only one patient developed a sterile gluteal abscess, which was drained, and healed.

Discussion

In spite of the antitumour effects recorded in various publications [5, 7–10,

Table IV. Marrow findings.

Treatment	Patient no.	Before treatment					After treatment				
		Overall cellularity	Red progenies	White progenies	R M/R[1]	Megalo[2] features	Overall cellularity	Red progenies	White progenies	R M/R[1]	Megalo[2] features
MPA	1	Good	42%	58%	1.3	+	Good	47%	53%	1.12	+ +
	2	Copious	33%	67%	1.93	+	Fair	52%	47%	0.90	+ +
	3	Copious	19%	81%	4.26	None	Good	44%	56%	1.27	+
	4	Copious	71%	29%	1.40	+ +	Not	done			
	5	Copious	29%	71%	2.44	+	Copious	36%	64%	1.77	+ +
	6	Good	38%	62%	1.63	+	Copious	52%	48%	0.92	+ +
	7	Copious	43%	57%	1.32	+	Good	49%	51%	1.04	+
	8	Good	42%	58%	1.38	None	Good	61%	37%	0.60	None
	9	Fair	46%	54%	1.17	+	Fair	41%	59%	1.43	+
	10	Good	47%	53%	1.12	+	Good	38%	62%	1.63	+
MPA + CT	1	Good	53%	47%	0.88	+	Good	49%	51%	1.04	+
	2	Scanty	15%	85%	5.66	None	Scanty	10%	90%	9.0	None
	3	Fair	53%	47%	0.88	+	Good	55%	45%	0.81	+ +
	4	Good	51%	48%	0.94	+	Good	59%	41%	0.69	+ +
	5	Fair	41%	59%	1.43	+	Fair	61%	39%	0.63	+ + +
	6	Scanty	20%	80%	4.0	None	Scanty	15%	85%	5.66	None
	7	Good	55%	45%	0.81	+ +	Good	62%	38%	0.61	+ +
	8	Scanty	26%	74%	2.84	None	Fair	32%	68%	2.12	+
	9	Scanty	39%	61%	1.56	None	Scanty	28%	72%	2.57	None
	10	Good	78%	22%	0.28	+	Good	33%	67%	2.03	None

[1] R M/R = ratio of myeloid to red precursors.
[2] Megalo. features = features of megaloblastic maturation.

+ : scanty
+ + : moderate
+ + + : severe

12, 14, 15], and speculation regarding its mode of action [2–6], MPA continues to be used empirically.

Thus it is not possible to identify a minimum effective dose, a maximum tolerated dose, a dosage regimen directed towards greater or lesser myeloprotection, useful in the case of combined hormonal therapy and chemotherapy, or the most desirable route of administration (oral or parenteral). Nevertheless, evidence is emerging that high parenteral doses are more effective in relation to remission rates in the treatment of breast cancer [15]. Although it is certain that high parenteral doses are associated with a high incidence of sterile abscesses or granulomas [2] these reactions diminish appreciably if a 5% solution is used.

Pellegrini et al. [13] have reported the corticoid-like effect of MPA, and the protection it accords to myelopoiesis, making it clear, moreover, that this effect is evident when MPA is used in combination with polychemotherapy [5, 6, 12, 13], and is not observed when MPA is used on its own. In this connection, our divergent findings (Table II and Fig. 3) may be attributable to the dosage regimen used. The employment of massive doses of parenteral MPA, which, in the study of Pannuti et al. amounted to 1,500 mg per day [12], does not improve the results obtained in our experience, and increases the percentage of side-effects (gluteal abscesses, hyperbilirubinaemia, and thrombosis).

Other authors compared parenteral MPA at a dose of 500 mg per day with parenteral MPA at a dose of 1,000 mg per day, in 2 groups of patients with metastatic breast cancer. The degree and duration of remission was similar for the 2 groups of patients, but the incidence of abscess, metrorrhagia and thrombophlebitis was greater with the higher MPA doses [15].

The improvement in clinical score measured according to the Karnofsky Index was 20 points in our study, and is in agreement with the improvement in general condition of patients recorded in other studies [5, 12, 15]. As far as effects on the bone marrow are concerned, no significant qualitative or quantitative changes could be demonstrated in either the red or white progenies. It may be presumed, nevertheless, that more prolonged dosage regimens would probably cause changes in marrow cellularity.

Our conclusion is that the regimen has shown itself to be safe, with virtually nonexistent morbidity.

The myelostimulant effects (group A) and myeloprotective effects (group B) of MPA could potentially reduce the incidence of infections associated with granulocytopenia secondary to otherwise myelosuppressive chemotherapy. The effect mentioned does not imply a dangerous medullary 'emptying'. The need to study maintenance regimens involving practicable doses and routes of administration tending to maintain the results obtained in treatments in which a combination of chemotherapy and hormonal therapy has been used for long periods, needs to be stressed. It is interesting to note that maintenance with oral MPA offers advantages in terms of patient comfort.

Acknowledgements

The author wishes to thank Miss L. Miras and Mrs. A. Gallo de Sacchi for their help in preparing the manuscript. The study was carried out with the cooperation of the Medical Directorate of Montedison Pharmaceuticals, Milan and Buenos Aires.

References

1. Babcock, Y.C., Gutsell, E.S. and Heve, N.H. (1958): 6-alpha-methyl-17-alpha-hydroxyprogesterone-17 acylates: a new class of potent progestins. *J. Am. Chem. Soc. 80,* 2904.
2. Ghione, M. (1977): Hormonoterapia con progestínicos y quimioterapia en oncología clínica. Paper read at Third Argentinian Congress on Clinical Oncology and Antineoplastic Chemotherapy, Buenos Aires, 1977.
3. Glick, J.H., Creech, R.H., Torri, S. et al. (1980): Tamoxifen plus sequential CMF chemotherapy versus tamoxifen alone in postmenopausal patients with advanced breast cancer. *Cancer 45*, 735.
4. Hortobagy, G.N., Gutterman, J.U., Blumenschein, G.R. et al. (1979): Combination chemoimmunotherapy of metastatic breast cancer with 5 fluorouracil, adriamycin, cyclophosphamide and BCG. *Cancer 43*, 1225.
5. Huys, J. and Van Vaerenbergh, P.M. (1975): Medroxyprogesterone and cytostatics in the treatment of advanced mammary carcinoma. Paper read at: Congress on functional explorations in senology, Liège, 1975.
6. Mascia, V., Massida, B. and Desogus, A. (1977): Polichemioterapia con o senza medrossiprogesterona acetato nel cancro avanzato della mamella. Paper read at: First International Symposium on Present Concepts on Treatment, Problems and Perspectives in some solid tumors, leukemia and lymphoma, Cagliari, 1977.
7. Ricciardi, I. (1975): MPA nella terapia dell'adenocarcinoma dell'endometrio. *Minerva Gynaecol. 27*, 744.
8. Stolbach, L., Begg, C., Hall, T. and Horton J. (1981): Treatment of renal carcinoma: A phase III randomized trial of oral medroxyprogesterone (Provera), hydroxyurea and nafoxidine. *Cancer Treat. Rep. 65*, 689.
9. Denis, L. and Declerq, G. (1976): Progestagens in Prostatic Cancer. Paper read at International Conference on Prostatic Cancer, Leeds, 1976.
10. Gercovich, F.G., Schieppati, E. and Rolnik, B. (1980): FAC-MPA en cáncer avanzado de mama. *Rev. Soc. Argentina de Cancerol. 18*, 51.
11. Gercovich, F.G., Rolnik, B. and Schieppati, E. (1977): Tratamiento combinado del cáncer avanzado de mama – comunicación personal. M.D. Anderson Hospital. Breast Service – Noviembre 30, 1977.
12. Pannuti, F., Martoni, A. and Lenaz, G.R. (1978): A possible new approach to the

treatment of metastatic breast cancer: Massive doses of medroxyprogesterone acetate. *Cancer Treat. Rep. 62*, 499.

13. Pellegrini, A., Mascia, V., Massida, B. et al. (1977): Il Trattamento del cancro metastatizzato della mamella con polichemioterapia e MPA. Risultati preliminari. Paper read at Tenth European Congress of the International College of Surgeons. Milan, 1977.
14. Rafla, S. and Johnson, R. (1974): The treatment of advanced prostatic carcinoma with medroxyprogesterone. *Curr. Ther. Res. 16*, 143.
15. Robustelli Della Cuna, G., Calciatti, A. and Strada, M.R.B. (1978): High dose medroxyprogesterone acetate (MPA) treatment in metastatic carcinoma of the breast: A dose response evaluation. *Tumori 64*, 143.
16. Blumenschein, G.R., Cardenas, J.O., Freireich, E.J. and Gottlieb, B.A. (1974): FAC chemotherapy for breast cancer. *Proc. Am. Assoc. Clin. Oncol. 15*, 193.
17. Sala, G., Camerino, B. and Cavallero, C. (1958): Progestational activity of 6-alpha-methyl-17-alpha-hydroxy-progesterone acetate. *Acta Endocrinol. 29*, 508.

Discussion

H. Brincker (Odense, Denmark): If we want to protect the patients against infection we are interested in having high granulocyte counts. However, I noticed nothing about granulocytes in Dr Gercovich's presentation, only the total leucocyte count being given.

Secondly, does he think that the augmentation of the leucocyte count proves that the patients can be protected against infection by giving MPA? I suggest that the granulocytes have merely been moved from the tissue pool to the blood pool, and that the total granulocyte pool is not larger than before treatment.

F.G. Gercovich: I believe that is true about the granulocyte count, but when we are dealing with such a high leucocyte count and with an average in all our patients of 60–70% granulocytes from the leucocyte count, the amount of granulocytes that the patients have is already known.

In answer to the second question, no clear-cut definition was really found with regard to change in cellularity of the red and white blood cells in the bone marrow. There were only trends found which did not clearly prove that.

A. Scanni (Milan, Italy): Why did Dr Gercovich use high doses of MPA? It is not yet known whether lower doses or half the doses that he used have a myeloprotective action. It is important to study that, and I hope he will go on investigating this. In my opinion, low doses may also have an important role here.

Finally, I am not sure whether all Dr Gercovich's patients had some infection during the study. He said that one patient had a gluteal abscess – so this patient was presumably taken out of the study – but how many other patients had some sort of infection or other problem? That is important to know.

F.G. Gercovich: First, the decision to use high-dose MPA, was made because it is supposed to be better than low-dose. Perhaps Dr Scanni can make his own decision whether or not to use low-dose MPA for this purpose.

Secondly, the infectious complications are an important point, but no such complications were in fact seen in this group of patients. However, the small number of patients does not allow us to make any final statement about that – which is why I did not mention it.

E. Robinson (Haifa, Israel): If I may make a suggestion to Dr Gercovich, some years ago we studied the effect of testosterone on the white blood count but, at that time, we did not study the bone marrow and the peripheral blood count. Typhoid vaccine or other pyrogen was injected into the patient to observe the release of the reserve. Would Dr Gercovich consider doing that in future experiments?

F.G. Gercovich: Actually, we have discussed doing that. A fifth group (that I did not mention because it is not in the study) will be given prothoate plus testosterone.

W.E. Hofmann (Zürich, Switzerland): I am worried about Dr Gercovich's study, because I do not think that the haematological questions have been addressed in the right way. First, a previous speaker suggested that pool tests should be performed – I think that is most important. Secondly, I see no sense in doing bone marrows on day one or day zero and day 29, that will do absolutely nothing.

Thirdly, it is possible that if there is a small infection in the gluteus, as an infection this could also produce a leucocytosis.

G. Robustelli Della Cuna: We have to remember that the same effect was also observed in patients treated orally.

A. Pellegrini (Cagliari, Italy): In 1974 we started chemohormonal treatment with other hormones but also with MPA, and we were about the first group to observe this kind of leucocyte protection. We studied many bone marrows (as has been said before), but nothing happened – nothing can be determined in such a study. In order to get the results that have not yet been obtained, we will have to use thymidine and so on. There may be a cortisone-like effect, with mobilisation of the peripheral reserve of leucocytes. This may be only one possible explanation.

Effects of high-dose medroxyprogesterone acetate on blood-clotting factors and platelet function

R. Rosso[1], F. Boccardo[1], L. Canobbio[1], M.A. Queirolo[2], D. Zarcone[2] and F. Brema[1]
[1]Scientific Institute for the Study and Treatment of Cancer, Oncology Institute, University of Genoa; and [2]Haematology Department, S. Martino Hospital, Genoa, Italy

Introduction

Medroxyprogesterone acetate (MPA) is a synthetic steroid related to progesterone, with a progestational action similar to that of progesterone [1]. During the last decade, high-dose MPA has been used in the treatment of breast and other hormone-dependent tumours to obtain increases over the response rates seen with low-dose progestins [2–4]. In a review of 450 cases reported in the literature, an overall response rate of 40% has been recorded [1]. Side-effects associated with high-dose MPA therapy most often take the form of abscess formation at the site of injection, weight gain, Cushingoid syndrome, mild tremor, vaginal bleeding, muscle cramps and thrombophlebitis [1]. The last-mentioned complication was encountered in 4 out of 571 breast cancer patients reported in the literature (11 publications) [3–13]. High-dose MPA has been employed in our Institute since 1977. A total of 154 breast cancer patients have been treated. Five of these (3.2%) developed thrombophlebitis.

Even though controversy still exists regarding the effects of progestational agents on blood-clotting factors and on platelet function, a number of studies have demonstrated that they induce thrombocytosis, modifications of thrombo-elastographic amplitude, decreases in fibrinolysis, reductions in partial thromboplastin time, decreases in factor II and decreases in collagen-induced platelet aggregation reaction time [14–16]. The inadequacy of data concerning the effects of high-dose MPA on blood coagulation, and the potential thrombo-embolic hazard related to treatment with this drug, prompted us to study coagulation factors and platelet function in metastatic breast cancer patients receiving high-dose MPA.

Patients and methods

An initial study has been carried out on 12 postmenopausal patients. Details concerning the patients, methods and results have been published elsewhere [17], but, in brief, the patients had advanced or disseminated breast cancer, without coagulation abnormalities, and were given 400 mg of MPA orally, twice daily, for at least 3 months, or until progression of disease. The following parameters were studied: prothrombin time (PT), partial thromboplastin time (PTT), liver PT, antithrombin III and fibrinogen levels, thromboelastogram (TEG), fibrinogen degradation products (FDP), platelet adhesiveness (according to Salzman), adenosine diphosphate (ADP) platelet aggregation, haematocrit (Hct), haemoglobin (Hb), red blood cell (RBC), white blood cell (WBC) and platelet counts, cholesterol levels, triglyceride levels, degree of lipaemia, and lipoprotein levels. The above parameters were measured prior to treatment with MPA, once weekly during the first month, and every 2 weeks during subsequent months. Student's *t*-test for unrelated samples was used to determine the significance of differences in the values found for various parameters before and during therapy. For each parameter, results for all patients prior to MPA therapy were pooled and were then compared with pooled results from assays carried out during treatment.

A second study has been carried out on 43 breast cancer patients. The main characteristics of these patients are summarized in Table I. Twenty patients (group I) were on oral MPA treatment (400–500 mg, twice daily) for at least 2 months. The median age in this group was 59 years (range 42–76). Twenty-three patients (group II) were studied prior to treatment with combination chemotherapy. The median age in this group was 61 years (range 38–77). The 2 groups were well matched as regards menopausal status, and predominant sites of metastasis. The blood clotting factors and platelet function

Table I. Patient characteristics.

	Group	
	I	II
Numbers of patients	20	23
Median ages (years)	59 (range 42–76)	61 (38–77)
Premenopausal	2/20 (10%)	4/23 (17%)
Postmenopausal	18/20	19/23
Locally advanced or recurrent disease	18/20	15/23
MPA dosage	400–500 mg, twice daily	nil

parameters assessed in both groups were PT, liver PT, PTT, fibrinogen levels, thromboplastin time (TT), antithrombin III levels [semiqualitative (functional) assay], platelet adhesiveness, platelet aggregation, circulating platelet aggregation (CPA), platelet counts.

Values obtained for group-I patients were compared with those obtained for group-II patients. Student's *t*-test for unrelated samples was used to check the statistical significance of differences.

Results

Table II summarizes the results of the first study. Only parameters significantly modified have been recorded. Significant increases in Ht, RBC counts, platelet adhesiveness and antithrombin III levels were observed. In addition, significant decreases in PTT and TEG amplitude were observed.

Results of the second study were similar (Table III). In particular, significant decreases in PTT and antithrombin III levels were observed, together with trends towards increases in fibrinogen levels, TT, and platelet adhesiveness and aggregation (in vitro as well as CPA). It is noteworthy that in both studies all parameters were normal, even though at the upper limits in all cases.

Discussion

Alterations in blood clotting processes and platelet aggregation during the administration of oral contraceptives are well established. A 2-year follow-up study of a progestogen-only contraceptive (chlormadinone acetate) revealed

Table II. Parameters affected in study in 12 postmenopausal patients with advanced or disseminated breast cancer.

Parameter	Mean difference	*P*
Hct	+2.9	<0.05
RBC	+1,590	<0.005
PTT	−4.5 sec	<0.01
TEGR	−3.1 mm	<0.01
TEGK	−1.7 mm	<0.05
Platelet adhesiveness	+11.9%	<0.005
Antithrombin III levels	+7.15 mg%	<0.005
Platelet count	+27,000	<0.2 >0.1 (not significant)

Table III. Parameters affected in comparative study in breast cancer patients.

	Group I	Group II	
	Median (range)	Median (range)	
PT (minutes)	12.5 (11.5–14.5)	12 (7.8–13.2)	ns
PTT (minutes)	23.9 (21.2–28.5)	27.7 (25.1–35.6)	$P<0.05$
Liver PT (%)	115 (80–150)	130 (85–170)	ns
Fibrinogen (mg/100 ml)	400 (215–550)	340 (150–530)	ns
TT (minutes)	19.5 (15.8–25.2)	18 (12–22)	ns
Antithrombin III (%)	56.5 (47–63)	60 (57–68)	$P<0.05$
Platelets (10^3/ml)	160×10^3 ($50\times10^3-250\times10^3$)	160×10^3 ($85\times10^3-230\times10^3$)	ns
Platelet adhesiveness (minutes)	78 (45–83)	69 (20–94)	ns
CPA	0.63 (0.5–0.83)	0.66 (0.2–1.04)	ns
Platelet aggregation (%)	72.5 (40–91)	70 (30–83)	ns

ns = not significant.

no increase in factors VII and X, in contrast to findings with oestrogen-progestogen contraceptive combination products. Changes in the TEG were, however, recorded, and platelet aggregation was significantly accelerated [16].

Baele et al. studied blood coagulation changes during the parenteral administration of MPA for contraceptive purposes, and reported significant decreases in PTTs after 4 and 7 months of treatment and significant increases in PTs after 4 months [15]. However, factor II levels decreased after 7 months of treatment, and levels of factors V, VII, VIII and X remained unchanged. The reaction time for collagen-induced platelet aggregation decreased significantly after 4 and 7 months of treatment.

The only study in which blood-clotting parameters have been investigated during high-dose MPA therapy did not reveal any effect on blood-clotting processes [18].

Our studies indicate that high-dose MPA induces a condition of slight hypercoagulability as a result of significant changes in both intrinsic platelet functions (increases in platelet aggregation and adhesiveness), and liver-dependent functions (decrease in PTT, increase in liver PT and in fibrinogen levels, decrease in antithrombin III activity).

In our first study, antithrombin III levels increased during high-dose MPA treatment. However, when overall antithrombin III activity was assessed, a significant decrease was noted. This finding is in accordance with the decrease in other liver-dependent functions.

In view of the observations described above, the effects of high-dose MPA on blood clotting do not appear to differ substantially from those induced by low dose progestins.

Thrombo-embolic complications in cancer patients represent a major problem, since they often necessitate discontinuation of antineoplastic treatment. The hypercoagulability induced by cancer itself, in patients with advanced disease in particular, must be taken into account [19]. In addition, numerous factors, such as age, menopausal status, number of pregnancies, congenital or acquired thrombo-embolic and metabolic disorders, and prior treatment with combination oral contraceptives and/or other drugs conducive to thrombosis can contribute to the development of thrombo-embolic disease. Finally, almost all antineoplastic therapy, including cytotoxic chemotherapy [20–22] and antioestrogen therapy [23], can induce hypercoagulability.

The changes observed during treatment with high-dose MPA are not likely to increase the thrombotic risk in cancer patients significantly, in the absence of additional risk factors. However, we recommend that possible thrombotic risks be carefully evaluated in cancer patients before commencing MPA treatment.

Acknowledgements

The authors are indebted to staff nurse Mrs. G. Spanu and staff physicians Dr M. Merlano and Dr D. Guarneri for their help in collecting blood samples, to Dr E. Campora for reviewing the manuscript, and to Dr L. Bonelli for statistical assistance.

References

1. Ganzina, F. (1979): High dose medroxyprogesterone acetate (MPA) treatment in advanced breast cancer. A review. *Tumori 65*, 563.
2. Bonte, J., Decoster, J.M., Iole, R. et al. (1974): Progestogens in endometrial cancer. In: *Recent Prog. Obstet. Gynaecol.,* pp. 285–297, Eds: V.L.S. Persianivo and T.V. Chervacove, Excerpta Medica, Amsterdam.
3. Pannuti, G., Martoni, A., Lenaz, G.R. et al. (1978): A possible new approach to the treatment of metastatic breast cancer: massive doses of medroxyprogesterone acetate. *Cancer Treat. Rep. 62*, 493.
4. Robustelli Della Cuna, G., Calciati, A., Bernardo Strada, M.R. et al. (1978): High dose medroxyprogesterone acetate (MPA) treatment in metastatic carcinoma of the breast: a dose-response evaluation. *Tumori 64*, 143.
5. Martino, G. and Ventafridda, V. (1976): Effetto antalgico dell'alcoolizzazione ipofisaria, del medrossi-progesterone acetato ad alte dosi e della loro associazione nel carcinoma mammario in fase avanzata. *Tumori 62*, 93.
6. Amadori, D., Ravaioli, A. and Barbanti, F. (1976): L'impiego del medrossi-progesterone acetato ad alti dosaggi nella terapia palliativa del carcinoma mammario in fase avanzata. *Minerva Med. 67*, 1.
7. Amadori, D., Ravaioli, A., Ridolfi, R. et al. (1979): Il medrossiprogesterone ad alte dosi: esperienza su 21 pazienti trattate con somministrazione per via orale. *Chemioterap. Oncol. 3*, 219.
8. Pannuti, F., Martoni, A., Fruet, F. et al. (1979): Hormone therapy in advanced breast cancer: high dose medroxyprogesterone acetate (MPA) vs. tamoxifen (TMX). Preliminary results. In *Breast Cancer: Experimental and Clinical Aspects,* pp. 93–98. Eds: H.T. Mouridsen and T. Palshof, Supplement to the *Eur. J. Cancer.* Pergamon Press, Oxford.
9. Pannuti, F., Martoni, A., Di Marco, A.R. et al. (1979): Prospective, randomized clinical trial of two different high dosages of medroxyprogesterone acetate (MPA) in the treatment of metastatic breast cancer. *Eur. J. Cancer 15*, 593.
10. De Lena, M., Brambilla, C., Valagussa, P. and Bonadonna, G. (1979): High dose medroxyprogesterone acetate in breast cancer resistant to endocrine and cytotoxic therapy. *Cancer Chemother. Pharmacol. 2*, 175.
11. Bernardo Strada, M.R., Imparato, E., Aspesi, G. et al. (1980): Il medrossiprogesterone acetati (MPA) ad alte dosi per via orale nel trattamento delle fasi avanzata del cancro mammario ed endometriale. *Minerva Med. 1*, 1.
12. Cavalli, F., Goldhirsch, A., Jungi, F. et al. (1981): Low versus high dose medroxyprogesterone acetate (MPA) in the treatment of advanced breast cancer. In: *Proceedings of the IInd International Symposium on the Role of Medroxy-progesterone Acetate in Endocrine-related Tumours,* Rome, 1981. (In press.)

13. Mattsson, W. (1978): High dose medroxyprogesterone acetate treatment in advanced mammary carcinoma. *Acta Radiol. Oncol. 17*, 387.
14. Cantwell, B.M.S., Begent, R.H.S. and Rubens, R.D. (1979): Augmentation of vincristine-induced thrombocytosis by norethisterone. *Eur. J. Cancer 15*, 1065.
15. Baele, G., Vermeulen, A. and Thiery, M. (1974): Blood coagulation and platelet-function parameters before and during parenteral administration of medroxyprogesterone acetate as a contraceptive agent. *Thromb. Diathesis Haemorrhagica 32*, 346.
16. Poller, L., Thompson, J.M., Thomas, W. and Wray, C., (1971): Blood clotting and platelet aggregation during oral progestogen contraception: a follow-up study. *Br. Med. J. 1*, 705.
17. Brema, F., Queirolo, M.A., Canobbio, L. et al. (1981): Hematologic parameters during treatment with high dose medroxyprogesterone acetate. *Tumori 67*, 125.
18. Anzivino, F., Pollutri, E., Andollina, A. et al. (1977): High dose medroxyprogesterone acetate in oncology: Effects on the main parameters involved in blood clotting. *IRCS Med. Sci. 5*, 577.
19. Neri Serneri, G.G. (1981): Le alterazioni dell'emostasi nella malattia neoplastica (ad eccezione delle emoblastasi). In: *Malattie emorragiche e trombotiche*, Chapter 42, pp. 566–577, Società Editrice Universo, Rome.
20. Weiss, R.B., Tormey, D.C., Holland, J.F. and Weinberg, V.E. (1981):Venous thrombosis during multimodal treatment of primary breast carcinoma. *Cancer Treat. Rep. 65*, 677.
21. Klener, P., Kubisz, P. and Suranova, J. (1977): Influence of cytotoxic drugs on platelet functions and coagulation in vitro. *Thromb. Haemostasis 37*, 53.
22. Canobbio, L. (1982): (Personal communication.)
23. Enck, R.E., Cunningham, V.M. and Rios, C.N. (1981): Tamoxifen treatment of metastatic breast cancer and antithrombin III levels. *Proc. Am. Soc. Clin. Oncol. 22*, 354 (Abstract 85).

Adverse events during high-dose medroxyprogesterone acetate therapy for endocrine tumours

F. Ganzina[1] **and G. Robustelli Della Cuna**[2]
[1] R. & D. Therapeutic Research Department, Farmitalia Carlo Erba, Milan; and [2] Division of Oncology, Clinica del Lavoro Foundation, Pavia, Italy

Introduction

A major goal of cancer therapy is the improvement of the relationship between desired and undesired effects of a given treatment. When dealing with cytotoxic drugs the borderline between unacceptable damage to normal tissues and successful cure is, in most circumstances, small. With hormonal agents the pattern of toxicity is completely different since endocrine therapy is selective for target tissues, and even in the case of minor response it does not damage normal tissues. This report will deal with the undesired effects that are usually encountered with the use of high-dose medroxyprogesterone acetate (HD-MPA) when given by parenteral route in the treatment of advanced breast cancer, endometrial carcinoma and prostatic cancer.

Analysis and discussion

Since a substantial increase in response rate has been shown in the treatment of advanced breast cancer with the high daily doses now generally used [1], several large randomized studies, comparing different dose-schedules, namely 500 mg/day, 1 g/day, 1.5 g/day and the 1 g/week schedule, have been activated in order to select the best treatment schedule in terms of the risk to benefit ratio [2–8].

These studies have shown that in advanced breast cancer patients, using a dose-schedule of 500 mg/day intramuscularly (i.m.) for 4 weeks it was possible to reduce the frequency of undesired effects without compromising antitumour activity. From these studies it appeared that the incidence of some adverse events was related to the unit dose as well as the cumulative dose.

Moreover, the frequency of one adverse reaction, for example the occurrence of gluteal abscess, was related mostly to the pharmaceutical preparation used.

HD-MPA when administered by the intramuscular route is characterized by a slow but long lasting absorption from the site of injection. Recent pharmacokinetic studies carried out using radio-immunoassay have shown that daily administration of either 500 mg or 1 g produces, in the space of 3–4 weeks, fairly high drug blood levels which remain elevated for long periods of time after the interruption of treatment, resulting in a continuation of the drug's action upon tissues [9]. This aspect, which is useful from a therapeutic point of view, has to be taken into consideration in particular with regard to the predictability and to the management of the undesired effects of HD-MPA treatment.

The oral route of administration is characterized by rapid absorption and high drug blood levels, if the drug is taken on a daily schedule and on a long-term basis [10]. Several authors have attributed a variety of major and minor side-effects to the use of HD-MPA and this report will analyze some therapeutic trials [2–8, 11, 12] with particular regard to the dose-schedule employed and the disease involved. Tables I, II, III, IV, V and VI report the incidence of adverse events according to the daily HD-MPA by the i.m. route and the particular type of disease.

Table VII is a summarized analysis of adverse effects of HD-MPA therapy

Table I. Local toxicity following i.m. HD-MPA in breast cancer patients [8].

Adverse events (%)	Dose (mg/d)		
	500	1,000	1,500
Gluteal abscess	6	7.6	22

Table II. Cardiovascular toxicity following i.m. HD-MPA in breast cancer.

Adverse events (%)	Dose (mg/d)		
	500	1,000	1,500
Heart failure	—	2.1	—
Increased blood pressure (10/D–20/S mm Hg)	19	25	54
Thrombo-embolic (phlebitis)	—	2.6	1

Table III. Cardiovascular toxicity following i.m. HD-MPA in endometrial cancer.

Adverse events (%)	Dose (500 mg/d)
Increased blood pressure	31
Thrombo-embolic (phlebitis)	4.8

Table IV. Cardiovascular toxicity following i.m. HD-MPA in prostatic cancer.

Adverse events (%)	Dose (3 × 500 mg/week)
Heart failure	6
Thrombo-embolic	6
Water retention	6

Table V. Water retention and lipid metabolism following i.m. HD-MPA in breast and endometrial cancer.

Adverse events (%)	Dose (mg/d)		
	500	1,000	1,500
Cushing-like syndrome (moon face)	8	16	16
Body weight increase (2–10 kg)	30–100*	14–62	43
Water retention	33*	—	—

*Endometrial cancer.

Table VI. Other adverse effects following i.m. HD-MPA in breast cancer.

Adverse events (%)	Dose (mg/d)		
	500	1,000	1,500
Vaginal bleeding	2	3–20	6–20
Muscle cramps	2	20	19
Light tremors	12	—	20
Sweating	2	—	15

Table VII. Adverse events in 643 patients during i.m. HD-MPA therapy, for breast and endometrial cancer.

Adverse events (%)	Dose (mg/d i.m.)		
	500 (n = 137)	1,000 (n = 360)	1,500 (n = 146)
Gluteal abscess	6	7.6	22
Heart failure	0	2.1	0
Thrombo-embolic	1.4*	2.6	1
Increased blood pressure (10/D–20/S mm Hg)	19–31*	25	54
Cushing-like syndrome (moon face)	8	16	16
Body weight increase (2–10 kg)	30–100*	14–62	43
Vaginal bleeding	2	3–20	6–20
Muscle cramps	2	20	19
Light tremors	12	—	20
Sweating	2	—	15
Water retention	33*	—	—

*Endometrial cancer.

at different dose levels in breast cancer and endometrial cancer patients. The total patient population analysed was 707; 602 with breast cancer, 64 with prostatic cancer and 41 with endometrial cancer. Prostatic cancer patients have been analyzed separately (see Table IV).

Formation of gluteal abscess following intramuscular route

As shown in Table I the frequency of gluteal abscess is correlated with the dose, a higher frequency being observed with the 1.5-g/day dose schedule.

Since a new formulation containing 200 mg/ml of MPA has been available, the incidence of abscess has dramatically decreased. Large clinical trials, as the one carried out by the SAKK Swiss Cooperative Group on 165 patients [8], have confirmed this low incidence. No case of abscess had been observed. However, in 5% of the cases the i.m. route had been switched to the oral formulation because of poor compliance by the patient to the injection.

The modalities of the injection are obviously important in order to minimize the occurrence of this local toxicity and in particular a deep i.m. injection and an appropriate site of injection.

Cardiovascular complications

Thrombo-embolic disorders (phlebitis, pulmonary embolism) may occur with a frequency ranging from 0–6% if clinical trials in breast cancer, endometrial cancer and prostatic cancer are analyzed (see Tables II, III and IV); however, no correlation appears to exist between frequency and dose, but rather the different distribution of patients with pre-existing or predisposing risk factors seems to play a role.

In fact, the analysis of incidence by disease, shows that risk factors for cardiovascular complications are more prominent in one disease than in another.

In a series of 41 patients with endometrial cancer [13] treated with 500 mg/day, thrombophlebitis occurred in 4.8% of the patients (Table III) as opposed to the 0% incidence in breast cancer patients treated with the 500-mg/day dose schedule.

In an EORTC Urological Group protocol (No. 30761) comparing prospectively, in a randomized fashion, diethylstilboestrol vs MPA and cyproterone acetate in advanced prostatic cancer, an unusually high frequency of cardiovascular adverse reactions has been reported; in particular, out of 64 patients on the MPA regimen, 6% incidence of thrombo-embolism and 6% incidence of heart failure has been observed (Table IV) [11]. Cases of cardiac insufficiency have been reported by Amadori et al. [5] and Becher et al. [14] who used MPA in breast cancer at the dose of 1 g/day i.m. One case of pulmonary embolism has been reported by Gorins in breast cancer patients treated with 1 g daily (Table II) [12].

The occurrence of cardiovascular adverse reactions which is not unusual with other hormones employed in the treatment of neoplasms, could be correlated with the results of a study on the profile of haemocoagulative variables carried out in advanced breast cancer patients under HD-MPA treatment at a daily dosage of 800 mg/day by the oral route for at least 3 months [15]. The authors found that both platelet adhesiveness and some coagulation parameters* underwent statistically significant changes tending towards hypercoagulability, although, on average they did not exceed the upper normal range. These results suggest that in patients already at increased risk for pre-existing thrombo-embolic disorders the addition of HD-MPA might further predispose to venous thrombo-embolic complications.

The finding that thrombo-embolic disorders were mostly observed in patients with prostatic cancer and endometrial cancer [11, 13] (while in advanced

*Thromboelastogram, partial thromboplastin time.

breast cancer these adverse reactions occurred occasionally only at the high doses of 1 g and 1.5 g) could be explained by the fact that some predisposing factors (age for prostatic cancer; borderline hypertension, obesity and length of treatment for endometrial cancer) are present in a higher incidence in one population than in another. Hypertension, diabetes and previous thrombo-embolic disease, appear, as with other sexual hormones employed in therapy, to be additional risk factors for venous thrombo-embolism.

Increase in blood pressure

Increase in blood pressure appears to be dose-related (Tables II and III), its frequency being higher with the 1.5-g daily schedule. In patients with endometrial cancer a 31% frequency of increase in blood pressure has been reported and this high incidence could well be explained not only by the length of treatment but also by pre-existing risk factors in this series, like obesity, diabetes and alterated blood pressure values. In breast cancer patients treated with the 500 mg/day dose schedule the frequency of this event is lower (19%). Usually the increase in blood pressure is gradual and tends to manifest 1–2 months after the interruption of the loading dose and is usually reversible a few months after medication is discontinued; an appropriate pharmacologic treatment coupled with diuretics can easily control this side-effect. In this case too, pre-existing cardiovascular disease plus hypertension, impairment of carbohydrate metabolism and obesity appear additional risk factors for the patients if HD-MPA therapy is started.

When using high doses (1.5–2.0 g/day i.m.) Pannuti et al. reported that the diastolic value increased significantly on average from 88–99 mm/Hg and the systolic value on average from 150–169 mm/Hg [3]. After 6 months the systolic values tended to return to baseline values, while the diastolic values were still elevated. Usually with the 500 mg to 1 g daily schedule in patients with normal blood pressure, there is a moderate and temporary increase in blood pressure which can be easily controlled, and with a slow return to basal values after the interruption of treatment. There is no proved theory which can explain the mechanism by which MPA produces changes in blood pressure even if the occurrence of water retention could play a role in enhancing changes in blood pressure during treatment.

It is worthy of note that the increase in blood pressure is not an effect attributable exclusively to the high doses since a rise of both diastolic and systolic values has also been reported when MPA is used for contraceptive purposes [16, 17].

Water retention and lipid metabolism

Retention of water appears with a frequency of 6% in prostatic cancer (Table IV; [11]) to 33% in endometrial cancer (Table V; [13]) during HD-MPA administration and accounts for a portion of the gain in weight which is observed in about 50% of all patients. Water retention is clearly undesirable in patients with pre-existing or concomitant heart failure, renal disease and hypertension. Weight gain and water retention can be controlled by dietary measures and diuretics.

Taking into consideration the fact that MPA is a derivative of 17α-hydroxyprogesterone one should expect some action typical of corticosteroids; and this is the case with another typical undesired effect of MPA, the Cushing-like syndrome (Table V). The deposit of fat at the back of the neck and the 'moon face' are well-known examples. Weight gain, in addition to the corticosteroid-like effect, could be explained by an inhibitory effect of MPA on the hypothalamic/pituitary appetite control centre. In fact, an increase in appetite has been observed in the great majority of cancer patients treated with HD-MPA.

Carbohydrate metabolism

The diabetogenic-like action of MPA is another undesired effect which has been reported by some investigators, and which is more frequent in patients predisposed to diabetes. Ylöstalo described the increase in blood sugar and the impairment of glucose tolerance test in a series of patients with endometrial carcinoma after 12 months' treatment with i.m. MPA at the dose of 100 mg/day [18]. This adverse effect is in accordance with the diabetic-like status which occurs when glucocorticoids are given for a long period of time at large doses: glucose in the plasma tends to be elevated, glucose tolerance is decreased and increased resistance to insulin is observed. On the other hand the diabetogenic effect of MPA has also been observed by several authors who employed long-term MPA for contraception (150 mg i.m. for 3 months) [16].

Other adverse effects

Other adverse effects, such as vaginal bleeding, muscle cramps, light tremors and sweating, have been reported by several authors (Table VI).

Conclusion

The pattern of undesired effects of HD-MPA is, at least partly, the same as that observed with other hormonal agents such as corticoids, oestrogens and androgens. Generally, some of the adverse events encountered during HD-MPA treatment are similar in type to those that are usually reported when the drug is used as a contraceptive at doses of 150 mg for 3 months.

The frequency of HD-MPA adverse reactions and their severity are in some instances dependent on the dose and the length of treatment as well, and become relevant when very high doses of the drug are given for palliation in neoplastic diseases. However, with the dose schedule of 500 mg/day for 4 weeks, these side-effects are rarely severe, usually reversible, and only occasionally necessitating treatment interruption.

In order to prevent and minimize possible adverse effects, baseline clinical and laboratory assessment are important to allow the identification of patients who are likely to develop undesired effects if HD-MPA treatment is to be started. Particularly in patients with hypertension, obesity, diabetes, history of myocardial infarction, thrombo-embolic disorders and impaired hepatic function the risk/benefit ratio should be carefully evaluated. The extent of this evaluation is itself depending on many factors, including the availability of alternative therapies, and the assessment of the variables which are likely to increase the toxicity of the regimen.

References

1. Ganzina, F. (1979): High-dose medroxyprogesterone acetate (MPA) treatment in advanced breast cancer. A review. *Tumori 65,* 563.
2. Pannuti, F., Martoni, A., Di Marco, A.R. et al. (1979): A prospective randomized clinical trial of two different high dosages of medroxyprogesterone acetate (MPA) in the treatment of metastatic breast cancer. *Eur. J. Cancer 15*, 593.
3. Pannuti, F., Martoni, A., Lenaz, G.R. et al. (1978): A possible new approach to the treatment of metastatic breast cancer: massive doses of medroxyprogesterone acetate. *Cancer Treat. Rep. 62*, 499.
4. Robustelli Della Cuna, G., Calciati, A., Bernardo Strada, M.R. et al. (1978): High dose medroxyprogesterone acetate (MPA) treatment in metastatic carcinoma of the breast: a dose response evaluation. *Tumori 64*, 143.
5. Amadori, D., Ravaioli, A. and Barbanti, F. (1977): L'impiego del medrossiprogesterone acetato ad alti dosaggi nella terapia palliativa del carcinoma mammario in fase avanzata. *Minerva Med. 68,* 3967.
6. De Lena, M., Brambilla, C., Valagussa, P. and Bonadonna, G. (1979): High dose medroxyprogesterone acetate (MPA) in metastatic breast cancer previously treated with chemotherapy. *Cancer Chemother. Pharmacol. 2,* 175.
7. Mattsson, W. (1978): High dose medroxyprogesterone acetate treatment in ad-

vanced mammary carcinoma. A phase II investigation. *Acta Radiol. Oncol. 17,* 387.

8. Cavalli, F., Goldhirsch, A., Kaplan, E. and Alberto, F. for Swiss Group of Clinical Research (SAKK) (1981): High versus low dose medroxyprogesterone acetate in advanced breast cancer. In: *UICC Conference on Clinical Oncology, Lausanne (Switzerland) 28–31 October,* Abstract No. 03-0407.
9. Cavalli, F., Ganzina, F., Kiser, J. et al. (1981): Serum level profile of medroxyprogesterone acetate in breast cancer patients treated with two different dose-schedules by i.m. route. In: *13th International Congress of Chemotherapy, Florence (Italy), 19–24 July,* p. 101. Abstract No. 270.
10. Martin, F. and Adlercreutz, H. (1977): Aspects of megestrol acetate and medroxyprogesterone acetate metabolism. In: *Pharmacology of Steroid Contraceptive Drugs,* pp. 99–115. Eds: S. Garattini and H.W. Berendes. Raven Press, New York.
11. Pavone-Macaluso, M., Ingargiola, G.B., La Piana, E. et al. and the EORTC Urologic Cooperative Group (1981): La terapia ormonale del carcinoma della prostata. Risultati attuali delle ricerche cliniche del Gruppo Urologico dell'EORTC. Communication at the *'Ottavo Corso di Aggiornamento in Oncologia Clinica',* p. 285. Syllabus, vol. I, AIOM ed., Perugia, Italy, 6–10 October.
12. Gorins, A., Mignot, L., Gisselbrecht, C. et al. (1981): Preliminary results of a French multicenter study on the treatment by medroxyprogesterone acetate (MPA) of advanced breast cancer. In: *12th International Congress of Chemotherapy, Florence (Italy), 19–24 July,* p. 102. Abstract No. 271.
13. Battelli, T. and Saccani F. (1979): Il tumore dell'utero: il trattamento della fase avanzata. In: *La Chemioterapia dei Tumori Solidi, 2° Corso Nazionale dell'Ospedale Malpighi,* pp. 672–696. Patron, Bologna.
14. Becher, R., Firusian, N., Höffken, K. and Schmidt, C.G. (1981): High dose medroxyprogesterone acetate (MPA) in advanced breast cancer. In: *UICC Conference on Clinical Oncology, Lausanne, 28–31 October 1981,* p. 33. Abstract No. 03–0423.
15. Brema, F., Queirolo, M.A., Canobbio, L. et al. (1981): Hematologic parameters during treatment with high-dose medroxyprogesterone acetate. *Tumori 67,* 125.
16. Nash, H.A. (1975): Depo Provera®: A review. *Contraception 12,* 377.
17. Leiman, G. (1972): Depo-medroxyprogesterone acetate as a contraceptive agent: its effect on weight and blood pressure. *Am. J. Obstet. Gynaecol. 114,* 97.
18. Ylöstalo, P., Vehaskari, A., Kauppila, A. and Sotaniemi, E. (1974): Effects of high dose medroxyprogesterone acetate treatment given for endometrial carcinoma on carbohydrate metabolism and liver function. *Ann. Chir. Gynaecol. Fenniae 63,* 93.

Discussion

A. Pellegrini: We have been talking about the side-effects of MPA for a long time. If we look carefully, we can discover them, especially an increase in blood pressure. Certainly, there is water retention, and perhaps increase in blood volume in the left ventricle that works against the systolic gradient.

We still have to discuss the doses. This is very important too in considering the quality of life that is given to the patients.

S. Parboo (London, England): When Professor Rosso mentioned the incidence of thrombophlebitis, was this superficial thrombophlebitis or deep-vein thrombosis? The clinical assessment of deep-vein thrombosis is difficult and inaccurate.

Secondly, has he any personal experience of assessing these patients using radioactive fibrinogen, or does he know of any studies in which this has been carried out in patients on MPA? It is important: if the patient just develops superficial thrombophlebitis, it is a nuisance to the patient but it is not clinically important, whereas if it is deep-vein thrombosis, of course this contributes a morbidity. As far as I know, the impression is that breast cancers, unlike other cancers, have a low incidence of deep-vein thrombosis.

E.G. Giralt (Paris, France): We can confirm Dr Ganzina's data. We have treated more than 500 breast cancer patients with MPA, and the incidence of thrombo-embolic problems has been between 2 and 3%, with an increase in weight occurring in more than 30% of the patients. I do not understand why many groups never find toxicity – perhaps the Argentinian patients are very resistant and some others are not. In our experience, for instance, increase in weight in the female patients is a very important problem.

M. Fiorentino (Padua, Italy): There is a problem about the selection of the patients in Professor Rosso's first study. To my knowledge, it is quite uncommon to find normal coagulation data in disseminated breast cancer. If he had 12 patients with normal clotting parameters at the beginning of the study, from what larger series of patients with disseminated breast cancer was he able to find those 12 with a normal coagulation profile?

I think that he must have screened a large population in order to find 12 with a normal coagulation profile before starting the study.

R. Rosso: On one of my slides I showed the eligibility criteria: one of them was the absence of coagulation abnormalities. Another criterion was that any variation observed, if statistically significant, was within the range of normality. We did not select a particular population.

K. Landys (Gothenburg, Sweden): Professor Rosso talked about locally-advanced disease or recurrent disease in breast cancer. How does he define those – because most of these breast cancer patients have occult bone marrow dissemination? Were random bone marrow biopsies determined in all the patients?

R. Rosso: No, they were not done.

Pharmacokinetics and bioavailability of medroxyprogesterone acetate in cancer treatment

I.R. Hesselius
Department of Gynaecological Oncology, University Hospital, Uppsala, Sweden

Introduction

Medroxyprogesterone acetate (17-α-acetoxy-6-α-methyl-4-pregnene-3,20-dione; MPA) was first synthesized in 1958 [1, 2], and has been widely used since then in the treatment of several types of cancer. MPA has been found to cause regression in a considerable proportion of advanced cases of endometrial cancer [3, 4], and to destroy the tumour completely, in many cases, in the early stages of the disease [5]. The MPA doses used were, and in some places still are, moderate (150–400 mg/week, administered orally (p.o.) or intramuscularly (i.m.) [3–6]. However, as proposed by Bonte and others, several clinics subsequently began to use weekly doses of 1 g, i.m. [7, 8].

MPA was introduced for the treatment of breast cancer via clinical studies performed in the 1960's. The dosages employed ranged from 40–400 mg/daily, p.o., and from 100 mg/daily to 1.6 g weekly by the i.m. route [9]. Better clinical results were reported by Pannuti et al. with high dose MPA treatment in a clinical trial of 2 such regimens, 1.5 g/day i.m. and 2.0 g/day i.m. [10, 11]. The activity of high-dose MPA in advanced breast cancer has been confirmed in a number of clinical studies [12–15].

MPA has also been used in the treatment of renal, prostatic and ovarian carcinomas [16].

Blood concentrations of MPA were first measured after low MPA doses, given for contraceptive purposes [17–19]. Recently, there have been reports on blood levels of MPA given as treatment for cancer. In some studies, MPA blood levels have been monitored to assess the relationship between blood levels and therapeutic efficacy [6, 15, 16, 20–25].

Determinations of concentrations of MPA in blood

MPA levels have, in most studies, been determined by radio-immunoassay (RIA). Various RIA methods have been developed and modified [17–19, 26, 27]. In other studies, MPA has been determined by gas liquid chromatography (GLC) [22, 23]. The plasma levels found in studies using RIA and GLC methods of determination of MPA, or even different RIA procedures, are not strictly comparable. Because of the presence of metabolites, there is always a difference in the blood levels recorded as between GLC and RIA methods, while among RIA methods themselves there are variations in the antisera used, and in the extraction methods.

Pharmacokinetics

MPA administered p.o. is rapidly absorbed. Peak levels are reached 2–3 hours after drug administration, and the drug is rapidly eliminated. An oral dose of 100 mg of MPA given to each of 9 women with advanced endometrial cancer resulted in a peak level of 10 ng MPA/ml (Fig. 1). In 6 healthy women

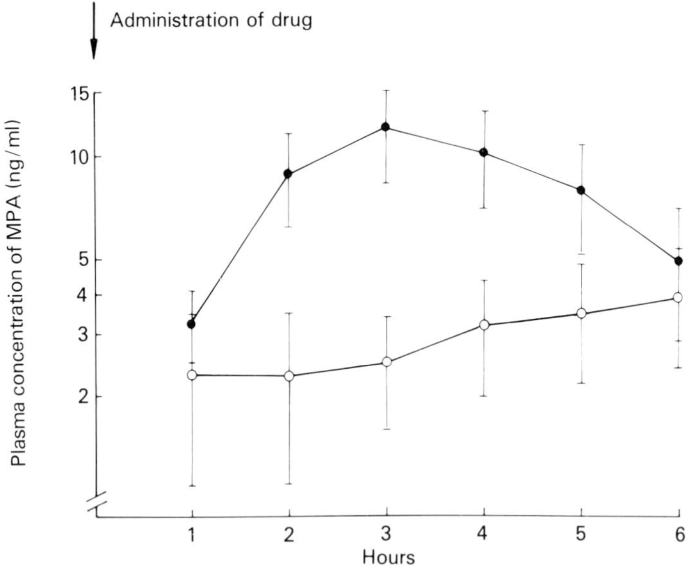

Fig. 1. Plasma concentrations of MPA after administration of a single dose of 1 g of MPA, i.m. (○———○), to 14 patients and of 100 mg of MPA, p.o. (•———•), to 9 patients. (Means ± standard errors of means.)

a dose of 200 mg of MPA, p.o., resulted in a mean peak value of nearly 15 g/ml plasma (Fig. 2). The interindividual differences were considerable, and were most pronounced in the group of 9 women with advanced endometrial cancer. There is a linear correlation between the dose administered and the plasma levels obtained. This is shown by a study of Loeber et al. [14] (Fig. 3). In this study, single i.m. injections of 100, 400, 800 and 1,200 mg were given to patients in each of 4 groups. After these doses of MPA, plasma levels remained steady during a one-week observation period, at 2, 4, 6 and 10 ng/ml, respectively.

A single dose of 1 g of MPA i.m. produced slowly increasing plasma values during the first few hours (Fig. 1). After 8–12 hours a level of 10–15 ng/ml was reached, and this level was maintained throughout the 72 hours studied (Fig. 2). The interindividual differences were even more pronounced in the patients to whom MPA was administered i.m. than in patients dosed p.o.

Since single oral doses of MPA produce much higher peak blood levels than those attained after i.m. administration of the same amount, it might be concluded that administration of equivalent doses would lead to higher blood

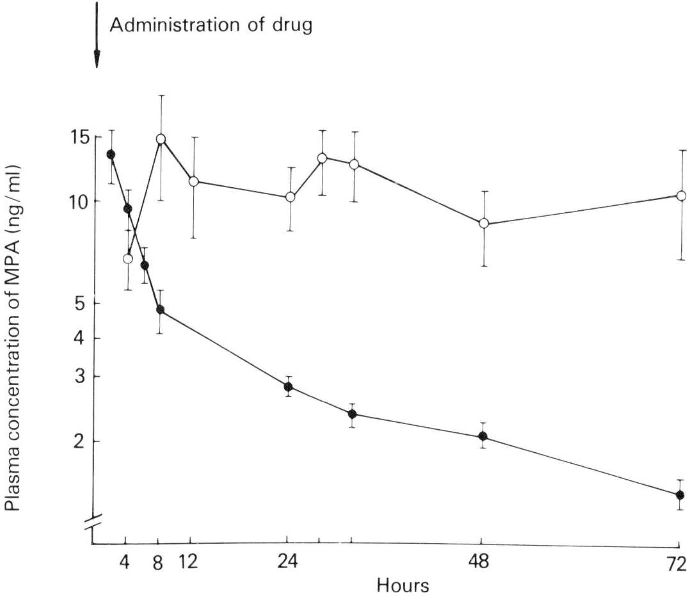

Fig. 2. Plasma concentrations of MPA after administration of a single dose of 1 g of MPA, i.m. (○——○), to 13 patients and of 200 mg of MPA, p.o. (•——•), to 6 healthy women. (Means ± standard errors of means.)

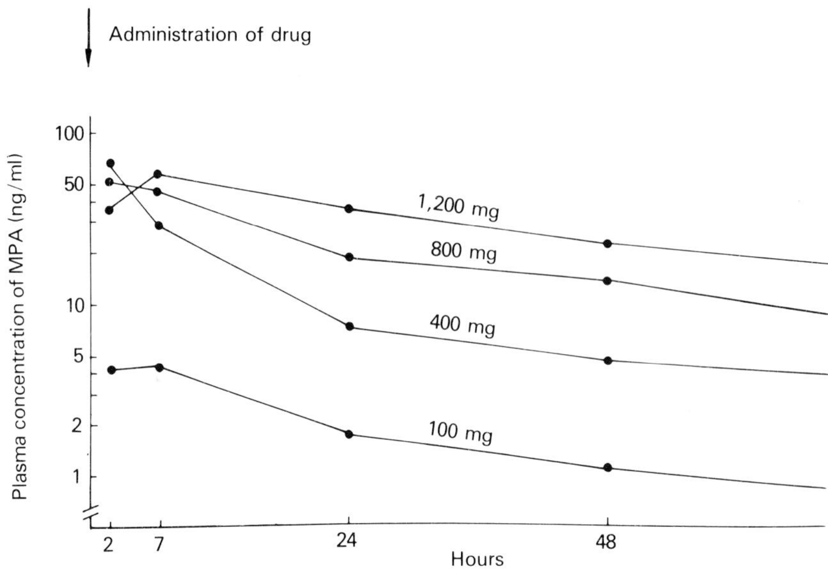

Fig. 3. Plasma concentrations of MPA after single oral doses of 100 mg, 400 mg, 800 mg and 1,200 mg to 5, 5, 5 and 4 patients, respectively. Data from Loeber et al. [24].

levels overall if the oral route were used. However, when MPA was administered i.m. once a week, steadily increasing plasma levels of MPA were obtained, whereas daily oral administration led to a steady state [25]. With MPA given i.m., release of the drug from the injection site has been shown, by monitoring of blood levels of MPA, to occur for up to 9 months [17]. From published data [17, 19], Tamassia has estimated the plasma half-life to be about 6 weeks [28]. In a long-term plasma level study of different MPA treatment regimens there were striking differences between findings after oral and i.m. administration of MPA [25]. In a group of 10 patients on 100 mg of MPA tablets twice daily, p.o., (1.4 g/week), a level of around 20 ng of MPA per ml of plasma was reached within about 4 weeks, and maintained through a follow-up period of one year. I.m. injections of 1 g of MPA once weekly produced higher blood levels than those following oral administration of 1.4 g of MPA per week (Fig. 4) from the first week. At the end of the one-year study, blood levels in the 10 patients treated orally remained at around 20 ng/ml. In the group of 10 patients in whom administration of MPA was by the i.m. route, a plasma level of around 100 ng/ml was attained after one year. This cumulative effect following the i.m. administration of MPA has also been reported by Maskens et al. [22].

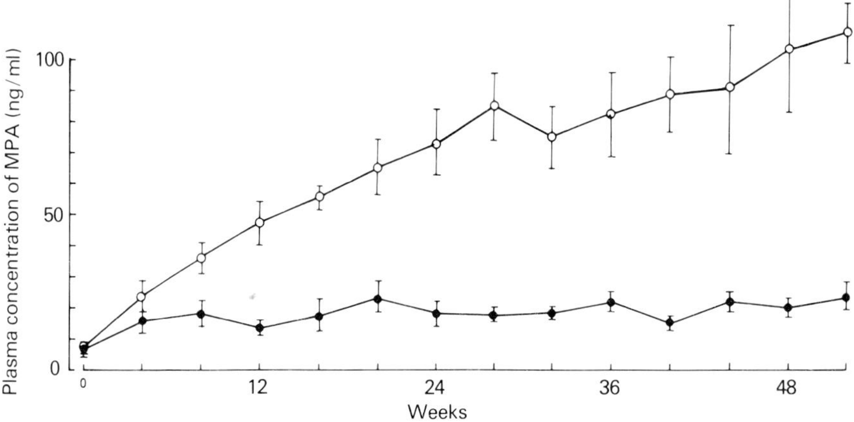

Fig. 4. Plasma concentrations of MPA in 10 patients treated with 1 g of MPA i.m. once a week for one year (○——○), and in 10 patients treated with 200 mg of MPA, p.o., daily for one year (●——●). (Means ± standard errors of means.)

Dosage schedules

Using the oral route of administration, higher blood levels of MPA can, obviously, be obtained by increasing the daily dosage. Using the i.m. route, higher blood levels can be obtained either by increasing each individual dose, or by increasing the number of administrations. By means of daily i.m. dosage it is possible to obtain increases in blood levels to the desired values in a few weeks which would take several months to reach using a weekly dosage schedule. A weekly schedule is satisfactory for maintenance therapy.

From several recent clinical reports, conclusions can be drawn as regards the MPA dosages adequate for the treatment of various types of cancer. Bonte obtained excellent results in advanced cases of endometrial cancer of stage I, as well as in MPA prophylaxis, using MPA doses, administered i.m. or p.o., of 1 g weekly [20, 21]. Bonte found, what he considered, adequate serum levels of MPA within 10 days of starting oral MPA treatment, and after 5 weeks of starting i.m. treatment. In the treatment of breast cancer, higher doses are currently used, because they are considered necessary for an optimal response rate. Pannuti et al. introduced high dose MPA treatment, using 1.5 g and 2.0 g i.m., daily, for 30 days [10, 11]. Robustelli Della Cuna et al. [13] found no differences in the clinical outcomes in 2 groups treated with 500 mg or 1 g of MPA daily, i.m., for 2 months. Cavalli et al. have reported significant differences between clinical results in 2 groups of advanced breast cancer patients treated with 1 g MPA i.m. daily for 5 days a week, over a 4 week period, or 500 mg i.m. twice weekly, for 4 weeks [14]. In both groups, maintenance treatment was 500 mg of MPA i.m., once weekly. It is, therefore, possible to determine appropriate dosages of MPA by means of clinical trials. Because there are considerable interindividual differences in MPA blood levels with any given dosage schedule, monitoring of MPA blood levels is necessary to allow adequate interpretation of the clinical results, and to allow an optimal dosage schedule to be devised.

As already mentioned, MPA administered p.o., daily, rapidly produces plasma levels which will be maintained as long as the same dose is administered daily. MPA injected daily, i.m., produces a continual increase in plasma levels, which can subsequently be maintained by weekly i.m. administration. The levels obtained by i.m. administration are considerably higher than those following oral administration. Long-term data have already been cited, but the effect is seen in the short-term also. Daily doses of 1 g i.m. for 14 days gave plasma levels of 90–100 ng/ml, as against levels of around 30 ng/ml following the oral administration of 1 g of MPA daily (Fig. 5). To achieve similar clinical effects, therefore, it is necessary to give considerably higher oral than i.m. doses. In many clinics, oral administration is preferred, because it is easier and more convenient for patients. Some clinical studies have been begun, and preliminary reports presented. Izuo et al. have reported encouraging preliminary clinical results in a series of patients treated with 1.2

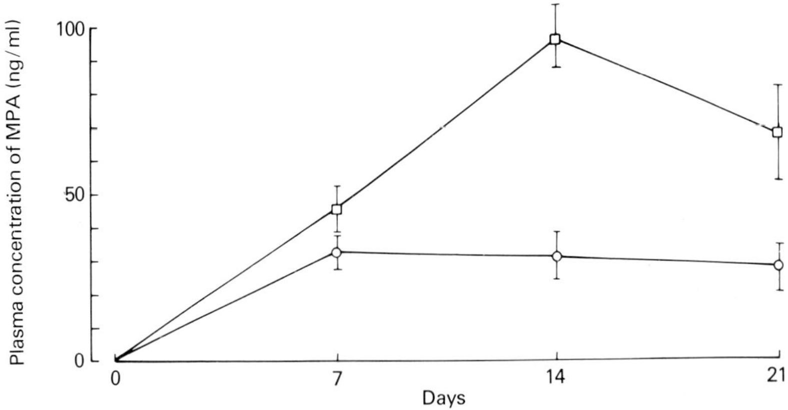

Fig. 5. Plasma concentrations of MPA in 14 patients treated with 1 g of MPA daily, i.m., for 14 days (□——□), and in 5 patients treated with 1 g of MPA daily, p.o., for 21 days (○——○). (Means ± standard errors of means.)

g of MPA daily, p.o. [15]. These investigators are also monitoring MPA blood levels, which will be valuable in assessing the results.

To achieve therapeutic plasma levels of MPA rapidly, a combination of oral administration followed by i.m. maintenance doses might be considered, offering some of the advantages of both routes of administration. This procedure has been proposed by Tamassia [28].

References

1. Babcock, Y.V., Gutselle, S., Heve, N.H. et al. (1958): 6-alpha-methyl-17-alpha-hydroxyprogesterone-17-acetylates: a new class of potent progestins. *J. Am. Chem. Soc. 80,* 2904.
2. Sala, G., Camarino, B. and Cavallero, C. (1958): Progestional activity of 6-alpha-methyl-17-alpha-hydroxyprogesterone acetate. *Acta Endocrinol. (Copenhagen) 29*, 508.
3. Anderson, D.G. (1965): Management of advanced endometrial adenocarcinoma with medroxyprogesterone acetate. *Am. J. Obstet. Gynecol. 92*, 87.
4. Bonte, J., Drochmans, A. and Ide, P. (1966): 6-alpha-methyl-17-alpha-hydroxyprogesterone acetate as a chemotherapeutic agent in adenocarcinoma of the uterus. *Acta Obstet. Gynecol. Scand. 45,* 121.
5. Bonte, J., De Coster, J.M., Ide, P. and Billiet, G. (1978): Hormonoprophylaxis and hormonotherapy in the treatment of endometrial adenocarcinoma by means of medroxyprogesterone acetate. *Gynecol. Oncol. 6,* 60.
6. Sall, S., Disaia, P. Morrow, P. et al. (1979): A comparison of medroxyprogesterone serum concentrations by the oral or intramuscular route in patients with persistent or recurrent endometrial carcinoma. *Am. J. Obstet. Gynecol. 135,* 649.
7. Bonte, J. (1972): Medroxyprogesterone in the management of primary and recurrent or metastatic uterine adenocarcinoma. *Acta Obstet. Gynecol. Scand. Suppl. 19*, 21.
8. Piver, S., Barlow, J., Lurain, J. and Blumenson, L. (1980): Medroxyprogesterone acetate (Depot-Provera) vs. hydroxyprogesterone caproate (Delautin) in women with metastatic endometrial adenocarcinoma. *Cancer 45,* 268.
9. Ganzina, F. (1979): High-dose medroxyprogesterone acetate (MPA) treatment in advanced breast cancer. A Review. *Tumori 65*, 563.
10. Pannuti, F., Martoni, A., Pollutri, E. et al. (1976): Massive dose progestional therapy in oncology (medroxyprogesterone). Preliminary results. Proceedings of the 4th Symposium on the Locoregional Treatment of Tumours. St. Vincent 1973. *Panminerva Med. 18,* 129.
11. Pannuti, F., Martoni, A., Lenaz, G.R. et al. (1978): A possible new approach to the treatment of metastatic breast cancer: massive doses of medroxyprogesterone acetate. *Cancer Treat. Rep. 62,* 499.
12. Mattsson, W. (1978): High dose medroxyprogesterone acetate treatment in advanced mammary carcinoma. A phase II investigation. *Acta Radiol. Oncol. 17,* 387.
13. Robustelli Della Cuna, G., Calciati, A., Bernardo Strada, M.R. et al. (1978):

High dose medroxyprogesterone acetate (MPA) treatment in metastatic carcinoma of the breast: a dose response evaluation. *Tumori 64*, 143.

14. Cavalli, F., Goldhirsch, A., Jungi, F. et al. (1981): Low versus high dose medroxyprogesterone acetate (MPA) in the treatment of advanced breast cancer. In: *Proceedings of the 2nd International Symposium of the Role of MPA in Endocrine-related Tumors, Rome, 1981.* (In press.)
15. Izuo, M., Yuichi, I. and Keiichi, E. (1981): Oral high-dose medroxyprogesterone acetate (MPA) in the treatment of advanced breast cancer. *Breast Cancer Research and Treatment 1*, 125.
16. Proceedings of the International Symposium on Medroxyprogesterone Acetate, Geneva, 1982. Excerpta Medica, Amsterdam.
17. Jeppsson, S. and Johansson, E.D.B. (1976): Medroxyprogesterone acetate, estradiol, FSH and LH in peripheral blood after intramuscular administration of Depo-provera to women. *Contraception 14,* 461.
18. Victor, A. and Johansson, E.D.B. (1976): Pharmacokinetic observations on medroxyprogesterone acetate administered orally and intravaginally. *Contraception 14,* 315.
19. Ortiz, A., Hiroi, M., Stanczyk, F.Z. et al. (1977): Serum medroxyprogesterone acetate (MPA) concentrations and ovarian function following intramuscular injection of Depo-MPA. *J. Endocrinol. Metab. 44*, 32.
20. Bonte, J. (1980): Medroxyprogesterone acetate in the management of endometrial adenocarcinoma. In: *Progestogens in the Management of Hormone Responsive Carcinomas. Proceedings of an International Symposium, Royal College of Physicians, London, 1980,* pp. 35–49. Ed: R.W. Taylor. The Medicine Publishing Foundation, Oxford.
21. Bonte, J. (1980): Hormonal dependence of endometrial adenocarcinoma and its hormonal sensitivity to progestogens and antiestrogens. In: *Hormones and Cancer,* pp. 443–455. Eds: S. Iacobelli and A. Di Marco. Raven Press, New York.
22. Maskens, A., Hap, B., Kozyreff, V. et al. (1980): Serum levels of medroxyprogesterone acetate under various treatment schedules. *Proc. Am. Soc. Clin. Oncol. 21,* 165.
23. Laatkainen, T., Nieminen, U. and Adlercreutz, H. (1979): Plasma medroxyprogesterone acetate levels following intramuscular or oral administration in patients with endometrial carcinoma. *Acta Obstet. Gynecol. Scand. 58*, 95.
24. Loeber, J., Mouridsen, H.T., Salimtschik, M. and Johansson, E. (1981): Pharmacokinetics of medroxyprogesterone acetate administered by oral and intramuscular route. *Acta Obstet. Gynecol. Scand. Suppl. 101,* 71.
25. Hesselius, I. and Johansson, E.D.B. (1981): Medroxyprogesterone acetate (MPA) plasma levels after oral and intramuscular administration in a long-term study. *Acta Obstet. Gynecol. Scand. Suppl. 101,* 65.
26. Cornette, J.C. Kirton, K.T. and Duncan, G.W. (1971): Measurements of medroxyprogesterone acetate (Provera) by radioimmunoassay. *J. Clin. Endocrinol. Metab. 33,* 459.
27. Schrimanker, K., Saxena, B.N. and Fotherby, K. (1978): A radioimmunoassay for serum medroxyprogesterone acetate. *J. Steroid Biochem. 9,* 359.
28. Tamassia, V. (1981): Dose schedules of medroxyprogesterone acetate for breast cancer treatment: a pharmacokinetic approach. In: *Progesteron and Progestins, International Symposium, Paris, 1981.*

Round table: MPA pharmacokinetics

Chairman: I.R. Hesselius, Uppsala, Sweden

Panelists:

C. Blossey	(Göttingen, Federal Republic of Germany)
C.M. Camaggi	(Bologna, Italy)
V. Kozyreff	(Brussels, Belgium)
A.P. Maskens	(Brussels, Belgium)
V. Tamassia	(Milan, Italy)

I.R. Hesselius

During this round table discussion we will elucidate some different aspects of the pharmacokinetics and bio-availability of MPA.

V. Tamassia

One of the most important clinical applications of pharmacokinetics is the design of the drug dose schedules (dose, route of administration, dosage interval, dosage form) to be used in drug therapy.

This design is based on the following. 1. The knowledge of the pharmacokinetic and bio-availability parameters of the drug, which can be determined after a simple single-dose study. 2. The selection a priori of a drug blood level profile which fits in the best way with the mode of action of the drug and the aim of the medication. 3. The application of the pharmacokinetic theory of the dose regimen calculations. This theory allows the prediction of the drug blood level profile during repeated administration at any dose schedule on the basis of some kinetic parameters of the drug and on the simple assumption of linear pharmacokinetics.

I would like to discuss some practical applications of these general principles in the particular case of MPA.

With regard to the ideal or desirable blood level profile, it can reasonably be assumed that, with a hormonal treatment, 'effective' drug blood levels must be reached as quickly as possible and they must be maintained until progression of the disease.

With regard to the main pharmacokinetic parameters of MPA, they have been calculated from the results of a study carried out by Salimtschik et al. who investigated the MPA plasma level profile after single oral and intramuscular (i.m.) doses ranging from 100–1,200 mg [1].

This study demonstrated that, in the dose range tested, the plasma levels increased linearly with increasing doses, suggesting linear pharmacokinetics. After i.m. administration the plasma levels were very low – about 1 ng/ml for each 100-mg dose – and remained steady during the one-week observation period. After oral administration there was a rapid absorption with peak levels much higher than after the same doses given by i.m. injection. The plasma levels after oral administration decreased quite rapidly, with a plasma half-life of about 2 days.

The different plasma level profile is due to the different bio-availability properties of the drug from the gastro-intestinal tract and the injection site. In particular, the unusual behaviour of the drug given by i.m. injection is explained by a depot effect. This depot effect is extraordinarily long-lasting. Published data on the use of MPA as a contraceptive suggest that the plasma levels following a single injection decrease very slowly with an apparent plasma half-life of about 6 weeks. It appears, therefore, that with an injection of 500 or 1,000 mg of MPA, the rate of absorption can be estimated as only of a few mg/day.

The above-mentioned differences have important consequences for the MPA plasma level profile during repeated dose administration.

The mathematical equations which can be used to predict the plasma level profile of MPA during repeated administration, by oral or by i.m. route, have been recently discussed [2]. They simply represent the application to MPA of the dose regimen calculation theory which is used routinely by people involved in the pharmacokinetics. The equations of the dose regimen calculations are as follows:

$$C_n\,(t') = C_o \frac{1 - e^{-nK\tau}}{1 - e^{-K\tau}}\, e^{-Kt'}$$

i.m. MPA

- n = dose number; τ = dosage interval
- t' = time after the n th dose
- $K = 0.693/t\frac{1}{2} = 0.115$ week^{-1}
- C_o = 1 ng/ml for each 100-mg dose

$$\overline{C_{ss}} = \frac{AUC\,(\tau)_{ss}}{\tau} = \frac{AUC\,(\infty)_{sd}}{\tau}$$

Oral MPA

- $\overline{C_{ss}}$ = average steady-state plasma levels (after $5 \times t\frac{1}{2}$ = 5×48 h = 10 days)
- $AUC\,(\tau)_{ss}$ = area under curve in the dosage interval τ
- $AUC\,(\infty)_{sd}$ = total area under curve after single dose
- $AUC\,(\infty)_{sd}$ = 250 ng $\times$ h/ml for each 100-mg dose

Figure 1 shows the plasma level profile predicted during a dose schedule based on a weekly i.m. injection of 1,000 mg of MPA – the classical dose schedule used in the past for endometrial cancer. The continuous increase in MPA plasma levels up to a steady-state situation, which is reached after about

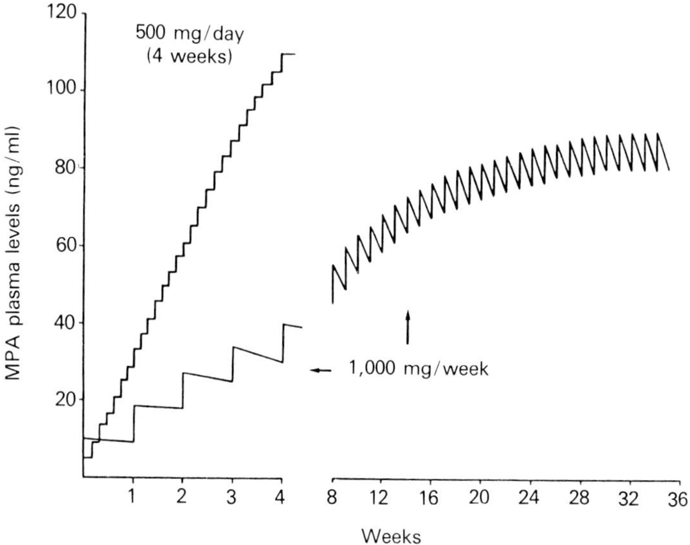

Fig. 1. *MPA plasma level profile predicted during repeated i.m. administration at the following dose schedules: 1,000 mg/week or 500 mg/day for 4 weeks.*

6–8 months of therapy, is a direct consequence of the long-lasting depot effect. The pharmacokinetic theory, in fact, predicts that steady-state levels will be reached after about 4–5 times the half-life of the drug. Since the half-life of MPA after i.m. administration is 6 weeks, 4–5 times 6 weeks means about 6–8 months. Moreover, the steady-state levels will be several times higher than those reached after the first dose. In this case, the theory predicts about 9 times higher – 90 ng/ml at steady state against 10 ng/ml after the first dose.

It appears that the dose schedules based on a weekly injection are not rational from the point of view of the plasma level profile. On the reasonable assumption that high, steady-state levels are necessary for therapy, it is possible to shorten the time interval required to reach these levels by adopting a loading phase with daily injections. As shown in Figure 1, 500 mg/day given i.m. for a period of 4 weeks gave about 100 ng/ml at the end of the loading period. These levels are of the same order of magnitude as those reached after 6–8 months of therapy with weekly injections of 1,000 mg of MPA.

The general principle is that we have to add the small contributions coming from many injection sites in order to obtain a higher dose absorbed and correspondingly higher blood levels.

However, the true amount absorbed every day and available for therapeutic efficacy represents only a negligible part of the cumulative dose administered (about 1–2%), the remainder being in the injection site from which it will be released very slowly.

Another consequence of these unusual bio-availability properties of MPA is that, after stopping the therapy, the drug plasma levels will decrease very slowly, with a plasma half-life of about 6 weeks (Fig. 2). A maintenance treatment with weekly injections of 1,000 mg is sufficient to counterbalance the amount of drug eliminated and to maintain indefinitely the plasma levels reached at the end of the loading phase. The proposed maintenance treatment with weekly injections is not strictly necessary on a short-term basis (a few weeks), but it is necessary if we want to maintain the plasma levels in the long-term (more than 2 months).

In conclusion, from the theoretical point of view, the dose schedules based on a loading phase with daily injections followed by a maintenance therapy with weekly injections are completely rational from the point of view of the plasma level profile.

With regard to the oral administration, the situation is completely different (Fig. 3). Owing to the relatively short plasma half-life (about 2 days), the plasma level profile during repeated daily oral doses is characterized by a

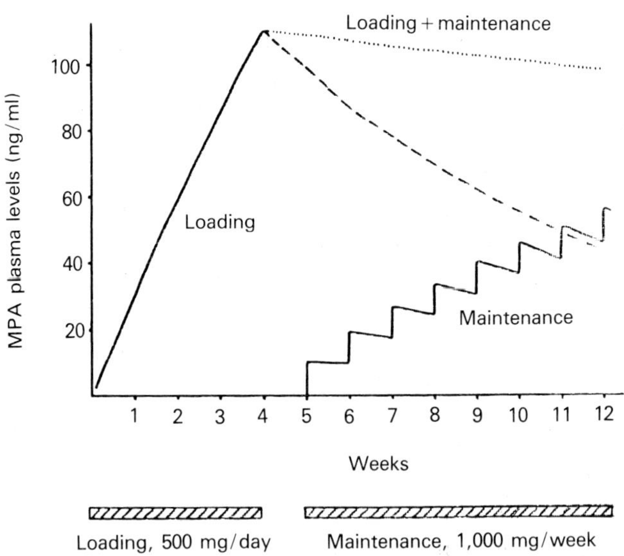

Fig. 2. MPA plasma level profile predicted during and after a loading i.m. phase (500 mg/day for 4 weeks) with (·····) or without (-----) a maintenance i.m. treatment with 1,000 mg/week.

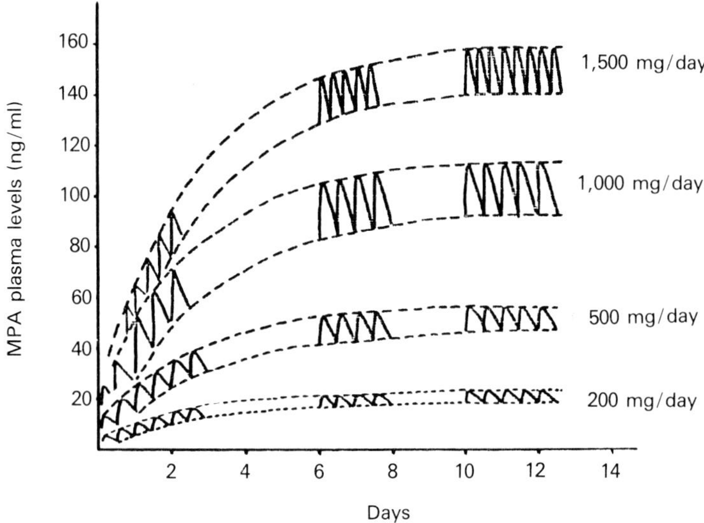

Fig. 3. MPA plasma level profile predicted during repeated oral administration at various dose schedules.

phase of build-up lasting about 10 days, followed by a steady-state situation. The average steady-state levels that are expected after oral administration are about 10 ng/ml for each 100-mg dose.

Obviously, any reduction in the daily dose will be followed by a rapid proportional decrease in the plasma level within 10 days as is shown in Figure 4.

Comparing the plasma level profile expected with oral and i.m. MPA, it appears that they are not bio-equivalent, i.e., the same daily dose does not produce the same blood level profile. However, it is possible to design equipotent dose schedules for the 2 routes of administration.

Taking as a reference the dose schedule for i.m. administration, the daily injections of 500 mg for 4 weeks followed by a maintenance therapy of weekly injections of 1,000 mg, a similar plasma level profile can be achieved by oral administration of 1,000 mg/day, without any dose reductions during the maintenance phase (Fig. 5). Other equipotent dose schedules can be calculated on the basis of the following rule: For oral administration, the steady-state levels will be about 10 ng/ml for each 100-mg/day dose. For the i.m. administration, each 1,000-mg cumulative dose will contribute about 8–9 ng/ml on a short-term basis (less than 4 weeks), whereas for the long-term treatment (more than 6 months) each 1,000-mg/week dose will contribute about 90 ng/ml. The plasma levels which can be achieved with various dose schedules are summarized in the Table.

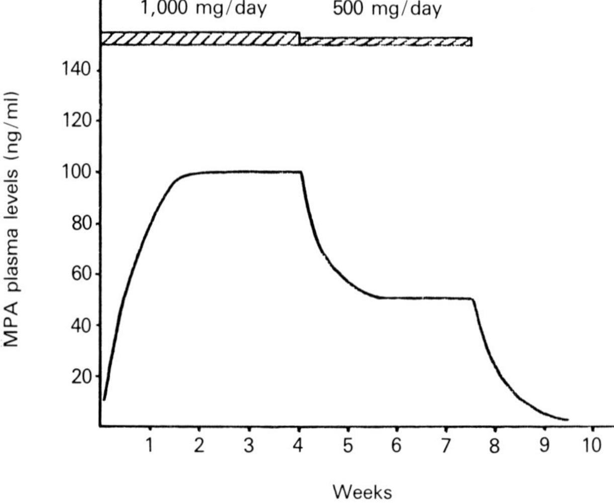

Fig. 4. MPA plasma level profile predicted during repeated oral administration at the following dose schedule: 1,000 mg/day for 4 weeks followed by 500 mg/day for 4 weeks.

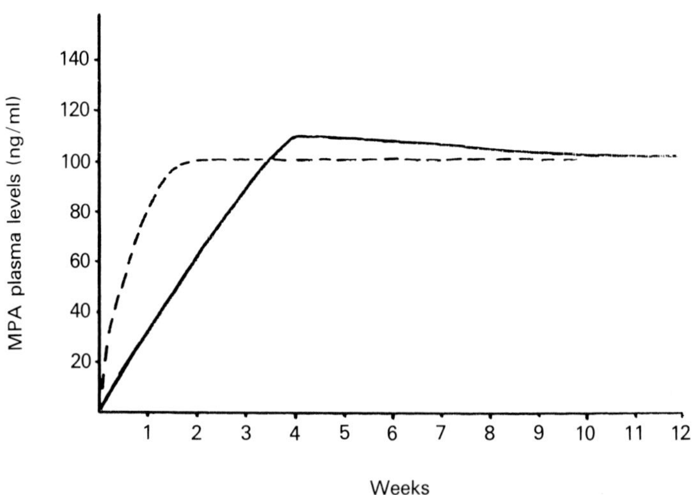

Fig. 5. MPA plasma level profile predicted following 2 equipotent dose schedules by oral and i.m. route; (———) = i.m. administration, 500 mg/day for 4 weeks + 1,000 mg/week; (-----) = oral administration, 1,000 mg/day.

Table. Relationship between MPA plasma levels and various drug dose schedules.

Dose schedule	Treatment	Plasma levels (ng/ml, radio-immunoassay)
Oral MPA		
200 mg/day	>10 days	~ 20
500 mg/day	>10 days	~ 50
1,000 mg/day	>10 days	~100
1,500 mg/day	>10 days	~150
I.m. MPA		
500 mg/day*	4 weeks	~110*
1,000 mg/day	4 weeks	~220
1,000 mg/week	4 weeks	~ 40
1,000 mg/week	>6 months	~ 90

*Or other dosage schedules equivalent in terms of cumulative loading doses ($\simeq$ 15 g in $\leq$4 weeks).

These data clearly indicate that the overall bio-availability of MPA after oral administration is lower than after i.m. administration, and that the difference is more evident during chronic treatment.

These predictions refer to average plasma levels (interpatient variations are expected) measured by the radio-immunoassay method employed by Salimtschik et al. [1]. The plasma levels measured by other analytical methods can be higher or lower than shown here, depending upon the specificity of the method used, but the general rules for selection of the dose schedules should remain valid.

References

1. Salimtschik, M., Mouridsen, H.T., Loeber, J. and Johansson E. (1980): Comparative pharmacokinetics of medroxyprogesterone acetate administered by oral and i.m. route. *Cancer Chemother. Pharmacol. 4,* 267.
2. Tamassia, V., Battaglia, A., Ganzina, F. et al. (1982): Pharmacokinetic approach to the selection of dose schedules of medroxyprogesterone acetate in clinical oncology. *Cancer Chemother. Pharmacol.* (In press.)

C.M. Camaggi

We routinely determine MPA plasma levels in advanced-cancer patients. Dr Tamassia's calculations are in qualitative agreement with the data obtained by us from a total of about 500 patients. Our analytical approach is different. In our opinion, gas chromatography is more accurate than radio-immunoassay and less prone to interference. To date, the metabolic pathways of MPA are almost unknown and, therefore, it is of course not possible to test the cross-reactivity.

In his opening lecture, Professor Pannuti extensively reported the results of single-dose pharmacokinetics. I would like to present in more detail our data on MPA plasma levels following multiple administration. Figure 1 shows the MPA plasma concentrations (ng/ml) determined during treatment involving daily i.m. administration of 500, 1,000 and 2,000 mg for a period of 30 days. For each curve data were obtained from at least 10 cancer patients. The important and more relevant features to note are: even with 2,000 mg/day of MPA, the plasma levels are relatively low; the steady-state concentration is reached slowly – in fact, it is not reached until after discontinuing the treatment; the steady state is maintained for a very long time.

Figure 2 shows the MPA plasma levels after multiple oral administration. Here again, the treatment was discontinued after 30 days. Even with the massive dose of 5,000 mg/day of MPA, the mean plasma levels did not exceed 400 ng/ml. In only 2 patients MPA levels of about 1 μg/ml were observed – and both patients, incidentally, had good objective remissions. Steady state after oral administration was reached rather quickly (as predicted by the theory presented by Dr Tamassia). After discontinuation of the treatment, the drug levels decayed exponentially. The dose dependency of MPA plasma concentrations is not so clear-cut here as it is following i.m. administration. I would like to emphasize that single-dose pharmacokinetics provided several indications of a rather low percentage of MPA absorption by the oral route. For instance, our (still unpublished) comparison of the areas under the time/concentration curve (AUC) relative to single oral and single intraperitoneal administration suggests that only about 1/500th of the dose given is absorbed when the drug is given orally. This fact is confirmed both by the low plasma levels obtained even after massive oral administration and by the interindividual variation in MPA bio-availability.

Figure 3 shows the MPA plasma levels observed after discontinuing the treatment for both the oral and i.m. route of administration (on a semilogarithmic scale). I.m. and oral MPA administration are definitely not equipotent. As I showed above, MPA plasma levels increase faster after oral administration, but with oral administration at least 3 times the original i.m. MPA dose must be given to obtain the same plateau of plasma concentration. In addition, after the last oral dose MPA concentration decays, with a half-life of about 2 days, whereas after i.m. treatment the plasma levels remain unaltered.

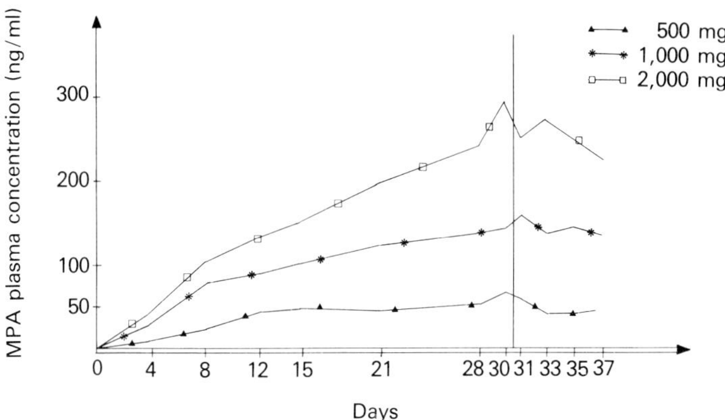

Fig. 1. *MPA high i.m. doses: plasma levels after multiple administration.*

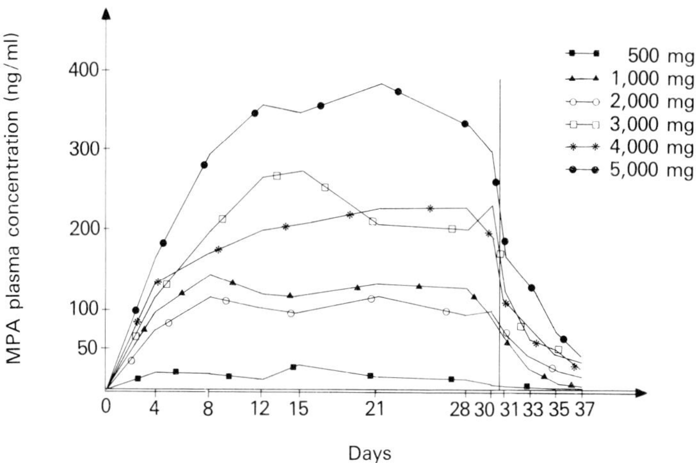

Fig. 2. *MPA high oral doses: plasma levels after multiple administration.*

Figure 4 shows the AUC observed for each patient treated with MPA. These areas are calculated in the 0–37 day's interval, and they are a good indication of the MPA bio-availability. In considering this scattergram, I must warn against the use of only moderate MPA doses with oral administration without checking the extent of the drug absorption. There are indications, at least for the treatment of breast cancer, that below a certain bio-availability of MPA the percentage of remission is quite unfavourable. In our opinion, if oral administration is used without routine MPA analysis, massive doses of

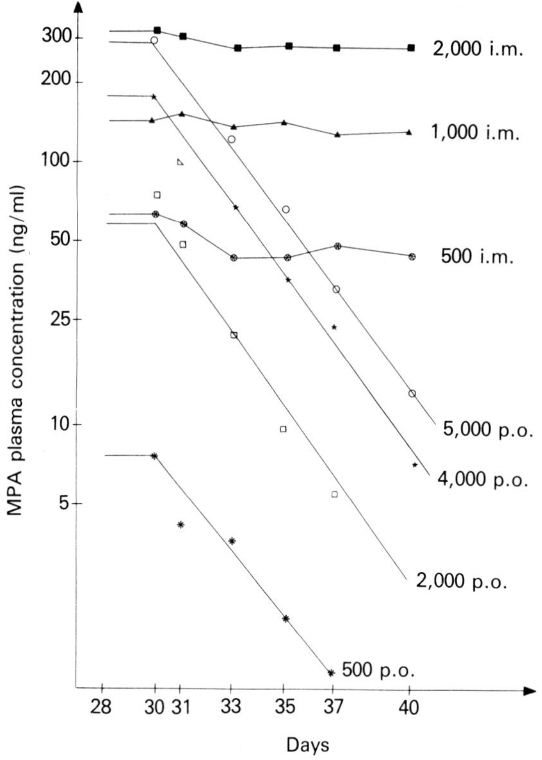

Fig. 3. MPA high oral (p.o.) and i.m. doses: plasma levels after discontinuing administration.

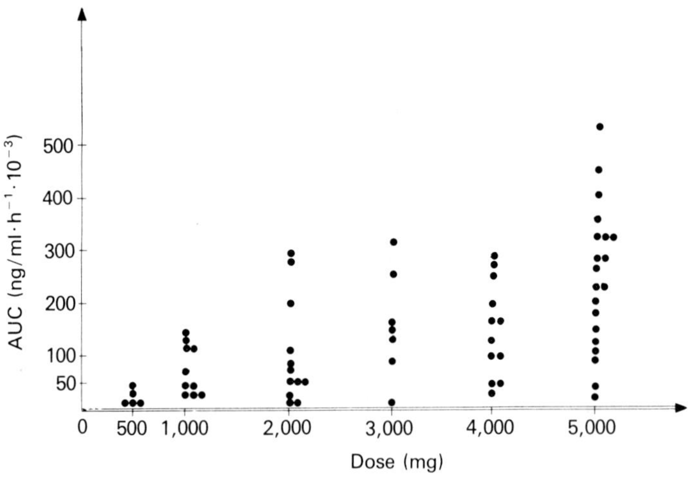

Fig. 4. MPA high doses: AUC after multiple administration.

MPA are necessary to achieve, and consistently maintain, a therapeutic MPA plasma level.

C. Blossey

I would only like to stress some important features of the oral form of high-dose MPA therapy.

Using the radio-immunoassay technique without extraction, MPA plasma levels appear in a higher concentration (μg/ml). The therapy schedule was 1,500 mg/day of MPA, p.o., continuously given. Under these conditions there is a rapid increase of the MPA plasma levels (Fig. 1). The plateau state is reached after about 5 days, indicated by the ranges and medians on the right-hand side of panel A. A subgroup of patients (about 20%) seems to have a delayed increase in MPA plasma levels reaching the plateau state after 10–14 days (panel B).

Within the plateau state there is a broad intra- and interindividual variation

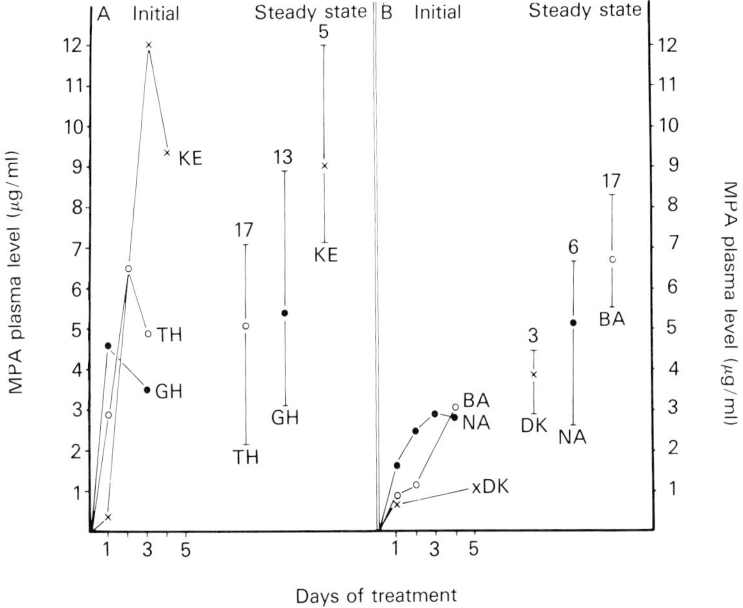

Fig. 1. Initial kinetics of MPA plasma levels in 6 patients in a therapy schedule of 1,500 mg (3 × 500 mg/day), p.o. Ranges and medians in the plateau state are seen on the right-hand side of the panels. The numbers on top of the ranges reflect the number of determinations in the plateau state.

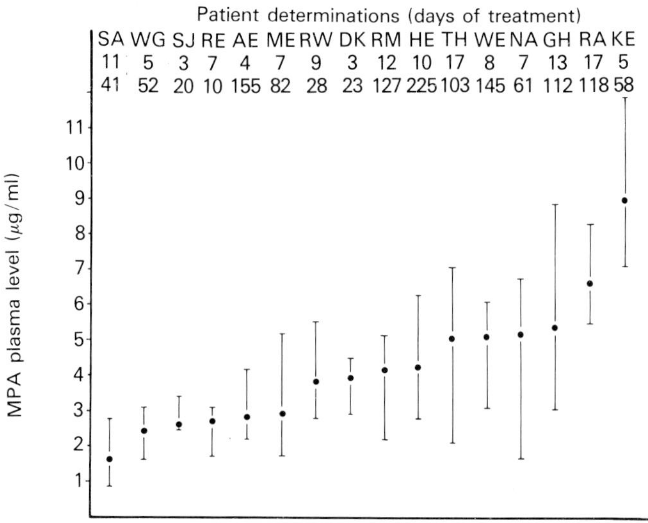

Fig. 2. Ranges and medians of MPA plasma levels in the plateau state in 16 patients. Apparently there is no correlation between the number of determinations or duration of treatment and the plasma levels.

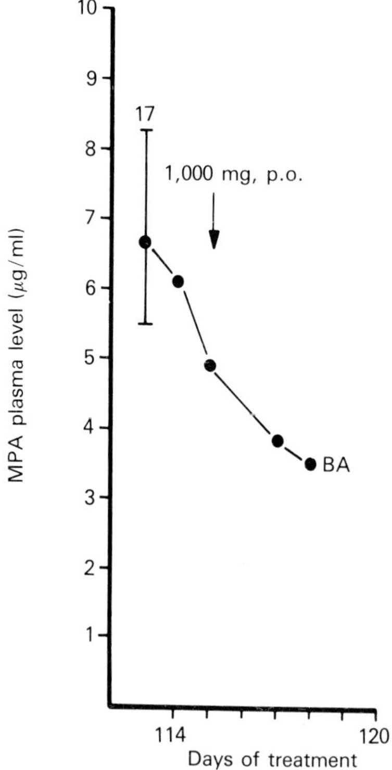

Fig. 3. Effect of MPA dose reduction, from 1,500 to 1,000 mg/day, on plasma level in one patient. For further details see text.

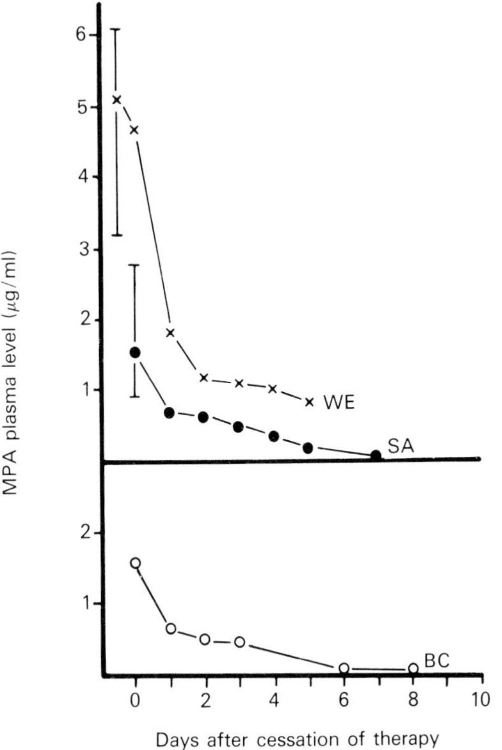

Fig. 4. Elimination kinetics of MPA in 3 patients. For further details see text.

of the MPA plasma levels possibly due to differences in absorption, distribution, metabolism, and excretion (Fig. 2).

The system is very sensitive to dose modifications. After MPA dose reduction from 1,500 to 1,000 mg/day, p.o., an immediate decrease in the plateau state is observed (Fig. 3). The same phenomenon is observed in the elimination kinetics. After cessation of therapy there is a rapid decrease in MPA plasma levels in a biphasic manner with half-times of 20 hours and 4 days, respectively (Fig. 4).

The main characteristics of the pharmacokinetics in oral (tablets) high-dose MPA therapy are: a rapid increase in MPA plasma levels; a broad intra- and interindividual variation of MPA plasma levels in the plateau state; a high sensitivity of MPA plasma levels in the plateau state to dose modifications; a rapid decrease in MPA plasma levels after cessation of therapy.

As a clinical consequence the regular ingestion of MPA tablets by the patients is crucial to maintain their individual plateau state.

A.P. Maskens

I will summarize the results from a pilot series, published in 1980 in cooperation with Dr Kozyreff. They are in complete agreement with the predictions of the theoretical model of Dr Tamassia and the findings presented by the other speakers, showing higher levels obtained with i.m. MPA treatment given on a chronic basis, and also demonstrating the depot effect of i.m. treatment.

Figure 1 shows the MPA serum levels in several subjects following long-term (more than 8 weeks) administration of the drug, comparing the oral with the i.m. route (full squares), as measured by the gas chromatography technique. The following treatment schedules were used:

1. Three different doses given by the oral route. The patients received 100, 200 or 500 mg of MPA daily for 7 days a week (a total weekly dose of 700, 1,400 or 3,500 mg).
2. Two different schedules by the i.m. route. The patients received either 500 mg twice a week or 500 mg 5 times a week.

There indeed exists a clear correlation between the administered dose and the serum level, but the linear regression coefficient is much greater for the i.m. than for the oral route, such that with a comparable weekly dose the

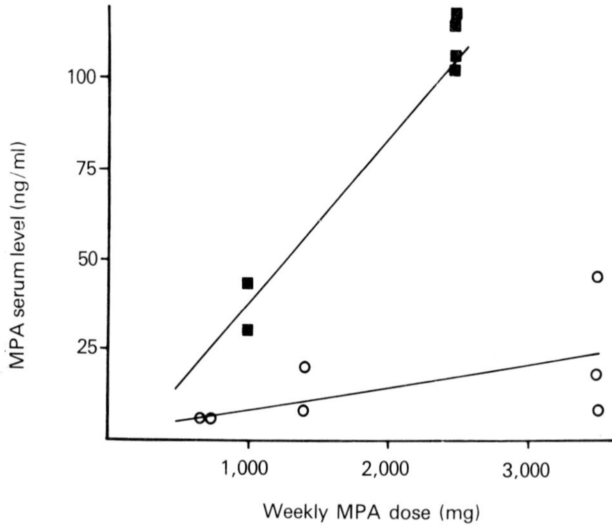

Fig. 1. Serum levels after long-term MPA administration, comparing the oral (○) with the i.m. (■) route.

serum level is considerably higher with the i.m. administration.

How these curves build up with time is shown in Figure 2 for several individual patients, 2 of whom received oral treatment and 5 of whom received i.m. treatment. Again, as the weeks go by, the serum levels become continuously higher with no interruption with i.m. treatment, although there is a plateau with oral treatment at a much lower level than is reached with i.m. treatment.

The 3 patients shown in Figure 3 had a loading daily dose of 500 mg of MPA, given i.m. for a period of 8 weeks, and were then changed to receiving twice-weekly injections as maintenance treatment. They have been followed for 4–12 months. The serum levels (given as percentages of the levels obtained after the loading phase) have remained high, indicating that with the maintenance dose it is possible to keep the serum levels high for as long as 300 days. The decline in the serum level using this maintenance treatment schedule is very slow, and the twice-weekly injections are able to maintain high serum levels.

The data from the single patient shown in Figure 4 illustrate that the difference between oral and i.m. treatment is true for individual patients. This patient with breast cancer was started on oral treatment, first on a loading dose (500 mg/day) which was then followed by a maintenance dose (200 mg/day). There is clearly no depot effect. As soon as the oral dosage is reduced, the serum level is reduced accordingly. Having not obtained good results with

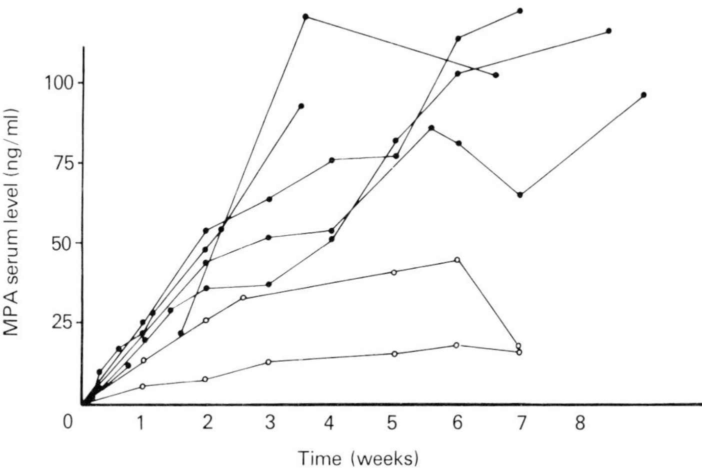

Fig. 2. Relationship between MPA serum levels and time comparing oral (○) with i.m. (•) treatment.

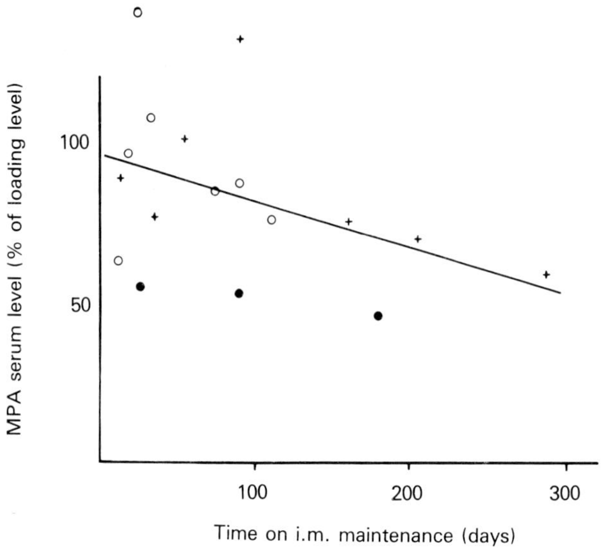

Fig. 3. MPA serum levels of 3 patients on i.m. maintenance treatment.

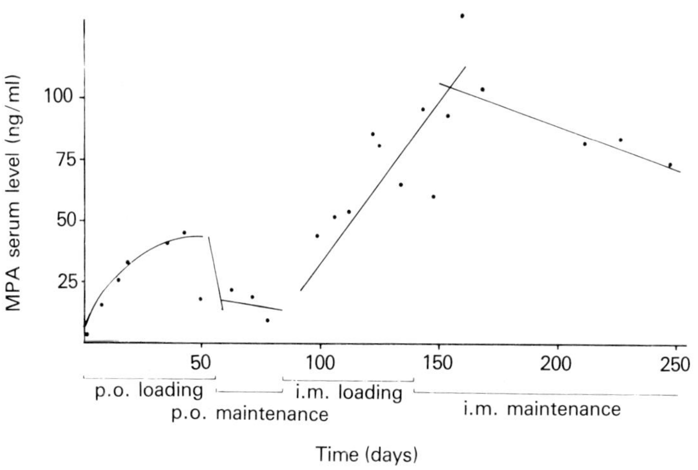

Fig. 4. MPA serum levels of a patient on oral and i.m. treatment.

this patient, she was then started on the classic loading schedule with i.m. treatment. In this same patient, the same dose, 500 mg/day, but now given i.m., resulted in a MPA serum level of more than 100 ng/ml. This high level was quite well maintained by the maintenance treatment of twice-weekly injections of 500 mg.

This result therefore illustrates the difference between oral and i.m. administration and of the depot effect of the latter route of administration.

Discussion

I.R. Hesselius: As has already been stated today, one important question is: What are the therapeutic blood levels of MPA? Obviously, there could be different therapeutic blood levels for different diseases – such a conclusion could be drawn from the results of different clinical trials.

Another question is whether the blood level is a discriminating factor predicting prognosis. To answer such a question it is necessary to monitor the blood levels of MPA in the clinical trials, because of the large individual differences.

What do you think about these questions, Dr Camaggi?

C.M. Camaggi: We have some preliminary data from a bio-availability/response study that is now in progress. We chose to examine the bio-availability/response relationship rather than the more generally-accepted dose-response relationship because, as we have shown earlier, the same dose of MPA can generate vastly different MPA plasma levels. MPA absorption by the i.m. route is extremely *slow,* whereas by the oral route it is extremely *low.* This behaviour is mainly due to the low solubility of the drug in plasma (about 2 μg/ml). The rate of absorption is primarily dependent on the available surface area of absorption between the body fluids and the administered drug and, after oral treatment, on the period of time it is maintained in the gastro-intestinal tract. These are highly variable parameters, as was demonstrated in the intersubject spread of the MPA levels previously documented.

Surprisingly enough, these facts seem to have been overlooked in the past by those people who did not realize that high doses of MPA are necessary to obtain only relatively low MPA plasma levels. For instance, shown in Figure 1 are the plasma levels of tamoxifen, of its major metabolite, N-desmethyltamoxifen, and of MPA in a patient following simultaneous treatment with 'high' doses of MPA (2,000 mg/day), and 'low' doses of tamoxifen (20 mg/day). After 20 days of treatment, tamoxifen and N-desmethyltamoxifen levels are more than twice the corresponding MPA levels, and are still increasing. Differences both in the proportion of the drug which is absorbed and in the half-life of each drug are responsible for this behaviour.

All the relevant clinical data and the MPA plasma levels of the patients under MPA therapy are now recorded in our data bank (Fig. 2). For this

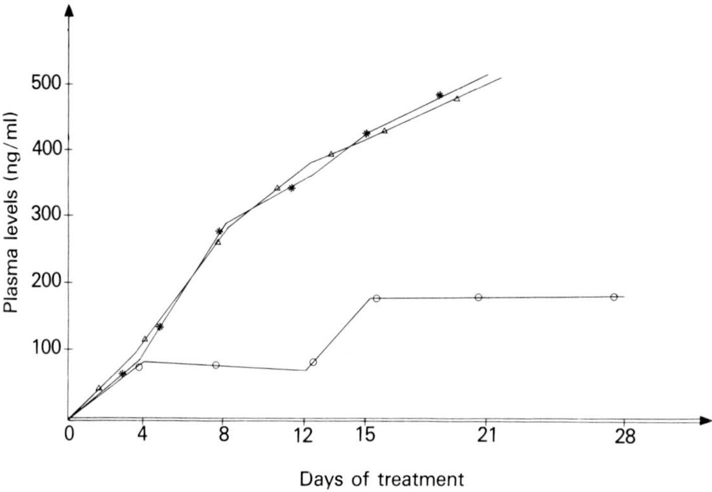

Fig. 1. Treatment with multiple oral doses of MPA (2,000 mg/day) and tamoxifen (20 mg/day): plasma levels of tamoxifen (△——△), N-desmethyl-tamoxifen (——*) and MPA (○——○).*

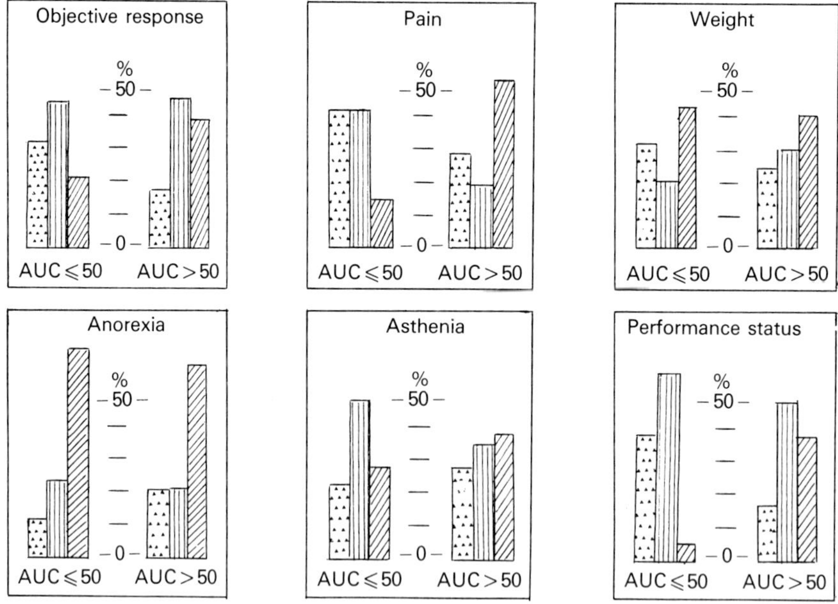

Fig. 2. MPA high doses in advanced cancer patients: clinical correlation with bioavailability (▦ = progression; ▥ = no change; ▨ = response).

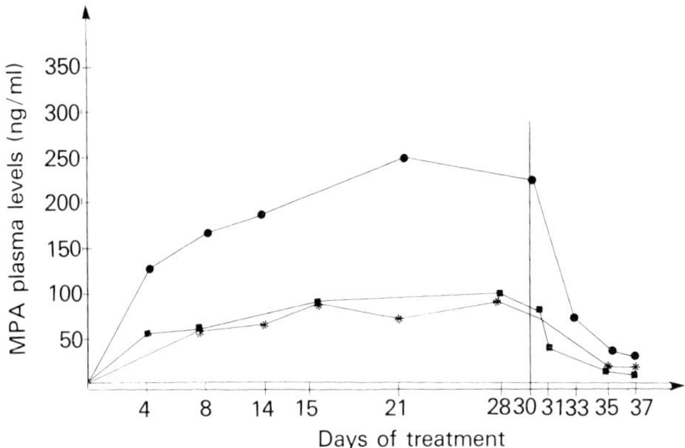

Fig. 3. MPA high doses in advanced cancer patients: MPA plasma levels for pain-response category ((•———•) = response; (———*) = progression; (■———■) = no change).*

study, the complete clinical history of 89 patients was available for any kind of univariate or multivariate analysis.

I would briefly like to review some preliminary results reported in Professor Pannuti's opening lecture.

First, the objective bio-availability/response correlation. Our patient sample was not sufficiently homogeneous and it was too limited (only 38 breast cancer patients) for extensive multivariate analysis to be undertaken. A definite trend towards better response was shown in the presence of better bio-availability, but it is not yet possible to define a therapeutic level. A better bio-availability/response correlation can be found in pain remission and in improvement in performance status.

Shown in Figure 3 are the means of the MPA plasma levels observed in patients with pain remission together with the corresponding levels for patients who showed no improvement. In this case it is possible to define a therapeutic range. The differences in the MPA plasma levels between the responders and the non-responders are statistically significant and were obtained in a random sample of 89 patients.

I.R. Hesselius: To be able to monitor the MPA levels during a clinical trial or otherwise in cancer treatment it is necessary to have laboratory facilities available. Could there perhaps be another way of drawing conclusions about the MPA treatment from the general endocrine effects?

C. Blossey: The definition of a 'therapeutic' plasma level of MPA seems to be very difficult. MPA is a hormone which is administered in g/day continuously – a unique feature of high-dose MPA therapy. There should be some endocrine reactions of the organism and we have tried to find out what correlations exist between the biological or endocrine response and the MPA plasma levels.

Since MPA is primarily a progestogen we have looked at the gonadotropins. Figure 1 shows the reaction of the gonadotropins in 3 patients with different endocrine situations. Depending on the increasing MPA plasma levels

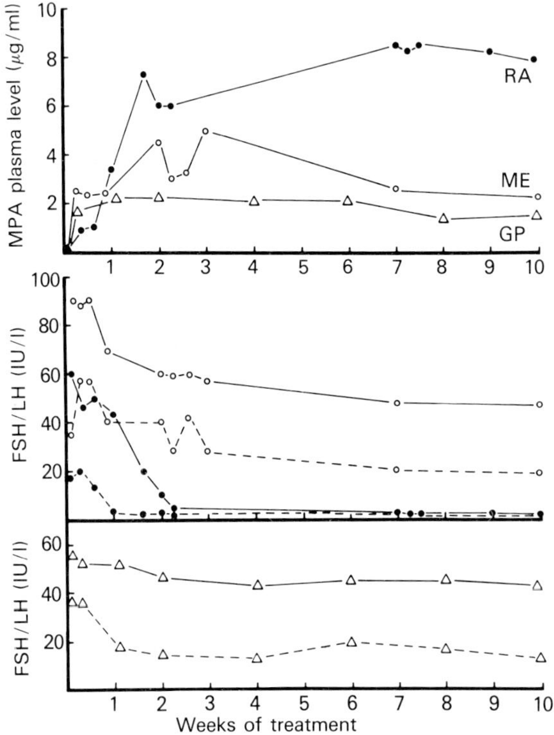

Fig. 1. Typical time course of MPA plasma levels, luteinizing hormone (LH), and follicle-stimulating hormone (FSH) in 3 patients with different endocrine situations. Upper panel: Initial kinetics and plateau state of MPA plasma levels. Middle and lower panels: Corresponding time courses of LH and FSH in a postmenopausal patient (•-----•/•———•); in an oöphorectomized patient (○-----○/○———○); and in a patient treated with MPA 1,500 mg/day, p.o., and aminoglutethimide 1,000 mg/day, p.o. (△-----△/△———△). The plateau state of MPA plasma levels in the patients is different, but in any case sufficient to suppress the gonadotropins.

(1,500 mg/day, p.o.) LH and FSH become typically suppressed. In the postmenopausal patients the gonadotropins are normally high and the suppression is complete after about 2 weeks of treatment. This situation remains stable also in long-term treatment without an escape phenomenon.

In the premenopausal oöphorectomized patients the suppressibility of the gonadotropins is markedly reduced. This phenomenon is more pronounced in the postmenopausal patients treated with the combination of MPA and aminoglutethimide, a non-steroidal, non-cytotoxic anticancer drug. One of the important pharmacological mechanisms of action of aminoglutethimide is the

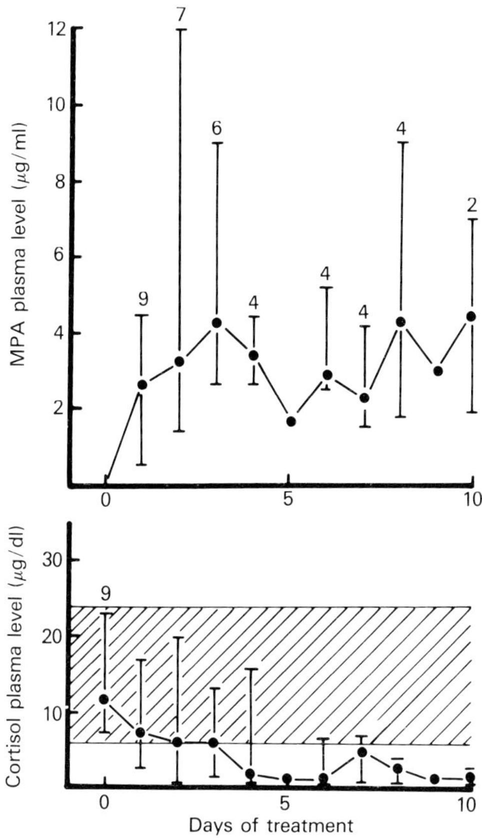

Fig. 2. Ranges and medians of the initial kinetics of MPA plasma levels and the corresponding cortisol plasma levels. Therapy schedule: MPA tablets 1,500 mg/day, p.o. The numbers on top of the ranges reflect the number of patients observed. The normal range of plasma cortisol in our laboratory is shown by the hatched area.

inhibition of the aromatase systems in the peripheral tissues. So there is a marked reduction in the circulating oestrogen levels mainly in the postmenopausal patients. A comparable oestrogen reduction is observed after oöphorectomy. The oöphorectomized patients and those treated with aminoglutethimide are both oestrogen-depleted very rapidly. In the sense of a regulatory mechanism on the pituitary level the sensitivity against progestogens seems to be modulated by the oestrogens. For the suppression of the gonadotropins by MPA a certain amount of oestrogens is apparently mandatory.

One of the predominant side-effects of MPA is based on its pronounced intrinsic glucocorticoid activity. Figure 2 shows the initial kinetics of high-dose MPA (1,500 mg/day, p.o.) in some patients. The corresponding ranges and medians of the endogenous cortisol secretion are given in the lower panel. The cortisol suppression is complete after about 5 days and remains stable even in long-term treatment with only a marginal basal secretion (Fig. 3).

Adrenocorticotropic hormone (ACTH) and, in consequence, cortisol are normally secreted in bursts periodically repeated every 30–60 minutes in a diurnal rhythm with a peak in the early morning. Figure 4 shows MPA plasma levels in the plateau state taken serially every hour. Plasma cortisol is nearly

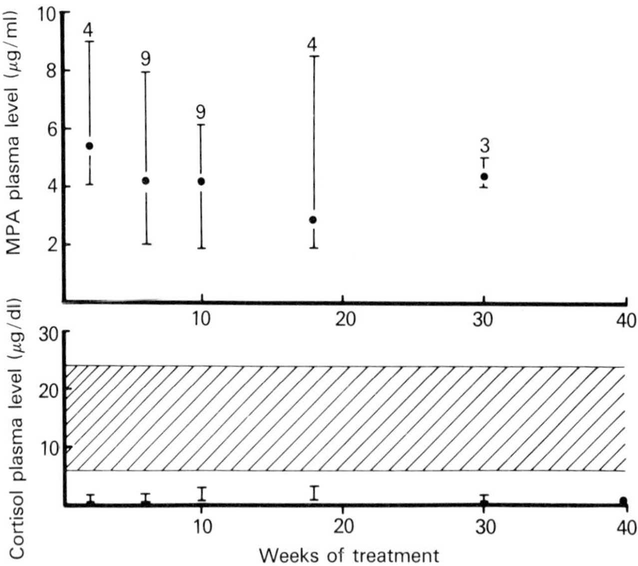

Fig. 3. Ranges and medians of MPA plasma levels and the corresponding cortisol plasma levels in long-term treatment (1,500 mg/day, p.o.). For details see legend to Fig. 2 and text.

completely suppressed with a minimal basal secretion and the basis for this is clearly the complete suppression of plasma ACTH. No burst or diurnal rhythm can be observed. The intrinsic glucocorticoid potency of MPA with the plasma levels shown here seems to be sufficient to replace endogenous cortisol production.

One of the central questions in high-dose MPA therapy is the relation between dosage and the 'therapeutic' plasma levels. With different therapy schedules and different forms of administration we looked at the endocrine response of the patients depending on the MPA plasma levels. Figure 5 shows

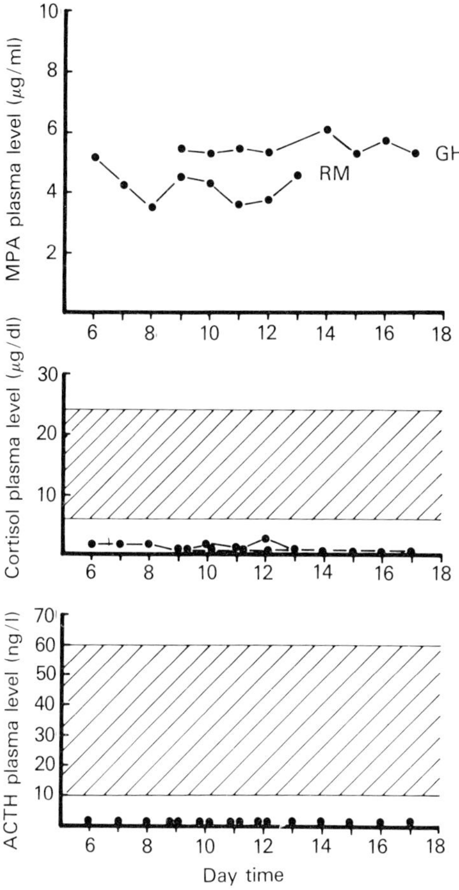

Fig. 4. MPA plasma levels in 2 patients in the plateau state and the corresponding plasma levels of cortisol and ACTH. Blood samples were taken serially.

the decrease of the MPA plasma levels after a dose reduction from 1,500 to 500 mg/day, p.o. (tablets). Correspondingly, the suppressibility of cortisol secretion is markedly diminished. In 3 patients, plasma cortisol is nearly normal and only in 2 patients the MPA plasma levels reached with 500 mg/day seem to be sufficient to suppress endogenous cortisol secretion. Two patients did not take their tablet regularly and the MPA plasma levels were low and plasma cortisol was normal. It is a great clinical problem to motivate the patients to ingest so many tablets for such a long time; we tried the oral administration of the crystal suspension normally used for the i.m. route. Figure 6 shows that the MPA plasma levels are somewhat lower than those reached with tablets, but they are more stable. The intra- and interindividual variability is not as large as can be observed during the therapy with the tablets. The endocrine response in terms of cortisol suppression is very efficient. The MPA plasma levels produced with 500 mg/day are not sufficient to suppress plasma cortisol. Within another therapy schedule MPA was administered by i.m. route. From the data given in Figure 7 it is absolutely clear that the MPA plasma levels are very low during this regimen and plasma cortisol is only marginally suppressed or mainly normal.

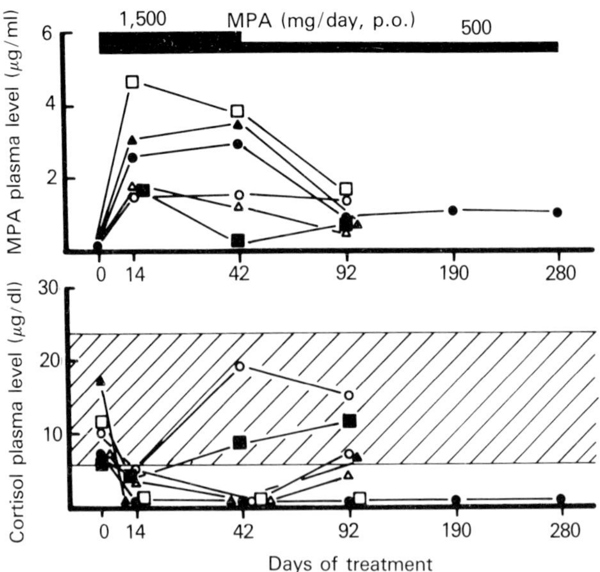

Fig. 5. MPA plasma levels and the corresponding cortisol plasma levels in a biphasic schedule. MPA was administered in tablets. Details are given in the legend to Fig. 2. Two patients (○——○, ■——■) did not take their tablets.

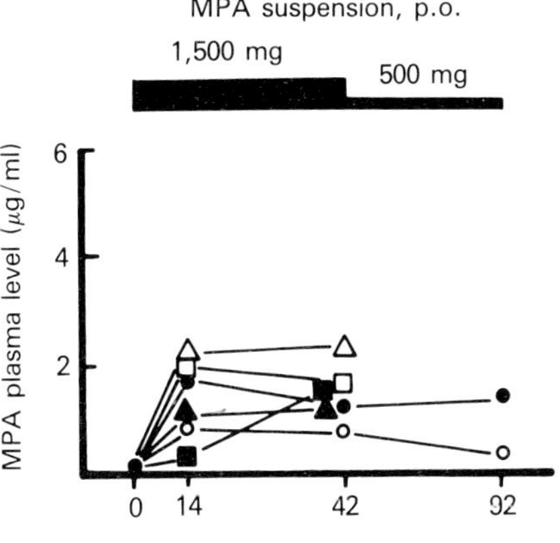

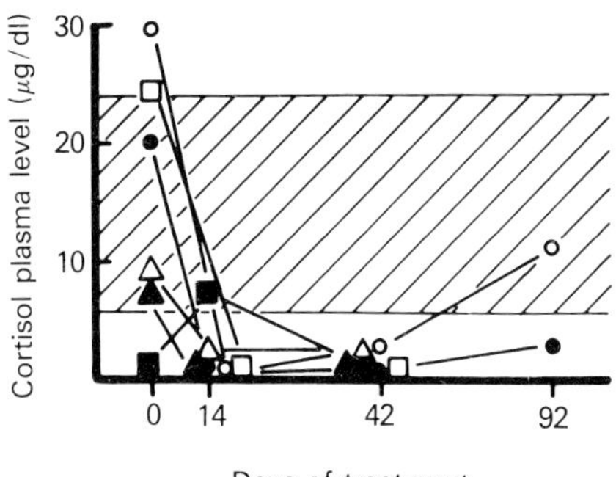

Fig. 6. MPA plasma levels and the corresponding cortisol plasma levels in a biphasic schedule. MPA was administered with the crystal suspension, p.o.

The crucial question is: What is the significance of cortisol suppression by MPA? We have the impression that the 'therapeutic' MPA plasma levels and the MPA levels for cortisol suppression are identical or at least closely related. Whether this is causative or just accidental is not clear. This may be an interesting aspect in the discussion of the mechanism of action of MPA.

The intrinsic glucocorticoid activity of MPA was used for the replacement of the obligate cortisol substitution in aminoglutethimide therapy. Briefly, aminoglutethimide blocks the 20,21 desmolase step in the adrenals which means the conversion of cholesterol to pregnenolone. Endogenous cortisol synthesis is impaired and a substitution therapy mandatory. Figure 8 shows that in MPA monotherapy (1,500 mg/day, p.o., tablets) cortisol and ACTH

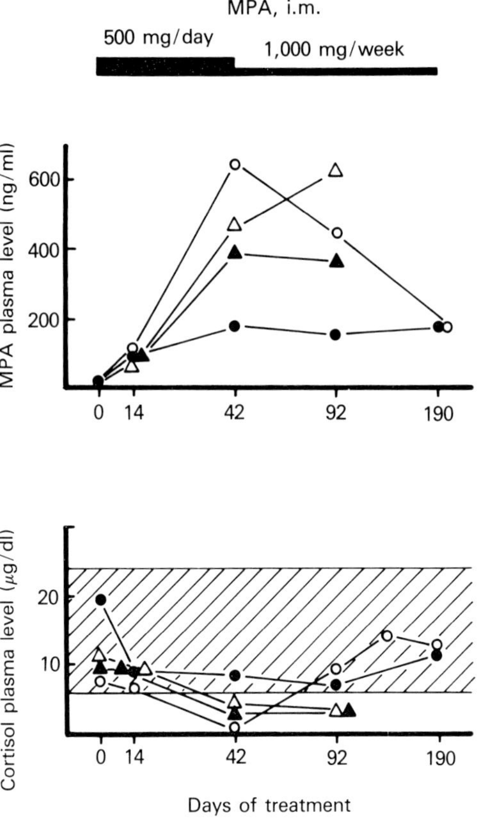

Fig. 7. MPA plasma levels and the corresponding cortisol plasma levels in a biphasic schedule. MPA was administered with the crystal suspension, i.m.

are suppressed. In the combination therapy, aminoglutethimide + MPA, endogenous ACTH and cortisol are normal with a broad variation. This is essentially what was found in the classical aminoglutethimide-hydrocortisone combination. So MPA can replace the obligate glucocorticoid in aminoglutethimide therapy, and the combination of the 2 non-cytotoxic anticancer drugs is possibly revealing additional antitumour activities.

The biological response of the organism in high-dose MPA therapy does reflect in a very reliable manner a certain, endocrinally-active plasma level of the drug. This may be another approach to evaluate the 'therapeutic' MPA plasma levels and may lead to a better understanding of the modalities and mechanisms of this therapy.

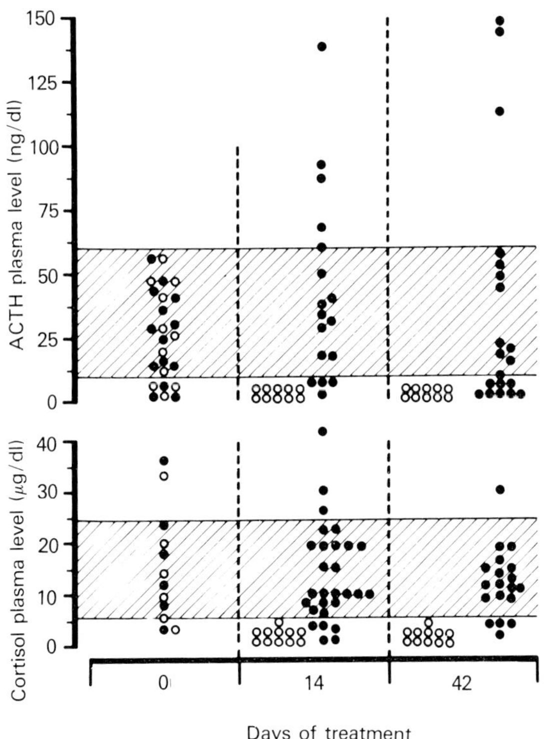

Fig. 8. Plasma ACTH and cortisol in MPA monotherapy ((○), 1,500 mg/day) and in the combination therapy with aminoglutethimide ((•), 1,000–1,500 mg/day).

I.R. Hesselius: In various reports the blood levels of MPA obtained after the same doses are different. Could such differences be due to different laboratory methods for MPA determination?

V. Kozyreff: Shown in Figure 1 is a follow-up study of the MPA serum levels obtained, using 2 different laboratory techniques. The patients received MPA, 500 mg twice a week, i.m. In each blood sample (taken at the times shown), MPA was determined in 2 separate laboratories. In our laboratory, a gas-liquid chromatography (GLC) method was used, and in the Farmitalia laboratory in Milan a radio-immunoassay (RIA) technique was used. The GLC method is a modification of that of Kaiser et al. [1], and the RIA technique is that described by Shrimanker et al. [2].

The literature contains studies that use various RIA methods. These differ from one another by the presence or absence of an extraction procedure, by the type of extraction, when present, and by the origin of the antibodies. As a consequence, many of the published RIA results are not directly comparable with others. It is accepted as a reasonable hypothesis that the difference between the GLC and the RIA results is related to the presence of metabolites which seem to occur in very high concentrations. They will be more or less extracted, depending on which method is used, and will more or less cross-react with MPA, depending on which antibodies are used.

In the present case, the 2 methods used give results that are in close agreement. The absolute values are highly comparable in the 2 curves, which are remarkably parallel – except for the end of the observation.

Several patients were studied in this way, using the 2 MPA determination methods.

Shown in Figure 2 is the correlation study of a sample of such paired determinations. The RIA values are represented as a function of the GLC values, and the regression line is given. The calculated linear correlation coefficient is 0.735, giving an r^2 value of about 0.5 – indicating thus that relatively little can be predicted from the individual RIA values if only the GLC value is given, and vice versa. The regression coefficient of 1.14 shows that the average agreement between the 2 sets of values is good.

We believe that some factors, specific to the patient, related to the moment at which the comparison is made in the course of treatment, or perhaps to the

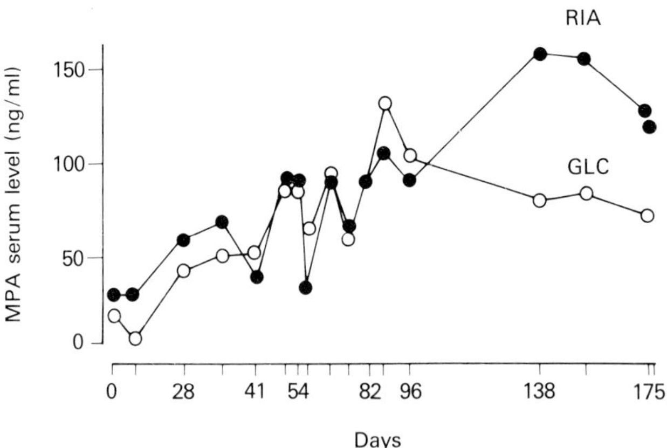

Fig. 1. MPA serum levels obtained with 2 different laboratory techniques – radio-immunoassay (RIA) and gas-liquid chromatography (GLC).

mode of MPA administration, could affect the ratio of the 2 values, GLC to RIA.

Figures 3–5 are illustrations of other parallel studies, done in collaboration with the group of Professor Mangioni, in Milan, in which Dr Landoni, of the Istituto Mario Negri was particularly active. In this work, MPA was given by the oral route. The corresponding curves suggest that the ratio between the 2 sets of values may be a function of the individual patient metabolism of the drug. It is remarkable that, although the ratio seems to vary from one patient to another, it seems to be much more constant for a given patient or for a given route of administration. As far as the latter is concerned, the present observations show a greater difference between the 2 groups of values in the cases where the drug was given orally, as though more metabolites were pres-

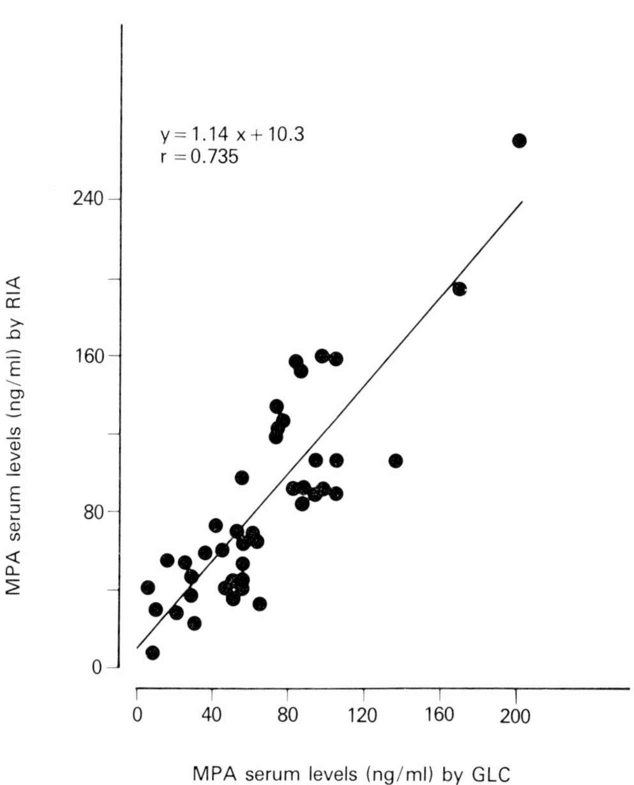

Fig. 2. Correlation between RIA and GLC values obtained from one sample.

ent. We think that this may reflect the personal way in which the patients react to the treatment, as far as the metabolism of the drug is concerned, and that the latter may be a function of time and of the route of administration.

If this hypothesis should be confirmed, it may appear that these mechanisms are to be taken into account, while studying or investigating the efficacy of the drug, and that more conclusive results will be obtained.

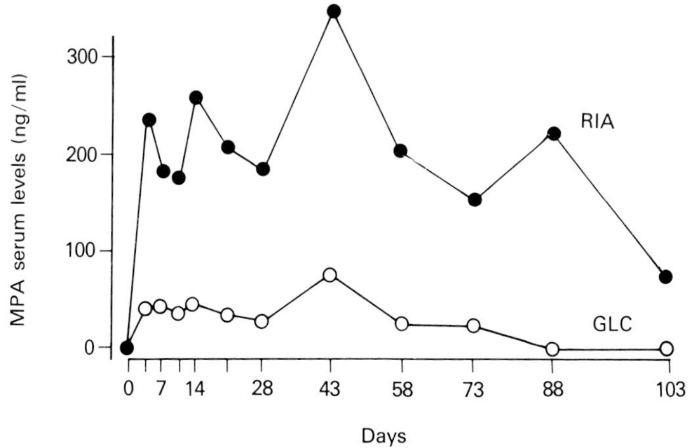

Fig. 3. MPA serum levels obtained with RIA and GLC; results from one patient.

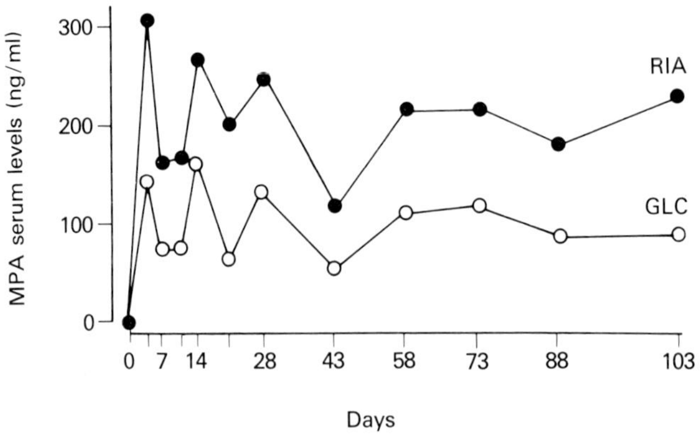

Fig. 4. MPA serum levels obtained with RIA and GLC; results from one patient.

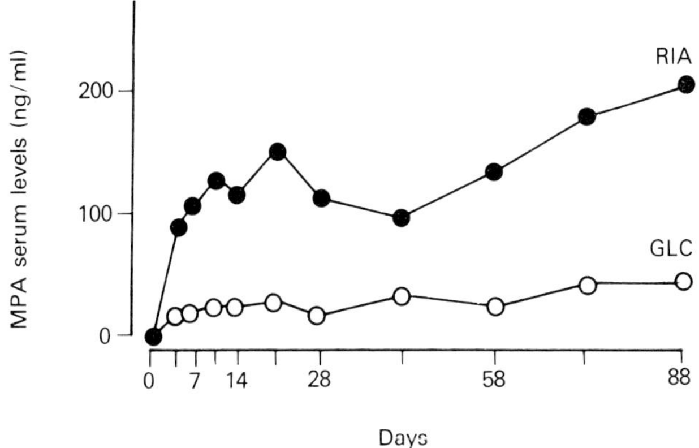

Fig. 5. MPA serum levels obtained with RIA and GLC; results from one patient.

References

1. Kaiser, D.G., Carlson, R.C. and Kirton, K.T. (1974): GLC determination of medroxyprogesterone acetate in plasma. *J. Pharm. Sci. 63,* 420.
2. Shrimanker, K., Saxena, B.N. and Fotherby, K. (1977): A radioimmunoassay for serum medroxyprogesterone acetate. *J. Steroid Biochem. 9,* 359.

I.R. Hesselius: The difference between oral and i.m. administration of MPA has been well elucidated during this session. The same doses give completely different blood levels.

As a final question to the panelists as well as to the audience: which is the best method of administration in order to obtain an optimal blood level of MPA in the treatment of cancer?

V. Tamassia: With regard to the problem of the dose schedule for i.m. MPA, Figure 1 shows that the one-month duration of the loading phase is not strictly necessary. Similar plasma levels at the end of the loading phase can be reached with 500 mg/day for one month, 1,000 mg/day for 2 weeks or 1,000 mg twice a day for one week because, on a short-term basis, the main determinant of the MPA plasma levels is the cumulative i.m. dose.

One may wonder whether and how the 2 routes of administration can be combined. From the plasma level profile point of view, there are combinations which should be avoided because they are not rational combinations. I mainly refer to the following: first, an initial treatment with oral daily doses,

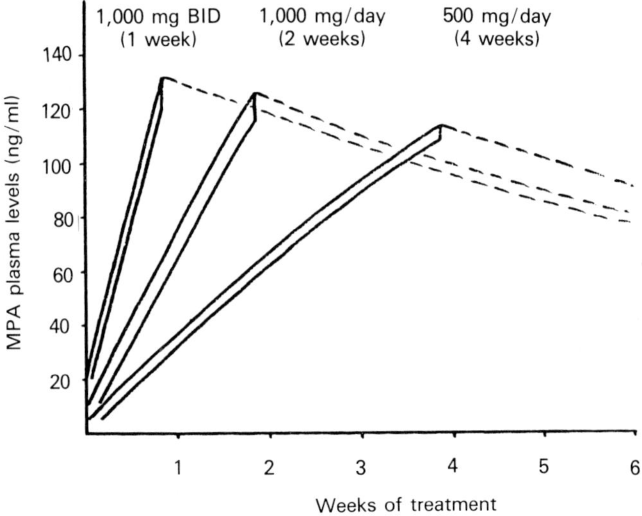

Fig. 1. *MPA plasma level profile predicted during 3 different loading i.m. treatments characterized by the same cumulative loading dose (14 g = 500 mg/day × 4 weeks = 1,000 mg/day × 2 weeks = 2,000 mg/day × 1 week).*

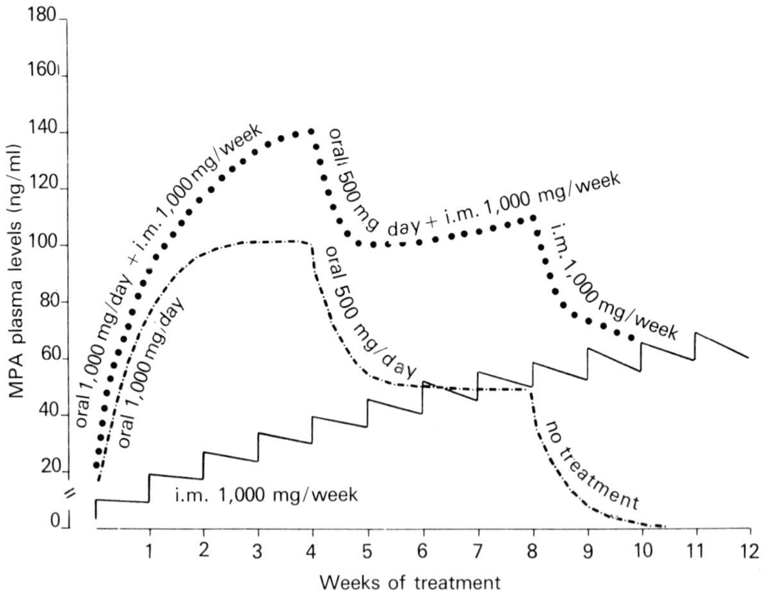

Fig. 2. *MPA plasma level profile during a combined oral and i.m. treatment.*

followed by maintenance therapy with weekly injections. This is irrational because the interruption of the oral daily dose will be followed by a rapid decrease of the plasma levels which will not be counterbalanced for several weeks because of the very low plasma levels achieved initially with weekly i.m. injections.

The second dose schedule to avoid is a loading treatment with i.m. daily doses, followed by maintenance therapy with oral daily doses. This is because, in the short term, the oral daily doses will simply increase the sustained plasma levels achieved after the loading i.m. treatment, whereas, in the long term, there will be only the contribution of oral MPA.

A possible rational combination of the 2 routes of administration is the following: a basic treatment with weekly injections (1,000 mg) to exploit the good maintenance properties of i.m. administration, plus an initial treatment with daily oral doses for one month (1,000 mg/day), followed by 500 mg/day for another month (Fig. 2). The plasma levels which can be achieved using this combined dose schedule are of the same order of magnitude of those achieved with the previously-shown equipotent oral or i.m. dose schedules.

C.M. Camaggi: There are well-defined clinical indications that i.m. treatment generally yields better results, and in particular better long-term results. Professor Pannuti reported his findings in this field extensively in his opening lecture.

The pharmacokinetics explain the results. After i.m. administration MPA is slowly but completely absorbed, and the plateau levels are higher than after oral administration and are maintained for a longer time.

On the other hand, i.m. administration has 2 main drawbacks: 1. The rather long time required to reach sufficiently-high plasma levels. 2. The impossibility to really discontinue the treatment because of lack of response. This is because even after the last dose the depot effect maintains high MPA plasma levels for some weeks.

In my opinion, oral treatment with massive MPA doses is more suitable for obtaining immediate high plasma levels, whereas i.m. administration is better suited for maintenance therapy. However, rather than suggesting a particular treatment schedule, I would like to propose that controlled clinical studies are performed in order to test the clinical relevance of the experimental data presented at this meeting. I.m. and oral treatments must be compared by taking into account the pharmacokinetic properties of both methods.

A controlled clinical study is now in progress in our institute, in which equipotent i.m. and oral treatments are used and the MPA plasma levels are monitored.

Session III: Breast cancer

Chairmen: R.A. Estevez – Buenos Aires, Argentina
F. Pannuti – Bologna, Italy

Introduction

We were fortunate to have had the opportunity yesterday to hear Professor Pannuti talking about the mechanism of action and the clinical uses of MPA. Professor Pannuti clearly stressed the questions and the problems in the use of MPA: the relationship (if there is one) between the doses used and the percentage of results achieved, the necessity to take into account the subjective results, in particular the improvement in weight and the lack of myelotoxicity which are really useful. For these reasons this session must include experts in different aspects of the use of MPA in advanced breas cancer.

R.A. Estevez

Treatment of advanced breast cancer with 2 different high doses of medroxyprogesterone acetate

H. Cortés Funes[1], M. Méndez[1], P.L. Madrigal[2] and A. Alonso[2]
[1]Hospital '1° de Octubre'; and [2]Hospital Oncologico Provincial, Madrid, Spain

Introduction

Medroxyprogesterone acetate (MPA) has been shown to be an effective drug in advanced breast cancer. At low dosages (less than 500 mg/day), response rates in terms of objective remission never exceeded 25%. In 1972, several investigators began studies on the use of doses equal to or greater than 500 mg/day. The maximum tolerable dose was identified as 1,500 mg/day, intramuscularly (i.m.), for 30 days [1]. Objective remission rates at these higher doses ranged from 30–50%. The improvement was attributable to several factors, which have been studied in recent years. They include the fact of higher dosage previous therapy, menopausal status, and response criteria.

In connection with dosage, there are 2 important controlled studies. Robustelli et al. compared a daily dosage of 500 mg with a daily dosage of 1,000 mg in 101 postmenopausal women who had not previously received chemotherapy [2]. There was effectively no difference between response rates in the 2 groups of patients: 43% of patients showed objective remission in the 500 mg group, and 41% showed objective remission with the 1,000 mg/day regimen. In this trial, cases with skeletal and soft-tissue metastases responded best. The mean durations of response were 8 months for the 500-mg regimen, and 9 months for the 1,000-mg regimen.

In the other study, Pannuti et al. treated 92 patients at random with 500 mg MPA/day or 1,500 mg of MPA/day, i.m., for 30 days [3]. These patients had also not previously been treated with combination chemotherapy. The overall response rate was 44%. There was no significant difference in response rates between the 2 regimens (43% and 54%, respectively). However, differences were noted as regards side-effects. The 500-mg/day regimen had less side-effects, and was better tolerated.

Three other investigators have studied the anti-tumour effect of high-dosage MPA, in patients previously treated with chemotherapy. Lower objective remission rates were obtained.

De Lena et al. treated 81 patients with 2 dosage regimens of MPA in an uncontrolled study [4]. Objective remission was obtained in 21% of patients treated with 1,500 mg/day, and in 32% of patients treated with 1,000 mg/day. The median durations of response were 5 months and 7.5 months, respectively.

Amadori et al. treated 74 patients with a dosage of 1,000 mg/day, and obtained a 45% objective remission rate [5]. All patients were postmenopausal, and had relapsed after previous combination chemotherapy and hormonotherapy.

In a group of 25 breast cancer patients studied by Mattson a remission rate of 28%, with a median duration of remission of over 5 months was obtained [6].

In an early study by our group, Mendiola et al. obtained a 22% remission rate, in 27 intensively pretreated patients, and a median duration of response of 6.5 months [7].

In the present study, we have tried to determine the effects of previous therapies in patients treated with 1,000 mg of MPA/day, and have compared the results with those in a similar group of patients treated with the standard high dose of 500 mg of MPA/day.

Material and methods

Patients with metastatic breast cancer, resistant, in most cases, to conventional therapy, were enrolled. Both pre- and postmenopausal women, with measurable and/or evaluable metastases, expectation of survival of up to 3 months, and a Karnofsky performance status index of up to 50% were eligible for enrolment.

Patients were treated in 2 institutions with doses of 500 mg or 1,000 mg of MPA administered daily, i.m., for 30 consecutive days. After this induction period, patients responding continued treatment at the same dosage, twice a week, until relapse. The characteristics of both groups are shown in Table I. The 2 groups of patients were similar in relation to predominant sites of metastases, previous therapy, menopausal status and age. There was a small difference of 6 months in the median disease-free interval.

When progressive disease was recorded, therapy different from that used previously was administered. The results were assessed every fourth week for 12 weeks by means of physical examination, determination of Karnofsky in-

Table I. Patient characteristics .

	Treatment		Total
	MPA 500 mg	MPA 1,000 mg	
Numbers	46	43	89
Median age (years)	56	59	575
Premenopausal patients	15	10	25
Postmenopausal patients	31	33	64
Disease-free interval (months)	31	25	28
Predominant site of metastases			
Soft tissues	22	20	42
Visceral	7	8	15
Osseous	12	12	24
Other	5	3	8
Previous treatment			
Chemotherapy alone	11	8	19
Hormonotherapy alone	8	9	17
Chemotherapy + hormonotherapy	18	14	32
None	9	12	21

dex, chest X-ray and laboratory investigations (complete blood count and biochemical profile-SMAC). Bone and liver isotope scans were repeated every 3 months. Oestrogen and progesterone receptor determinations were performed in some patients using the charcoal method, but the results were not used in analysing responses.

Therapeutic response was evaluated according to the following criteria:
a. Complete remission: disappearance of all disease, and radiological recalcification of lytic bone lesions.
b. Partial remission: more than 50% decrease in size of measurable lesions, and objective improvement in evaluable but nonmeasurable lesions, if no new lesions occurred.
c. Stabilization or no change: recorded when lesions were unchanged in size (by less than 50% or more than 25% in cases with measurable lesions).
d. Progressive disease: recorded when some lesions regress while others progress, or new lesions appeared, or when some or all of the lesions progressed and/or new lesions appeared.

Subjective improvement was also analysed, but was not used in evaluating response. Subjective improvement included relief of pain, improvement in asthenia, anorexia and performance status, and increase in weight.

Durations of remission and survival are recorded from the day of commencement of therapy.

Results

Analysis of the results failed to reveal any statistically significant difference between the 2 treatment groups.

Twenty-eight patients (31.5%) experienced objective responses, with 6 (6.7%) complete remissions and 22 (25%) partial remissions (Table II). Response overall was a little lower (28%) in patients treated with 500 mg as compared with that in patients treated with 1,000 mg (35%) but the incidence of complete responses was more than twice as great in the latter group (9% as against 4%). There was stabilization of the disease in 30% of the patients in the 500-mg group and in 26% of the patients in the 1,000-mg group.

The response by predominant metastatic site is recorded in Table III. Here also, there were no significant differences between the 2 groups in any subclass of patients. In patients with soft-tissue metastases the percentage response overall was 18% in the 500-mg group and 25% in the 1,000-mg group. In patients with bony metastases, the response rate was 50% in both groups of patients, and, in the group with predominantly visceral metastases, there was a small difference in favour of the higher dose (37% as against 28%).

In premenopausal patients, the response rate was 16%, lower than in postmenopausal patients, where it was 37%.

There were no differences in the average durations of remission between the subclasses of patients in the 2 treatment groups (range 2–23 months).

Table IV shows subjective remission in relation to dose. The significant reduction in pain in 65% of all cases is noteworthy. This effect was greater in patients receiving 1,000 mg (77%) than in patients receiving 500 mg (54%).

Table II. Response to therapy (numbers of patients (%)).

Response	Treatment			
	MPA 500 mg		MPA 1,000 mg	
Complete remission	2	(4)	4	(9)
Partial remission	11	(24)	11	(25)
Overall response	13	(28)	15	(35)
Stabilization	4	(30)	11	(26)
Progression	19	(41)	17	(39)

Table III. Response in relation to predominant metastatic site (numbers of patients (%)).

Metastatic site	Treatment													
	MPA 500 mg						MPA 1,000 mg						
	Numbers of patients	CR	+	PR[1]	NC[2]	P[3]	Numbers of patients	CR	+	PR[1]	NC[2]	P[3]
Soft tissue	22	1		3	9	9	20	2		3	7	8
			(18)		(41)	(41)			(25)		(35)	(40)
Visceral	7	—		2	2	3	8	1		2	2	3
			(28)		(28.5)	(43)			(37)		(25)	(37)
Osseous	12	1		5	3	3	12	1		5	2	4
			(50)		(25)	(25)			(50)		(17)	(33)
Other	5	—		1	—	4	3	—		1	—	2
			(28)			(80)			(33)			(67)
Totals	46	2		11	14	19	43	4		11	11	17
			(28)		(30)	(41)			(35)		(26)	(39)

[1]CR + PR = complete remission + partial remission;
[2]NC = no change;
[3]P = progression.

Subjective responses were otherwise very similar for both groups of patients.

Response in relation to previous treatment is shown in Table V. The response rate was slightly higher in patients without prior therapy (38%) than in those previously treated with chemotherapy (31%), hormonotherapy (35%) or both (25%). MPA did not appear to exhibit cross resistance in relation to these types of treatment.

Median duration of response was 6.8 months. There was effectively no difference between the 2 regimens (7.3 months and 6.4 months).

Clinical toxicity related to treatment is shown in Table VI. There was no difference in the incidence of side-effects between the 2 groups of patients.

Table IV. Subjective response (cases showing symptoms indicated (%)).

Subjective response	Treatment	
	MPA 500 mg	MPA 1,000 mg
Pain	54	77
Asthenia	39	44
Anorexia	52	56
Performance status impairment	37	42
Weight increase	67	72

Table V. Response in relation to previous treatment.

Prior therapy	Numbers of patients	Response to prior therapy (%)	Numbers of patients	Response to MPA (CR + PR)[1] (%)
Hormonotherapy (castration, antiandrogens, androgens, oestrogens)	17	22	6	(35)
Chemotherapy (CMF – CMFVP – CAF)	19	48	6	(31)
Hormonotherapy + chemotherapy	32	47	8	(25)
None	21	—	8	(38)
Totals	89	—	28	(31.5)

[1]CR + PR = complete remission + partial remission.

Table VI. Toxicity (incidence of side-effects indicated (%)).

Side-effects	Treatment	
	MPA 500 mg	MPA 1,000 mg
Gluteal abscess	10	11
Sweating	12	13
Cushingoid face	17	19
Tremor	13	12
Cramps	7	8
Vaginal bleeding	6	7
Thrombophlebitis	2	0

Gluteal abscess was the only side-effect which limited continuation of the treatment. It occurred in 10 and 11% of patients in the 2 groups. Other toxic effects, such as moon face, sweating, tremor and cramps, were tolerable and reversible.

Discussion

The results of this study confirm the therapeutic efficacy of high dosage of MPA in advanced breast cancer.

The global response rate is slightly higher (31.5%) than in our previous study (22%), probably because the performance status of the patients was better. There was a predominance of soft-tissue metastases (48%), as opposed to 26% osseous metastases and 16% visceral metastases. This could also explain the lower response rate obtained in this study than in the previous studies of Robustelli and Pannuti mentioned previously.

The overall response rate in patients treated with 1,000 mg/day was higher (35%) than in patients treated with 500 mg/day (28%), with 9% and 4% of complete remissions, respectively. This difference is not significant, but subjective improvement was much better in patients in the higher dose group, particularly as regards pain relief.

The analysis of response in relation to previous treatment shows that patients who had responded to hormonotherapy had a better response rate to MPA (35%) than patients previously treated with chemotherapy alone (31%) or combined with hormonotherapy (25%). Patients not previously treated had the best response rate (38%).

The remaining factor influencing response rate with high dose MPA is menopausal status. As with other hormonotherapies, premenopausal patients are less responsive to MPA than postmenopausal patients.

On the basis of these data, and reports in the literature, we conclude that high doses of MPA result in good objective response rates in patients with advanced breast cancer [8]. Response rates are directly related to the localization of metastases, previous treatment and menopausal status, but have no relation to dosage, if this is above 500 mg. A dosage of 1,000 mg of MPA/day has a better analgesic effect than 500 mg of MPA/day, with the same incidence of side-effects.

Further studies of MPA together with combination chemotherapy, or additional hormonotherapy, to clarify more precisely the role of MPA in the management of advanced breast cancer are desirable.

References

1. Pannuti, F., Martoni, A., Lenaz, G.R. et al. (1976): Management of advanced breast cancer with medroxyprogesterone acetate (MPA, F.I 5837, F.I.7001, NSC 26386) in high doses. In: *Functional Exploration in Senology,* pp. 243–265. European Press, Ghent.
2. Robustelli Della Cuna, G., Calciati, S., Bernardo-Strada, M.R. et al. (1978): High dose medroxyprogesterone acetate (MPA) treatment in metastatic carcinoma of the breast. A response evaluation. *Tumori 64,* 143.
3. Pannutti, F., Martoni, A., Di Marco, A.R. et al. (1979): A randomized trial of two different dosages of medroxyprogesterone acetate (MPA) in the treatment of metastatic breast cancer. *Eur. J. Cancer 15,* 593.
4. De Lena, M., Brambilla, C., Valagussa, P. and Bonadonna, G. (1978): High dose medroxyprogesterone acetate (MPA) in metastatic breast cancer. *Chemother. Pharmacol. 2,* 180.
5. Amadori, D., Ravaioli, A. and Barbanti, F. (1976): L'impiego del medrossiprogesterone acetato ad alti dosaggi nella terapia palliativa del carcinoma mammario in fase avanzate. *Minerva Med. 67, 1.*
6. Mattson, W. (1978): High dose medroxyprogesterone acetate treatment in advanced mammary carcinoma. A phase II investigation. *Acta Radiol. Oncol. 17,* 387.
7. Mendiola, C., Mañas, A., Ramos, A. et al. (1979): Medroxiprogesterone acetato (MPA) a altas dosis como tratamiento del carcinoma de mama avanzado resistente. *Oncología-80 3,* 21.
8. Ganzina, F. (1979): High-dose medroxyprogesterone acetate (MPA) treatment in advanced breast cancer. A review. *Tumori 65*, 563.

Discussion

M. Kjaer (Copenhagen, Denmark): Dr Cortes Funes said that he had a significant proportion of patients with stabilisation of their disease. What exactly does he mean by 'stabilisation'?

H. Cortés Funes: A response rate of less than 50% reduction of the tumour mass.

M. Kjaer: Dr Cortes Funes also said that he had a significant proportion of pain reduction. How was pain reduction measured? I know that it is very difficult to measure it...

H. Cortés Funes: It is enormously difficult. Sometimes the Scott-Huskisson system was used to measure pain, and sometimes it was only measured by questioning the patients.

Low- versus high-dose medroxyprogesterone acetate in the treatment of advanced breast cancer

F. Cavalli[1], A. Goldhirsch[2], W.F. Jungi[3], G. Martz[4] and P. Alberto[5]*

[1]Department of Oncology, San Giovanni Hospital, Bellinzona; [2]Institute for Medical Oncology, Insel Hospital, Berne; [3]Department of Oncology, Medical Clinic C, Cantonal Hospital, St. Gallen; [4]Department of Oncology, University Hospital, Zurich; and [5]Department of Oncology, Cantonal Hospital, Geneva, Switzerland

Introduction

Progestins, particularly medroxyprogesterone acetate (MPA), have been used for a relatively long time in the treatment of patients with disseminated breast cancer. In the literature, the response rate reported for MPA ranges from 0–36%, with a tendency for it to be below 20% in the larger series [1–6]. SAKK used MPA at a dose of 500 mg intramuscularly (i.m.), weekly, in a trial in which chemotherapy was compared with chemotherapy combined with hormonal therapy. This trial was not particularly suitable for evaluation of the role of MPA. Nevertheless, the results were somewhat disappointing [7]. However, in recent years, a renewed interest in MPA in the treatment of advanced breast cancer has been prompted by the data published by Pannuti et al. [8] and Robustelli et al. [9], who reported a response rate of over 40% using high doses of MPA (1 g per day or more).

We therefore decided to embark on a pilot study, treating 19 patients with far-advanced breast cancer, who had already been intensively treated, with 1 g MPA daily, for 4 weeks [10]. The promising results in this trial (6 partial remissions (PRs)) encouraged SAKK to set up a controlled trial to compare low and high doses of MPA in the treatment of advanced breast cancer. In this paper, we report the preliminary results of this trial, which, for some subsets of patients, has already been closed. As is usual in cooperative trials,

* (For the Swiss Group for Clinical Cancer Research (SAKK)).

much data still has to be reviewed. In addition, an independent review of most cases is currently being carried out.

Patients and methods

Selection of patients

All patients selected for this trial had advanced, measurable breast cancer. Osteoblastic bony metastases and malignant effusions were not considered to be evaluable lesions. All patients were postmenopausal. Patients below the age of 65 were accepted only if they had been pretreated with chemotherapy and/or hormones. Patients above the age of 65 could enter the study even if previously untreated. Patients with brain metastases, with a performance status >3 (Eastern Co-operative Oncology Group/SAKK scale) or with another life-threatening disease were excluded from the study.

Patients were allocated at random either to regimen A (1 g MPA i.m. daily, except Saturdays and Sundays, for 4 weeks, or to regimen B (500 mg MPA i.m. twice weekly for 4 weeks). The protocol called for treatment for 4 weeks unless life-threatening progression occurred earlier. The patients were evaluated at the end of the fourth week of treatment. Patients showing progression of disease then left the study. Patients responding, or those showing stabilization of the disease, at least, (i.e. no change (NC)) subsequently received maintenance treatment with 500 mg of MPA i.m., once weekly. This maintenance treatment was continued until a progression occurred. In defining PR, NC and progression of disease (PD), standard criteria were used [11].

Between September 1979 and November 1981, 181 patients were enrolled into the trial (91 regimen A, 90 regimen B). At the last evaluation (November 15th, 1981), 6 patients had not been on treatment long enough for a clinical assessment of antitumour activity (under 4 weeks of treatment). Twenty-three patients were not evaluable for various reasons. In 4 instances (2 cases in regimen A, 2 cases in regimen B) the patients refused to continue treatment. Twelve patients (7 on regimen A, 5 on regimen B) were excluded from analysis because of major deviations from protocol. These included poorly assessable or nonevaluable lesions, and transfer to oral MPA treatment during induction treatment. The remaining 7 cases were not evaluable because of death less than 4 weeks after starting the treatment. In most cases, these patients had a poorer performance status than that called for by the protocol.

Table I summarizes the main characteristics of the 152 remaining patients. The 2 treatment groups were fairly comparable in terms of mean age, mean disease-free interval, predominant site of disease, mean number of known

Table I. Pretreatment characteristics of evaluable patients.

	Dosage regimen	
	A	B
Numbers of patients	76	76
Mean age (years)	60.9 (40–85)	59.5 (27–83)
Mean disease-free interval (months)	33.7 (0–185)	28.3 (1–180)
Predominant site of metastases (numbers of patients)		
loco-regional	15	13
soft tissue	12	14
osseous	29	26
visceral	20	23
Mean number of metastatic sites	2.2	2.3
Previous chemotherapy and response (numbers of patients)		
no response	19	12
CR	12	15
NC	3	7
PD	24	21
not evaluable because of concurrent hormonal therapy	17	21
Previous hormone therapy and response (numbers of patients)		
no response	13	12
CR	19	25
NC	7	4
PD	24	26
not evaluable because of concurrent chemotherapy	13	9

metastatic sites, previous therapy, and response to previous treatment. Differences in respect of individual prognostic factors were minimal. It is nevertheless, interesting to note that there were somewhat more responders to previous chemotherapy or previous hormonal treatment among the patients allocated at random to the low-dose regimen. In about one-third of cases, the outcome of previous treatment could not be attributed to any one therapeutic modality, since the patients had received chemotherapy and hormonal therapy concurrently.

In the course of this trial, ancillary pharmacokinetic and endocrinological studies, which will be reported in detail elsewhere, were performed. In 10 patients, MPA blood levels were monitored up to the fourth month of treatment. Five of these patients were treated with the low-dose MPA, the other 5 with high-dose MPA. Blood samples were taken from 21 patients and luteinizing hormone (LH), follicle stimulating hormone (FSH), prolactin, androstenedione, sex hormone-binding globulin (SHBG), hydrocortisone and oestradiol (E_1) determined before treatment and 4 and 8 weeks after starting treatment.

Results

Table II shows the therapeutic results in the 2 groups receiving the different doses of MPA. While at this preliminary stage fewer than 20% of patients in either group showed stabilization of disease, the group treated with high-dose MPA shows significantly more remissions (24/76, 31%) than the group treated with low-dose MPA (8/76, 11%). This difference is statistically significant ($P<0.01$).

The median time to progression, calculated from the beginning of treatment, is 368 days for all patients responding. Progression of the disease was observed in all patients showing only NC after a median period of 157 days. The actuarial curves for both PR and NC are practically superposable for the 2 treatments.

Patients responding to treatment, or those showing stabilization of disease, at least, have yet to reach the median value on their survival curve: the median survival time is 220 days for patients progressing under treatment with MPA.

Table II. Therapeutic outcome.

Response	Treatment group	Numbers of patients showing response indicated	Numbers of patients in treatment group	Percentage of patients showing response indicated
PR	A	24	76	31
PR	B	8	76	11
NC	A	21	76	28
NC	B	18	76	24

Table III outlines the characteristics of the patients responding. With regard to the predominant site of the disease, therapeutic responses were mostly achieved in patients having loco-regional, osseous or soft-tissue lesions. In contrast, response was much less frequent in patients with visceral lesions. In addition, all responses in such patients were recorded in patients with lung metastases. None of the patients with lymphangitis carcinomatosa or liver involvement responded to the hormonal treatment.

Most patients with pain experienced improvement. A more exact evaluation of pain relief is now in progress. As regards previous treatment, patients previously unresponsive to chemotherapy were virtually unresponsive to low-dose MPA also, but a remarkable number of cases (6/28) responded to high doses of MPA. Even more astonishing are the results so far in relation to the outcome of previous hormonal therapy. Responders to previous hormonal treatment responded in 9 cases out of 19 (47%) to high-dose MPA, whereas only 3 out of 25 previous responders to hormonal therapy (12%) exhibited PR with low-dose MPA. High-dose MPA was able to elicit PR in 7 cases out of 31 (23%) who had been resistant to previous hormonal treatment. None of the 30 patients who were resistant to previous hormonal therapy responded to MPA at low dosage. Patients who had not previously received either cytotoxic drugs or hormonal treatment (most had not been treated at all) had a remission rate of around 55% in the case of the group treated with high-dose MPA, and around 20% in the case of the group treated with low-dose MPA. Almost all of these patients were women above the age of 65, most with a slow growing tumour.

Having regard to these results, the trial has been closed in the case of previously treated patients, who did not respond to either previous chemotherapy or to past hormonal treatment. The trial remains open in the case of previously untreated patients and those who responded to previous therapy.

Hormonal receptor status is known in less than 30% of patients, since most cases enrolled in this trial underwent mastectomy before the determination of hormone receptors became a routine procedure in our institutions. Table IV shows the correlation between receptor status and response to high and low doses of MPA. The receptor status is known in 40 patients, but it should be noted that in almost all cases this result arises from determinations relating to biopsy just before entering the trial described here. In only a few instances do the receptor values refer to determinations at the time of mastectomy.

The analysis of side-effects recorded in this trial has still to be completed. However, up to now, no major difference in the pattern of toxicity observed with the 2 regimens has emerged. Most patients exhibited an increase in body

Table III. Characteristics of patients responding.

	Treatment group A			Treatment group B		
	Numbers of patients responding	Numbers of patients in category indicated	Percentage response in category indicated	Numbers of patients responding	Numbers of patients in category indicated	Percentage response category indicated
Predominant site of metastases						
loco-regional	6	15	20	3	13	23
soft tissue	5	12	41	0	14	0
osseous	10	29	34	3	26	11
visceral	3	20	15	2	23	8
overall	24	76	31	8	76	11
Previous chemotherapy and response						
no response	11	19	57	1	12	8
CR	3	12	25	2	15	13
NC	1	3	33	1	7	14
PD	5	25	20	0	21	0
not evaluable	4	17	23	4	21	19
Previous hormonal therapy and response						
no response	7	1	53	3	12	25
CR	9	19	47	3	5	12
NC	4	7	57	0	4	0
PD	3	24	12	0	26	0
not evaluable	1	13	7	2	9	22

Table IV. Receptor status in relation to response (x = ER; y = P_gR; (y) = P_gR qualitatively +, but exact value unknown).

Receptor status (x/y)	Treatment group A		Treatment group B	
	Number of patients in whom receptor status known	Number of patients showing response indicated	Number of patients in whom receptor status known	Number of patients showing response indicated
+/+	7	5 PR, 2NC	3	
+/−	5	2PR, 1NC	5	1NC
−/+	1	1PR	1	1NC
−/−	7		6	1PR
+/(+)	1	1NC	4	1PR
Totals	21		19	

weight of the order of 3–10 kg. Almost all patients noticed a dramatic increase in appetite. Minor vaginal bleeding developed in 3 women. Muscle cramps were observed in about 20% of patients during treatment, and for a few weeks thereafter. In about 25% of the patients, a median increase of 15–20 mm Hg in the median value for systolic blood pressure was recorded. Two cases of gluteal abscess were observed in patients on high-dose MPA.

Discussion

What is presented here is an interim evaluation of results in our trial, which, in the case of some subsets of patients, is still in progress. It must be stressed that our current results are very preliminary. Within the framework of a cooperative trial, data can be properly assessed only when information is available from all participants. Final evaluation requires review of most cases by an external assessor.

Our preliminary data nevertheless suggest that high doses of MPA yield better results in the treatment of advanced breast cancer than conventional, low MPA doses.

In trials of hormonal treatment for advanced breast cancer, differences in results often reflect differences in patient selection (age, extent of disease, prior therapy) as well as varying criteria for the assessment of therapeutic results and nonuniform methods of reporting data. It is, therefore, not surprising that response rates in the literature for treatment of breast cancer with conventional doses of MPA range from 0–36%.

Our preliminary data are consistent with those published by De Lena et al. [12]. In their prospective, nonrandomized trial, MPA induced objective tumour response in about 30% of patients. This finding is very similar to the 31% remission rate in the group treated with high-dose MPA in the present trial. In the trial of De Lena et al., all patients had been intensively treated previously. In our study, about 20% of patients had not previously been treated, and this may account for some of the differences observed. In addition, De Lena et al. state that: '...patients with a disease-free interval of longer than 2 years who were postmenopausal and had lesions either in the soft tissue or in the lungs and pleura were the ones who benefited most from treatment with MPA'. In the De Lena et al. study, 25% of patients were premenopausal, whereas all those enrolled in our trial were postmenopausal. Another factor which explains why our cases were likely to respond favourably is the fact that patients over 65 were allowed to enter the study, even though they had not been pretreated. In the context of a cooperative trial that means, in essence, that physicians would enrol mainly older patients. This fact is reflected in the median age of the population treated. Such patients will tend to have fairly slow-growing tumours. De Lena et al. failed to observe any difference in therapeutic activity as between 500 mg i.m. daily for 30 days and 1 g i.m. daily for 30 days. Since the high-dose schedule used in our study (1 g i.m. daily, 5 days a week for 4 weeks) gives an average daily dosage of less than 700 mg if calculated over a 1-month period, it is easy to see why the results of the 2 trials are so similar. Having regard to results reported in the literature [1–6], the disappointing results obtained in our group treated with low-dose MPA cannot be considered as wholly surprising. The fact that we failed to observe responses with low-dose treatment in patients who had been resistant to previous therapy is noteworthy. Patients treated with high doses, in contrast, responded fairly frequently, even if they had previously been regarded as nonresponders. This fact is also in accordance with the findings of De Lena et al. [12], who reported a 32% response rate in patients who had not responded to previous hormonal treatment, and a 21% response rate in women previously resistant to cytotoxic drugs.

Of particular interest is the fact that patients previously responsive to hormonal treatment are fairly resistant to low doses of MPA (12% PR), whereas high doses of PMA elicited a 47% response rate in such patients. The data on the correlation between receptor status and therapeutic outcome, though limited, exhibits one striking feature. Whereas among patients treated with high doses of MPA there seems to be a 'conventional' pattern of correlation, results among cases receiving the low doses of MPA are much more erratic. In the latter group, receptor status seems to have almost no prognostic significance.

The data on receptor status, and the strikingly different results with the 2 regimens in those previously responding to hormonal therapy, could be interpreted on the basis that the dose used in the low-dose regimen was too low to be fully effective.

The fact that no major difference in the patterns of toxicity between the 2 treatment groups has been detected is also noteworthy. However, a more detailed analysis of the side-effects observed has still to be performed. The toxicity recorded in our trial is similar to the toxicity reported in previous studies.

It is possible that, in future, more appropriate uses for progestational agents in the palliative therapy of mammary carcinoma will be found, if results of hormone receptor determinations are available for all patients at the time when decisions on therapy are made. Even though, in our trial, results of hormone receptor determinations were available for fewer than 1 in 3 patients, we hope that the evaluation of our data will shed some light on the possible significance of hormone receptor status.

In conclusion, we feel that it is, at present, very difficult to decide whether high-dose MPA or tamoxifen should be regarded as the treatment of choice in postmenopausal women with breast cancer with characteristics of a kind which would justify trying hormonal therapy. A controlled trial of the 2 treatments, with the possibility of cross-over if one treatment fails, therefore appears to be indicated in postmenopausal women with receptor-positive tumours, or tumours of unknown receptor status, and no hepatic involvement.

Acknowledgement

We wish to thank Ms. O. Kraitova for preparing this manuscript.

References

1. Goldenberg, I.S. (1969): Clinical trial of △'-testolactone (NSC 23759), medroxyprogesterone acetate (NSC 26386), and oxylone acetate (NSC 47438) in advanced female mammary cancer. A report of the cooperative breast cancer group. *Cancer 23*, 109.
2. Klaassen, D.J., Rapp, E.E. and Hirte, W.E. (1976): Response to medroxyprogesterone acetate (NSC 26386) as a secondary hormone therapy for metastatic breast cancer in postmenopausal women. *Cancer Treat. Rep. 60*, 251.
3. Muggia, F.M., Cassileth, P.A., Ochoa Jr., M. et al. (1968): Treatment of breast cancer with medroxyprogesterone acetate. *Ann. Intern. Med. 68*, 328.
4. Segaloff, A., Cuningham, M., Rice, B.F. and Weeth, J.B. (1967): Hormonal therapy in cancer of the breast. XXIV. Effect of corticosterone or medroxy-

progesterone acetate on clinical course of hormonal excretion. *Cancer 20*, 1673.

5. Stoll, B.A. (1966): Therapy by progestational agents in advanced breast cancer. *Med. J. Aust. 1*, 331.
6. Stoll, B.A. (1967): Progestin therapy of breast cancer: comparison of agents. *Br. Med. J. II*, 338.
7. Brunner, K.W., Sonntag, R.W., Alberto, P. et al. (1977): Combined chemotherapy and hormonotherapy in advanced breast cancer. *Cancer 39*, 2923.
8. Pannuti, G., Martoni, A., Lenaz, C.R. et al. (1978): A possible new approach to the treatment of metastatic breast cancer: massive doses of medroxyprogesterone acetate. *Cancer Treat. Rep. 62*, 504.
9. Robustelli Della Cuna, G., Calciati, A., Bernardo Strada, M.R. et al. (1978): High dose medroxyprogesterone acetate (MPA) treatment in metastatic carcinoma of the breast: a dose response evaluation. *Tumori 64*, 143.
10. Castiglione, M. and Cavalli, F. (1980): Ergebnisse einer Pilotstudie mit hochdosiertem Medroxyprogesteron-Azetat in der Behandlung des metastasierenden Mammakarzinoms. *Schweiz. Med. Wochenschr. 110*, 1073.
11. *WHO Handbook for reporting results of cancer treatment*. WHO, Geneva, 1979.
12. De Lena, M., Brambilla, C., Valagussa, P. and Bonadonna, G. (1979): High-dose medroxyprogesterone acetate in breast cancer resistant to endocrine and cytotoxic therapy. *Cancer Chemother. Pharmacol. 2*, 175.

Discussion

J.G.M. Klijn (Rotterdam, The Netherlands): Has Dr Cavalli (or anybody else) any experience with abdominal pain because of the presence of gastric or duodenal ulcers as a side-effect of this treatment, and has he seen any gastro-intestinal bleeding, for example, in those patients who died early?

F. Cavalli: No.

W.L. McGuire: I am surprised that the suggestive statement can be made that the 1,000-mg dose is better than the 500-mg. I am not convinced that the groups are necessarily comparable. I must focus immediately on Dr Cavalli's receptor data. The first group seemed to correlate with what might be anticipated, whereas the second group did not make any sense. I can not imagine a biological principle concerned with receptors or endocrine dependence that would be different according to whether 1,000-mg or 500-mg therapy was given. It seems to me that, before at least some of us here could be convinced that there is a difference between those 2 doses, these studies will have to be much more tightly controlled with regard to the variables that we know how to measure, or think we know how to measure.

The numbers of patients are sufficiently small, and the characteristics are sufficiently different so that we may be comparing 'apples' and 'oranges' rather than identical subsets of patients.

F. Cavalli: First, I would like to stress that I concluded my presentation by saying that our preliminary data *tend to support...* I did not say that they *demonstrate...*

Secondly, now having studied more than 150 patients and having based my study on all the clinical characteristics that were possible to find and to analyse, I was unable to demonstrate any difference between the 2 groups.

Thirdly, the difference between the 2 regimens is probably slightly more marked in that we gave 1 g daily 5 times a week, for a 4-week period, versus 500 mg twice a week. It is not, therefore, 1 g versus 500 mg, but, if it is calculated on a monthly basis, in total this is 650 mg versus 135 mg daily – so that is about 5 times more.

I am also surprised by the receptor data – but the receptors are known, as I said, for about 25% of the patients, and those were the data found. Perhaps, with regard to receptors, we are not really dealing with 2 comparable populations at the moment. However, looking at the 2 different populations from the point of view of the clinical features, I can not see any difference between them – although there may be some.

W.L. McGuire: I do not mean to sound too critical. I am sympathetic with the studies that Dr Cavalli is trying to do – but it would be like designing an adjuvant trial and having lymph node status on only 25% of the patients. Would any of us feel good about that kind of study? I would not. It tends to be more of a 'no contest' study, because the parameters that are thought to be important to measure are not being measured. Why not do the study properly in the first place, measuring those parameters that should be measured, making sure that the groups are in fact comparable, and then we can obtain some definitive information and get an answer? I do not mean this in a personal sense – but I am very disappointed.

F. Cavalli: I do not think that in the end we shall have a final conclusion as regards the correlation between receptors and response. I can see the point Professor McGuire is making – and that is the reason for continuing the study. However, I think that there might be a possibility of having 2 comparable groups of patients when we have, say, 125 or 150 patients in each treatment arm, based on the philosophy of the randomised clinical trial, and taking into account that even now there are no differences in the clinical prognostic features between the 2 groups.

W.L. McGuire: I disagree. The clinical features to which Dr Cavalli refers have not usually stood the test of time. If they had, we would not continue to search for more objective measurable parameters to help us compare groups A and B. Dr Cavalli is interpreting my remarks as saying that receptors are the answer to hormonal therapy – that is not what I mean. I just want to see him measure receptors in more than 25% of the patients and to be sure that both groups, A and B, have the same number of receptor-positive patients, both for oestrogen receptors and progesterone receptors. If differences are then observed, to me they would be interpretable.

F. Cavalli: That is our aim too, but when the study was started 2 years ago, many of the patients had been operated previously and it was impossible to check their receptors. Now, we do check the receptors in any case where that is possible.

On the other hand, I think that the clinical prognostic factors are still of some importance, and all groups use them too, for the time being, in order to stratify the patients if the receptors are unknown. I do not think Professor McGuire's criticism should be so straightforward.

W.L. McGuire: Again, nothing personal – but this is 1982. The clinical factors have now been known for 10 or 15 years – and where has that got us? Not very far. We now have some parameters to measure. They may be far from perfect, but at least they can be measured and quantified, and we can ensure that they are equal in 2 groups of patients which we are trying to compare.

I appreciate Dr Cavalli's comments that when the study was first started receptors were not available – which is why I say my comments are not personal. However, without measuring those parameters, it is not possible to make the conclusive statements that we want to be able to make at this sort of a meeting. I am willing to argue for ever that anybody who is unwilling to make those measurements is not doing a scientific study in the way it should be done in the 1980's.

F. Cavalli: On the basis of the clinical prognostic facts, we have learned something, and I am not convinced that since it has been possible to measure the receptors we have learned a great deal more.

Treatment of generalized carcinoma of the breast with high parenteral doses of medroxyprogesterone acetate given daily for 90 consecutive days*

D.V. Razis, L. Stamogiannou, K. Gennatas and D. Sionis
Piraeus Cancer Institute (Metaxas Memorial), Piraeus, Greece

Introduction

High (500 mg/day) parenteral doses of medroxyprogesterone acetate (MPA) have elicited high rates of therapeutic response in breast cancer, in all age groups. Higher doses (1 g/day or more), did not, however, yield better results with regard to either response rate or duration of response [1–5]. We felt that the therapeutic effect of MPA might be enhanced by increasing the duration of dosing to maintain high blood levels of MPA for longer periods. Up to now, the longest period of MPA administration has been 50 days [6]. On September 1st 1979 we began a study of the effectiveness and toxicity of 500 mg of MPA daily, intramuscularly (i.m.), for 90 consecutive days, followed by maintenance therapy with MPA. Patients were admitted to the trial up to November 30th 1980, and the results have been analysed up to December 31st 1981.

Material and methods

Selection of patients

Patients enrolled into this study were suffering from histologically-proven, advanced cancer of the breast, clinically evaluated as slow growing. These patients were no longer responding to current established hormonal and chemotherapeutic manipulation, or such types of manipulation were contra-indicated. There had been more than 4 weeks without any specific treatment

*This study was supported by Farmitalia Carlo Erba Hellas.

in the case of all patients previously treated with other hormonal and/or chemotherapeutic medication, before MPA treatment began. Previous or concomitant palliative treatment involving surgery or irradiation did not exclude a patient from the study. Palliative and symptomatic treatment with analgesics, sedatives and corticosteroids was also permitted. There were measurable masses for objective evaluation of therapeutic outcome in all patients, and each patient entering the study was estimated as likely to survive for more than 3 months.

Forty-four patients (40 female, 4 male) have been admitted to the study. The principal characteristics of these patients are listed in Table I. The mean age of the patients was 52 (range 35 to 82). The dominant sites of metastatic disease were soft tissues (27 patients), bones (12), and viscera (5).

Two patients were premenopausal (at least one menstrual period during the last year), 4 perimenopausal (last menstrual period 1–5 years previously) and 14 postmenopausal (last menstrual period more than 5 years before admission to trial). Twenty patients had been sterilized, either by surgery or irradiation. The disease-free interval was less than one year in 18 patients and more than one year in 12 patients. There had been no disease-free interval in 14 patients with stage IV disease when first diagnosed. The performance status was grade

Table I. Principal patient characteristics.

Males	4
Females	40
Mean age (range) (years)	52 (35–82)
Dominant site of metastases (number of patients)	
Soft tissue	27
Bones	12
Viscera	5
Menopausal status (number of patients)	
Premenopausal	2
Perimenopausal	4
Postmenopausal	14
Sterilized	20
Previous treatment (number of patients)	
Hormonotherapy	3
Chemotherapy	3
Chemotherapy + hormonotherapy	32
None	6

0 in one patient, grade 1 in 11 patients, grade 2 in 13 patients and grade 4 in 7 patients. Three patients had previously received hormonotherapy, 3 chemotherapy, 32 both chemotherapy and hormonotherapy, and 6 patients had not received any treatment before the administration of MPA.

The therapeutic regimen followed was 500 mg of MPA daily, i.m., for 90 consecutive days, followed by maintenance treatment consisting of 500 mg of MPA, i.m., twice weekly, or 500 mg per os (p.o.) daily. Patients were allocated at random to the 2 types of maintenance treatment.

Admission and follow-up

A full range of clinical and laboratory studies, including haematological and biochemical investigations, X-rays, carcino-embryonic antigen (CEA) tests and myelograms were performed in all patients on admission. The investigations were repeated at regular intervals, as indicated in Table II. The

Table II. Schedule of clinical and laboratory investigations.

Investigation	During first month of treatment	After first month of treatment
History	Once weekly	
Clinical examination		
Blood count and differential blood count		Every 4 weeks
Sedimentation rate		Every 2 weeks
Platelets-reticulocytes		
Blood calcium		
Blood urea, fasting blood sugar		
Serum creatinine		
Serum phosphorus		
Serum alkaline phosphatase		
Serum glutamic oxaloacetic transaminase, serum glutamic pyruvic transaminase, γ-glutamic acid transaminase		
Serum bilirubin	Every 4 weeks	Every 4 weeks
Serum cholesterol		
Prothrombin time		
Serum proteins		
Urinalysis		
Serum carcino-embryonic antigen		
Electrocardiogram		
Chest X-ray		
Skeletal survey	Every 12 weeks	
Myelogram	Only if indicated	

parameters for objective evaluation of response were determined during the first examination. Responses and toxicity were evaluated monthly. Response was evaluated strictly regarding to Union International Contra le Cancrum (UICC) criteria [7]. In cases of improvement or no progression, treatment was continued. In cases of deterioration, treatment was discontinued.

Results

Overall twenty-five out of the 44 patients (56.8%) responded, 4 with complete and 21 with partial remission. Best results were achieved after the third month of treatment (Table III). There were no cases of complete remission after the first month of treatment. Thirteen patients (29.5%) exhibited partial remission. In 20 patients (45.5% of the original 44), the disease remained static, and in 11 (25%) it got worse. After the second month of treatment, 20 patients (45.5% of the original 44) exhibited partial remission, in 8 (18.2%) the disease remained static, in 2 (4.5%) it got worse, and one patient died. By the third month of treatment, 54.5% of the original 44 patients had responded (3 complete remissions, 21 partial remissions).

Table III. Results of treatment; numbers of patients (percentages of original 44 patients).

Month	Total no. of patients	Complete remission	Partial remission	Static disease	Deteri-oration	Deaths
1	44	0	13 (29.5 +)	20 (45.5)	11 (25)	
2	31	0	20 (45.5)	8 (18.2)	2 (4.5)	1
3	26	3 (6.8)	21 (47.7)	0	2 (4.5 +)	
4	24	3 (6.8)	18 (40.8)	0	2	1
5	20	3 (6.8)	13 (30)	0	3	1
6	15	4 (9)	8 (18)	0	2	1
7	8	3	5	0	0	
8	7	2	5	0	0	
9	6	1	5	0	0	
10	6	1	3	0	1	1
11	4	1	3	0	0	
12	2	1	1	0	0	
13	1	1	1	0	0	
14	1	1	1	0	0	
18	1	0	1	0	0	

+ 2 Cases classified as partial remissions after the first month of treatment were classified as having deteriorated after 3 months of treatment.

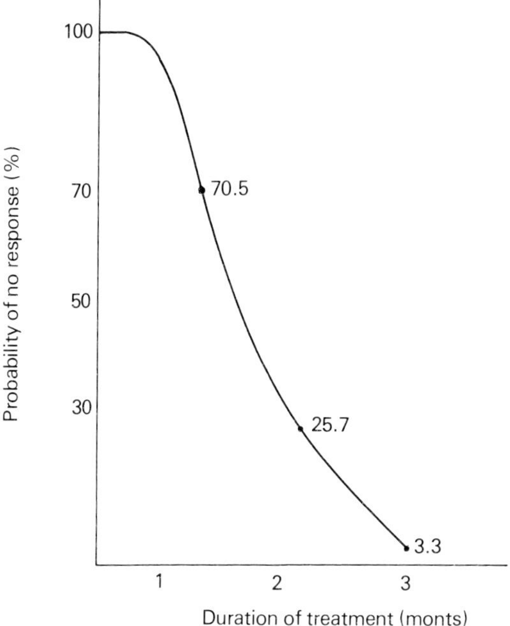

Figure. Probability of no response in relation to duration of treatment.

Table IV. Expectation of response in relation to duration of treatment.

Duration of treatment (months)	No. of patients	Expectation of response indicated		
		Positive	Negative	
			Monthly	Cumulatively
0–1	44	0.295	0.705	0.705
1–2	33	0.646	0.364	0.257
2–3	29	0.872	0.128	0.033

As shown in Figure 1 and Table IV, after completion of one month's treatment, 70.5% of the patients did not show remission. Of the patients who started a 2nd month of treatment 36.4% did not show remission. Finally, the patients who continued and completed 3 months' treatment had a probability of only 12.8% of not showing remission. Thus, patients who managed to complete 3 months' treatment have an additive probability of only 3.3% of not exhibiting remission. The difference in response rates after one month and

Table V. Responses to treatment in relation to sites of metastases; numbers of patients (percentages).

Month	Site of metastases								
	Soft tissue			Bones			Lungs		
	Complete plus partial remission	Complete remission	Partial remission	Complete plus partial remission	Complete remission	Partial remission	Complete plus partial remission	Complete remission	Partial remission
1	10 (29.5)	1	9				1		1
2	6 (17.6)	3	3				2		2
3	6 (17.6)	3	3	13	2	11			
4							1		1
5									
6				1 +	1				
Total numbers of patients showing complete or partial remission		22			13			4	
Total numbers of patients treated		34			24			10	
Percentage response rate		64.7			54			40	

+ This patient, in complete remission after 6 months, was in partial remission after the third month. Some patients in this table are included more than once, as metastatic disease was not localized in one system.

3 months' treatment is statistically highly significant ($z=3.56$, $P<0.001$) using the Greenwood method of statistical analysis.

Few patients who experienced partial remission, or whose disease remained static after the first month of treatment, progressed to complete remission by the third month. There was a slow but progressive decline in rates of therapeutic response after the third month (47.6% of the 44 original patients showing complete or partial remissions by the fourth month, 36.8% after the fifth month, etc). However, one patient, who was in partial remission after the third month exhibited complete remission by the sixth month while on maintenance treatment with MPA (500 mg i.m., twice weekly). There were no differences in the rates or durations of response as between patients on i.m. or p.o. maintenance therapy with oral MPA. There were 5 deaths during the first 10 months of treatment.

Table V illustrates response rates in relation to dominant site of metastases. The best response rates were obtained in cases of soft tissue metastases (64.7% partial or complete remissions). The percentage response rate was 54% in cases of bony metastases, and 40% in cases of pulmonary metastases. The response rates in cases of soft tissue metastases were 29.5% after the first month, 47.1% after the second month, and 64.7% after the third month. This may indicate that one month of treatment with MPA is not enough. All patients with bony metastases were evaluated for objective response not before the third month of treatment. One patient in partial remission by the third month demonstrated complete recalcification of bones after 6 months of treatment. The bone marrow infiltrated by metastatic disease in 2 patients cleared completely, and the haematological picture was restored to normal after the third month of treatment.

As shown in Table VI, postmenopausal and sterilized patients responded better than patients in other categories. As would be expected, patients not previously treated with hormonotherapy, and patients with more than one year of disease-free interval responded better than other types of patient. The response rate in patients with a disease-free interval of more than one year was more than 90%.

The duration of objective response (partial or complete remission) was over 6 months. A few patients are still in remission and are still taking MPA, though no longer in the trial. The longest duration of remission is more than 18 months, in a patient with a very satisfactory partial remission, who remains in the trial.

In 18 out of 26 patients (69%) pain was controlled satisfactorily with MPA. Improvement of performance status was also observed in all patients responding to treatment.

Table VI. Response rates in relation to menopausal status, disease-free intervals and previous treatment.

	No. of patients	Complete plus partial remission (no. of patients)	Percentage responses
Last menstrual period			
0–1 year before trial	2	–	
1–5 years before trial	4	1	25
5 years or more before trial	14	10	71
Sterilization	20	13	65
Disease-free interval			
nil	14	5	36
1 year	18	9	50
>1 year	12	11	91.7
Previous treatment			
None	6	5	83
Hormonotherapy	3	1	33
Chemotherapy	3	2	66
Hormonotherapy plus chemotherapy	32	17	53
Totals	44	25	56.8

Finally, the response of male breast cancer to MPA was very satisfactory. Three out of 4 patients responded, one with complete remission, 2 with satisfactory partial remissions. The complete response was both impressive and lasting.

Toxicity

The toxicity of MPA in this study was acceptable, and always reversible. Side-effects were manifested by 23 patients (52%) (Table VII). Increases in body weight and moon-faces were observed in 16 patients (38.8%). Weight increased by 4–10 kg, or 57–130 mg/kg of body weight.

In 20.5% of patients, diabetes developed, or pre-existing diabetes became worse. Of the 9 patients concerned, the diabetes developed de novo after MPA treatment in 6, and in 4 of these insulin treatment was necessary.

In 6 patients (13.5%), electrolyte abnormalities, mainly hypernatraemia and hyperkalaemia were observed. The mean arterial pressures increased by 10–20 mm Hg in 4 patients (9%).

Table VII. Toxicity.

Side-effect	No. of patients showing side-effect indicated	Percentages of patients showing side-effect indicated
Increase in body weight, moon-face	17	38.6
Diabetes or worsening of pre-existing diabetes	9	20.5
Electrolyte disturbances	6	13.5
Increase in arterial blood pressure	4	9
Metrorrhagia	2	4.5
Fine tremor of the extremities	2	4.5
Hypercalcaemia	1	2.3
Visual disturbances	2	4.5
Thrombophlebitis	1	2.3
Totals	23	52

Metrorrhagia occurred in 2 patients (4.5%). In one of these it was necessary to use intravaginal radium therapy in order to control bleeding. Tremor of the extremities, which interfered with patients' ability to perform fine movements, was observed in 2 patients (4.5%).

Hypercalcaemia was also observed in one patient (2.3%), visual disturbances in 2 patients (4.5%) and thrombophlebitis in one patient (2.3%), but in these cases MPA may not have been the only cause, since other factors (generalized cancer, immobilization) also predispose to such complications.

Gluteal abscess did not occur in any patient, nor was it necessary to discontinue treatment because of toxicity in any patient. The most troublesome side-effects were the increases in body weight, and the appearance of moon-face. The most interesting was the appearance of diabetes or worsening of pre-existing diabetes.

Discussion

This was the first study in which high daily doses of MPA have been administered parenterally for 90 consecutive days. High daily doses of MPA have given higher response rates than low doses. Pannuti and other investigators have reported impressive results with high doses of MPA, and a mean duration of response of 7–8 months [1, 5, 6, 8, 9]. Most investigators have administered the drug for 30 days. A few investigators have given the drug for 40–50 days. Amadori et al., using 1 g daily for 40–50 days, achieved a 56.8% response rate [6, 8].

In administering the drug for 90 days, we hoped to keep blood levels high for longer periods, and thus to enhance the therapeutic effect. Response rates were highest after the third month of treatment. The differences between response rates after the first and third months of treatment were statistically highly significant. Higher response rates were observed in postmenopausal women and in sterilized women than in women not in these categories (71% and 65%, respectively). This is in agreement with other reports in the literature (De Lena et al. [1], Robustelli et al. [5]). It is, however, not in agreement with one study by Pannuti et al. who reported a 93% response rate in premenopausal women [10]. Response rates were also better in patients with soft tissue and bony metastases, and in patients with disease-free intervals of more than one year, than in patients not in these categories. The response rate in patients with disease-free intervals of more than one year was 91.7%. The number of patients was, however, small. The reports in the literature concerning response rates in patients with soft tissue metastases are not all in agreement, but there is agreement concerning the relationship between response rates and disease-free intervals [1]. In our trial, however, it was only after administration of the drug for 3 months that the maximum number of remissions was achieved in patients with soft tissue metastases. Bony metastases responded in 54% of instances. Response rates recorded in the literature in cases of bony metastases vary from 13–67%. Pulmonary metastases responded in 40% of cases. This is in agreement with the figure in the reports of De Lena et al. (41%) [1]. The effects of MPA on pain were somewhat less in our trial than in other trials [3]. It is interesting that 53% of cases resistant to customary hormonal and chemotherapeutic combinations responded. This is in line with reports in the literature [1, 5]. Only 6 out of the 44 patients in the study had not had any treatment prior to administration of MPA.

Finally, we would draw attention to the high response rate in the group of male patients with breast cancer. The case in which there was complete remission was striking and the remission lasting. Though the number of patients is very small, the results are impressive, and further evaluation of the treatment of male breast cancer with progesterone is clearly indicated.

Toxicity was within acceptable limits, and always reversible. The most troublesome side-effect in our patients was the body weight increase, which occurred in 38.8% of instances. Incidences of side-effects reported in the literature vary from 56–77% [1, 3, 15]. The effects of MPA in causing or worsening diabetes are not fully explicable at present. It is possible that the hyperglycaemic action of MPA may be explained by the 6,21-dihydroxylated MPA metabolite, which seems to have corticosteroid-like activity [11, 12]. Electrolyte disturbances (mainly hyperkalaemia and hypernatraemia) have been reported in the literature. In our trial there were only modest increases in serum levels of K and Na, similar to those recorded in the literature [13, 14]. In a few patients, increased arterial blood pressures, metrorrhagia, muscular tremor, hypercalcaemia, thrombophlebitis and visual disturbances were recorded. Higher incidences of increased blood pressure, metrorrhagia and tremor, have been recorded in the literature [3, 15]. Hypercalcaemia and thrombophlebitis are regarded as typical complications of MPA therapy. Visual disturbances are rare [3].

None of our patients developed gluteal abscesses, a side-effect reported by some investigators to be the commonest side-effect with MPA therapy. This is probably explained by the relatively low daily dose, use of MPA in the form of the commercial preparation Farlutal®, in a syringe, ready to use, and the care taken by our nursing personnel.

The percentages of complications were, generally, low. This is partly attributable to the moderate doses used. A similar finding has been recorded by Pannuti et al. [4] and Robustelli et al. [5].

Acknowledgement

We are grateful to Professor G. Papaevangelou for help with the statistical analysis of our results and for designing Figure 1 and Table VI.

References

1. De Lena, M., Brambilla, C., Valacussa, P. and Bonadonna, G. (1979): High-dose medroxyprogesterone acetate in breast cancer resistant to endocrine and cytotoxic therapy. *Cancer Chemother. Pharmacol. 2*, 175.
2. Pannuti, F., Martoni, A. and Piana, E. (1977): Higher doses of medroxyprogesterone acetate in the treatment of advanced breast cancer. *IRCS Med. Sci. 5*, 54.
3. Pannuti, F., Martoni, A., Lenaz, G.R. et al. (1978): A possible new approach to the treatment of metastatic breast cancer: massive doses of medroxyprogesterone acetate. *Cancer Treat. Rep. 62*, 499.
4. Pannuti, F., Martoni, A., Di Marco, A.B. et al. (1979): Prospective, randomized clinical trial of two different high dosages of medroxyprogesterone acetate (MPA) in the treatment of metastatic breast cancer. *Eur. J. Cancer 15*, 593.
5. Robustelli Della Cuna, G., Calciati, A., Bernardo Strada, M.R. et al. (1978): High doses medroxyprogesterone acetate (MPA) treatment in metastatic carcinoma of the breast: a dose response evaluation. *Tumori 64*, 143.
6. Amadori, D., Ravaioli, A. and Barbanti, F. (1976): High-dose medroxyprogesterone acetate in the palliative therapy of advanced breast carcinoma. *Minerva Med. 67*, 1.
7. Hayward, J.L., Carbone, P.P., Heuson, J-C. et al. (1977): Assessment of response to therapy in advanced breast cancer. *Cancer 39*, 1289.

8. Amadori, D., Ravaioli, A. and Barbanti, F. (1977): The use of medroxyprogesterone acetate in high doses in palliative treatment of advanced mammary carcinoma (Clinical experience with 44 cases). *Minerva Med. 68*, 3967.
9. Pannuti, F., Martoni, A., Pollutri, E. et al. (1974): Medroxyprogesterone acetate (MAP): Effects of massive doses in advanced breast cancer. *IRCS Med. Sci. 2,* 1605.
10. Pannuti, F., Martoni, A., Piana, E. and Fruet, F. (1977): Metastatic breast cancer in premenopause with medroxyprogesterone acetate (MAP) in massive doses. *IRCS Med. Sci. 5,* 49.
11. Helmreich, M.L. and Huseby, R.A. (1962): Identification of 6,21-dihydroxylated metabolite of medroxyprogesterone acetate in human urine. *J. Clin. Endocrinol. Metab. 22*, 1018.
12. Sala, G. and Castegnaro, E. (1964): Biotransformation of 21-methyl into 21-methoxy steroids. In: *Structure and Metabolism of Corticosteroids.* pp. 95–102. Academic Press, London and New York.
13. Falconi, G., Gardi, R., Bruni, C. and Ercoli, A. (1961): Studies on steroidal enol ethers: an attempt to dissociate progestational from contraceptive activity in oral oestrogens. *Endocrinology 69*, 638.
14. Kraay, R.J. and Brennan, D.M. (1963): Evaluation of chlormadinone acetate and other progestogens for foetal masculinization in rats. *Acta Endocrinol. 43*, 412.
15. Pannuti, F. (1977): Prospects in the treatment of the breast cancer and its metastases. Medroxyprogesterone in massive doses, an alternative to polychemotherapy. *Minerva Chir. 32,* 1.

Discussion

E. Gercovich: My question is not closely related to the subject of Dr Razis' paper. We see a lot of statistics and figures, but the basic question to ask is: When someone is switched to hormonal therapy, on what basis are hormones given? If it is simply on the basis of 'let's give hormones and see what happens in the future', that is not a very scientific attitude towards either the patient or the therapy.

With regard to the receptors, I think that the only way to judge whether a neoplasia is hormone-responsive and not hormone-dependent, is on the basis of receptors. I believe that, first, we have to have a clear idea about receptors – or at least about the extent of hormonal responsiveness or hormonal dependence of the neoplasia. Otherwise, hormones are only being given on an empirical basis.

D.V. Razis: It might take a long time to answer the question about when to give hormonal therapy in breast cancer. I think that it is perfectly ethical to treat a patient with MPA (which is not a drug with high toxicity) when that patient is resistant to established hormonal and chemotherapy, and when there is clinically a slowly growing disease. Of course, we do not have many patients in whom the receptors are known – it is less than 25% in our group. It is not easy, and sometimes even impossible, in patients with a generalized disease, to take a piece of tissue and search for oestrogen and progesterone receptors. Not only from the research point of view, but also from the point of view of our duty to the patients. I think that it is perfectly all right to go ahead, even without knowledge of the receptors, and to give MPA to this particular group of patients.

M. Kjaer: Dr Razis stated in the abstract to his paper that after 90 days the patients were randomized between an oral-treatment schedule, and an intramuscular-treatment schedule. I do not think anything was said about that in the presentation that we have just heard.

D.V. Razis: In the small group remaining in the protocol after 3 months, there was no difference between the oral administration of 500 mg daily and the intramuscular administration 500 mg twice weekly, as regards their response.

Oral high-dose medroxyprogesterone acetate therapy in advanced breast cancer: clinical and endocrine studies

Research Group for the MPA Treatment of Breast Cancer in Japan: M. Izuo (Chairman)[1], Y. Iino[1], T. Tominaga[2], Y. Nomura[3], O. Abe[4], K. Enomoto[4], O. Takatani[5] and K. Kubo[6]

[1]Department of Surgery, Gunma University Hospital, Gunma; [2]Department of Surgery, Tokyo Metropolitan Komagome Hospital, Tokyo; [3]Department of Surgery, National Kyushu Cancer Centre Hospital, Fukuoka; [4]Department of Surgery, Keio University Hospital, Tokyo; [5]Department of Internal Medicine, Defence Medical College Hospital, Tokorozawa; and [6]Department of Surgery, National Nagoya Hospital, Nagoya, Japan

Introduction

The objectively-assessed response rate to medroxyprogesterone acetate (MPA) in cases of advanced breast cancer did not exceed 20% with doses below 500 mg/day in earlier studies [1]. Following a study of doses of over 500 mg/day by Pannuti [2], however, the response rates achievable went up to over 40% [3–5], and no serious toxic effects were observed. As the drug was given daily by intramuscular (i.m.) injection, therapy occasionally resulted in local side-effects such as gluteal abcesses and indurations [4–7].

In order to avoid such side-effects, we in the Research Group for the MPA Treatment of Breast Cancer in Japan have evaluated the effect of oral, high-dose MPA treatment in patients with advanced breast cancer [8, 9]. This paper describes the clinical results, and reports on the effects of therapy on the various hormones of the pituitary-gonadal and pituitary-adrenal axes.

Material and methods

Clinical studies

All patients selected for this trial were postmenopausal women with advanced breast cancer, or a recurrence of breast cancer. Patients were selected on the basis of Union Internationale Contre le Cancer (UICC) criteria [10]. The number of patients taking part in this trial was 120. Treatment took place in one or other of the 6 institutions participating in the Japanese Research Group for the MPA Treatment of Breast Cancer. Results relating to 110 patients were capable of analysis.

MPA was given orally, as 200-mg tablets in all cases. Daily dosages ranged from 600 mg to 2,400 mg. A dosage of 1,200 mg was most frequently used.

Treatment was continued for at least one month. No other drug that might affect the results was given concomitantly. All cases were assessed clinically before and after treatment, according to UICC criteria [10]. Side-effects and body weight changes were also assessed. Clinical tests were carried out before and during therapy, and included routine blood counts and determinations of serum glutamic oxaloacetic transaminase (SGOT) and serum glutamic pyruvic transaminase (SGPT) levels, serum alkaline phosphatase (SAP) values, and calcium and phosphorus levels in serum.

Endocrinological studies

Determinations of hormone levels in patients in the 1,200-mg group treated at Gunma University Hospital were made. Blood samples were taken at 8 a.m., before the first dose of MPA each day. Levels of luteinizing hormone (LH), follicle stimulating hormone (FSH), prolactin (PRL), growth hormone (GH), adrenocorticotrophic hormone (ACTH), thyroid-stimulating hormone (TSH), hydrocortisone, oestrogens and progesterone were measured in blood samples from 12 patients before and during treatment. In addition, the urinary excretion of 17-ketosteroids (17KS) and 17-hydroxycorticosteroids (17OHCS) was studied.

Results

Clinical studies

The main characteristics of the 110 patients for whom results capable of analysis were available are summarized in Table I according to dosage levels. Distribution of patients between the 4 groups was fairly even in terms of mean age, mean cancer-free interval, time since menopause, predominant site of disease, and previous therapy.

The overall objective responses to MPA in relation to dosage are shown in Table II. Results were evaluated according to UICC criteria [10]. The results

Table I. Pretreatment characteristics of patients.

Dosage (mg/day)	600–1,000	1,200	1,600–2,400	Varied	Total/ overall mean values
Numbers of patients	42	55	7	6	110
Mean age (years)	54.3	56.2	51.0	52.7	54.9
Mean duration of response (months)	32.2	41.5	19.0	29.5	35.9
Mean period elapsing since menopause (years)	9.2	10.2	6.1	5.2	9.3
Predominant site of lesions					
Soft tissues	13	15	4	2	34
Bones	14	28	2	2	46
Viscera	15	12	1	2	30
Previous therapy					
Chemotherapy	32	39	6	6	83
Ablative endo-crinological	25	23	4	1	53
Additive endo-crinological	25	29	3	3	60

analysed related to patients treated for 4 weeks or more. The 1,200-mg per day group showed a significantly higher ($P<0.05$) response rate, (21/55, 38.2%) than the groups treated with lower doses (7.7 to 18.2%). The groups receiving doses of 1,600 mg or more did not show any consistent tendency to a further increase in response rate. Subsequently, 3 groups of results were formed, corresponding to the group of patients who received 600–1,000 mg of MPA per day, the group of patients who received 1,200 mg of MPA per day, and the group of patients who received 1,600–2,400 mg of MPA per day.

The duration of response (defined as the mean time to recommencement of progression in cases which responded) is shown in Table III. Response was taken to begin from the start of treatment. The mean duration of response in all those responding was 41.1 weeks. The mean duration of response in the 600–1,000-mg per day group was 49.5 weeks. In the 1,200-mg per day group it was 40.0 weeks. The difference in mean durations of response between the 2 groups is not statistically significant. Each group included several cases who were still responding at the time of assessment of results, as indicated in Table III.

Table II. Objective response to MPA in relation to dosage.

Dosage (mg/day)	Response		None	Progress of disease	No. of responders/no. of patients treated	Response rate (%)	
	Complete	Partial					
600	1	1	5	4	2/11	18.2	6/42 (14.3%)*
800	1	2	8	7	3/18	16.7	
1,000		1	8	4	1/13	7.7	
1,200	2	19	15	19	21/55	38.2*	
1,600			1		0/1		2/7 (28.6)
1,800		2		3	2/5	40.0	
2,400				1	0/1		
Dose changed		3	1	2	3/6	50.0	
Total	4	28			32/110	29.1	

* Difference significant, $P<0.05$ (χ^2 test).

Table III. Duration of response in those responding.

Dosage (mg/day)	Numbers responding		Mean duration of response (weeks)	Numbers of cases still responding at time of analysis of data
	Completely	Partially		
600–1,000	2	4	49.5	3
1,200	2	19	40.0	5
>1,200	–	2	13.5	0
Totals/ overall mean value	4	25	41.1	8

Table IV is a comparison of response in relation to the predominant sites of lesions in the 3 dosage groups. The predominant sites of lesions were categorized as soft tissues, bones or viscera. The 1,200-mg per day group showed higher response rates than the lower dosage group for all 3 categories of site; 46.7% (7 out of 15 patients) for soft tissue sites, 39.3% (11/28) for

Table IV. Response to MPA according to predominant site of lesions.

Predominant site of lesions	Dosage (mg/day)	Numbers of patients responding completely or partially/number of patients treated	Response rate (%)
Soft tissues	600–1,000	3/13	23.1
	1,200	7/15	46.7
	>1,200	1/4	
Bones	600–1,000	1/14	7.1*
	1,200	11/28	39.3*
	>1,200	1/2	
Viscera	600–1,000	2/15	13.3
	1,200	3/12	25.0
	>1,200	0/1	

* Difference significant, $P<0.05$ (χ^2 test).

Table V. Relationship between response to previous therapies and response to MPA therapy.

Previous therapies	Numbers of patients responding to MPA/numbers of patients treated	Response rate (%)
None	6/14	42.9
Ablative endocrine therapy		
Responders	9/14	64.3*
Failures	0/24	0 *
Additive endocrine therapy		
Responders	7/21	33.3
Failures	10/37	27.0
Chemotherapy		
Responders	8/31	25.8
Failures	10/41	24.4

* Different significant, $P < 0.05$ (χ^2 test).

Table VI. Relationship between presence or absence of ER and response to MPA.

ER	Number responding		Number responding/number treated	Response rate (%)
	Completely	Partially		
(+)		8	8/21	38.1*
(−)	1	1	2/20	10.0*
Unknown	3	20	23/68	33.8

* Difference not significant.

Table VII. Side-effects of MPA in relation to dosage.

Side-effect	Dosage (mg/day)			
	600–1,000	1,200	>1,200	Total numbers of cases showing side-effect indicated
Moon face	3	9	3	15
Vaginal spotting	4	6		10
Rash		4		4
Pruritus		3		3
Aggravated diabetes mellitus	1	2		3
Acne		1		1
Excessive sweating	1			1
Nausea		1		1
Hypertension		1		1
Abnormal glucose tolerance	2	1	1	4
Abnormal liver function			1	1
Body weight gain greater than 5 kg	6	15	2	23
Total numbers of cases treated	42	55	7	104

bony sites and 25.0% (3/12) for visceral sites. The difference in response rates to the 3 dosages was most marked in the case of bone metastases (1,200-mg per day group: 39.3% (11/28 patients); 600–1,000-mg per day group: 7.1% (1/14)). The difference was statistically significant ($P<0.05$).

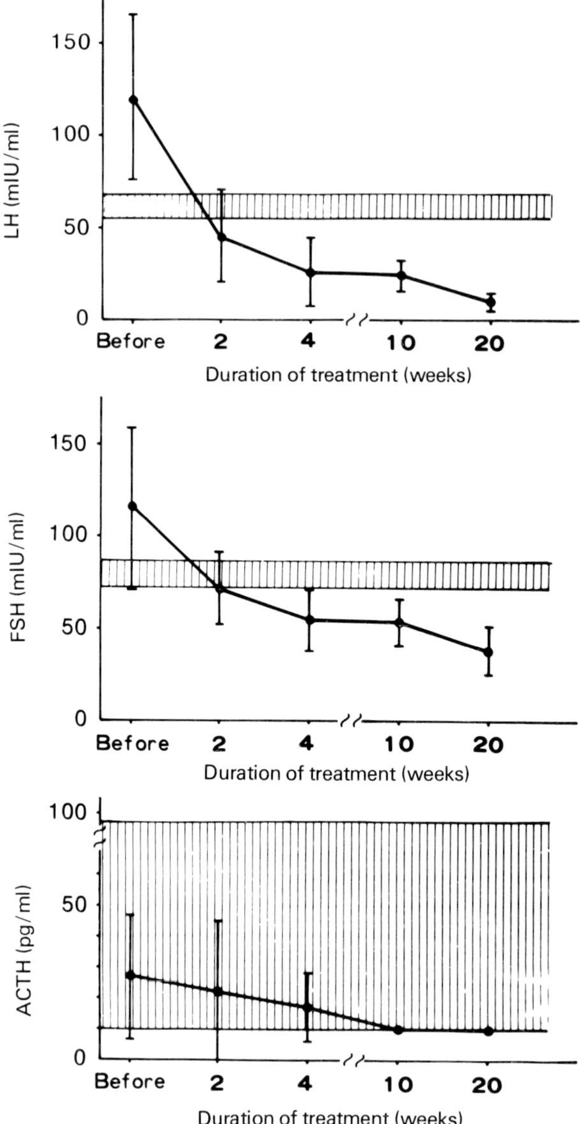

Fig. 1. Serum levels of LH, FSH and ACTH during MPA treatment.

Table V shows the relationship between response to previous therapies and response to MPA therapy. MPA tended to be more effective in new cases. In cases where there had been previous ablative endocrine therapy, the effectiveness of MPA in those responding to the previous therapy was high (9/14

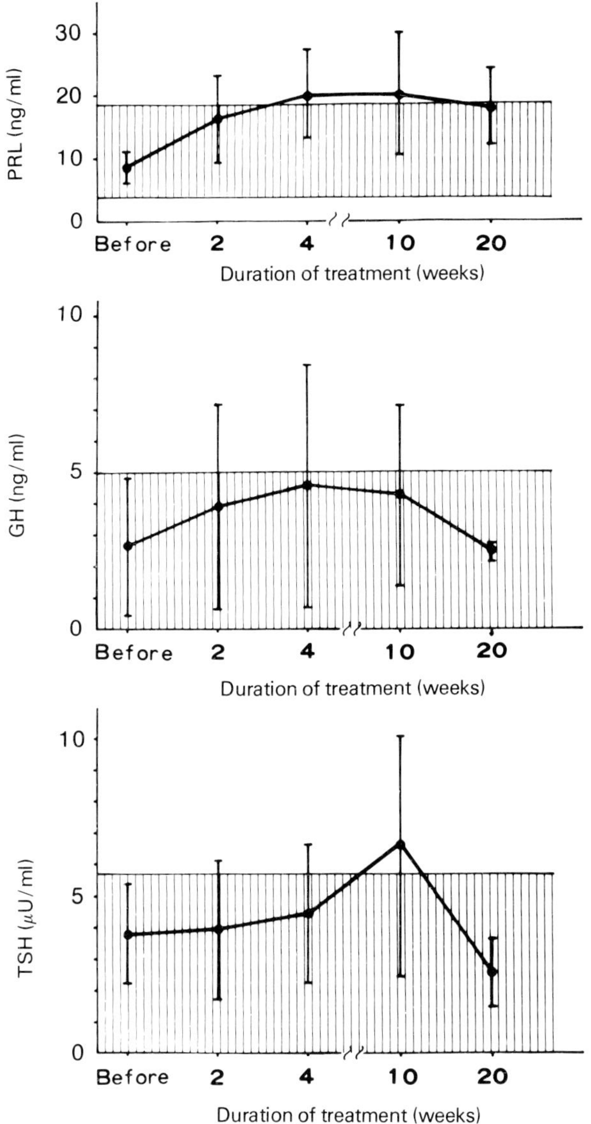

Fig. 2. Serum levels of PRL, GH and TSH during oral, high-dose MPA treatment.

patients, 64.3%). None of the 24 patients who had not responded to previous ablative therapy responded to MPA therapy. The difference was statistically significant ($P<0.01$). With additive endocrine therapy and chemotherapy, however, there was no significant difference in rates of response to MPA as

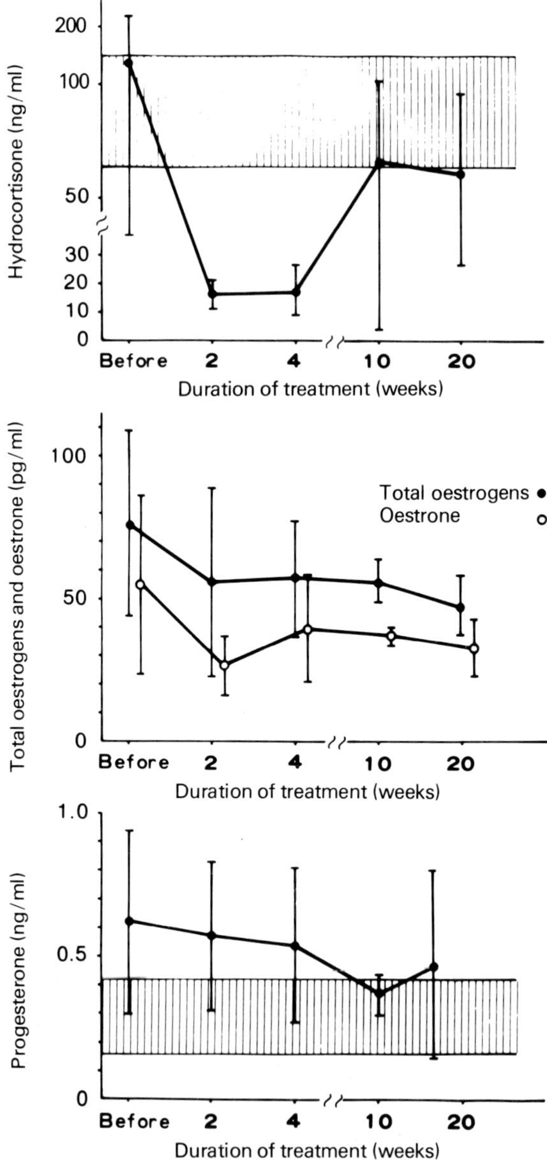

Fig. 3. Serum levels of hydrocortisone, oestrogens and progesterone during oral, high-dose MPA treatment.

between those responding to previous therapy and those not responding.

Table VI shows the relationship between oestrogen receptor (ER) status and response to MPA therapy. There were 8 responders to MPA therapy in 21 ER-

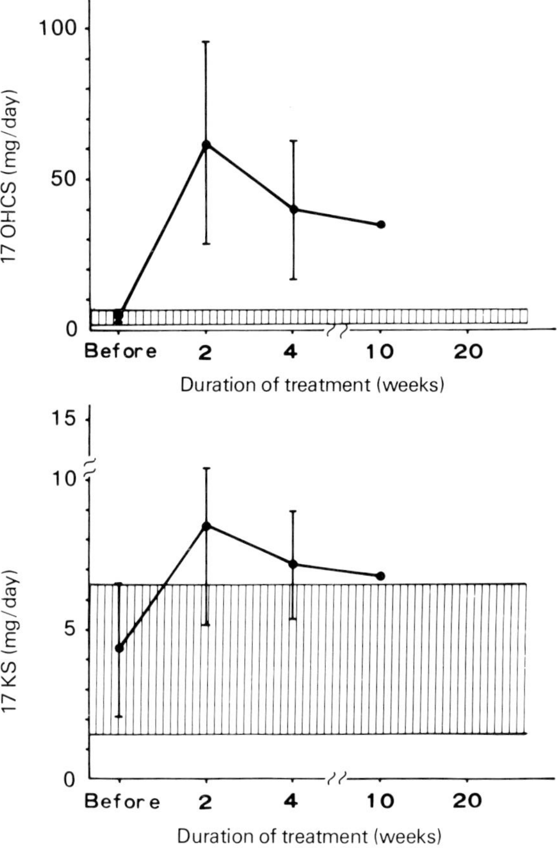

Fig. 4. Levels of 17OHCS and 17KS in urine during oral, high-dose MPA treatment.

positive cases, as against 2 responders in 20 ER-negative cases. The difference is not statistically significant.

Side-effects during MPA therapy are listed in Table VII together with their frequencies of occurrence. Moon face occurred in 15 cases, vaginal spotting in 10, rash in 4, pruritus in 3 and aggravation of diabetes in 3. Among the cases in which there were abnormal clinical chemical results there were 4 with abnormal glucose tolerance. An increase in body weight of more than 5 kg was noted in 23 out of 104 cases (22.1%). Two cases apart, side-effects were tolerable within the context of treatment.

Endocrine studies

The hormonal patterns in the pituitary-gonadal and pituitary-adrenal axes were investigated during treatment with oral, high-dose MPA.

LH, FSH and ACTH serum levels decreased significantly once treatment had begun, and remained low throughout the period of administration (Fig. 1).

Figure 2 shows the serum values of PRL, GH and TSH. The levels of these hormones showed no significant change overall, although there was a slight tendency for PRL and GH levels to increase.

As shown in Figure 3, serum levels of hydrocortisone, oestrogens and progesterone decreased significantly, in correspondence with the changes in ACTH and gonadotropin levels, during MPA treatment. The change in total oestrogen levels seemed to be mainly attributable to changes in oestrone levels. These observations indicate that high dosages of MPA have an intensive inhibitory effect on the pituitary-adrenal and pituitary-gonadal axes.

Figure 4 shows urinary levels of 17OHCS and 17KS over a 24-hour period. The levels of 17OHCS were increased throughout the period of MPA administration. The increases in 17KS levels were less than the increases in 17OHCS levels. We believe that the rises are attributable to increases in the quantities of metabolites of MPA in the urine.

Discussion

MPA treatment for advanced breast cancer was introduced in the early 1960's. When the drug was used at doses of 40–300 mg/day, objective regression was found in not more than 17% of cases, on average [11]. After doses of over 500 mg/day, i.m., began to be administered, response rates increased to over 40% [2, 3] but treatment sometimes led to gluteal abcesses or indurations [4–7].

To simplify administration and avoid side-effects related to injection, we used oral, high-dose MPA in Japanese patients with advanced breast cancer. The treatment seemed, in this preliminary, open study, to be adequate to obtain clinical responses comparable to those previously attained using i.m. administration [3–7].

In the trial described in this paper, the overall response rate in the 110 patients for whom results capable of analysis were available was 29.1%, on average, over the entire range of dosages (600–2,400 mg/day). However, the response rate in the 1,200-mg group was 38.2%, significantly ($P < 0.05$) higher than that in the group receiving 600–1,000 mg/day (14.3%). Although no other trials of oral, high-dose MPA have been reported, 2 studies comparing 2 i.m. dosage regimens have been published [4, 5]. The authors concerned observed no appreciable difference in response rates between 500 mg and 1,000 mg (Robustelli) or 1,500 mg of MPA (Pannuti) daily. The latter author, however, regarded the 1,500-mg/day regimen as superior to the 500-mg/day regimen, on the basis of response rates and subjective improvements. Accordingly, 1,200 mg of MPA per day would seem likely to be a suitable dose.

Regression in the present study lasted for more than 40 months, irrespective of dosage. The values found are comparable to those reported previously [4, 5, 7].

High response rates for lesions in soft tissues and bones have previously been reported [1, 11]. We also found response to be best when lesions in these sites predominated. Some degree of correlation was observed between the response to oral, high-dose MPA therapy and previous therapies, and ER status as reported by other authors [6, 7, 12], but it is interesting to note that there were some exceptions.

Side-effects were observed in this study, as in previous studies, but they were, in most cases, well tolerated. With i.m. injection, the most frequent side-effects were abscess or induration at the site of injection [4–7]. However, the most frequent side-effect in the study described here was moon face in the groups receiving the higher dosages. Weight gain was also a side-effect regularly observed. It most probably resulted from increased appetite and fluid retention [1]. No serious abnormalities in clinical chemical findings, including those relating to liver function, were observed.

The mechanism of action of MPA is an important factor to be taken into account in considering these results. Progesterone and progestational steroids are believed to affect breast tumours in several ways [1]. One possible mechanism is antagonism by progesterone of the action of oestrogen, as suggested by Clark et al. [13] and Hsueh et al. [14]. In a previous report [8], we recorded that an in vitro study relating to human breast cancer showed that MPA acted as an oestrogen antagonist at oestrogen receptor sites by competitive inhibition. As long as there is more than a certain concentration of MPA in the blood it can act as an anti-oestrogen, and this effect can be used in the treatment of cancer.

MPA may also affect hormone levels in the pituitary-gonadal and pituitary-adrenal axes.

In the endocrinological studies reported here, marked inhibitory effects of MPA on gonadotropin (FSH, LH) levels and ACTH levels were observed. Consequent effects on oestrogens, progesterone and hydrocortisone levels were also observed. Decreases in gonadotropin and ACTH levels following MPA administration have already been recorded [15–18]. Serum levels of

PRL and GH showed no marked changes in the present study. Conflicting results have been recorded in relation to these 2 hormones. Danguy, in a study of MPA treatment of dimethylbenzanthracene-induced mammary tumours in rats, observed that PRL blood levels were lowered by 10 and 100 mg/kg of MPA [19]. In a study of MPA treatment in human beings, however, Sala et al., like us, observed no significant changes in PRL blood levels [20]. In the same paper, serum GH levels are recorded as tending to decrease, in contrast to our findings. These discrepancies may be a result of differences in dosage or route of administration. Further investigation is needed.

MPA may also have a direct inhibitory action on the proliferation of cells via an effect on DNA or RNA synthesis, which has been shown in many experiments [21–23].

Summing up, the results in the clinical studies recorded here indicate that oral, high-dose MPA therapy can produce useful clinical effects. A daily dose of 1,200 mg (400 mg $\times$ 3) would seem best as regards therapeutic outcome and side-effects. MPA caused appreciable suppression of FSH, LH, ATCH, oestrogen, progesterone and hydrocortisone levels. Oral dosage is more acceptable to the patient than daily i.m. injections, and is particularly convenient for the treatment of out-patients.

References

1. Ganzina, F. (1979): High-dose medroxyprogesterone acetate (MPA) treatment in advanced breast cancer. A review. *Tumori 65*, 563.
2. Pannuti, E., Martoni, A., Pollutri, E. et al. (1974): Medroxyprogesterone acetate (MPA): effect of massive doses in advanced breast cancer. *IRCS Med. Sci. 2*, 1605.
3. Amadori, D., Ravaioli, A. and Barbanti, F. (1976): L'impiego del medrossiprogesterone acetato ad alti dosaggi nella terapia palliativa del carcinoma mammario in fase avanzata. *Min. Med. 67*, 1.
4. Pannuti, F., Martoni, A., Lenaz, G.R. et al. (1978): A possible new approach to the treatment of metastatic breast cancer: massive doses of medroxyprogesterone acetate. *Cancer Treat. Rep. 62*, 499.
5. Robustelli Della Cuna, G., Carciati, A., Bernardo Strada, M.R. et al. (1978): High dose medroxyprogesterone acetate (MPA) treatment in metastatic carcinoma of the breast: a dose-response evaluation. *Tumori 64*, 143.
6. De Lena, M., Brambilla, C., Valagussa, P. and Bonadonna, G. (1979): High-dose medroxyprogesterone acetate in breast cancer resistant to endocrine and cytotoxic therapy. *Cancer Chemother. Pharmacol. 2*, 175.
7. Mattsson, W. (1978): High dose medroxyprogesterone-acetate treatment in advanced mammary carcinoma. A phase II investigation. *Acta Radiol. Oncol. 17*, 387.
8. Izuo, M., Iino, Y. and Endo, K. (1981): Oral high-dose medroxyprogesterone acetate (MAP) in treatment of advanced breast cancer: A preliminary report of

clinical and experimental studies. *Breast Cancer Res. Treat. 1*, 125.

9. Tominaga, T., Izuo, M., Abe, O. et al. (1981): Oral high dose medroxyprogesterone acetate (MAP) in treatment of advanced breast cancer. XIIth International Congress of Chemotherapy, Florence, Abstract No. 272.
10. Hayward, J.L., Carbone, P.P., Heuson, J.C. et al. (1977): Assessment of response to therapy in advanced breast cancer. *Eur. J. Cancer 13*, 89.
11. Pannuti, F., Di Marco, A., Martoni, A. et al. (1980): Medroxyprogesterone acetate in treatment of metastatic breast cancer: seven years of experience. In: *Role of Medroxyprogesterone in Endocrine-Related Tumors,* pp. 73–92. Eds: S. Iacobelli and A. Di Marco. Raven Press, New York.
12. Bumma, C., Serra, M.C., Zaccara, F. et al. (1978): Correlazione tra risposta terapeutica e presenza di recettori ormonali in pazienti trattate con alte dosi di MAP. Riunioni Integrate di Oncologia, Florence, Abstract No. 93.
13. Clark, J.H., Anderson, J.N. and Peck, E.J. (1974): Oestrogen receptors and antagonism of steroid hormone action. *Nature 251*, 446.
14. Hsueh, A.J.W., Peck, E.J. and Clark, J.H. (1975): Progesterone antagonism of the oestrogen receptor and oestrogen-induced uterine growth. *Nature 254*, 337.
15. Kupperman, H.S. and Epstein, J.A. (1962): Medroxyprogesterone acetate in the treatment of constitutional sexual precocity. *J. Clin. Endocrinol. Metab. 22*, 456.
16. Laron, Z. and Rummey, H. (1965): Treatment of precocious sexual development by medroxyprogesterone acetate. *Acta Endocrinol. 49*, (Suppl. 101), 27.
17. Mathews, J.H., Abrams, C.A. and Morishima, A. (1970): Pituitary-adrenal function in ten patients receiving medroxyprogesterone acetate for true precocious puberty. *J. Clin. Endocrinol. Metab. 30*, 653.
18. Sadoff, L. and Lusk, W. (1974): The effect of large doses of medroxyprogesterone acetate (MPA) on urinary estrogen levels and serum levels of cortisol, T4, LH and testosterone in patients with advanced cancer. *Obstet. Gynecol. 43*, 262.
19. Danguy, A., Legros, N., Devleeschouwer, N. et al. (1980): Effects of medroxyprogesterone acetate (MPA) on growth of DMBA-induced rat mammary tumors: Histopathological and endocrine studies. In: *Role of Medroxyprogesterone in Endocrine-Related Tumors*, pp. 21–28. Eds: S. Iacobelli and A. Di Marco. Raven Press, New York.
20. Sala, G., Castegnaro, E., Lenaz, G.R. et al. (1978): Hormone interference in metastatic breast cancer patients treated with medroxyprogesterone acetate at massive dose: preliminary results. *IRCS Med. Sci. 6*, 129.
21. Nordvist, S. (1970): Survival and hormone responsiveness of endometrial carcinoma in organ culture. *Acta Obstet. Gynecol. Scand. 49*, 275.
22. Nordvist, S. (1972): Effect of progesterone on human endometrial carcinoma in different experimental systems. *Acta Obstet. Gynecol. Scand. 19*, 25.
23. Anderson, D.G. (1972): The possible mechanisms of action of progestins on endometrial carcinoma. *Am. J. Obstet. Gynecol. 113*, 195.

Discussion

M. Kjaer: In his last sentence, Professor Izuo said that he continued with the randomized trial – but this was not a randomized trial.

M. Izuo: That is right – it was not randomized.

Medroxyprogesterone acetate plus chemotherapy versus chemotherapy alone: 3 randomized clinical trials

A. Pellegrini[1], G. Robustelli Della Cuna[2], B. Massidda[1], B. Bernardo[2], V. Mascia[1] and L. Pavesi[2]
[1]*Institute of Clinical Oncology, Cagliari University Medical School, Cagliari; and* [2]*Division of Oncology, Clinica del Lavoro Foundation, University of Pavia, Pavia, Italy*

Introduction

Hormonal manipulation of advanced breast cancer has reached a plateau in terms of both response rate and overall duration of survival. Treatment based on monitoring of receptor status has almost doubled the response rate but without any evident increase in duration of response, or survival period.

Notwithstanding the high rate of response achieved with polychemotherapy [1], the duration of survival in women with clear evidence of tumour regression has, in fact, remained at 18–24 months (in contrast to 8–10 months for those not responding [2, 3].

In the 1970's, combined chemotherapy and hormonal therapy was considered, on the basis that it might be a more aggressive means of treatment of disseminated breast cancer. The rationale for combined treatment was essentially the different tumour cell sensitivity to hormones and cytotoxic drugs [3]. This therapeutic approach seemed to fulfil the prerequisites for any worthwhile combination: each component was active on its own, the components acted via different mechanisms, and the maximum effective dose of each component could be administered without cumulative manifestations of toxicity.

By 1975, our groups had begun a number of controlled clinical trials comparing polychemotherapy alone versus the identical chemotherapy plus high doses of medroxyprogesterone acetate (HD-MPA).

The first 2 trials (cyclophosphamide + doxorubicin + methotrexate + fluorouracil (CAMF) ± MPA, and fluorouracil + doxorubicin + cyclophosphamide (FAC) ± MPA) have already reached follow-up periods of 5 and 4 years, respectively. MPA was administered by the oral (p.o.) and/or parenteral route. A third trial (vincoisine + doxorubicin + cyclophosphamide (VAC) ± MPA) with a follow-up period, so far, of only 18 months, was conducted administering MPA only by the parenteral route.

The main objectives of the trials were:

a. to compare response rates, duration of response, duration of survival, and other clinical parameters, relating to a polychemotherapy schedule, with or without p.o. MPA (CAMF ± MPA).

b. to evaluate possible differences in response between p.o. and parenteral routes of administration of MPA (FAC ± MPA).

c. to compare response rates etc. as in a. and b. using a chemotherapy protocol, having a cross-over maintenance schedule not involving doxorubicin, to save the latter drug for treatment of subsequent relapses, and to maintain the possibility of adding high-dose methotrexate in case of induction failure.

Material and methods

In the first trial, 50 patients with disseminated breast cancer were allocated at random to treatment with combined chemotherapy with CAMF, with or without oral MPA; when a total doxorubicin dose of 480 mg/m^2 was reached, chemotherapy was continued using vincristine, cyclophosphamide, methotrexate and fluorouracil (VCMF) (Table I) [4]. At the 5-year follow-up period, 45 patients were evaluable, 24 in the CAMF group and 21 in the CAMF + MPA-treated group. Patient characteristics are summarized in Table II. Fifteen cases had received short-term chemotherapy at least 2 months before entering the trial. All patients were spontaneously or surgically postmenopausal. Clinical and laboratory evaluations were conducted twice monthly, and complete restaging was carried out every 4 months, or more often, depending on clinical requests. Evaluation of response followed the criteria recommended by Hayward et al. [5].

The second trial was a 3-branch prospective controlled study [6], in which 120 patients, most previously untreated, with metastatic progressive disease were allocated at random to receive:

a. FAC.

b. FAC plus HD-MPA, intramuscularly (i.m.).

c. FAC plus HD-MPA, p.o.

When a total dose doxorubicin of 480 mg/m^2 was reached, chemotherapy was continued with cyclophosphamide, methotrexate and fluorouracil (CMF) or CMF + MPA (Tables III and IV). The main characteristics of the evaluable patients are summarized in Table V. Clinical and laboratory evaluations were

Table I. CAMF (VCMF) + MPA trial: dose schedule.

Therapy	Dosage and route of administration	Days of treatment													
CAMF		1	2	3	4	5	6	7	8	9	10	11	12	13	14
ADM	40 mg/m^2 i.v.	×													
EDX	125 mg/m^2 p.o.			×	×	×	×	×	×						
MTX	15 mg/m^2 i.v.			×					×						
5-FU	400 mg/m^2 i.v.			×					×						
VCMF															
VCR	1.4 mg/m^2 i.v.	×													
EDX	100 mg/m^2 p.o.	×	×	×	×	×	×	×	×	×	×	×	×	×	×
MTX	30 mg/m^2 i.v.	×							×						
5-FU	500 mg/m^2 i.v.	×							×						
MPA	600 mg/day/p.o.	continuous administration to patients allocated at random to receive it													

ADM = doxonicin; EDX = cyclophosphamide; MTX = methotrexate; 5-FU = fluorouracil; VCR = vincristine.

Table II. CAMF (VCMF) trial: patient characteristics.

	CAMF	CAMF + MPA
Numbers of patients evaluable/total numbers of patients treated	24/25	21/25
Median age (years)	51	49
Numbers of postmenopausal patients/numbers of patients evaluable	24/24	21/21
Spontaneous menopause	8	7
Ovariectomy	16	14
Predominant sites of metastases (numbers of patients)		
Soft tissue	9	14
Visceral	15	8
Osseous	16	14
Mixed	13	13
Prior treatment (numbers of patients)		
Radical mastectomy	21/24	18/21
Radiotherapy	14/24	7/21
Chemotherapy + hormonal therapy	10/24	5/21

Table III. FAC (CMF) ± MPA trial: treatment scheme.

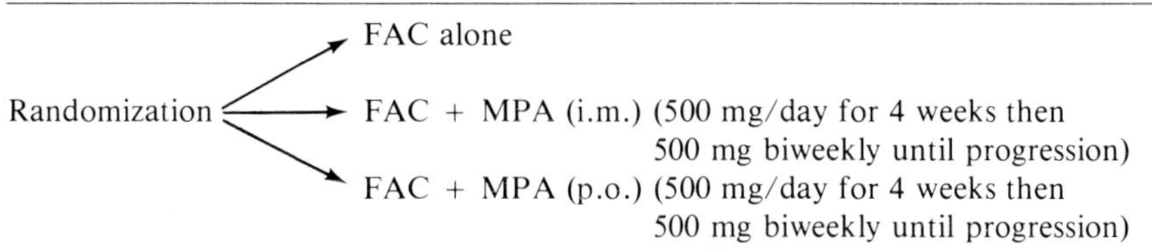

FAC treatment was changed to CMF treatment if there was progression, and, in cases of complete remission, partial remission or no change after 8 cycles of treatment.

Table IV. FAC (CMF) ± MPA trial: dose schedule.

Drugs	Days of treatment		Rest period (days)
F: 500 mg/m², i.v.	1	8	
A: 50 mg/m², i.v.	↑	↑	8–28
C: 500 mg/m², i.v.	↑		
C: 400 mg/m², i.v.	↑	↑	
M: 40 mg/m², i.v.	↑	↑	8–28
F: 400 mg/m², i.v.	↑	↑	

carried out in a manner similar to that previously described, using the same criteria.

The third trial was a multicentre controlled clinical trial involving 10 institutions in Argentina, Brazil, Chile, Italy, Spain and Mexico (Table VI). Two hundred and sixty patients with advanced breast cancer were enrolled into the study, and were randomly allocated to chemotherapy with VAC, with or without parenteral MPA. After 4 induction cycles, patients experiencing complete or partial response or stabilization of disease underwent an additional consolidation cycle, then switched to a vincristine, cyclophosphamide, fluorouracil (VCF) schedule, as maintenance treatment. In cases of initial failure or subsequent relapse, patients were treated with VAC plus methotrexate (VACM). Subjects in whom disease still progressed, or who relapsed on VACM were also given parenteral MPA (Figure; Tables VII and VIII). Clinical and laboratory evaluations were carried out as before. The same criteria of response were also used. At the last analysis (15th September 1981), the median follow-up time was 18 months, and 87 patients were evaluable in respect of the VAC regimen and 92 in respect of the VAC + MPA treatment.

Table V. FAC (CMF) ± MPA trial: patient characteristics (numbers of patients).

	FAC alone	FAC + MPA 500 i.m.	FAC + MPA 500 p.o.
Numbers of patients evaluable	40	40	40
Median age (years)	54	52	55
Premenopausal	5	4	5
Postmenopausal	35	36	35
Predominant site of metastases			
Soft tissue	6	7	5
Visceral	10	10	9
Osseous	15	14	15
Mixed	9	9	11
Disease-free interval (years)			
0 – 1	15	13	13
1 – 5	20	22	21
> 5	5	5	6
Previous therapy			
Chemotherapy	2	3	1
Hormonotherapy	3	1	2
Karnofsky rating			
≥ 60	34	35	35
< 60	6	5	5

Results and discussion

CAMF combination chemotherapy alone gave a response rate of 45.8%, made up of complete remissions (4.2%) and partial remissions (41.6%). The median duration of response was 11 months. The median duration of survival in responders was 31 months. The overall survival period was 21.5 months. The CAMF + MPA-treated group gave a response rate of 62%, made up of 19% of complete remissions, and 42.8% of partial remissions. The median duration of response was 22.5 months, the median duration of survival of responders was 33 months, the overall median survival period was 28 months (Table IX). Even though all results seemed to favour the combination of chemotherapy and hormonal therapy, the only statistically significant difference related to the longer median duration of response in patients receiving such therapy.

Table VI. VAC ± MPA trial: participants and accrual of patients up to October 15, 1981.

Participants	Numbers of patients enrolled	Treatment	
		VAC	VAC + MPA
Argentina			
Prof. Estevez	100	46	54
Brasil			
Prof. Junqueira	10	6	4
Chile			
Prof. Arraztoa	19	7	12
Italy (CA)			
Prof. Pellegrini	29	18	11
Italy (PV)			
Prof. Robustelli	40	21	19
Spain			
Dr Cortes Funes	17	8	9
Argentina			
Dr Luchina	20	11	9
Mexico			
Prof. Lira Puerto	25	12	13
Totals	260	129	131

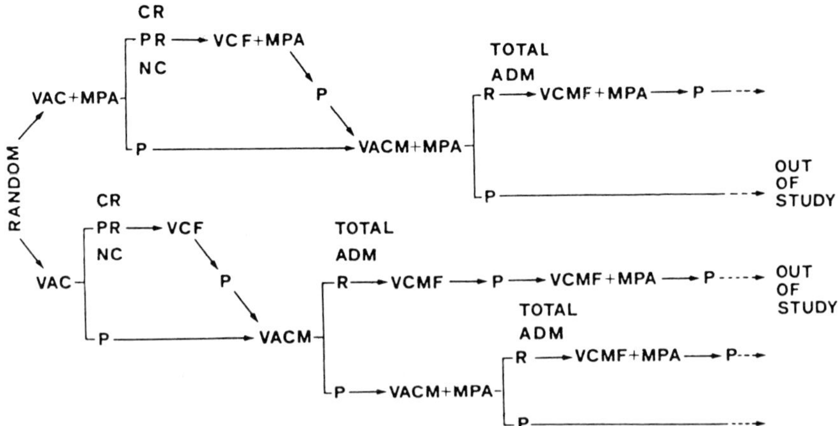

Figure. VAC + MPA trial: study design (CR = complete remission; PR = partial remission; NC = no change; P = progression; Total ADM = total doxorubicin dose 500 mg/m²; VCMF = vincristine cyclophosphamide, methotrexate, fluorouracil).

Table VII. VAC ± MPA trial: dose schedule (I).

Drug	Dosage	Route of administration	Day(s) of administration
V	1 mg	i.v.	1
A	50 mg/m^2	i.v.	1
C	100 mg/m^2	p.o.	1–8
V	1 mg	i.v.	1
A	50 mg/m^2	i.v.	1
C	100 mg/m^2	p.o.	1–8
M	200 mg	i.v. +	
	15 mg × 3	p.o.	8
MPA	500 mg	i.m.	1–15
	500 mg	i.m.	Twice weekly after 15 days of treatment

Table VIII. VAC ± MPA trial: dose schedule (II).

Drug	Dosage	Route of administration	Day(s) of administration
V VCR	1 mg	i.v.	1
C EDX	100 mg/m^2	p.o.	1–8
F 5-FU	750 mg/m^2	i.v.	1
V VCR	1 mg	i.v.	1
F 5-FU	750 mg/m^2	i.v.	1
C EDX	100 mg/m^2	p.o.	1–8
M MTX	200 mg	i.v. +	
CF	15 mg × 3	p.o.	8
MPA	500 mg	i.m.	1 to 15
	500 mg	i.m.	Twice weekly after 15 days of treatment

This first study was not completely homogeneous as far as the distribution of metastatic sites between the 2 groups was concerned, but it would also seem worth stressing that the response to combined treatment with chemotherapy and hormonal therapy was better, but still not significantly, in the case of pleural, soft tissue, breast and nodal metastases than to chemotherapy alone.

Both treatments were well tolerated, and side-effects related mainly to mild

Table IX. Results of the CAMF (VCMF) ± MPA trial (5 year follow-up).

	CAMF	CAMF + MPA
Overall response (complete remissions + partial remissions) (%)	46	62
Median duration of response (months)	11	22.5
Overall median survival period (months)	21.5	28
Median survival period of responders (months)	31	33
Numbers of patients still alive/total	3/24	4/21
Numbers of patients treated (%)	(12%)	(19%)
Numbers of patients still alive/numbers of patients responding (%)	1/11 (9%)	3/13 (23%)

nausea, alopecia, and bone marrow toxicity. Leukopenia was significantly less frequent in the chemotherapy plus MPA-treated group than in the group treated with chemotherapy alone. Hyperglycaemia, slight increases in blood pressure, moon-face, and slight tremors were observed rarely in the chemotherapy plus MPA-treated group. They were obviously related to hydrocortisone-like activity of MPA. However, hormonal treatment never needed to be stopped. Patients treated with combined chemotherapy and hormonal therapy experienced greater improvement in their general condition, sense of well-being, increase in body weight and pain relief than those on chemotherapy alone.

In the second trial (FAC ± MPA), in which the follow-up period was 48 months, there was a 55% response rate, made up of 15% of complete remissions and 40% of partial remissions, with a median duration of response of 9 months (Table X). The survival period in responders and the overall survival period were 20 and 16 months, respectively. In the group treated with chemotherapy plus p.o. MPA, a 65% response rate (47% partial remissions, 17% complete remissions) was achieved, with a median duration of response of 13 months. In responders, the survival period was 24 months. The overall survival period was 22 months. The patients treated with chemotherapy plus parenteral MPA showed a 75% response rate (52% partial remission, 22% complete remission), with a median duration of response of 19 months. The overall survival period and the survival period in responders were 28 and 31.5 months, respectively. Though all results favour combined chemotherapy and hormonal treatment, only the differences in durations of response and in the survival periods in responders were significantly better with the combination with parenteral MPA than with FAC alone. Considering both trials (CAMF and FAC) together, it would seem that only parenteral MPA administration

Table X. Results of FAC (CMF) ± MPA trial (4-year follow-up).

	FAC alone	FAC + MPA (i.m.)	FAC + MPA (p.o.)
Overall response (complete remissions + partial remissions (%))	55	75	65
Median duration of response (months)	9	19	13
Overall median survival period (months)	16	28	22
Median survival period of responders (months)	20	31.5	24
Numbers of patients still alive/ total numbers of patients treated (%)	4/40 (10%)	9/40 (22%)	5/40 (12%)
Numbers of patients still alive/ numbers of patients responding (%)	2/22 (9%)	7/30 (23%)	4/26 (15%)

$P < 0.001$ $P < 0.05$ (Log rank test).

makes the difference in the survival period in responders statistically significant. This may be related to a higher specific activity of MPA when administered by the i.m. route. Recent pharmacokinetic studies have revealed higher plasma levels of MPA following parenteral administration than after p.o. administration of the same dose [7].

The second trial has also shown that the incidence of leukopenia and thrombocytopenia in chemotherapy plus MPA-treated groups is significantly lower than in patients who received chemotherapy alone. The addition of MPA to the FAC regimen resulted in an increase in body weight (60%) and performance status (50%), together with marked pain relief (50%). These favourable side-effects were greatest in the group of patients treated with parenteral MPA. Adverse reactions such as moon face, muscle cramps, or vaginal bleeding occurred in a small percentage of patients, treated parenterally or p.o. with MPA. In the patients treated with MPA i.m. there was a 15% incidence of gluteal abscess.

The third trial (VAC ± MPA) has reached only the 18-month follow-up stage. The first extramural review is still in progress. It is not possible to draw any definite conclusions. Eighty-seven patients are evaluable in the case of chemotherapy alone, and 92 in the case of the combined treatment. The response rate was 48.2% (14.9% of complete remissions and 33.3% of partial remissions) in the first-mentioned group, as compared with 50% (8.7% of complete remissions, 41.3% of partial remissions) in the other group, i.e. a higher percentage of minor responses was observed, in patients receiving both chemotherapy and hormonal therapy. While the median time to progression was 9 months in the VAC-treated group, the median value had not been reached at 18 months in VAC plus MPA-treated patients. The protection afforded by MPA against bone-marrow toxicity in patients receiving chemotherapy is evident, as are other favourable side-effects (increased body weight and performance status, pain relief). The relatively short duration of follow-up and the correspondingly high number of patients at early stages following admission do not allow any more profound analysis.

Conclusions

Combined chemotherapy and hormonal therapy results in higher percentages of remissions and longer durations of response than chemotherapy alone in metastatic breast cancer. Results in the VAC ± MPA trial are, however, not yet fully evaluable. Complete remissions are more frequent with the combined treatment. The survival periods overall and in responders alone, after 5 (CAMF ± MPA) and 4 (FAC ± MPA) years of follow-up were fairly similar. Patients responding, who have a longer duration of response on the chemotherapy plus MPA schedule than patients on chemotherapy alone, also have a better quality of life than patients treated with chemotherapy alone. It can be argued that the higher response rate and longer duration of response achievable with combined chemotherapy and hormonal therapy is likely to be related to the 'protective' effect of MPA against the bone marrow toxicity induced by the prolonged use of cytotoxic drugs. Such an effect could allow stricter adherence to the therapeutic dosage schedule. Even although a statistically significant difference in requirements for dose reduction between the combined regimens and chemotherapy alone was not evident in our studies, the above-mentioned hypothesis cannot be excluded. The VAC ± MPA trial may help to provide an answer to this question.

The FAC trial allowed comparison between p.o. and parenteral MPA administration. The observed difference in response rate in favour of the i.m. route was not statistically significant. However, the p.o. route also seems suitable for high-dose administration and is acceptable to the patients. There are, obviously, no abscesses, and this contributes towards continuity of treatment. Finally on the basis of our studies with CAMF and FAC there does not seem to be any difference as regards either remission rate or duration of response between the groups of patients treated with 500 mg and 600 mg doses of the 2 schedules.

In our opninion, treatment with a combination of chemotherapy and hormonal therapy represents a more aggressive strategy, with the possibility of achieving higher response rates, and longer durations of response. Longer survival periods than with chemotherapy alone are rare. It is not at present known (no convincing evidence is available in the literature) whether the concurrent use of chemotherapy and hormones leads to longer survival periods and a better quality of life than conventional sequential treatment.

MPA seems to be a useful hormonal component in combinations of the type described above, mainly because of its favourable side-effects. However, combinations of MPA and chemotherapy cannot be recommended routinely until the optimum doses, and sequences of administration of this progestin and cytotoxic regimens are clearly defined.

References

1. Carbone, P.P., Bauer, M., Band, P. and Tormey, D.C. (1977): Chemotherapy of disseminated breast cancer: current status and prospects. *Cancer 39,* 2916.
2. Lloyd, R.E., Jones, S.E. and Salmon, S.E. (1979): Comparative trial of low-dose adriamycin plus cyclophosphamide with or without additive hormonal therapy in advanced breast cancer. *Cancer 43,* 60.
3. Robustelli Della Cuna, G., Pellegrini, A. and Ganzina, F. (1980): *Chemotherapy and Hormonal Treatment of Advanced Breast Cancer.* Farmitalia Carlo Erba, Milan.
4. Pellegrini, A., Massidda, B., Macia, V. et al. (1980): CAMF versus CAMF + MPA nel carcinoma mammario avanzato: valutazione a 42 mesi. *Tumori 66 (Suppl.)*, 99.
5. Hayward, J.L., Carbone, P.P., Heuson, J.C. et al. (1977): Assessment of response to therapy in advanced breast cancer. *Eur. J. Cancer 13,* 89.
6. Robustelli Della Cuna, G. and Bernardo-Strada, M.R. (1980): High dose medroxyprogesterone acetate (HD-MPA) combined with chemotherapy for metastatic breast cancer. In: *Role of Medroxyprogesterone Acetate (MPA) in Endocrine-Related Tumors,* p. 53. Editors: S. Iacobelli and A. DiMarco. Raven Press, New York.
7. Tamassia, V., Battaglia, A., Ganzina, F. et al. (1982): Pharmacokinetic approach to the selection of a dose of schedule for medroxyprogesterone acetate in clinical oncology. *Cancer Chemother. Pharmacol.* (In press.)

A trial of tamoxifen versus high-dose medroxyprogesterone acetate in advanced postmenopausal breast cancer. A final report

W. Mattsson[1], F. von Eyben[2], L. Hallsten[2] and L. Tennvall[2]
[1]*Department of Oncology and Radiotherapy, Central Hospital, Karlstad; and* [2]*Department of Oncology and Radiotherapy, General Hospital, Malmö, Sweden*

Introduction

Interest in endocrine treatment in advanced breast cancer has revived during the 1970's. There has been a growth in knowledge about endocrine-related tumour growth. More specific anti-oestrogenic agents have been introduced clinically [1–3], and pharmacological adrenalectomy has also been practised [4]. The concept of heterogeneity of tumour cell populations has led to studies involving combinations of drugs with different modes of action. Combinations of different types of endocrine therapy, and of endocrine therapy and cytotoxic chemotherapy have been examined [5–10], with conflicting initial results, however.

Another trend has been towards the re-evaluation of older drugs. Progestins in metastatic breast cancer have previously been reported to give a response rate of 10–35% after low or moderate doses (50–400 mg) [11, 12]. Higher remission rates have been recorded in patients treated with high-dose medroxyprogesterone acetate (HD-MPA) [13, 14]. Progestins can act as anti-oestrogens, both directly on tumour cells, by inhibiting binding of oestradiol to receptors, and indirectly, by reducing the amount of oestrogen available to the tumour cells through increase in oestrogen catabolism, decrease of the conversion of androgens to oestrogens and suppression of the hypophyseal release of LH and FSH [15].

The biological actions of progestins and the initial results with HD-MPA therapy led us to carry out a trial in patients with advanced breast cancer who had previously undergone intensive treatment [16]. The efficacy of HD-MPA, its good clinical tolerance, and, above all, the subjective improvements which it produces in severely ill patients were confirmed. Consequently, we proceeded to a further trial in which HD-MPA was compared with tamoxifen, regarded as the drug of choice in advanced breast-cancer patients in whom endocrine therapy was indicated. The initial results have been reported previously [17].

Material and methods

Between November 1977 and February 1980, all patients with advanced postmenopausal breast cancer who were referred to the Department of Oncology and Radiotherapy at Malmö General Hospital were enrolled in this trial if they fulfilled the following criteria;

1. Measurable and/or evaluable metastases.
2. Karnofsky index ≥50.

3.1 Oestrogen receptor-rich tumours (tamoxifen 10 patients, HD-MPA 8 patients). (First line therapy.)

3.2 Oestrogen receptor status of tumour unknown, patients older than 70. (First line therapy.)

3.3 Oestrogen receptor status of tumour unknown, patients younger than 70 when clinical resistance to cytotoxic chemotherapy had occurred.

Sixty-three patients have been enrolled. All are evaluable. The characteristics of the 2 treatment groups were very comparable (Table I). There were no significant differences between groups in relation to median

Table I. Patient characteristics.

	Tamoxifen	HD-MPA
Numbers of patients	33	30
Age (median) (years)	64	65
Age range (years)	40–79	42–80
Disease-free interval		
Median (months)	28	25
Range (months)	0–150	0–146
Predominant location of metastases (numbers of patients)		
Soft tissue	1	1
Bone	9	9
Viscera	23	20
Previous therapy of metastases		
VAC/VACM (3) (no. of patients)	15	13

V = vincristine, A = doxorubicin, C = cyclophosphamide, M = methotrexate.

disease-free intervals, pretreatment Karnofsky indices (median value 80 in both groups) or median age. Fifteen patients in the tamoxifen group had previously been treated with doxorubicin-based regimes, and 13 patients in the HD-MPA group. The distribution of sites of metastases was similar in both groups. Visceral sites were the most common. Patients shown to have liver metastases were not enrolled because of the insignificant effect which endocrine therapy has on such metastases.

Before each patient was included in the study, the extent of disease was assessed by means of clinical and gynaecological examinations, chest and skeletal radiography, isotope-scanning of the liver, and fine needle aspiration biopsy of accessible metastases in the skin, lymph nodes, lungs and liver. When clinically indicated, these examinations were supplemented by mammary radiography, ultrasonic examination of the abdominal and pelvic cavities, computerized tomography of the suspected diseased organ, and isotope-scanning of the brain and of the skeleton. Laboratory investigations included haemoglobin determination, erythrocyte, leukocyte and differential counts, platelet count, serum electrolyte status, serum creatinine determination, and liver function tests serum aspartate aminotransferase, alanine aminotransferase and alkaline phosphatase. Electrophoresis and the carcinoembryonic antigen test were also performed. Symptoms were recorded by means of the Karnofsky performance scale.

Patients who had measurable or evaluable metastases were allocated at random, using a stochastic array of numbers, closed envelop system, to treatment with either tamoxifen, 10 mg orally, 3 times daily, or HD-MPA, 1 g intramuscularly (i.m.) daily for 30 days. Patients were then assessed, and, if progression of the disease could not be established, treatment with tamoxifen was continued as before, and treatment with HD-MPA with 1 g, i.m., once a week, until evidence was found of progression of disease or relapse. If progression of disease was established, the possibility of cross-over to the other treatment existed, and cross-over was executed in 30 patients. Patients with rapidly progressing metastases were excluded from cross-over.

Results were assessed every fourth week for 12 weeks by means of physical examination, calculation of the Karnofsky index, chest and skeletal X-ray, and isotope-scanning of the liver. Other investigations performed in order to establish remission were ultrasonic examination of the abdominal and pelvic cavities, isotope-scanning of the brain and bones, and mammary radiography. After the first 12 weeks of treatment, follow-up was individualized, but, at intervals of 3 months, at most, remissions were assessed by physical examination, calculation of the Karnofsky index, chest and skeletal X-ray and isotope-scanning of the liver.

The criteria used to judge remission were those recommended by the Union International Contra le Cancrum [18]. Complete remission (CR) was disappearance of all established disease. In the case of lytic bone metastases, radiography had to show that the lesions had calcified. Partial remission (PR) was a decrease of 50% or more in the size of measurable lesions, with objective improvement of evaluable but nonmeasurable lesions, and no new lesions. No change (NC) was recorded when the size of measurable lesions decreased by less than 50%, or increased by less than 25%. Progressive disease (PD) was when some lesions regressed, others progressed, or new lesions appeared, or when some or all lesions progressed, or new lesions appeared. The durations of remission and survival were recorded from the day of starting therapy.

Results

The overall response rates were 55% in the tamoxifen group and 70% in the HD-MPA group. The median durations of remission did not differ significantly ($P>0.1$, log rank test) (Table II). There was a significant difference in durations of remissions as between patients in whom there was CR and those in whom there was PR (Table III). Periods of NC were significantly shorter than durations of CR and PR. The median survival time tended to be longer in patients who received tamoxifen initially, but the difference was not statistic-

Table II. Remissions following tamoxifen and HD-MPA.

	Tamoxifen	HD-MPA
CR + PR (no. of patients)	17/33	21/30
Duration of remission (months)		
Median	24	15
Range	3 to 42+	4 to 43+
Still alive (number of patients)	18	10

Table III. Median durations of remissions (months).

	Tamoxifen	HD-MPA
CR	33+	25+
PR	16	15
NC	8	8

Table IV. Median survival (months).

	Tamoxifen	HD-MPA
CR	42+	25+
PR	27+	17
NC	8	25+
PD	6	3

Table V. Objective response in relation to dominant site of metastases (no. of patients).

Site of metastases	Tamoxifen	HD-MPA
Bone	4/9	7/9
Viscera	13/23	14/20

ally significant (Table IV). The objective response rates in relation to site of metastases did not differ (Table V). Patient numbers are small. The high rate of objective response in patients with bone metastases is noteworthy. The response rates were high when the metastases were rich in oestrogen receptors (tamoxifen 6/10 patients, HD-MPA 7/8 patients).

Treatment with tamoxifen or with HD-MPA was effective in patients in whom combination chemotherapy had failed, or in patients on combination chemotherapy who had suffered a relapse. Thus, 4 out of 15 patients treated with tamoxifen, and 9 out of 13 patients treated with HD-MPA showed an objective response when treatment was instituted in patients clinically resistant to doxorubicin-based regimes.

Both treatments were well tolerated. Treatment did not have to be discontinued in any patient because of side-effects. In patients treated with tamoxifen, 5 experienced hot flushes, and 2 patients had slight nausea for 2–5 weeks. One patient complained of headache. Two patients had vaginal symptoms. The injections of HD-MPA caused a degree of swelling in the buttocks in 8 patients. Nineteen patients had local infiltration, but these did not cause the patients any discomfort. Sterile abscesses were not observed. Increased appetite was noted in almost all patients, and 22 exhibited weight gain during HD-MPA therapy. Moon face, as in Cushing's disease, occurred in 5 HD-MPA patients, but no other adverse effects of an adrenocorticoidal nature could be detected. Vaginal bleeding occurred in 2 patients treated with HD-MPA.

The subjective improvement as measured by the Karnofsky index was 0–30 points (median 10 points) in the tamoxifen group, and 10–40 points (median 20 points) in the HD-MPA group.

Discussion

These results for treatment with tamoxifen and HD-MPA, correspond to results reported elsewhere [1–3, 13, 14, 16, 19, 21, 22], and compare favourably with those obtained with other endocrine treatments [3, 19, 23].

Both tamoxifen and MPA act at receptor sites [20, 21]. MPA depresses the level of oestradiol as a result of enzymatically accelerated catabolism of oestrogen, and, in consequence of increased androgens reduces the amounts of androgen converted to oestrogens [15]. Since blood levels of oestradiol have been found to be increased in patients not responding to treatment with tamoxifen [22], it seems reasonable to suppose that HD-MPA decreased the amounts of oestrogens available to the tumour cells, and thus modified the effects of oestrogens on cell replication, in patients responding to HD-MPA after cross-over therapy. This latter supposition might indirectly be supported by our findings in relation to the oestrogen-progestogen ratio as assessed by protein analysis using Laurell's rocked method in patients treated with tamoxifen [3]. Normal levels were restored when HD-MPA was administered. On the other hand, only a few patients have responded to treatment with tamoxifen after progression of disease or relapse was observed during treatment with HD-MPA.

The effectiveness of tamoxifen and HD-MPA was probably not reduced by previous cytotoxic chemotherapy. This confirms our earlier findings [3]. The somewhat lower response rate of 28% recorded in our earlier study [3] results from the selection of very advanced cases in that trial.

Three controlled trials have evaluated the effects of different doses of HD-MPA [24–26]. It seems reasonable to conclude that 500 mg of MPA a day for 30 days, to begin with, and 500 mg a week as subsequent continuous therapy in responders are the most effective dose levels. This conclusion is also supported by the results of a pharmacological study conducted at the same time as one of the controlled trials [24]. If results from various studies in which MPA has been used are compared, a dose-response relationship seems to emerge. A dose-response relationship has also been reported for oestrogens [23] and androgens [3]. So far, no significant differences in response rates after treatment with tamoxifen at different dosages (20–200 mg/day) have been established [2]. On the other hand, there is an upper dose limit at which the effect of additive endocrine therapy levels off. About the same results were obtained, for example, with 15 mg/day of diethylstilboestrol as with higher doses [23]. Oral testolactone at a dosage of 1 g per day induced an objective response in about 15% of patients as compared with a response rate of 12% when 2 g a day was used [27].

There is general agreement concerning the relationship between the receptor-content of tumours and their response to endocrine therapy. In the present study the response rates for tamoxifen and HD-MPA correlated with the presence of oestrogen receptors in the tumours.

An objective response to previous cytotoxic chemotherapy correlated significantly with remission resulting from subsequent treatment with tamoxifen or HD-MPA. Since breast cancer tissue may contain a mixture of hormone-dependent and hormone-independent tumour cells, these results may be interpreted as indicating that previous chemotherapy has decreased the number of oestrogen receptor-poor tumour cells, and that at the relapse stage, a more oestrogen receptor-rich tumour cell population has developed.

This explanation is supported by findings of a high growth rate in oestrogen receptor-poor tumours and a high level of glucolytic enzymes, which indicates a favourable response to cytotoxic chemotherapy [3]. Kiang and Kennedy [28] found a higher median oestrogen receptor content in oestrogen receptor-rich tumours in patients previously treated with chemotherapy.

Clinical studies have shown the effectiveness of tamoxifen after failure of previous ablative endocrine surgery, or relapse after such treatment. Older additive hormonal measures were rarely effective in such cases. In this study, and in previous studies [3], the effectiveness of tamoxifen in situations of this kind has been confirmed, and the effectiveness of treatment with HD-MPA has also been established.

In elderly patients with advanced breast cancer, and in postmenopausal patients with proven oestrogen receptor-rich metastases, tamoxifen and HD-MPA must both be considered as therapeutic agents of first resort. The main advantage of tamoxifen over HD-MPA is that it can be given by mouth. On the other hand, HD-MPA therapy has such important subjective benefits as increase of appetite, weight gain, and improved feelings of well-being. HD-MPA therapy is therefore recommendable for patients in whom relief of symptoms is important. We are currently studying sequential treatment with tamoxifen and HD-MPA, as well as endocrine treatment together with combination chemotherapy.

References

1. Ward, H.W.C. (1973): Antiestrogen therapy for breast cancer: a trial of tamoxifen at two dose levels. *Br. Med. J. I,* 13.

2. Mouridsen, H., Palshof, T., Patterson, J. and Battersby, L. (1978): Tamoxifen – a review of its efficacy in advanced breast cancer. *Cancer Treat. Rev. 5,* 131.
3. Mattsson, W. (1979): *Endocrine Treatment and Combination Chemotherapy in Metastatic Postmenopausal Breast Cancer*, Thesis, Gotab, Malmö, Sweden.
4. Santen, R.J., Worgul, T.J., Samojlik, E. et al. (1981): A randomized trial comparing surgical adrenalectomy with aminoglutethimide plus hydrocortisone in women with advanced breast cancer. *N. Engl. J. Med. 305*, 545.
5. Mouridsen, H.T., Elleman, K., Mattsson, W. et al. (1979): Therapeutic effect of tamoxifen versus combined tamoxifen and medroxyprogesterone acetate in advanced breast cancer in postmenopausal women. *Cancer Treat. Rep. 63,* 171.
6. Tormey, D.C., Simon, R.M., Lippman, M.E. et al. (1976): Evaluation of tamoxifen dose in advanced breast cancer: a progress report. *Cancer Treat. Rep. 60,* 1451.
7. Dogliotti, L., Mussa, A. and di Carlo, F. (1978): Human breast cancer responsiveness to a new chemotherapeutic association. In: *Proceedings of the 10th International Congress of Chemotherapy,* Vol. II, p. 1287. Eds: W. Siegenthaler and R. Lüthy. American Society for Microbiology, Washington DC.
8. Settatree, R.S., Butt, W.R., London, D.R. et al. (1978): Treatment with tamoxifen versus tamoxifen combined with bromocriptine in metastatic breast cancer. In: *Proceedings of 12th International Cancer Congress, Buenos Aires.* (Abstract.)
9. Brunner, K.W., Sonntag, R.W., Alberto, P. et al. (1977): Combined chemo- and hormonaltherapy in advanced breast cancer. *Cancer 39*, 2923.
10. Robustelli della Cuna, G. and Bernardo-Strada, N.R. (1979): High dose medroxyprogesterone acetate combined with chemotherapy for metastatic breast cancer. In: *Role of Medroxyprogesterone in Endocrine-Related Tumours.* p. 53. Eds: S. Iacobelli and A. di Marco. Raven Press, New York.
11. Ansfield, F.J., Davis Jr., H.C., Ellerby, R.A. and Ramereg, G. (1974): A clinical trial of megesterole acetate in advanced breast cancer. *Cancer 33,* 907.
12. Muggia, F.M., Cassileth, P.A., Ochoa Jr., M. et al. (1968): Treatment of breast cancer with medroxyprogesterone acetate. *Ann. Intern. Med. 68*, 528.
13. Pannuti, G., Martoni, A., Lenaz, G.R. et al. (1978): Management of advanced breast cancer with medroxyprogesterone acetate in high doses. *Cancer Treat. Rep. 62*, 499.
14. Amadori, D., Ravaioli, A. and Barbanti, F. (1976): L'impiego del medrosiprogesterone acetato alti dosaggi nella terapia palliativa del carcinoma mammario in fase avanzato. *Minerva Med. 67,* 1.
15. Gurpide, E. (1976): Hormones and gynecologic cancer. *Cancer 38*, 503.
16. Mattsson, W. (178): High dose medroxyprogesterone acetate treatment in advanced mammary carcinoma. *Acta Radiol. Oncol. 17*, 387.
17. Mattsson, W. (1980): A phase III trial of treatment with tamoxifen versus treatment with high dose medroxyprogesterone acetate in advanced postmenopausal breast cancer. In: *Role of Medroxyprogesterone in Endocrine Related Tumours,* pp. 65–71. Eds: S. Iacobelli and A. di Marco. Raven Press, New York.
18. Hayward, J.L., Carbone, P.P., Heuson, J.C. et al. (1977): Assessment of response to therapy in advanced breast cancer. *Eur. J. Cancer 13,* 89.
19. Stoll, B.A. (1977): Palliation by castration or by hormone administration. In: *Breast Cancer – Early and Late,* p. 133. Ed: B.A. Stoll. William Heinemann Medical Books, London.

20. Hsveh, A.J.W., Peck, E.J. and Clark, J.H. (1975): Progesterone antagonism of the estrogen receptor and estrogen induced uterine growth. *Nature (London) 254,*337.
21. Jordan, V.C. (1976): Antiestrogenic and antitumour properties of tamoxifen in laboratory animals. *Cancer Treat. Rep. 60*, 1409.
22. Willis, K.J., London, D.R., Ward, H.W.C. et al. (1977): Recurrent breast cancer treated with the antiestrogen tamoxifen. Correlation between hormonal changes and clinical course. *Br. Med. J. I,* 425.
23. Carter, A.C., Sedransk, N., Kelley, R.M. et al. (1977): Diethylstilbestrol: recommended dosage for different categories of breast cancer patients. Report of the Co-operative Breast Cancer Group. *J. Am. Med. Assoc. 237,* 2079.
24. Cavalli, G., Goldhirsch, A., Kaplan, E. and Alberto, P. (1981): Swiss group for clinical cancer research (SAKK): high versus low dose medroxyprogesterone acetate in advanced breast cancer. In: *UICC Conference on Clinical Oncology, Lausanne 28–31 October,* p. 32.
25. Robustelli della Cuna, G., Calciati, A., Strada, M.R.B. et al. (1978): High dose medroxyprogesterone acetate treatment in carcinoma of the breast: a dose response evaluation. *Tumori 64*, 143.
26. Pannuti, F., Martoni, A., di Marco, A.R. et al. (1978): A randomized trial of two different dosages of medroxyprogesterone acetate in the treatment of metastatic breast cancer. In: *Proceedings of the Seventh Congress on Cancer, Buenos Aires.* (Abstract.)
27. Volk, H., Deupree, R.H., Goldenberg, I.S. et al. (1974): A dose-response evaluation of delta 1-lactone in advanced breast cancer. *Cancer 33,* 9.
28. Kiang, D.F. and Kennedy, B.J. (1977): Factors affecting estrogen-receptors in breast cancer. *Cancer 40*, 1571.

Clinical experience with medroxyprogesterone acetate in advanced breast cancer

G. Beretta, D. Tabiadon and G. Luporini
Department of Medical Oncology, San Carlo Borromeo Hospital, Milan, Italy

Introduction

This report summarizes and updates the results of a trial which has previously been described [1–3] and records results currently available relating to the more recent use of medroxyprogesterone acetate (MPA) treatment in our department. Two studies have been performed recently, one comparing oral MPA and tamoxifen citrate (TAM), the other involving investigation of intramuscular (i.m.) MPA.

Material and methods

The dosage schedules used in the trials, and the characteristics of patients taking part, are summarized in Table I.

Patients who had completed induction treatment (30 days), at least, were regarded as evaluable. Responses were classified according to the more recent World Health Organization criteria [4], and were also categorized according to the sites of metastatic disease.

Patients were admitted consecutively to each study, even if they had previously been treated with chemotherapy and/or subjected to hormonal manipulation. The oestrogen or progestogen receptor status was determined in less than 10% of patients.

Results

Table II summarizes the therapeutic results obtained up to now in adequately-treated patients. Future findings may be different as a result of late

Table I. Patient characteristics.

Therapy	Induction (mg/day)	Maintenance	Total numbers of patients	Median age (years)	Age range (years)	Percentage aged between 50 and 70	Percentage previously untreated
Intramuscular MPA	500	1,000 mg/week	39	60	39–77	65	28
Oral MPA	600	400–600 mg/day	42	62	31–80	60	19
zoral TAM	20	20 mg/day	43	64	37–78	69	23

Table II. Therapeutic response.

Therapy	Numbers of evaluable patients	Percentage of patients experiencing complete* or partial remission	Percentage of patients experiencing no change	Percentages of patients with metastases in sites indicated experiencing complete or partial remission		
				Soft tissue	Bone	Viscera
Intramuscular MPA	39	25.6	51.2	33	42	16
Oral MPA	42	26.2	47.6	50	15	20
Oral TAM	43	28.1	48.7	35	9	33

*Percentage of complete remissions no greater than 5 in each series.

recalcification of bone lesions but are not likely to alter substantially. Late recalcification is a phenomenon which can be observed even one year after the start of treatment, as we have previously pointed out [3]. The results recorded following i.m. MPA are still likely to be modified considerably since it is not long since results were obtained.

The durations of response and of survival are recorded in Table III in relation to the various treatments and therapeutic responses. Although a trend towards better results following the anti-oestrogenic substance TAM is observable, the differences are not, at present, significant, within the small, prognostically-homogeneous subsets of patients. In forming these subsets, the prognostic factors principally taken into account were the site of the predominant lesion, the numbers of metastatic sites, previous treatments and responses to previous treatments, the disease-free interval between surgery and relapse, the time elapsing since the menopause etc.

The important finding, in our view, is that we have observed true progression (a greater than 25% increase in pre-existing lesions and/or the appearance of new lesions) in about 25% of treated cases without any selection of patients. We regard the fact that 75% of cases treated experienced stabilization, at least, of previously progressive disease for a considerable period of time as indicative of therapeutic success.

Other findings emerging from our studies are:

a. At present, no substantial difference has been detected between oral (p.o.) and i.m. MPA, with the dosage schedules used, though a somewhat higher response rate is evident following i.m. administration in cases of bone metastases than is evident following p.o. administration.

b. We have not so far observed any withdrawal reaction following p.o. or i.m. MPA, but such a reaction has been reported following TAM, in one case with soft-tissue metastases [3].

c. It is possible to induce further therapeutic response by cross-over to treatment with either MPA or TAM. In particular, a 17% response rate (complete or partial remissions) has been observed following MPA in patients previously treated with TAM, and a 19% objective response rate following TAM in patients previously treated with, but resistant to, p.o. MPA. No patient resistant to i.m. MPA responded to subsequent TAM. The response rate to MPA in TAM-resistant patients was greater (30%) in cases not previously responsive to TAM than in cases previously responsive to TAM.

Side-effects were similar in incidence and type to those reported elsewhere [1,5,6]. A 10% incidence of gluteal abscess was observed following i.m. MPA. The better tolerance observed with hormonal therapy than with conventional chemotherapeutic regimes is well known.

Table III. Response and survival.

Therapy	Median duration of response (months) in patients experiencing		Median duration of survival (months) in patients experiencing		
	Complete or partial remission	No change	Complete or partial remission	No change	Progressive disease
Intramuscular MPA	10	5	13	9	4
Oral MPA	7	4.5	15.7	12	7
Oral TAM	10	6	18	12	10

Discussion and conclusions

We believe that both the hormonal treatments studied are very effective in inducing response in subjects with advanced postmenopausal breast carcinoma. MPA and TAM, given p.o. at the doses administered in our studies, appear to be equally active, and capable of prolonging survival, especially in patients responding.

Continuous daily high p.o. doses of MPA are probably as active, are certainly easier to administer, and are better tolerated than traditional high-dose i.m. treatment.

Prospective studies will need to be undertaken to clarify the response rate to high p.o. doses of MPA, and its influence on survival. Particular attention will have to be paid to correlations between the oestrogen and/or progestogen receptor contents of the various tumour lesions and response. There will need to be studies on the optimization of induction and maintenance dosage schedules for both p.o. and i.m. MPA, on the best role for MPA in the complex strategy for treatment of pre- and postmenopausal patients suffering from locally-advanced, inoperable and/or metastatic disease, and on whether MPA has a role in treatment of patients who have undergone therapy for a $T_{1-3}N+$ resected tumour, at high risk of relapse.

References

1. Beretta, G., Tabiadon, D., Tedeschi, L. and Luporini, G. (1982): Hormonotherapy of advanced breast carcinoma: comparative evaluation of tamoxifen citrate versus medroxyprogesterone acetate. In: *The Role of Tamoxifen in Breast Cancer*, pp. 113–120. Eds: S. Iacobelli and M.E. Lippman. Raven Press, New York.
2. Luporini, G., Beretta, G., Tabiadon, D. et al. (1981): Comparison between oral medroxyprogesterone acetate (MPA) and tamoxifen (TMX) in advanced breast carcinoma. In: *Proc. AACR/ASCO 22,* 434-abs C-398.
3. Beretta, G., Luporini, G., Clerici, M. et al. (1981): Tamoxifen versus medroxyprogesterone acetate in the treatment of metastatic breast carcinoma. In: *12th International Congress of Chemotherapy, Florence, July 19–24, 1981,* Abstract 267.
4. Miller, A.B., Hoogstraten, B, Staquet, M. and Winkler, A. (1981): Reporting results of cancer treatment. *Cancer 47,* 207.
5. Ganzina, F. (1979): High-dose medroxyprogesterone acetate treatment in advanced breast cancer. A review. *Tumori 65,* 563.
6. Iacobelli, S. and Di Marco, A. (eds.) (1980): *Role of Medroxyprogesterone Acetate in Endocrine Related Tumors.* Raven Press, New York.

High-dose medroxyprogesterone acetate in metastatic breast cancer. A critical review

G. Robustelli Della Cuna[1], M.R. Bernardo-Strada[1] and F. Ganzina[2]
[1] Division of Oncology, Clinica del Lavoro Foundation, University of Pavia, Pavia and [2] Department of Therapeutic Research, Farmitalia Carlo Erba S.p.A., Milan, Italy

Introduction

Medroxyprogesterone acetate (MPA) (6-α-methyl-17-α-hydroxprogesterone acetate), a synthetic C-21 progestin dating from 1958 [1, 2], was widely used in the late 1960's, mainly for the treatment of endometrial adenocarcinoma, in both an adjuvant and palliative context [3].

Clinical findings at the same period in advanced breast cancer, using a variety of doses and routes of administration, gave disappointing results, with the consequence that progestins in general, and MPA in particular, came to be considered as drugs of minor value in the treatment of metastatic breast cancer [4–6].

In 1973, Pannuti's group in Bologna started to employ high doses of MPA in advanced breast carcinoma [7]. Pannuti's pilot studies demonstrated the possibility of giving MPA at high dosage (1,500 mg intramuscularly (i.m.) daily), or at very high dosage (2,000 mg i.m. daily). These doses were associated with acceptable systemic toxicity and an encouraging rate of objective response (40–45%). Subsequently, many investigators in Italy [8–12], and some in other countries [13, 14] set out to verify the results reported by Pannuti's group. The initial trials confirmed the therapeutic efficacy of high doses of MPA, but left a number of problems, mainly concerning the exact role of MPA in the therapeutic strategy of advanced breast cancer (optimal dose and route of administration, criteria for selecting patients eligible for treatment, use of MPA as primary or second line hormonal therapy) unresolved.

Since high dose MPA is currently employed in the treatment of advanced breast cancer in many countries, notwithstanding the above mentioned uncertainties, which persist, an up-to-date critical analysis of published data on this topic seems opportune.

Patient population

We have analysed all papers dealing with high dose MPA in advanced breast cancer. The clinical trials regarded as suitable for review had to meet the following criteria:

1. At least 15 evaluable patients with advanced, histologically-proven breast cancer.
2. All patients treated with high-dose MPA, by the i.m. route only.
3. Clearly defined response criteria (see below).
4. Clearly documented data on the characteristics of patients treated (age, disease-free interval, menopausal status, dominant site of disease, previous treatments, performance status), on adverse reactions, and on side-effects related to treatment.

Response criteria

The major difficulty encountered in reviewing the clinical trials with high-dose MPA in advanced breast cancer is that different criteria have been employed by different investigators for evaluating response. While taking such differences into account, we felt it reasonable to assume good agreement between responders (R) and partial responders (PR), as defined by the Union International contre le Cancer (UICC) [15] and Cooperative Breast Cancer Group (CBCG) [16] criteria used by some investigators [8, 9, 11, 12], and between no change (NC) and minimal response (MR) as defined by UICC and Pannuti [7]. On this basis (Table I), we analysed the results of 17 clinical trials [7–14, 17–25] in an endeavour to answer the following series of questions on the clinical use of MPA in metastatic breast cancer.

Questions

1. Did MPA really result in response rates of 40% or over in advanced breast cancer?

Two controlled clinical trials, carried out by Mattsson in Sweden [13], and by Bonadonna's group at the National Cancer Institute in Milan [10], though involving only a limited number of cases, apparently failed to confirm previously published results, calling in question the high response rate with high-dose MPA therapy, and allowing the suggestion that there were no differences between low and high doses, at least in terms of response rates. A detailed analysis of the 2 clinical trials mentioned above clearly shows that the

Table I. Comparison of criteria for assessment of response employed in clinical trials on medroxyprogesterone acetate in advanced breast cancer.

CBCG		UICC		Pannuti
--		CR	=	CR
R	? → CR = → PR			
		PR	=	PR
			? → MR	MR
NC	=	NC		
			= → NC	NC
P		P		P
4 trials		9 trials		4 trials

R = response; CR = complete response; PR = partial response; MR = minimal response; NC = no change; P = progression.

patients studied had been intensively pretreated, and were resistant to all conventional treatments.

In such a subset of patients the therapeutic efficacy of MPA has, in our opinion, been clearly stated as indicating a response rate of around 30%. These and other clinical trials [14, 17] confirmed the beneficial effects of MPA previously reported in relation to quality of life, pain relief and feelings of well-being. In addition, these clinical trials first drew the attention of investigators to the characteristics of patients eligible for treatment. With MPA best results may be expected in previously untreated patients. This statement remains true even when the results recently presented by the Schweizerische Arbeitsgruppe für Klinische Krebsforschung (SAKK) [18] are taken into account. The overall results obtained using i.m. MPA to date, irrespective of previous systemic treatment, are summarized in Table II. The overall response rate to therapy was 41.6% (range 21–62%).

2. Does a dose-response relationship exist with MPA?

Opinions regarding the existence of a dose-response relationship with MPA have been formed on the basis of early clinical studies [7]. At that time, it seemed likely that an increase in response rate could be obtained by increasing dosage. In fact, it would seem more appropriate to refer to therapeutically effective doses, rather than to low or high doses, i.e. to consider the matter in

Table II. High-dose medroxyprogesterone acetate in advanced breast cancer. Results up to 1982.

Dose (mg i.m./day)	Authors	No. of responders/ No. of patients treated	%
500	Robustelli Della Cuna [12]	22/50	
	Bumma [9]	23/55	
	Pannuti [24]	20/46	
	Cortes Funes [19]	13/46	
	Mendiola [14]	6/27	
	Estevez [20]	108/238	41.5
		192/462	
1,000	Robustelli Della Cuna [12]	21/51	
	De Lena [10]	17/53	
	Mattsson [13]	7/25	
	Mattsson [22]	14/26	
	Castiglione [17]	6/19	
	Madrigal [21]	9/21	
	Amadori [8]	51/82	
	Cortes Funes [19]	15/43	
	Cavalli [18]	27/76	42.1
		167/396	
1,500	Pannuti [7]	20/45	
	De Lena [10]	6/28	
	Pannuti [24]	19/44	
	Pannuti [23]	21/46	40.4
		66/163	
Totals		425/1021	41.6

terms of therapeutic efficacy. Low conventional doses are not effective. High doses are effective. This concept is now supported by clinical and pharmacokinetic data. As Table II clearly shows, the response rate using the i.m. route does not seem to depend on dose, provided that the minimum effective dose of MPA ($\geq$ 500 mg i.m. daily) is given. On the reasonable assumption that serum plasma levels of MPA ranging from 120 to 200 ng/ml are required for effective treatment of advanced breast cancer [26], the optimal dose is of the order of 500–1000 mg i.m. daily, for more than 3 weeks (induction), followed by maintenance therapy using weekly injections. Even although no conclusive data are available on the correlation between MPA plasma levels and response rates in advanced breast cancer [18, 26, 27], it seems more reasonable to consider as optimal the dose capable of producing plasma levels of MPA suitable for effective therapy, rather than to differentiate arbitrarily between low and high doses, in seeking a dose-response relationship with this compound (Table III).

3. What does high-dose MPA really mean?

This is still debated. However, it seems clear, from both clinical and pharmacokinetic data, that the optimal high dose schedule for MPA administration is 500 mg i.m. daily for 4 weeks, followed by maintenance doses of 500 mg i.m., twice weekly. This conclusion is supported by results of 2 controlled clinical trials specifically designed to compare intermediate doses (500 mg i.m.) and high doses (1,000 and 1,500 mg i.m.) of MPA [12, 24]. The results obtained (Table IV) show an almost exact correspondence in terms of both response rates and median durations of response. The same conclusion can be reached by analysing the results available up to December 1981 [4, 7–14,

Table III. MPA plasma levels predicted during treatment with various dose-schedules of a parenteral formulation (modified from [27]).

Route of administration	Dosage schedule	Duration of treatment	Plasma levels* (ng/ml)
Intramuscular	1,000 mg/week	<6 months	~ 90
	1,000 mg/week	4 weeks	~ 40
	500 mg/day	4 weeks	~ 110
	1,000 mg/day	4 weeks	~ 220

* mean steady-state.

Table IV. High versus intermediate doses of MPA in advanced breast cancer.

Authors	Dose (mg i.m./day)	No. of evaluable patients	Complete response	Complete response + partial response (%)	Median duration (months)
Pannuti et al. [23]	R* → 500	46	–	43.5	6
	R* → 1,500	46	1	45.6	6
Robustelli Della Cuna et al. [12]	R* → 500	50	–	44	8
	R* → 1,000	51	–	41	8

*R = randomized.

17–25, 28, 29]. No difference can be demonstrated between intermediate and high doses in relation to overall response rates (Table II), type of response, response by predominant site of metastases, median durations of response, or survival (Tables, V, VI, VII, VIII). The clinical findings are confirmed by pharmacokinetic data obtained by comparing the theoretical predictions with actual drug serum levels in patients with advanced breast cancer receiving intermediate doses of MPA, i.m. [26, 27]. During the loading period, there was a progressive increase in MPA serum levels, up to 80 ng/ml after 3 weeks,

Table V. High-dose MPA in advanced breast cancer: type of response in relation to different dose schedules (for references see Table II). (Numbers of patients (%)).

Dose (mg i.m./daily)	No. of patients treated	Complete response	Partial response	No change	Progression
500	407	42 (10)	127 (31)	108 (26)	130 (32)
1,000	396	20 (5)	147 (37)	98 (25)	131 (33)
1,500	163	2 (1)	64 (39)	44 (27)	53 (32)

Table VI. High-dose MPA in advanced breast cancer: response rate by dominant site of lesions in relation to different dose schedules (for references see table II). (Numbers of patients responding/numbers of patients treated (%)).

Dose (mg i.m./daily)	Soft tissues	Bone	Viscera
500	40/123 (32)	109/204 (53)	41/133 (31)
1,000	55/137 (40)	72/141 (51)	50/139 (36)
1,500	17/59 (29)	42/74 (57)	9/55 (16)

Table VII. High-dose MPA in advanced breast cancer: duration of response (months) in relation to daily doses administered (for references see Table II).

Dose (mg i.m./daily)	No. of patients	Median	Range
500	407	7.5	6–9
1,000	307	8.0	6–13
1,500	163	7.0	5–7

Table VIII. High-dose MPA in advanced breast cancer: duration of survival (months) in relation to different dose schedules (for references see Table II).

Dose (mg i.m./daily)	No. of patients	Overall		Complete response + partial response	
		Median	Range	Median	Range
500	123	16	9–18	22	12–24
1,000	130	13.5	12–18	24	22–24
1,500	163	12.5	11–18	20	15–24

followed by steady state serum levels maintained by biweekly administration. More recently, a prospective controlled clinical trial by the SAKK confirmed the clinical and pharmacokinetic data on MPA [18]. This study was designed to compare high versus low doses of this progestin in a series of unselected women with advanced carcinoma of the breast. Patients were allotted at random to treatment with either 1,000 mg of MPA, i.m., daily, 5 days a week (not Saturdays or Sundays), for one month (equivalent to a daily dose of about 650 mg) or 1,000 mg of MPA, i.m., weekly, for one month (equivalent to a daily dose of about 140 mg). After one month of therapy, all patients received 500 mg of MPA, i.m., weekly, until progression. The data from the SAKK study revealed a statiscally significant difference in favour of high-dose MPA, as far as response rate and median duration of response were concerned, and a higher incidence of responders among previously untreated patients (65%) than in previously treated patients (27%). In conclusion it seems that the regimen based on the administration of 500 mg of MPA, i.m., daily, for 4 weeks, followed by biweekly maintenance treatment can be recommended.

4. What is the local and systemic tolerability to i.m. MPA?

The tolerance of high-dose MPA (500 mg, i.m. daily, or more) appears fairly good. The major untoward occurrence connected with the parenteral administration of MPA which sometimes led to interruption of treatment, was the occurrence of gluteal abscess (Table IX). An objective evaluation of this adverse reaction must take into account not only the dose schedule used and the pharmaceutical dosage form, but also the degree of experience of the nurses administering the injections. In fact, the greatest incidence of abscesses (36.6%) in the early work with high dose MPA occurred when the drug was available only at a concentration of 50 mg/ml, i.e. when, for a dose of 1,500 mg of MPA, i.m. daily, a volume of 30 ml had to be injected. In addition, the greatest number of abscesses occurred in the first series of women treated by Pannuti's group [7]. There were 15 abscesses in the first 22 consecutive patients. Since a new formulation containing 200 mg of MPA/ml has become available, the incidence of such local complications had dramatically decreased. In the SAKK trial on 165 patients, no cases of gluteal abscess were, in fact, observed. The intramuscular route was abandoned in favour of the oral route because of the poor compliance in only 5% of cases [18]. As shown in Table IX, some of the adverse reactions with high-dose MPA are dose related. With doses from 500 mg i.m. to 1,000 mg i.m. daily the incidence of gluteal abscess is below 10%. It is greater than 20% with doses over 1,000 mg i.m. per day. Another adverse reaction related to parenteral MPA administration is phlebitis. This adverse reaction, which is not very common (incidence less than 2%), has been shown not to be dose-dependent, reversible, and easily controllable by withdrawing medication and undertaking appropriate treatment. A dose related increase in blood pressure has been described, mostly in women over 60, or in patients with pre-existing mild or stabilized forms of hypertension. Such increases in blood pressure are the consequence of MPA-induced fluid retention and/or the corticosteroid-like effect of MPA. Cushing-like 'moon' face, muscular cramps, slight tremor, sweating, vaginal bleeding and hot flushes are other adverse effects occasionally observed dur-

Table IX. High-dose MPA in advanced breast cancer: adverse events in relation to daily doses administered (for references see Table II).

Adverse event	Dosage					
	500 mg (n = 462)		1,000 mg (n = 396)		1,500 mg (n = 163)	
	No.	%	No.	%	No.	%
Gluteal abscess	45	9.7	34	8.5	36	22
Gluteal infiltration	9	1.9	28	7.0	3	1.8
Cushing-like face	29	6.2	63	15.9	26	16
Muscular cramps	11	2.3	27	6.8	18	11
Vaginal spotting	13	2.8	19	4.7	13	8.0
Slight tremors	41	8.8	36	9.0	33	20.8
Sweating	19	4.1	21	5.3	26	16
Thrombophlebitis	7	1.5	4	1.0	3	1.8
Increased blood pressure (10 mm Hg diastolic, 20 mm Hg systolic)	74	16	84	21.2	79	48.4

Table X. High-dose MPA in advanced breast cancer: side-effects in relation to daily doses administered (for references see Table II).

Effect	Dosage (i.m., daily)					
	500 mg (n = 462)	%	1,000 mg (n = 396)	%	1,500 mg (n = 163)	%
Increased appetite	334	72	354	89	135	83
Increased Karnofsky-Burchenal index	291	63	286	72	126	77
Increased body weight (2–10 kg)	185	40	174	44	83	51
Pain relief (< 2 points)	252	55	206	52	143	88

ing long-term MPA treatment. Finally, a series of other side-effects (Table X) have been reported in the majority of patients undergoing high-dose MPA therapy. These are increase in appetite, weight gain, improvement in performance status, pain relief and increase in leukocyte count. All of these effects undoubtedly contribute towards improving the quality of life and feelings of well-being of patients with disseminated disease. The observation of an increase in circulating leukocytes during MPA treatment is of interest, especially in combined treatments, where the possibility of controlling cytopenia allows cytotoxic drugs to be administered without dose reduction [4].

5. What are the roles of MPA and tamoxifen (TAM) in advanced breast cancer?

TAM has an anti-oestrogenic effect, and acts by competing for cytoplasmic oestrogenic binding sites. It may lower circulating prolactin levels through inhibition of oestrogenic stimulation of hypophyseal prolactin-producing cells. TAM antagonizes prostaglandins, probably via inhibition of prostaglandin synthetase. As a consequence of its partial oestrogen-like effect, TAM can stimulate replenishment of the cytoplasmic progesterone receptor (PgR) [30, 31].

Even although its mechanism of action has not yet been completely elucidated, MPA is known to act [28, 31–33] via its antiandrogenic activity, by interfering with androgen binding sites. The antiandrogenic effect is related to a lowering of testosterone plasma levels through increase in the rate of androgen catabolism (enhanced hepatic androgen-reductase), reduction of testicular steroidogenesis, and interaction with androgen receptors [34]. MPA has an anti-oestrogenic effect. This has been shown in vitro [32, 35], by inhibition of oestradiol binding to oestradiol-specific receptors, by blockade of hypophyseal release of gonadotropins, by lowering of intracellular levels of oestradiol (E_2), through its ability to induce and increase the activity of E_2-dehydrogenase, and by induction of a hepatic 5-α-reductase which, by accelerating enzymatic androgen catabolism, reduces the transformation of androgens into oestrogens.

As a result of the specific mechanisms of action outlined above, TAM and MPA would not appear to be self-excluding in the therapy of advanced breast cancer. They can, in fact, be used sequentially or alternatively, depending on the patient's clinical characteristics and on the receptor status of the tumour. At the moment, definitive results from prospective, controlled clinical trials specifically designed to compare the therapeutic efficacies of MPA and TAM are few. Only one controlled study has been carried out, in Sweden [22]. Although the number of cases was small, the results in this study showed a trend in favour of MPA-treated patients, as far as response rate was concerned (Table XI). This trial, however, produced further interesting results. After cross-over following progression, MPA was effective in 6 out of 10 patients who had failed to respond to TAM. No response was observed using TAM after cross-over in women failing to respond to MPA. This finding is in agreement with both experimental [35] and clinical observations [36] which have shown that MPA is responsible, in human breast cancer, for inhibition of oestrogen receptor (ER) and reduction in PgR levels. TAM can induce PgR, thus preparing the cell for the action of MPA given sequentially (Table XII). This interference at the receptor level, with consequential reciprocally depressed specific activity, may explain the reported [37] lower therapeutic efficacy of TAM + MPA as compared with TAM alone in the therapy of metastatic

Table XI. High-dose MPA versus TAM in advanced breast cancer [22]. (Numbers of patients showing response indicated/number of patients treated (%).)

	First line therapy	Complete response + partial response	Crossover	Complete response + partial response
R*	TAM: 30 mg Daily p.o.	17/32 (47)	→ MPA	6/10 (60)
	MPA: 1000 mg Daily i.m.	14/26 (54)	→ TAM	0/10 (1 no change lasting 4 months)

*R = randomized.

Table XII. Response rates to TAM, high-dose MPA in oestrogen receptor-rich advanced breast cancer [9, 22, 30].

Treatment	No. of patients	Complete remission + partial remission	%
TAM	308	150	49
High-dose MPA	39	23	59

breast cancer. Although evaluated in a number of cases clearly in favour of the anti-oestrogen, response rates with TAM and MPA were similar when correlated with the oestrogen receptor content of tumour specimens [9, 22, 30]. Similar results were also attainable in unselected patients of unknown receptor status. The results suggest that MPA may be more effective than TAM as primary treatment. Similar response rates have been reported for both TAM and MPA in previously treated cases [4].

Even though MPA and TAM have fairly similar therapeutic effects, from several points of view, their place in the management of advanced breast cancer can be summarized by saying that TAM should be used as primary treatment in low risk women, both premenopausal (including women who have undergone oophorectomy) and postmenopausal, with oestrogen receptor-rich tumours, and in patients with unknown receptor status, at risk of non-neoplastic illness (diabetes, hypertension, cardiovascular disease). In such cases, TAM seems preferable to MPA, in order to avoid side-effects relating to metabolism and water-electrolyte balance. TAM should be used in combination with chemotherapy in high risk women with receptor-rich, rapidly-growing tumours (in such cases, MPA can also be used). TAM can be used as second line therapy on the occasion of a recurrence after chemotherapy, or conventional endocrine treatment, in women with moderately aggressive disease.

Medroxyprogesterone acetate should be employed as primary treatment in high risk, postmenopausal or premenopausal women (including women in relapse after previous response to oophorectomy) with positive or unknown receptor status, and an aggressive tumour, in an attempt to profit from its multiple mechanisms of action which may interfere with a number of events responsible for cancer cell growth. MPA should also be used in far advanced cases with known or unknown receptor status, suffering from pain. In the latter type of patient, MPA is particularly suitable for treatment because of its ability to relieve pain, increase performance status and improve feelings of well-being. MPA should also be used in combination with chemotherapy in high risk patients with aggressive disease, irrespective of receptor status. In such patients, MPA must be preferred over TAM because of its protective effect on bone marrow which allows full doses of cytotoxic drugs to be administered, and improves compliance with chemotherapy. MPA should, in addition, be used as second line therapy in all cases of advanced disease initially responding but subsequently failing to respond to TAM treatment; sequentially with TAM in patients failing to respond after previous response to conventional endocrine treatments, and in far advanced cases with serious clinical conditions, as a hormonal third-line procedure after primary or secondary failure to respond to chemotherapy or other endocrine manipulations. The choice between the 2 above-mentioned hormonal treatments must be part of a decision-making process in which each physician selects the best therapeutic strategy for each patient.

6. Does concurrent MPA therapy and chemotherapy produce better results than chemotherapy alone in advanced breast cancer?

Although some clinical findings favour combination of chemotherapy and hormonal therapy, most results so far obtained in disseminated breast cancer are equivocal [38, 39]. High-dose MPA has been used in combination with different chemotherapeutic regimens with encouraging preliminary results. In a controlled clinical trial involving mostly previously untreated postmenopausal women with advanced disease [38], the concurrent use of MPA (500 mg i.m., daily) and chemotherapy (fluorouracil (FAC), doxorubicin, and cyclophosphamide-FAC) resulted in a higher response rate than FAC alone (75% versus 55%) and a significantly longer median duration of survival in patients responding (29.5 months versus 18.5 months). In another controlled prospective study [34], combined treatment with cyclophosphamide, adriamycin, methotrexate and fluorouracil (CAMF) was compared with the same regimen plus oral MPA (600 mg daily) in 50 previously untreated patients with advanced carcinoma of the breast. The response rate with CAMF alone was 45.8% (median duration of response 10.9 months, overall median duration of survival 21.5 months). A 61.9% response rate (median duration 22.5 months, overall median duration of survival 28.5 months) was observed in the CAMF plus MPA group. In these studies, also, MPA produced an improvement in performance status, and induced pain relief, and a feeling of well-being. A 'protective' effect on chemotherapy-induced leukopenia, has also been observed. This 'protective' effect of MPA on bone marrow has not yet been explained. However, the ability of this progestin to bolster bone marrow reserve would seem to allow the administration of higher doses of cytotoxic drugs. Despite these findings, no definitive conclusions can so far be drawn. Only by identifying subsets among women eligible for treatment will it be possible to define the exact role of MPA-chemotherapy combinations in the therapy of advanced breast cancer. The results currently available cannot be regarded as conclusive, and doubt still remains as to whether the initially increased response rate and prolongation of the time to progression might not subsequently be offset in relation to increased survival. For this reason, it does not currently seem possible to recommend MPA and chemotherapy in combination as routine treatment for metastatic breast cancer. In our opinion, such a combined approach should be adopted only in selected patients, with rapidly growing tumours, or if other conventional therapies have failed.

Conclusions

The findings in trials involving more than 1,000 patients treated with parenteral high-dose MPA allow the following conclusions to be reached:

1. Parenteral MPA at the intermediate dose of 500 mg/day appears to be among the most effective of hormonal treatments, in both previously untreated and previously treated patients with advanced breast cancer.
2. A daily dose of 500 mg of MPA can be considered as the optimal dose, from the points of view of both therapeutic efficacy and tolerance.
3. Local toxicity (gluteal abscess) can be markedly decreased or completely avoided if injections are carefully performed by experienced nurses.
4. Some treatment-related side-effects proved valuable in women with advanced painful disease and in a poor general condition.
5. The protective effect of MPA in chemotherapy-induced leukopenia, may be useful in patients being treated with chemotherapeutic agents. The effect requires further study.
6. In future trials, the highest priority might be assigned to evaluation of the effectiveness of MPA in oestrogen receptor-rich tumours, and to definition of the optimum dosage schedule for the administration of oral and i.m. MPA.

References

1. Babcock, Y.V., Gutselle, S., Heve, N.H. et al. (1958): 6-alpha-methyl-17-alpha-hydroxyprogesterone-17-acylates: a new class of potent progestins. *J. Am. Chem. Soc. 80,* 2904.
2. Sala, G., Camerino, B. and Cavallero, C. (1958): Progestational activity of 6-alpha-methyl-17-alpha-hydroxyprogesterone acetate. *Acta Endocrinol. 29*, 508.
3. Bonte, J., Drochmans, A. and Ide, P. (1966): 6-alpha-methyl-17-alpha-

hydroxyprogesterone acetate as a chemotherapeutic agent in adenocarcinoma of the uterus. *Acta Obstet. Gynaecol. Scand. 45*, 121.

4. Robustelli Della Cuna, G., Pellegrini, A. and Ganzina, F. (1980): *Chemotherapy and Hormonal Treatment of Advanced Breast Cancer*, pp. 51–59. Farmitalia Carlo Erba, Milan.
5. Stoll, B.A. (1967): Progestin therapy of breast cancer: comparison of agents. *Br. Med. J. 3*, 338.
6. Tagnon, H.J. (1976): Role of hormones in the modern treatment of advanced breast cancer. In: *Breast Cancer: Trends in Research and Treatment*, p. 187. Eds: J.C. Heuson, W.H. Mattheim and M. Rozenweig. Raven Press, New York.
7. Pannuti, F., Martoni, A., Lenaz, G.R. et al. (1975): Nuovo protocollo di trattamento del cancro della mammella in fase avanzata a base di medrossiprogesterone (MAP) a dosi massive. *Osped. Vita 2*, 4.
8. Amadori, D., Ravaioli, A., Ridolfi, R. et al. (1979): Il MPA ad alte dosi nella terapia del carcinoma della mammella in fase avanzata. *Chemioter. Oncol. 3*, 44.
9. Bumma, C., Serra, M.C., Zaccara, F. et al. (1977): Correlazione tra risposta terapeutica e presenza di recettori ormonali in pazienti trattate con alte dosi di MAP. Atti Riunioni Integrate di Oncologia, Firenze, 15–16 giugno, 1977. (Abstract no. 93.)
10. De Lena, M., Brambilla, C., Valagussa, P. and Bonadonna, G. (1979): High-dose medroxyprogesterone acetate (MPA) in breast cancer resistant to endocrine and cytotoxic therapy. *Cancer Chemother. Pharmacol. 2*, 175.
11. Martino, G. and Ventafridda, V. (1976): Effetto antalgico dell'alcoolizzazione iposifaria, del medrossiprogesterone acetato ad alte dosi e della loro associazione nel carcinoma mammario in fase avanzata. *Tumori 62*, 93.
12. Robustelli Della Cuna, G., Calciati, A., Bernardo-Strada, M.R. et al. (1978): High-dose medroxyprogesterone acetate (MPA) treatment in metastatic carcinoma of the breast: a dose-response evaluation. *Tumori 64*, 143.
13. Mattsson, W. (1978): High dose medroxyprogesterone acetate treatment in advanced mammary carcinoma. A phase II investigation. *Acta Radiol. Oncol. 17*, 387.
14. Mendiola, C., Manas, A., Ramos, A. et al. (1979): Medroxyprogesterone acetato (MPA) a altas dosis como tratamiento del carcinoma de mama avanzado resistente. *Oncologia 80*, 21.
15. Hayard, J.L., Carbone, P.P., Heuson, J.C. et al. (1977): Assessment of response to therapy in advanced breast cancer. *Eur. J. Cancer 13*, 89.
16. Cooperative Breast Cancer Group (1964): Results of studies of the Cooperative Breast Cancer Group, 1961–1963. *Cancer Chemother. Rep. 41* (Suppl. 1), 1.
17. Castiglione, M. and Cavalli, F. (1980): Ergebnisse einer Pilotstudie mit hochdosiertem Medroxyprogesterone-acetat in der Behandlung des metastasierenden Mammakarzinomas. *Schweiz. Med. Wochenschr. 110*, 1073.
18. Cavalli, F., Goldhirsch, A., Jungi, F. et al. (1982): Low versus high dose medroxyprogesterone acetate (MPA) in the treatment of advanced breast cancer. In: *Role of Medroxyprogesterone Acetate (MPA) in Endocrine-Related Tumors*. Eds: L. Campio, G. Robustelli Della Cuna and R.W. Taylor. Raven Press, New York. [In press].
19. Cortes Funes, H., Madrigal, P.L., Perez Mangas, G. and Mendiola, C. (1982): Medroxyprogesterone acetate at two different doses for the treatment of advanced

breast cancer. In: *Role of Medroxyprogesterone Acetate (MPA) in Endocrine-Related Tumors.* Eds: L. Campio, G. Robustelli Della Cuna and R.W. Taylor. Raven Press, New York. [In press].

20. Estevez, R.A. (1981): MAP altas dosis en cancer avanzado de mama: experiencia argentina. Paper read at: International School of Pharmacology, VIth Course. Advances in Cancer Chemotherapy, Erice, 1981.
21. Madrigal, P.L., Alonso, A., Manga, G.P. and Modrego, S.P. (1980): High doses of medroxyprogesterone acetate (MPA) in the treatment of metastatic breast cancer. In: *Role of Medroxyprogesterone Acetate (MPA) in Endocrine-Related Tumors*, p. 93. Eds: S. Iacobelli and A. Di Marco. Raven Press, New York.
22. Mattsson, W. (1980): A phase III trial of treatment with tamoxifen versus treatment with high dose medroxyprogesterone acetate in advanced postmenopausal breast cancer. In: *Role of Medroxyprogesterone Acetate (MPA) in Endocrine Related Tumors*, p. 65. Eds: S. Iacobelli and A. Di Marco. Raven Press, New York.
23. Pannuti, F., Martoni, A., Fruet, F. et al. (1979): Il tumore della mammella: il trattamento della fase avanzata. In: *La Chemioterapia dei Tumori Solidi*, p. 439. Ed.: F. Pannuti. Patron, Bologna.
24. Pannuti, F., Martoni, A., Di Marco, A.R. et al. (1979): Prospective randomized clinical trial of two different high dosages of medroxyprogesterone acetate (MAP) in the treatment of metastatic breast cancer. *Eur. J. Cancer, 15*, 593.
25. Pannuti, F., Di Marco, A.R., Martoni, A. et al. (1980): Medroxyprogesterone acetate in treatment of metastatic breast cancer: seven years of experience. In: *Role of Medroxyprogesterone Acetate (MPA) in Endocrine-Related Tumors*, p. 73. Eds: S. Iacobelli and A. Di Marco. Raven Press, New York.
26. Hesselius, I. (1982): Pharmacokinetics of medroxyprogesterone acetate and plasma levels in long term treatment. In: *Role of Medroxyprogesterone Acetate (MPA) in Endocrine-Related Tumors.* Eds: L. Campio, G. Robustelli Della Cuna and R.W. Taylor. Raven Press, New York. [In press.]
27. Tamassia, V., Battaglia, A., Ganzina, F. et al. (1982): Pharmacokinetic approach to the selection of dose schedules of medroxyprogesterone acetate in clinical oncology. *Cancer Chemother. Pharmacol.* [In press.]
28. Robustelli Della Cuna, G. (1979): *Il medrossiprogesterone acetato (MPA): caratteristiche, risultati ed indicazioni in oncologia*, pp. 10–11. Il Pensiero Scientifico Editore, Rome.
29. Robustelli Della Cuna, G., Imparato, E. and Bernardo, G. (1981): High dose medroxyprogesterone acetate (HD-MPA) in advanced breast cancer: update 1981. *Med. Biol. Environmental 9*, 527.
30. Furr, B.J., Patterson, J.S., Richardson, D.N., Slater, S.R. and Wakeling, A.E. (1979): Tamoxifen. In: *Pharmacological and Biochemical Properties of Drug Substances*, pp. 371–373. Ed.: M.E. Goldberg. American Pharmaceutical Association, Washington.
31. Pellegrini, A., Massidda, B., Mascia, V. and Ionta, M.T. (1982): Medroxyprogesterone acetate and tamoxifen: two different drugs in alternate or sequential modality treatment. In: *Role of Medroxyprogesterone Acetate (MPA) in Endocrine-Related Tumors.* Eds: L. Campio, G. Robustelli Della Cuna and R.W. Taylor. Raven Press, New York. [In press.]
32. Di Carlo, F., Pacilio, G. and Conti, G. (1975): Sul meccanismo d'azione dei

progestinici nella terapia dei tumori mammari ormonodipendenti. *Tumori 61*, 501.

33. Necco, A., Dasdia, T. and Di Marco, A. (1979): The antagonistic action between MAP and estradiol in a hormone-responsive human cancer cell line (MCF-7). *Cancer Treat. Rep. 63*, 1174.
34. Pellegrini, A., Massidda, B., Mascia, V. et al. (1980): CAMF vs. CAMF+MPA nel carcinoma avanzato della mammella: valutazione a 42 mesi. *Tumori 66 (Suppl.)*, 99.
35. Iacobelli, S., Natoli, C. and Sica, G. (1982): Inhibitory effects of medroxyprogesterone acetate on the proliferation of human breast cancer cells. In: *Role of Medroxyprogesterone Acetate (MPA) in Endocrine-Related Tumors.* Eds: L. Campio, G. Robustelli Della Cuna and R.W. Taylor. Raven Press, New York. [In press.]
36. Namer, M., Lalanne, C. and Beaulieu, E.E. (1980): Increase of progesterone receptor by tamoxifen as a hormonal challenge test in breast cancer. *Cancer Res. 40,* 1750.
37. Mouridsen, H.T., Palshof, T. and Rose, C. (1980): Therapeutic effect of tamoxifen alone versus tamoxifen in combination with gestagen and oestrogen in advanced breast cancer. In: *Endocrine Treatment of Breast Cancer*, p. 169. Eds.: B. Henningsen, F. Linder and C. Steichele. Springer-Verlag, Berlin-Heidelberg-New York.
38. Robustelli Della Cuna, G., Cuzzoni, Q., Preti, P. and Bernardo, G. (1982): Concurrent hormonal and cytotoxic treatment for advanced breast cancer: In: *Role of Medroxyprogesterone Acetate (MPA) in Endocrine-Related Tumors.* Eds: L. Campio, G. Robustelli Della Cuna and R.W. Taylor. Raven Press, New York. [In press.]
39. Robustelli Della Cuna, G. (1980): Current concepts of endocrinotherapy for advanced breast cancer. *Med. Biol. Environmental 8*, 371.

Round table: MPA in breast cancer

Chairman: K. Brunner, Bern, Switzerland

Panelists:

C. Blossey	(Göttingen, Federal Republic of Germany)
R.D. Chacón	(Buenos Aires, Argentina)
M. De Lena	(Bari, Italy)
E. García-Girált	(Paris, France)
W. Mattsson	(Karlstad, Sweden)
G. Robustelli Della Cuna	(Pavia, Italy)

K. Brunner

We have decided to discuss in this round table 4 different topics:
1. What is the optimal dose schedule of MPA? Is there a dose-dependency?
2. Is combined MPA and chemotherapy better than chemotherapy alone, or what is the optimal sequence of using chemotherapy and hormonal therapy?
3. Is there any advantage in the use of combined (i.e., simultaneous or sequential) hormonal therapy? We have heard this morning that some laboratory data suggest that tamoxifen and MPA given sequentially may be useful.
4. Probably the most important question is what is the real place of MPA in the management of advanced breast cancer in postmenopausal patients?

We will start with the first topic, the optimal dose schedule of MPA.

G. Robustelli Della Cuna

It seems to be proven, from clinical and pharmacokinetic data now available, that the optimal dose schedule of MPA administration is 500 mg daily, intramuscularly (i.m.), for a period of 4 weeks, followed by a maintenance treatment of 500 mg i.m. twice a week. Such a conclusion may be drawn from an analysis of all reports published up to December 1981. Such an analysis clearly shows that there are no differences in the overall response rates between an intermediate daily dose and higher daily doses of MPA given i.m. (500 mg = 41.5%, 1,000 mg = 42.1%, 1,500 mg = 40.4%). The same holds true from a detailed analysis of the type of response in a patient where comparable criteria of response evaluation have been employed. If the response rate is analysed by dominant site of the disease, there are no differences between 500 mg and the higher doses 1,000 and 1,500 mg. If the same cases are analysed in terms of duration of response, there is no difference between the intermediate and the higher doses. Finally, the same happens if duration of survival, both for overall survival and survival of the responders, is considered. Such conclusions, furthermore, are supported by pharmacokinetic data obtained in patients with disseminated breast cancer treated with MPA.

Taking those data into consideration, it can be concluded that the optimal plasma levels necessary for an effective treatment of advanced breast cancer are in the range of 100–200 ng/ml. With regard to the route of administration, the steady-state plasma levels of the same order of magnitude can be reached with both routes of administration provided that oral MPA is given in daily doses twice as large as the i.m. doses of MPA during an induction period and continued during the maintenance phase.

With regard to the dose-response relationship for MPA, my own opinion (supported by clinical data) is that rather than talking about 'high' or 'low' MPA doses it would be better to refer to the therapeutically-effective doses of this compound. On the basis of previously-shown clinical and pharmacokinetic evidence, such a dose ranges between 500 and 1,000 mg daily, i.m., for a period of 4 weeks, followed by a maintenance treatment of 1,000 mg weekly, i.m.

Professor Brunner asked me another question about the duration of induction therapy with MPA and the optimal maintenance therapy. I think that these topics have not yet been clearly defined. If we look at the results that have been shown, and the comments that we have heard today, and talking in terms only of i.m. MPA, the conventional high-dose MPA schedule is 500 mg i.m., for a period of 4 weeks, followed by maintenance therapy. As far as oral administration is concerned, there are no conclusive data to clearly support a well-defined dose schedule.

Last but not least, what is the basis of the improved remission rate with high-dose MPA? What is the mechanism of action by the hormone receptor? Is high-dose MPA effective in oestrogen receptor (ER)-negative or in low ER-positive tumours?

As regards the question of the mechanism of action of MPA, at the moment I do not know whether it is strictly correlated with response, but it has been clearly defined this morning. I think that we have to look at some of the MPA-related effects (anti-oestrogenic, anti-androgenic) together with the capacity of this compound to compete with ER and, finally, at the direct cytotoxic action of MPA, clearly demonstrated some years ago by Swedish and Italian authors, in tissue cultures from endometrial carcinoma.

As far as the activity of MPA in ER-negative or low ER-positive tumours is concerned, I can only give my own experience. I have treated 40 patients with metastatic breast cancer, 11 of whom had ER-poor tumours (less than 10 fmol/mg ER). With the earlier-mentioned schedule (i.e., 500 mg/day, i.m. for 4 weeks, and then twice a week), no significant results were observed except for a 8% response rate.

Discussion

K. Brunner: As I understand it, Professor Robustelli Della Cuna's recommendation is not to use doses of MPA higher than 500 mg daily, i.m., during an induction period of 4 weeks, followed by 500 mg twice weekly. Does anybody question this practical proposition? Why is it 4 weeks, and not 3 or 2 weeks?

G. Robustelli Della Cuna: I can not really answer this question – other than to say that the experience available up to now seems to demonstrate that this is the best way to give MPA. In the trial, conducted with Professor Pellegrini and other people all over the world, we tried to give the same dosage for only 2 weeks, but unfortunately there are no pharmacokinetic data on that dosage. During the round table on MPA pharmacokinetics Dr Tamassia showed us a very interesting pharmacokinetic model (pp. 179–185). I would like to hear him state clearly his opinion about whether there is a relationship between plasma level and response in breast cancer.

V. Tamassia (Milan, Italy): This morning a lot of evidence was shown, perhaps in an unusual way, that there is a blood level response curve. To have an answer to the question, about 1,000 patients would be required, with all the pharmacokinetics. Perhaps in the future, at a next congress, such data could be presented.

The basic dose schedule is 500 mg daily, i.m., for a period of 4 weeks – but this period of 4 weeks is not necessary. The same results could be obtained even with only one day's treatment, provided that it was possible to administer the same cumulative dose. I suggest the possibility of attaining such blood levels in 2 weeks by giving 1,000 mg/day for a period of 2 weeks (or even more rapidly than that). What is important is to give about 1,500 mg during the loading phase.

I feel that in his paper Dr Cavalli has clearly demonstrated that the response is lower using a dosage lower than the standard dose schedules (pp. 224–233). I will not discuss the difference between statistical significance and clinical significance, but the difference was so impressive that I feel that in the future none of us would treat patients with 1,000 mg/week.

The problem has been solved in part. There is clinical evidence that, with doses higher than 500 mg/day for a period of 4 weeks, there is no substantial improvement in the response, whereas with doses lower than 500 mg/day for a period of 4 weeks there is the risk of a reduced response rate.

K. Brunner: Is there a place for an oral loading dose combined with i.m. administration – i.e., starting with an oral dose to reach an early high plasma level as soon as possible, and at the same time starting i.m. dosing?

V. Tamassia: This is exactly what is planned and Professor Robustelli Della

Cuna is involved in the project. We plan to investigate a dose schedule based on the weekly i.m. treatment plus a loading phase with oral doses for one month. This model will be checked through pharmacokinetic studies and through comparative clinical trials. We should be able to give the answer during the next few months.

K. Brunner: Does anyone else wish to comment on this proposition of 500 mg daily, i.m. for a period of 4 weeks, followed by the same dose twice weekly?

A. Pellegrini (Cagliari, Italy): I am afraid that we are confusing something. Professor Pannuti and Professor Robustelli Della Cuna started 10 years ago on the clinical basis; by giving a certain amount of MPA they obtained a certain response. On the basis of that experience, that went on for about 8 years, they stated that 500 mg a day, i.m., followed by 500 mg twice a week, should be a convenient dose schedule because, using that schedule, there is a response rate of about 43%. This is only the clinical situation and only a clinical observation. Pharmacokinetic knowledge, however, is far from exhaustive, and I think a further step can be taken – from what Professor Robustelli Della Cuna has told us. Also, Professor Brunner is right in saying that we now know that giving MPA i.m. means that the plasma levels increase very slowly, perhaps because of the compartmental distribution of the drug. If the oral route of administration is used, however, the MPA plasma level grows very rapidly. So we could start by using both routes of administration at the same time in order to reach a very high plasma level in a very short period of time. I would like to suggest something like that. We need to think about it, and to make an appropriate schedule.

K. Brunner: Another question which I would like to discuss is that there is still a 15–20% response rate to low-dose MPA. What kind of patients respond to the low dose, and is there any possibility of selecting those patients who really need high-dose MPA to achieve the reported remission rate of between 30–40%? On what basis could patients not needing high-dose MPA be selected? Is there a response relationship with ER content?

This question has to be studied carefully, not only from the point of view of cost but also of convenience to the patients. It is not an easy matter to give 5 or 7 injections per week to a patient.

A. Pellegrini: In answer to Professor Brunner's question about how to select those patients who will show a 15–50% response to low-dose MPA, it must always be kept in mind that if a hormone is used in physiological doses it works through its own receptors – it needs those receptors. But when hormones are given in very high doses (such as we are now doing with MPA), they also work through non-specific receptors. It is known that MPA acts through the dihydrotestosterone and glucocorticoid receptors.

J.C. Heuson (Brussels, Belgium): With regard to i.m. versus oral administration, this is a problem that is faced with any kind of endocrine treatment. It is impossible to know whether certain endocrine treatments do not stimulate growth in some cases of breast cancer. We all know cases of flare-up, for example, with tamoxifen. I have some data – anecdotal, because they relate to only one case – demonstrating a distinct stimulation, with a very nice dose-response curve in one case of breast cancer using the clonogenic assay.

Therefore, there is the possibility that in some patients MPA could stimulate growth. Then there is the question of whether it is reasonable to give the i.m. depot preparations. If there is such a stimulation, we cannot recognize it – other than observing progression of disease in the patient. Perhaps the progression of the disease is greatly accelerated – so treatment is stopped, but the drug is still there and continues to stimulate. I think, therefore, that we should consider selecting the oral route of administration rather than the i.m. route.

K. Brunner: That is a very important remark. What is interesting about MPA is that hypercalcaemia, which usually occurs with every additive hormonal treatment, has never been observed. The question remains open whether there is any possible tumour stimulation by MPA – the answer is unknown. I have asked all the panelists whether they had ever observed hypercalcaemia after MPA – and no one had. Have you, Professor Heuson?

J.C. Heuson: No, I have not. I do not think that hypercalcaemia means growth stimulation of a cancer cell; it may simply be a metabolic effect of the hormone on the cancer cell that is accompanied by the release of calcium from the bone. Therefore, the lack of observation of hypercalcaemia with MPA does not mean that it does not accelerate growth of some breast cancers.

W. Mattsson: It is very seldom that a progressive disease is seen in which it is possible to imagine that the tumour growth has been promoted, or accelerated, by high-dose MPA. I have never seen it, and I have now treated about 100 patients with that type of therapy. However, of course, we must always be aware that this might happen but, from our experience, there must be a very low risk for the patients.

P. Bastit (Strasbourg, France): I have seen one case of possible stimulation in vivo in a 72-year-old patient with an endometrial carcinoma treated with MPA. After 3 months of this treatment a double breast cancer appeared (on the right and the left side). Unfortunately, it was not possible to study the receptors of these tumours because the patient refused surgical removal. Only a fine-needle biopsy could be performed in order to confirm the diagnosis.

K. Brunner: What makes you assume that this was a stimulation and not a natural course of disease?

P. Bastit: I have only said that it was a possible stimulation after a 3-month treatment.

K. Brunner: The next topic of discussion is whether combined MPA and chemotherapy is better than chemotherapy alone. We have heard some important data presented by Professor Pellegrini together with Professor Robustelli Della Cuna. Professor Pellegrini has already pointed out that this may not be *the* important question. The really important question may be whether sequential hormonal chemotherapy is better or worse than simultaneous hormonal chemotherapy. If we have a patient, especially in the postmenopausal age group, who is a candidate for hormonal therapy (from the receptor content), I have difficulty in understanding why such a patient should receive chemotherapy from the beginning in addition to the hormonal therapy. Only when we can define special risk factors in a subgroup of patients, for which the delay of chemotherapy during the hormonal therapy trial would result in inferior results of the later chemotherapy, simultaneous hormonal chemotherapy may be justified.

We will now review some other data about MPA and chemotherapy versus chemotherapy alone, bearing in mind that this may not be the important question. Dr Chacón will present his data on hormonal chemotherapy versus chemotherapy alone.

R.D. Chacón

The aim of our two-arm trial was to evaluate a combined modality protocol (hormonochemotherapy) as induction regimen, followed by hormonal maintenance, which would possibly facilitate re-induction chemotherapy. Such a programme would be consistent with the concept of continuing hormonotherapy with chemotherapy on relapse, especially for initially-complete responders.

In neither arm of the trial were receptor assays performed. All patients who entered the trial were postmenopausal women with advanced breast cancer. Average age, prior treatments and dominant metastases were similar in both arms.

In arm A, 50 patients, 38 of whom were evaluable, received the combination chemotherapy, vincristine + doxorubicin + cyclophosphamide (VAC) recycled every 3–4 weeks, plus 500 mg of MPA, intravenously twice a week. In arm B, 21 patients, 17 of whom were evaluable, were given VAC only. Clinical response was assessed after completing 3 chemotherapy courses. In arm A, the complete responders were continued on oral MPA, 400 mg daily, alone, while most partial responders were changed onto vincristine + cyclophosphamide + 5-fluorouracil (VCF) chemotherapy, and only a few received maintenance oral MPA. In arm B there were no complete responders. The partial responders were either continued on VCF, or left without any further treatment (mere observation).

As regards the results, in arm A the complete-remission (CR) rate was 29%, rising to 34.2% if patients with exclusively bone metastases are included, in whom, however, CR is hardly ascertained. The partial-remission (PR) rate was 38.3%. In arm B, there was no CR, but there was a PR rate of 53.8%. Whereas the overall response rate showed no statistically significant difference, such a difference is obvious if only CR is considered. Concerning the free interval, one should notice that 3 months (corresponding to induction period) have to be added to the response duration. In arm A, the complete responders showed an average free interval of 18.9 months (11 months if patients with skeletal metastases are included), versus 12 months for the partial responders achieving CR after change-over to VCF.

For the patients showing progression or no change on MPA, improvement only lasted about 4 months. In arm B, improvement was short-lasting, namely 3 months in the patients without any further treatment, and 5.5 months in those who continued with chemotherapy.

For most tumour types, CR is associated with prolonged free interval and sometimes survival, and for some neoplasms even cure, the latter obviously being not the case for advanced breast cancer. For breast cancer patients showing CR, the therapeutic decision is difficult – discontinuation of treatment until relapse occurs: chemo- or hormonotherapy? Most currently-employed regimens allow 15–25% CR, with a free interval averaging 9–12 months. Our trial, too, emphasizes the critical relevance of CR to prolongation of remission.

Simultaneous hormonochemotherapy appeared to yield the highest CR rates. On the other hand, the role of maintenance hormonotherapy as such would require further evaluation in the light of poor outcome in the partial responders. Selection of receptor-positive patients for this combined modality treatment would be reasonably expected to yield even better results.

K. Brunner: On the basis of this randomized trial, conducted on a limited series, as well as of data reported by Professor Pellegrini, we may agree that there is possibly some advantage in administering combined hormonal (MPA) and chemotherapy in patients with an unknown receptor status. The next logical question would be whether this applies specifically to MPA, or holds true for any simultaneous hormonochemotherapy. Dr García-Girált will tackle this topic, on the basis of his group's trials of different combined modalities.

E. García-Girált

I will present some data from the Curie Foundation showing results quite different from those of Dr Chacon, and also somewhat different from those of Professor Pellegrini, as a stimulation to further debate. A total of 320 patients received the following treatment variants: 1) chemotherapy (doxorubicin + cyclophosphamide + 5-fluorouracil) plus tamoxifen; 2) chemotherapy plus tamoxifen and MPA; 3) chemotherapy alone; 4) tamoxifen plus MPA; and 5) chemotherapy plus MPA.

Survival did not significantly differ for the different treatment groups, but higher response rates were obtained with any combined modality. However, the results did not vary with single- versus 2-agent hormonotherapy combined with chemotherapy.

Interpretation of such an outcome proved to be rather difficult. Two basic points are to be made. First, the patients treated with chemotherapy alone do receive hormonotherapy on relapse, which may give a second or third remission. Secondly, in our opinion, simultaneous hormonochemotherapy is inadequate on account of several reasons, the most important being probably that such a schedule may prevent the chemotherapy-induced increase of receptor content, and hence response to hormonal treatment. Sequential chemo- and hormonal therapy, as discussed by Professor Pellegrini, is likely to prove more rewarding to this purpose.

Furthermore, when the patients were selected on the basis of receptor assays, the receptor-positive women did not reach a median survival time (MST) at 36 months, as opposed to a MST of 14 months for the receptor-negative subjects. Here, we are dealing with two clearly-distinct patient populations, in terms of both prognosis and treatment; receptor-negative women are requiring a different and more aggressive therapy programme.

Discussion

W.L. McGuire (San Antonio, U.S.A.): There are a number of points to be made. Dr García-Girált has mentioned a couple of them, which I would like to re-emphasize.

To start at the beginning, this is what I think should happen when we want to do a study of combined endocrine chemotherapy. First, if we take all the patients and do not measure the receptors, almost by definition two-thirds of those patients are not endocrine-responsive. That means that for two-thirds of our groups it is 'no contest'; we are not testing anything because they cannot have the inherent possibility of responding to endocrine therapy in the first place. Therefore, in a non-selected group, two-thirds of the patients are not even evaluable because they do not have the potential for responding.

Secondly, if the receptors are measured, or if the thought that the receptors are not important for the mechanism of MPA response is the reason for not measuring them, then we should pay attention to what has just been shown (and has been published on very many occasions), namely that ER-negative patients have a worse survival than ER-positive patients. If we are going to compare two things, it is important to be sure that the same number of ER-negative and ER-positive patients are present in the same group, even if the receptors have nothing to do with the endocrine therapy.

Thirdly, about one year ago there was a conference in San Antonio entirely on combined chemo-endocrine therapy. All these matters were discussed, dealing, I must admit, more extensively with tamoxifen and chemotherapy. The point is that we are re-learning what is now becoming well known for chemotherapy: that 2 drugs are better than one and that 3 drugs may be better than 2, in terms of the complete or partial response rate. If overall survival is measured, however, using those 3 or 4 drugs sequentially, there is no difference in survival in the treatment of advanced breast cancer. That has been published recently, and it was also published a long time ago. Therefore, this should not be forgotten while considering combined chemo-endocrine therapy.

In order to do a proper combined chemo-endocrine therapy, which I have not seen today, chemotherapy plus MPA or plus tamoxifen or plus whatever must be used – but to those patients who receive only chemotherapy, an opportunity must be given at a later date to respond or fail to that endocrine therapy. In other words, the patients in both groups must receive the same drugs, and only then it is possible to compare survival. I do not think (unless I missed it) that fact has been taken into consideration in the trials so far.

In summary, if we are going to do a combined chemo-endocrine trial, we have to ensure that the patients are stratified with regard to receptor negativity and positivity and that both groups receive the same chemotherapy and the same endocrine therapy, even though in one instance it may be combined.

K. Brunner: Professor McGuire's comments are absolutely to the point. As I mentioned before, the relevant question is not chemotherapy versus combined MPA/chemotherapy, but MPA followed by chemotherapy versus combined hormonal and chemotherapy.

MPA may have one special quality which may make it interesting for use in those patients who are not candidates for hormonal therapy alone, in that there may be some non-specific bone marrow protection effects, or other non-tumour-specific actions, of MPA.

It is conceivable that even the patients who are candidates for primary chemotherapy, on account of negative receptors or other risk factors, may benefit from adding MPA to chemotherapy because of such non-tumour-specific effects of MPA. Dr Blossey will comment on such effects and interactions with chemotherapy.

C. Blossey

We have some experience with 2 therapeutic regimens: 1. VAC in combination with high-dose MPA; and 2. mitomycin C in combination with high-dose MPA.

The combination of high-dose MPA and cytotoxic polychemotherapy (such as cyclophosphamide + methotrexate + 5-fluorouracil (CMF), 5-fluorouracil + doxorubicin (adriamycin) + cyclophosphamide (FAC), doxorubicin + vincristine (AV)) in metastatic breast cancer has been reported by Professor Robustelli Della Cuna and also today we have heard similar results from Professor Pellegrini. The real problem is what is 'additional antitumour activity'? This was claimed for the above-mentioned 3 combinations. In our experience, the combination with VAC does not show a clear additional effect; however, as far as the combination with mitomycin C is concerned an additional antitumour activity has been observed in terms of a higher response rate, but not clearly in terms of survival. The problem is that all the patients were highly selected in the sense of previous therapy and in most patients receptor determination was not available because they underwent surgery at a time when, at least in Germany, receptor assays were not usually performed.

Another matter which may be very interesting from the point of view of the patients is the mitigation of chemotherapy-related side-effects. All people working with high-dose MPA have probably noticed that the performance status (PS) of the patients is generally better with than without MPA. We do not know whether an increase in body weight is always such a good thing, but there is a group of patients with poor PS who will benefit from high-dose MPA in the sense that they feel better, they gain weight, and are perhaps slightly euphoric, which may be due to the corticoid-like activity of MPA. Pain relief, which has been mentioned several times today, is quite clear. There is also a possible bone marrow protection; this has been claimed for the combinations with FAC, AV and VAC, but it is not so clear for Mitomycin-C or CMF. In our experience, this effect was very impressive by combining MPA with VAC therapy.

The combined treatment has no effect on the development of alopecia. Unfortunately, there is a possible increase in toxic side-effects in the combination with Mitomycin-C. This drug, as is well known, is associated with lung toxicity, and it is feared that there are some patients in whom this side-effect was increased in the presence of MPA. At the moment, it is not known whether there was an actual causative relationship or this happened simply by chance. In conclusion, with regard to the well-being of the patients, there may be advantages in the combination of high-dose MPA and cytotoxic drugs. It is still unclear whether there is any enhancement of survival, or whether it is better than without MPA. We must be very careful, and pay attention to untoward effects.

Discussion

K. Brunner: There are 2 possible effects in combining MPA with chemotherapy: 1. A synergistic effect on possibly 2 different cell populations – this has not been confirmed with other hormonal chemotherapy; 2. A non-specific bone marrow-protective effect, so that higher doses of chemotherapy can be given with, as a consequence, better results. That is the other explanation.

There is, however, a third possibility which should be investigated and which has also been described in the literature: a possible antagonistic effect of combined MPA and chemotherapy. As may be known, some years ago, using *low-dose* progesterone therapy, Rubens published results showing that he could detect a bone marrow-protective effect of progesterone but accompanied by worse therapeutic results. The explanation is that low doses of hormones may trigger tumour cells into the G1-G0 phase and render them less sensitive to chemotherapeutic agents. I do not suggest that this is a reality in every case, but possible adverse effects from combining hormonal and chemotherapy must be studied.

I think that probably we have now said all that can be said at the moment about combined MPA and chemotherapy versus chemotherapy alone. Is there anybody who has anything to add to that subject?

A.T. van Oosterom (Leiden, The Netherlands): When we are giving MPA combination chemotherapy in order to raise the performance status of the patient, I suggest that we go back and see what Cooper, and later Canellos, prescribed, namely 30 mg of prednisone, which I think is at least one-tenth or one-twentieth of the cost. When social security and health are already so expensive, I think that it is better to prescribe prednisone if a patient needs improvement.

K. Brunner: That has to be considered. There are other possibilities to improve the tolerance of chemotherapy. It has been demonstrated by the Eastern Co-operative Oncology Group and by the Swiss group that prednisone, and possibly androgens, improve tolerance to chemotherapy.

A. Pellegrini: I agree with Professor Brunner and I already said that, in my opinion, hormonochemotherapy has to be considered to be still investigational. However, the bone marrow-protective activity shown by MPA (we do not know its mechanism) is absolutely not the only reason to use MPA in the combined modality treatment; it rather may be considered as a toward side-effect of a *per se* antitumoral agent. Our main objective is not at all to give high-dose MPA to improve the patient's performance status but, as I told, to try to get higher response rates, longer response duration and a better quality of life. We cannot compare MPA with prednisone: they both have some similar activities (cortisol-like effects of MPA), but MPA has a specific antitumour and endocrine activity that prednisone does not possess at all. Moreover, it has been demonstrated that prednisone, and possibly androgens, improve tolerance to chemotherapy, but it is also known that the combination with androgens may decrease the response rate; for MPA, to my knowledge and according to the schedule we spoke about, this has never been demonstrated. However, I still repeat that we do not know the best sequences, schedules and timing of the combined modality approach and that, considering these pilot trials, in the next studies the eligibility of the patients has to be monitorized through receptor analysis.

K. Brunner: All we are trying to do, Professor Pellegrini, is to try to draw conclusions on the present state of the art – what is not known should be clearly defined and studied further. But we also have to define what recommendations can be given to the medical community based on present knowledge, which is one of the purposes of this symposium and of this round table. We will now turn to the third topic: the combination of hormonal therapies either sequentially or simultaneously. Dr Girált has data on this topic – especially on the sequential use of tamoxifen and MPA. Laboratory data have already been presented by Dr Iacobelli earlier during this symposium.

E. García-Girált

Everybody knows that if a patient is given chemotherapy, this destroys the receptors for progesterone and for oestrogen. If oestrogenic therapy is given, for instance diethylstilbestrol, oestrogen receptors are increased.

A compound like tamoxifen will increase the number of progesterone receptors, and a compound like MPA decreases the numbers of both progesterone and oestrogen receptors. If MPA is given continuously, no receptors will remain and the anticancer action disappears. That was the reason for introducing a sequential administration of tamoxifen and MPA for hormone-resistant patients, in our group only. By doing so, we obtained a 75% response in non-responsive patients using associated sequential administration of the same regimen that had no effect when given simultaneously.

This result is in accordance with the results obtained by Dr Beaulieu and Dr Martin following the modification of receptors after several hormonal or chemotherapeutic agents.

Discussion

K. Brunner: I may show some rather interesting data later on from Dr Pouillart's group.

We will now discuss the possibilities of combining different hormonal therapies – MPA or other combinations. Is it rational to do that? What does Professor McGuire think about such possibilities, from a theoretical point of view?

W.L. McGuire: It depends on whether we are talking about advanced disease or about adjuvant therapy.

K. Brunner: We are talking about advanced disease.

W.L. McGuire: Then, I think that the situation does not matter. Everybody knows that if the patient responds to one endocrine therapy, the chances are good that that patient will respond to another, and perhaps even to a third. Probably the person who carries this out the longest is Pearson, in Cleveland. He will start with tamoxifen, then go to androgen, then perhaps to hypophysectomy and then to who knows what, perhaps MPA. In advanced disease I think that it is a matter of palliation, continuing treatment and so on.

It is very different in the adjuvant situation where we are trying to decrease tumour burden rapidly, and there we should combine everything to get the equivalent of a complete response.

In answer to Professor Brunner's question, I do not think that good definitive randomized studies have been done where everyone is given the same therapy, the receptor levels are clear and so on.

K. Brunner: Is there any theoretical basis for combining the hormonal procedures or using them sequentially in adjuvant therapy? What is your opinion about that?

W.L. McGuire: Absolutely. For example, in a premenopausal woman, if we really want to do an endocrine ablation or remove oestrogen, would it not be nice to do an oöphorectomy plus giving her tamoxifen? It is well known that patients given oöphorectomy for advanced disease will have a response followed by a recurrence of their disease. Why does the disease recur? It is because of the adrenal androgen/oestrogen precursors. These precursors can now be treated with tamoxifen or aminoglutethimide and the patients will have another response.

If we are talking about adjuvant therapy and cure, let us eliminate all those potential possibilities, combining it with effective chemotherapy. I think that the rationale is very different.

K. Brunner: Do you know of any results with this combination in adjuvant therapy?

W.L. McGuire: No.

V. Tamassia: I am afraid that from the pharmacokinetic point of view it will be quite difficult to obtain a true sequential therapy with MPA and tamoxifen. The biological half-life of tamoxifen is about 5 days. If MPA is given i.m., it will be absolutely impossible to obtain a true sequential therapy.

I am curious to know the experimental details of the studies just presented. Was there oral administration, what kind of dosages were given and so on?

K. Brunner: These would be important factors to consider. I assume that not i.m. administration of progesterone would be used to achieve such an effect, but oral – probably even low – doses

G. Beretta (Milan, Italy): I have some complementary data showing that it is possible to have a response after tamoxifen as well as MPA.

From the study fully reported elsewhere in this volume it appeared that after tamoxifen there was a response rate to MPA of 17%. Some patients were treated with MPA after being treated with tamoxifen. There was the same response rate (19%). It is interesting to see that there was a response only after oral MPA, and not following i.m. MPA. This is in agreement with Dr Tamassia's opinion.

K. Brunner: I would like to have dose data later because we now turn to the last, and in my opinion the most important, topic of this round table: what is the place of MPA – especially high-dose MPA – in the general management of the advanced breast cancer patients? The questions to be answered are the following. 1. Is MPA a better first-line treatment than any other hormonal treatment – anti-oestrogens, oestrogens or whatever? 2. In which patients should MPA be used as a first-line treatment? 3. In which patients is it justified to wait to give high-dose MPA until the patients either are primarily non-responsive to other hormonal procedures or have relapsed after remission?

These are the questions we want to address. We are now trying to define the place of high-dose MPA in the management of advanced breast cancer.

M. De Lena

In the National Cancer Institute, Milan, we have treated two groups of patients with metastatic breast carcinoma with MPA. The first group was treated with two different i.m. dosages: 1,500 mg/day for 27 consecutive days (total dose: 40,500 mg), or 1,000 mg/day for 40 consecutive days (total dose: 40,000 mg). This retrospective study was carried out between March, 1975 and November, 1977.

On the contrary, the second study was a controlled randomized trial using low mean dosages of MPA. Thirty-eight women were treated with MPA, 500 mg/day, i.m., for 30 consecutive days, and 36 patients were treated with MPA, 100 mg thrice a week, by oral route.

The main characteristics of the patients were the following. The median age was similar in the two groups, also the number of soft tissue and bone metastases. The group given the low mean dosages of MPA included fewer women with visceral involvement than the high-dose group (14 and 28, respectively). Most of the patients in both groups were in the postmenopausal. Oestrogen receptors were determined only in the low mean-dose MPA group, and were found to be positive in 32 women, negative in 8 and borderline in 2.

Most of the patients had been treated previously with cytotoxic and endocrine therapy (not progesterone, of course). In the high-dose MPA group, 79 were treated with various forms of combination chemotherapy, generally CMF or AV, and also therapy with endocrine manipulation, generally oöphorectomy, oestrogens and anti-oestrogens. In the low mean-dose MPA group, 67 women had been treated previously with cytotoxic therapy, and 46 with endocrine manipulation. Whereas all the women in the first group were also evaluable for successive high-dose MPA treatment, only 46 out of 67 and 34 out of 46 of the second group were also evaluable for low mean MPA dosage response.

Out of the 34 women evaluable for previous endocrine therapy and MPA, who had been treated with low mean MPA dosages, 13 had responded to previous endocrine therapy and 7 of them (54%) to subsequent MPA administration. Twenty-one did not have regression with previous hormonal treatment, and only 3 (14%) obtained regression with subsequent MPA low-dose adminstration.

Of the 30 women treated with high-dose MPA, 5 obtained regression with previous endocrine treatment and in 2 of them (40%) there was a new regression with MPA. Twenty-five had no regression with previous endocrine treatment, but 8 (32%) of them obtained regression with MPA.

In all 64 evaluable women, MPA induced a regression in 50% of the patients responsive to previous endocrine therapy, and in 24% of the women not responsive to previous endocrine therapy.

Considering the previous cytotoxic treatment, there was no difference between the low mean- and high-dose groups. In fact, in patients previously responsive to cytotoxic therapy 30% and 34%, respectively, tumour regression was observed in the two groups, and there was tumour regression in 19% and 21%, respectively, in the two groups of patients not previously responsive to chemotherapy.

In conclusion, MPA was effective in primary and secondary endocrine-resistant patients. With regard to the choice of the best therapeutic dose to employ, there is a trend in favour of the high-dose MPA, but the small number of patients evaluable and the different types of study (retrospective in the high-dose group, and a controlled randomized study in the low mean-dosage group) do not provide a definitive answer on the usefulness of high-dose MPA. Finally, the previous response to cytotoxic therapy does not seem to influence the response to subsequent MPA administration.

K. Brunner: Two figures should be remembered from Dr De Lena's presentation: first, he has a 28% overall remission rate and, secondly, when MPA is given after previous hormonal-therapy failure (primary failure – patients who never responded to any hormonal treatment) it induces an additional remission in 32%. These figures are very important in a discussion of the possible place of high-dose MPA in the hormonal management of advanced breast cancer.

Professor Mattsson will now present his data on a direct comparison between tamoxifen and MPA, and also on cross-over results.

W. Mattsson

In the mid-'70s I became interested in high-dose MPA when I heard about the very encouraging results reported by Professor Pannuti et al. Therefore, we initiated a phase-II trial and were able to confirm his data in very far advanced patients. As a result, we carried out a randomized trial, comparing tamoxifen (TMX), which is considered to be the drug of choice in postmenopausal breast cancer patients, versus high-dose MPA.

This trial was started in October, 1977 and rather strict criteria were taken for inclusion in the trial. Important exclusion criteria included patients with liver metastases – because I have never seen a patient respond when liver metastases were present.

The patients were randomly allocated to TMX, 10 mg t.i.d., or MPA, daily 1,000 mg i.m. for 30 days, and were treated until progression of the disease. The treatment was stopped after 30 days, after which patients who showed no change or high remission rate at that time were continued on TMX at the same dose, i.e. 10 mg t.i.d., and MPA, weekly 1,000 mg, until progression or relapse.

During almost three years of the study, 33 patients had been included in the TMX group and 30 in the MPA group. They were well balanced in both groups. The response rate was 72% for TMX and 70% for high-dose MPA, and obviously no statistically significant difference existed.

It is important to note that in such a selected group of patients the duration of remission can be very long indeed. CR lasted for 2 and 3 years in patients receiving MPA and TMX, respectively, while PR lasted almost 18 months. The patients in the 'no change' category (which, from the clinical point of view, is very useful) avoided cytotoxic chemotherapy for more than 6 months;

so this treatment might be very good for many patients.

There are some interesting data about the cross-over treatment at the time of relapse. All patients were supposed to be crossed over, if possible, except for those with advanced visceral disease, progressive liver metastases and life-threatening vital conditions. Patients who had high-dose MPA as a second-line treatment responded, with 10 out of 17 having a new remission. Six of these 10 responders had previously failed to TMX. Undoubtedly, therefore, high-dose MPA can induce useful remission in patients unresponsive to TMX. On the contrary, it is strange that when patients no longer responsive to high-dose MPA are treated with TMX they very seldom have a new remission. Only 2 out of 13 patients crossed over from MPA to TMX had a new remission. Both patients had previously had a remission on high-dose MPA.

In conclusion, high-dose MPA is as good as TMX as a first-line treatment. In patients resistant to combination chemotherapy high-dose MPA induced remission at the same rate as TMX. Furthermore, useful clinical remissions were obtained by high-dose MPA in TMX-resistant patients, both those who previously responded and who failed to TMX.

Discussion

K. Brunner: As we have heard, two randomized studies have been presented which show no statistically significant differences between the remission rate on TMX and on high-dose MPA. There is one important difference in the cross-over. Dr Beretta demonstrated that TMX given after oral MPA is as effective as vice versa, and Professor Mattsson has shown that TMX given after i.m. MPA is not as effective as vice versa. This suggests that TMX given after i.m. MPA may be less effective because there is a high MPA plasma level maintained over a longer period of time, so that TMX can not work.

Having heard all these data, the question to ask is whether high-dose MPA is indicated as the primary hormonal treatment in advanced postmenopausal breast cancer or whether it is a second-line 'rescue' therapy. I do not think that this question can be answered today definitely. But, in my view, there is definite evidence for recommending high-dose MPA treatment in advanced breast cancer. It is possible that a subpopulation of breast cancer patients exists, for which high-dose MPA is the therapy of choice. But this subpopulation still has to be defined. I do not think we can generally recommend high-dose MPA as first-line hormonal therapy.

In order to support this view, I will summarize the data presented at this symposium. Professor Mattsson showed that TMX given after i.m. MPA is less effective than vice versa. Dr De Lena demonstrated that MPA given after previous primary hormonal therapy failure (i.e., in patients who have not responded to previous hormonal therapy) is effective in 32%. Dr García-Girált also showed that high-dose MPA was effective in 26% (not large numbers – 4 out of 15 patients) of patients who had not responded to previous hormonal therapy. The Swiss group showed that 23% (7 out of 31) of patients who had not responded to previous hormonal therapy or had no change responded to high-dose MPA, but no patients of this group responded to low-dose MPA.

These data support the conclusion that MPA is quite an effective 'rescue' therapy after failure of previous endocrine treatment. Twenty years or more ago the dogma was held that when a patient did not respond to hormonal manipulation (on very careful objective evaluation), it was useless to try other hormonal treatments. It might be possible that this is different for high-dose MPA. High-dose MPA may be effective in patients who fail on other hormonal treatment – not fail in the sense of relapse after response, but as primary non-responders. Such patients have perhaps a 20–30% chance of responding to high-dose MPA.

I would like to open the discussion on this point.

W. Mattsson: There is one subgroup in advanced breast cancer: the patients with a lot of symptoms, such as pain from skeletal metastases and similar disorders. High-dose MPA might be a first-line treatment in them. For the past 2 years most oncologists in Sweden (and, in fact, throughout Scandinavia) have used high-dose MPA in that subgroup. That gives the patients a good symptomatic relief of the type we have heard today.

W.L. McGuire: If I were to play the devil's advocate, I would say that for most of our advanced diseases high-dose therapies are roughly equivalent in the response rate – at least, it is difficult to show major differences. It may be asked what is the cost per day of diethylstilboestrol. In the U.S.A. it is measured in cents. What is the cost of TMX per day? It is $ 1.40. What is the cost of high-dose MPA?

W. Mattsson: I would like to comment. In Scandinavia, taken over a couple of months – perhaps 6 months, it is almost cheaper to give high-dose MPA than to give TMX. There is no other argument.

K. Brunner: Professor McGuire, I have discussed this topic earlier with the panelists and it seems that the situation is totally different in every country. I do not think that we can go into this problem in detail, but we have to limit ourselves to the clinical research data. I would still like to have my view challenged that there is no firm basis for generally recommending high-dose MPA as a first-line treatment.

W.L. McGuire: Let us forget about cost and talk science. I am not sure I agree with Professor Brunner. Why not use MPA as a first-line treatment? Is it inferior to TMX? I am not sure about those cross-over studies – the same case could be made for aminoglutethimide.

K. Brunner: In Switzerland it is undoubtedly a question of cost.

W.L. McGuire: Let us talk science: let us pretend that the company can reduce the cost. If the cost were equal, why should MPA not be used as a first-line therapy?

K. Brunner: There is a possible reason, which has not yet been confirmed in clinical studies. Patients have to be maintained on i.m. MPA. When these patients have progressive disease there might be less chance of a response to other hormonal therapy after high-dose MPA. If other hormonal therapies, such as oestrogens or TMX, are used first, this problem does not arise. That is one possible reason.

W.L. McGuire: That could be circumvented, though. What I am really saying is that it should not necessarily be said that MPA has to be a second-line therapy – I am not convinced that it has to be.

K. Brunner: I am not convinced either. All I am saying is that it is not possible to make the general recommendation that high-dose MPA be used as a first-line therapy, based on the present data.

G. Beretta: I will not enter into the problem of first- or second-line treatment with MPA. In our randomized study, it was demonstrated that oral MPA is similar to oral TMX, so we could choose between those two drugs.

I would like to stress something that Professor Mattsson showed. In my experience, there were higher response rates after MPA in patients not responding to previous TMX than in patients who had responded to previous TMX. This is in agreement with the data shown by Professor Mattsson. It is important because it means that after failure on the first hormonal treatment, MPA could give another opportunity for treatment.

K. Brunner: How often, in Professor McGuire's experience, is a second-line hormonal therapy effective in patients who did not respond to previous hormonal therapy? That, to me, is the interesting aspect about MPA.

W.L. McGuire: Pearson has published on the sequence of TMX and androgen therapy – which might be somewhat analogous. In the TMX responders, the patients did very well on the androgen therapy. In the TMX failures, I think that the response rate was about 10% – which is very low.

M. Spittle (London, England): First, it seems to me that when one has to choose a hormone to give to patients with advanced disease, if there is no difference in the response to the hormones that have been mentioned so far, it is chosen on the side-effects they cause and the patients' tolerance as regards the way in which the treatment is given. This must make MPA a second-line drug, in comparison with an oral, fairly non-toxic drug which is available.

Secondly, on the point of view where patients have not responded to previous hormone therapy and then respond in vast numbers to MPA, is this not a rather painful and expensive way of giving steroids?

K. Brunner: I think that during this round table we have covered all the questions outlined initially quite extensively. We have come to a tentative conclusion about optimal dosage of high-dose MPA during induction and maintenance therapy. We have reviewed the data on combined MPA and chemotherapy versus chemotherapy alone, keeping in mind, that the more important question is the sequence of hormonal and cytostatic therapy, i.e., simultaneous versus sequential hormonal and chemotherapy. We have looked at some possibly non-specific beneficial effects of MPA when combined with chemotherapy, and a few possible adverse effects. Finally, we have not reached a definite conclusion about the question whether high-dose MPA is the first-line endocrine treatment in all breast cancer patients developing metastatic disease or whether it should rather be used as a second-line hormonal 'rescue' therapy after failure of other hormonal manipulations. This question cannot entirely be separated from economic considerations.

We certainly have learnt a lot about laboratory and clinical data concerning the effects and the optimal use of MPA. But, as in other areas of intensive investigation, many questions still remain unanswered and open to further studies.

Session IV: Endometrial cancer

Chairmen: J.P. Wolff–Villejuif, France
G. De Palo–Milan, Italy

Endometrial cancer: correlations between oestrogen and progestin receptor status, histopathological findings and clinical responses during progestin therapy

P.M. Martin
Experimental Cancerology Laboratory, Faculty of Medicine, University of Marseille, Marseille, France

Introduction

The administration of progestins to patients with endometrial carcinoma has led to inhibition of tumour growth in about 33% of cases. In those with well-differentiated tumours the response rate is higher [1–4]. The present study had 2 objects. The first was to examine the effect of progestin therapy on the concentrations of oestrogen receptors (ER) and progestin receptors (PR), in the cytosol and at the nuclear level. It has previously been demonstrated that variations in receptor levels occur in normal endometria in premenopausal women as the menstrual cycle progresses [5–15]. There are also variations in receptor levels in normal endometria in postmenopausal women, reflecting variations in oestrogenic influence, and in neoplastic endometria in postmenopausal women reflecting degrees of tumour differentiation. The second object of this study was to compare events at the molecular level with clinical responses in patients undergoing progestin therapy. The results were studied to investigate whether an improved selection procedure for patients likely to respond to endocrine therapy could be devised. The factors examined were the simultaneous presence of ER and PR, and the degree of differentiation of the carcinoma.

Material and methods

Collection of neoplastic endometria

The study involved patients with histopathologically-proven endometrial cancer, ranging in grade from well-differentiated (Grade I) to undifferentiated (Grade IV) [16–18], and 2 patients with vaginal recurrences of well-differentiated endometrial carcinomas. A total of 65 postmenopausal women, none of whom had undergone hormone therapy, but some of whom had received radiation treatment, took part in the trial. Eight patients were examined after daily treatment for 4 weeks with 5 mg of demegestone and 10 patients after daily treatment for 4 weeks with 150 mg of medroxyprogesterone acetate (MPA). In 2 cases, surgery was performed 4 hours after administration of 1 mg of demegestone, and in one case, 8 hours after MPA intramuscularly (i.m.). The tissues were washed in ice-cold isotonic NaCl solution. A sample weighing of 50 mg was kept for histological examination. The remainder was frozen and stored in liquid nitrogen for a maximum of one month.

Collection of normal endometrial specimens

Normal endometrial specimens were obtained from pre- and postmenopausal women. The premenopausal women, aged 25–39, were either healthy volunteers or patients who were sterile because of tubal occlusion. These patients had normal cycles, and no ovarian or uterine pathology. The postmenopausal women were hysterectomy patients undergoing surgery for gynaecological reasons other than endometrial disease. In 90 premenopausal women, of whom 78 fulfilled the above criteria, rectal temperature was recorded throughout the cycle, and endometrial biopsy material was examined histopathologically. In 40 of these women, oestradiol and luteinizing hormone (LH) radioimmunoassays (RIA) were performed on days 10, 12 and 14 of the cycle and progesterone RIA on days 12, 14, 16 and 18 of the cycle. On the basis of the findings, a common 28-day cycle could be constructed, permitting comparison of results. The status of the 42 postmenopausal women was judged by results of follicle-stimulating hormone (FSH), LH, oestradiol, oestrone and progesterone RIA [19]. These women were classified according to the degree of oestrogenic influence observed on histological examination of endometrial biopsy material. Blood levels of steroids were measured by RIA after celite chromatography [20]. LH and FSH determination were performed using French Atomic Energy Commission RIA kits.

The endometrial biopsy material was always taken from the same place in the uterine cavity. Biopsy was carried out in either the luteal or the follicular phases in 55 women, and in both phases within the same cycle in 23 women. The second biopsy of the uterine wall was performed at a site exactly opposite that used in the first biopsy. Biopsy yielded 150 mg of tissue in the luteal phase and 250 mg in the follicular phase. The tissues were treated as described for neoplastic endometrium.

For Scatchard analysis, single point assay gradient sucrose analysis and specific analysis we used techniques previously described, without any modification [22–24].

Recently, we have also used a new technique, involving simultaneous incubation for ER and PR followed by chromatographic separation. These techniques, established following collaborative work between H. Magdelenat (Institut Curie, Paris) [21], P. Kelly (CHUL, Quebec) and the author is described in the round table on hormone receptors (see pp. 544–546).

Results

ER and PR in normal endometrial specimens

The variations in levels of cytoplasmic ER and PR in normal endometrial specimens throughout the menstrual cycle are shown in Figures 1 and 2, respectively. Two different buffers were used in preparing cytosols, GTEM buffer and sucrose buffer. ER and PR levels with sucrose buffer tended to be

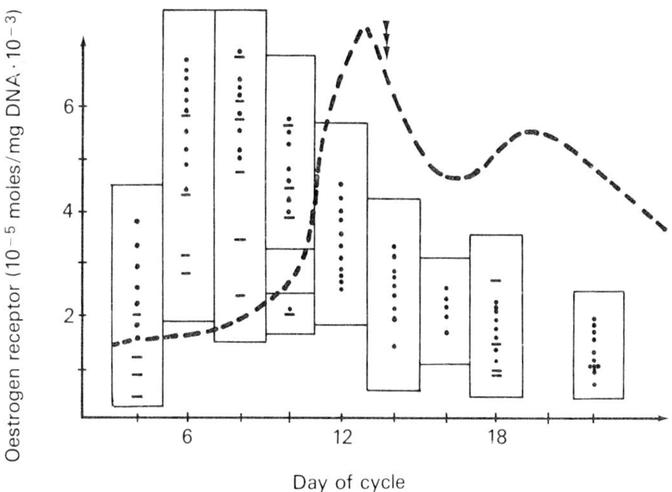

Fig. 1. Cytoplasmic oestrogen receptor levels in normal endometrium during the cycle. The dotted line represents the variation in circulating oestradiol. LM peak is shown. Two buffers were used to prepare cytosol – GTEM buffer (•) and sucrose buffer (—). The rectangles show the confidence interval of the date of biopsies (± 1 day) and receptor content (± SEM).

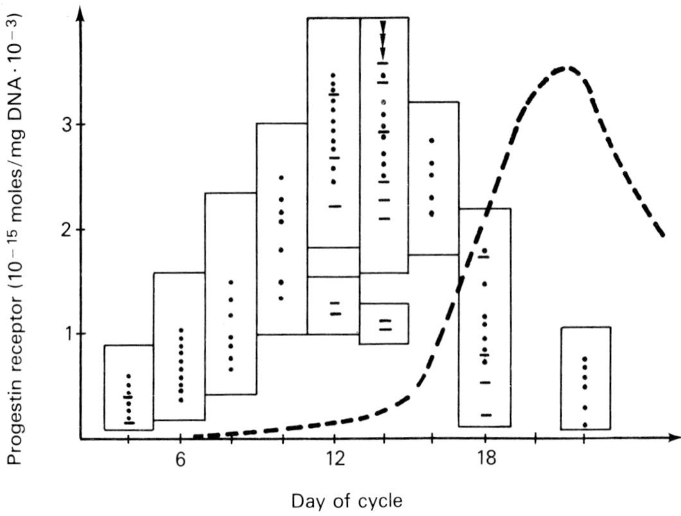

Fig. 2. Cytoplasmic progestin receptor levels in normal endometrium during the cycle. For explanation of symbols see the legend of Figure 1.

lower and more variable than those with GTEM buffer, but the differences were not statistically significantly different. In the following paragraphs, all values refer to GTEM buffer results.

The levels of ER are low at the beginning of the cycle, but increase rapidly to reach a maximum (5,392 ± 1,392 femtomoles (= moles × 10^{-15} = fmol)/mg DNA on day 8 (n = 14)) towards day 6–8, returning to initial levels at the time of the LH peak. The follicular phase is characterized by low ER levels. The variability of the values in this phase is small compared to that of the values recorded in the luteal phase. The lowest levels (1,230 ± 361 fmol/mg DNA on day 22 (n = 11)) were recorded towards the end of the cycle, and were significantly different ($P<0.01$) from the highest values. The levels of PR were lowest at the beginning (337 ± 178 fmol/mg DNA on day 4 (n = 8)) and at the end (491 ± 274 fmol/mg DNA on day 22 (n = 6)) of the cycle. These values were not statistically significantly different. PR levels reached a maximum at mid cycle (2,696 ± 706 fmol/mg DNA on day 12 (n = 16); 2,593 ± 729 fmol/mg DNA on day 14 (n = 16)). The curve of PR levels versus time, unlike the curve of ER levels versus time, is symmetrical over the cycle.

Table I shows the mean cytoplasmic ER and PR levels in normal endometria from postmenopausal women. The biopsy findings were grouped according to the degree of oestrogenic influence observed on histological ex-

Table I. Cytoplasmic levels of oestrogen and progestin receptors in normal endometria of postmenopausal women.

Histopathological assessment	Number of tumours studied	Mean ER levels ± standard errors of means (fmol/mg DNA)	Number of ER-positive tumours	Mean PR levels ± standard errors of means (fmol/mg DNA)	Number of PR-positive tumours
No oestrogenic influence	21	110 ± 50	21	—	0
Oestrogenic influence	9	700 ± 270	9	70 ± 10	5
Cystic glandular hyperplasia	12	1,800 ± 220	12	< 100	12

amination. In the absence of oestrogenic influence, ER levels were significantly lower (110 ± 50 fmol/mg DNA (mean of 21 subjects) than the lowest values recorded in premenopausal women ($P<0.01$), and PR could not be detected in the sucrose gradient assay. In cases in which oestrogenic influence was evident, ER were present in all 9 specimens examined, at an average level of 700 ± 270 fmol/mg DNA. In 5 of these specimens, PR were also present (70 ± 10 fmol/mg DNA). In 12 cases of cystic glandular hyperplasia, the mean ER level reached 1,800 ± 220 fmol/mg DNA. PR were always present, but at levels below 100 fmol/mg. The mean ER level was statistically significantly higher than that recorded in the 9 biopsy specimens showing signs of oestrogenic influence, taken from postmenopausal women.

In biopsy specimens of normal endometria from premenopausal women, maximum ER levels occurred just before the oestradiol peak with which a decrease in ER levels was associated. In pre- and postmenopausal women, a high PR level was never associated with a high ER level, although in postmenopausal women, PR were only detected when ER levels were high, and when there was histological evidence of oestrogenic influence. Our observations are in agreement with those in the literature [5–11]. In the first days of the menstrual cycle, ER levels are very low. They reach a maximum level within the first third of the proliferative phase, although oestrogen levels continue to rise in plasma. ER levels in endometria then decrease progressively, to reach their lowest values in tissues showing decidual reactions or disintegrating secretory changes. These results, and the relationship between histological evidence of oestrogenic influence and ER levels in normal endometria from postmenopausal women suggest that oestradiol plays a role in the induction of its own receptor, although the possibility of some other regulatory factors must also be taken into account [8, 9, 25]. The rise in PR levels occurs later than the rise in ER levels but before the rise in plasma progesterone concentrations. PR levels continue to increase slowly up to the end of the proliferative phase, and then fall sharply during the secretory phase, even though plasma progesterone levels continue to increase. These changes in the receptor levels are in agreement with a 3-stage mechanism in the sex hormone receptor (SR) system: induction of SR, nuclear stabilization, and prevention of replenishment of cytoplasmic SR. The regulation of the SR system is discussed later.

In endometrial carcinoma, a correlation between the numbers of cytosolic progestin binding sites and degree of differentiation of the tumour has been reported [7]. We have obtained evidence that both the presence and levels of PR are related to degree of differentiation. We have also been able to show that, in PR-positive carcinomas, ER levels are higher, the lower the degree of differentiation. These results are analogous to our findings in normal endometria, in which the presence of high levels of ER corresponds to the proliferative phase and hyperplasia, and the presence of high levels of PR to the secretory phase. We believe these findings indicate that the endometrium is a tissue containing the components necessary for responses to oestradiol and progesterone, which appear to have major regulating roles on cell growth and differentiation respectively [26–28].

ER and PR levels in neoplastic endometria before therapy with progestins

Tables II and III show ER and PR levels in cytoplasm from neoplastic endometria in postmenopausal women with stage I carcinoma before therapy with progestins. The results obtained with different assay buffers were significantly different ($P<0.01$). PR were detected more often when GTEM buffer was used, and levels of both types of receptors were higher when this buffer was used. ER were detectable in all classes of endometrial cancer examined, but levels varied according to the degree of histological differentiation. They were highest in moderately well-differentiated carcinomas and well-differentiated carcinomas. The levels found were below those recorded during the menstrual cycle in normal endometria. In contrast, PR were present in only 3 out of 12 undifferentiated carcinomas, but in 27 out of 29 well-differentiated carcinomas analysed.

ER and PR levels in neoplastic endometrium after therapy

Following radiation treatment, no PR were detected in 2 undifferentiated and 3 well-differentiated carcinomas, and ER levels were very low. The effect of daily administration of 5 mg of demegestone or 150 mg of MPA for 4 weeks on cytoplasmic PR levels is shown in Table IV. In 5 undifferentiated carcinomas, ER levels remained virtually unchanged, and PR were undetectable before and after therapy. In 5 moderately well-differentiated carcinomas, ER levels remained virtually unchanged and PR were undetectable before as well as after therapy. In 5 other moderately well-differentiated carcinomas, ER levels fell in cases in which PR had been detected initially. In 7 well-differentiated carcinomas, PR levels during therapy became undetectable, and ER levels became very low. The decrease in receptor levels with time is shown in Figure 3 (2 well-differentiated carcinomas (nos. 56 and 29 of Table IV). PR disappeared completely after one week of demegestone therapy and ER levels fell progressively over 2 months. Both vaginal recurrences (nos. 41 and 42) underwent remission during progestin therapy.

Table II. Cytoplasmic oestrogen and progestin receptor levels in endometrial carcinomas.

Degree of differentiation of tumour	Number of tumours studied	Mean ER levels ± standard errors of means (fmol/mg DNA)	Number of ER-positive tumours	Mean PR levels ± standard errors of means (fmol/mg DNA)	Number of PR-positive tumours
Undifferentiated	12 (A)	220 ± 110	6	87 ± 24	3
Moderately differentiated	18 (A)	450 ± 302	16	78 ± 21	14
	6 (B)	380 ± 280	5	197 ± 102	4
Well-differentiated	17 (A)	1370 ± 750	17	690 ± 113	15
	12 (B)	980 ± 350	12	267 ± 98	12

(A) = Cytosol prepared in GTEM buffer.
(B) = Cytosol prepared in sucrose buffer.

Table III. Oestrogen and progestin receptors in endometrial carcinoma.

Histopathological assessment	Number of tumours studied	Mean ER receptor levels (fmol/mg DNA)	Mean PR receptor levels (fmol/mg DNA)
Undifferentiated	2 (B)	2,686	104*
		312	< 10
Moderately differentiated	3 (A)	1,536	< 10
		510	308**
		207	180**
Papillary adenocarcinoma	2 (A)	1,880	90
		960	120
Vaginal recurrences	2 (A)	780	220***
		510	40

(A) = Cytosol prepared in GTEM buffer.
(B) = Cytosol prepared in sucrose buffer.
* = undifferentiated carcinoma with positive clinical response to MPA therapy.
** = moderately differentiated carcinoma with positive clinical response to MPA therapy.
*** = vaginal recurrences with positive clinical response to MPA therapy.

To determine whether the decrease in ER and PR levels during progestin therapy was a result of nuclear stabilization of receptors, nuclear and cytosolic ER and PR contents in 8 of the above mentioned well-differentiated carcinomas were assayed. The results (Table V) show nuclear stabilization of PR 4–8 hours after treatment. In addition, nuclear receptor analysis revealed that, in well-differentiated endometrial carcinomas before progestin therapy, nuclei contained low levels of PR. In contrast, oestrogen-specific binding sites were detected in the purified nuclei while ER levels remained the same after therapy (low level) in the nuclei but slowly decreased in the cytosol fraction.

Clinical results

It is not the main object of this paper to report clinical results. However, clinical responses to progestin therapy were recorded. A positive response was regarded as corresponding to the appearance of secretory and/or acanthomatous changes in the tumours, and changes in cells to a benign morphology. Findings in this respect are shown in Table IV. There was a very

Table IV. *Effects of progestin therapy on PR levels in endometrial carcinomas, and correlations between receptor status and clinical response.*

Case number	Grade	Mean PR level before therapy indicated (fmol/mg DNA)	Mean PR level after 4 weeks of therapy (fmol/mg DNA)	Clinical response
4	IIIb-IV	<10 MPA	<10	–
7	IIIb-IV	<10 Demegestone	<10	–
8	IIIb-IV	<10 MPA	<10	+/–
45	IIIb-IV	13 Demegestone	<10	–
46	IIIb-IV	<10 Demegestone	<10	–
9	II-IIIa	320 Demegestone	<10	+
14	II-IIIa	840 MPA	<10	+
16	II-IIIa	<10 MPA	<10	–
17	II-IIIa	710 MPA	<10	+
54	II-IIIa	1,830 Demegestone	<10	+
55	I	1,980 Demegestone	<10	+
56	I	1,620 Demegestone	<10	+
29	I	960 Demegestone	<10	+
32	I	1,780 MPA	<10	+
60	I	1,820 Demegestone	<10	+
34	I	810 MPA	<10	+
36	I	450 MPA	<10	+
41	II	220 MPA	<10	+
42	II	40 MPA	<10	+

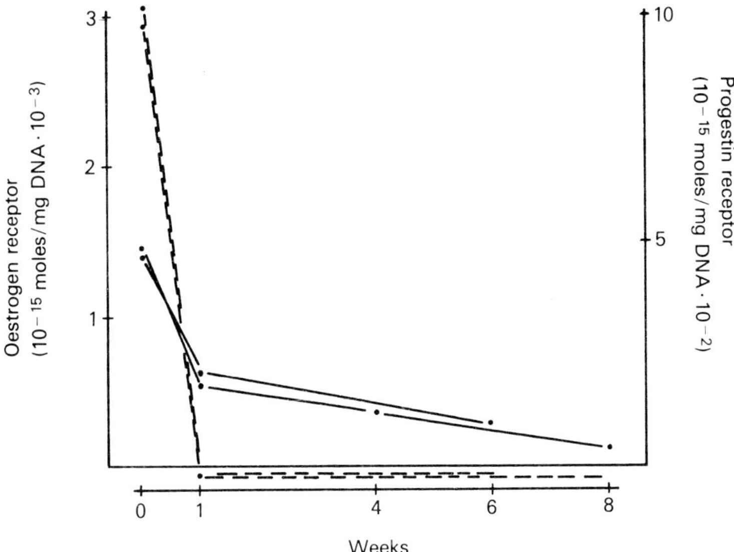

Fig. 3. Effect of progestin therapy on steroid receptor content. Two patients bearing well-differentiated endometrial carcinomas received progestin therapy for 4 weeks. Oestrogen and progestin receptors were measured by biopsies and micro-assays.

strong correlation between presence of PR and positive responses. All patients clinically responding were those with PR-positive lesions. In addition, the clinical response correlated well with decreases in receptor concentrations. The histological and radiological findings revealed a nonproliferative phase in the tumour cells but not cell death or lysis. No cytotoxic effects were ever observed. In the cases of vaginal recurrence, in which both ER and PR were present, complete remission occurred.

Since the growth of neoplastic cells is stimulated by oestrogen, and progestin induces histological differentiation associated with inhibition of the stimulant effect of oestrogen [29–35], it is reasonable to assume that some endometrial carcinomas, at least, have retained the physiological properties of the normal endometrium. Since steroid hormones exert their effects on target tissues via receptors [36], the relationship between the presence of PR and tumour differentiation (considered as consecutive events) supports the concept that the presence of PR and a high degree of differentiation of lesions may reflect potential hormonal sensitivity of these lesions. This correlation provides a basis for selection of patients for endocrine therapy.

At the molecular level, the effects of progestin therapy of endometrial car-

Table V. Nuclear and cytosolic receptor contents in well-differentiated endometrial carcinomas during progestin therapy.

Numbers of tumours studied	Therapy	Time from start of progestin therapy											
		0 minutes				4–5 hours		8 hours		4 weeks			
		Receptor levels (fmol/mg DNA)				Receptor levels (fmol/mg DNA)		Receptor levels (fmol/mg DNA)		Receptor levels (fmol/mg DNA)			
		PR		ER		PR		PR		PR		ER	
		cyto-solic	nu-clear	cyto-solic	nu-clear	cyto-solic	nu-clear	cyto-solic	nu-clear	cyto-solic	nu-clear	cyto-solic	nu-clear
1	Deme-gestone	255	0			65	98						
1	Deme-gestone	413	0			83	128						
5	Deme-gestone	650* ± 110 (5)	0	940* ± 170 (5)	5 to 7 (5)					5 to 7 (1)	6 to 8 (1)	141* ± 21 (3)	5 to 7 (5)
1	MPA	430	0					87	62				

*Means ± standard errors of means.
Numbers in parentheses are numbers of tumours containing receptors of type indicated.

cinomas on the SR system were to induce a fall in cytosolic PR to undetectable levels after less than one week, provided both ER and PR were initially present in the lesions. The first step was nuclear localization, detectable in vivo 4–8 hours after progestin treatment. The subsequent finding of very low cytosolic PR levels indicates that daily administration of progestin may result in continuous nuclear stabilization of PR. However, a concomitant fall in ER levels might also influence the cytosolic PR content. Progestogenic control of ER levels has been suggested [8, 9, 14, 15, 37–41]. This would correspond with the well known ability of progestins to modify and/or antagonize the action of oestrogens [32, 38, 42, 43]. On the other hand, oestradiol is presumably a major factor involved in ER induction in the early days of the cycle, and in postmenopausal women whose endometrium reveals oestrogenic influence [9, 44, 45]. Nuclear stabilization of ER-oestradiol complexes and lack of ER replenishment will result in the disappearance of cytosolic ER. The antagonistic effect of progestins on oestrogenic activity is mediated by interference with replenishment of ER. Since the rise in endometrial PR levels and plasma progesterone levels during the menstrual cycle occurs later than the rises in serum oestrogen and endometrial ER levels, this may explain the observed SR profiles in normal endometria in premenopausal women.

From the data reported here, we conclude that nuclear retention of PR results in a decrease in ER content of the cytosol, e.g., via ER-oestradiol complexes which are stabilized in endometrial cell nuclei. This phenomenon would correspond to the clinical response to progestin therapy, through which the oestrogen-dependent growth of neoplastic endometrial cells is reduced. It provides further evidence that the presence of PR indicates that ER in biopsy samples are functional. This can be a classical interpretation of our data. However, to study a subcellular compartmentalization of ER and PR in target tissue (i.e., human cell lines and rat uterus), we used several technical approaches: biochemical receptor determination in different conditions and autoradiography procedures. These determinations are made after incubation at 4° C and/or 37° C for a period of 5 minutes to 2 hours with specific receptor synthetic tags (such as R2858 for ER [46] and R5020 for PR).

The classical model for the mechanism of action of steroids holds that unbound receptors for steroids reside exclusively in the cytoplasmic compartment and that they undergo translocation to the nucleus when bound to steroids in a process which is temperature-sensitive. In our studies, when the tissue or cells were processed for autoradiography, the localization of steroid was nuclear and cytoplasmic [47, 48]. In contrast, when the tissue or cells were processed using the usual biochemical procedures, all binding activity appeared in the cytosolic fraction. In addition, when concentrated preparations of homogenized uteri as well as several nuclear preparations from cell lines were made, free receptor could be demonstrated in the crude nuclear preparations. Our data suggest that there are unbound receptors for oestrogen and progesterone in nuclei of the smooth muscle cells of myometrium as well as in nuclei of the several cell lines (ER+) [47–49]. We propose a new model for the distribution of ER in which unbound receptors are in equilibrium, partitioned between nuclei and cytoplasm according to the free water content of these intracellular compartments [50].

This new model for mechanism of action of steroids now needs to be considered for interpretation of the results obtained before and after therapy in human endometrium [50].

It should be noted that the induction of acanthomatous changes leads to development in a way different from normal. Progestin therapy may result in reduced oestrogen-dependent growth and in re-orientation of natural cell-differentiation. It has been suggested by Hsueh et al. that progestins redirect the cell's ability to respond to an oestrogen [39, 40]. It is not possible to determine whether reduced oestrogen-dependent growth and re-orientation of natural cell-differentiation results from an intrinsic effect of progestin or from a modified response to circulating oestrogen present in postmenopausal women [19]. The mechanism of this redirection of differentiation remains to be established.

References

1. Anderson, D.G. (1965): Management of advanced endometrial carcinoma with medroxyprogesterone acetate. *Am. J. Obstet. Gynecol. 92,* 87.
2. Kelley, R.M. and Baker, W.H. (1965): The role of progesterone in endometrial cancer. *Cancer Res. 25,* 1190.
3. Kistner, R.W. and Griffiths, C.T. (1968): Use of progestational agents in the management of metastatic carcinoma. *Clin. Obstet. Gynecol. 11,* 439.
4. Wentz, N.B. (1964): Effect of progestational agent on endometrial hyperplasia and endometrial cancer. *Obstet. Gynecol. 24,* 370.
5. Pollow, K., Lubbert, H., Boquoi, E. et al. (1975): Characterization and comparison of receptors for estradiol and progesterone in human proliferative endometrium and endometrial carcinoma. *Endocrinology 96,* 319.
6. Pollow, K., Lubbert, H., Boquoi, E. and Pollow, B. (1975): Progesterone metabolism in normal human endometrium during the menstrual cycle and in endometrial carcinoma. *J. Clin. Endocrinol. Metab. 41,* 729.
7 Pollow, K., Boquoi, E., Schmidt-Gollwitzer, H. and Pollow, B. (1976): The nuclear estradiol and progesterone receptors of human endometrium and endometrial carcinoma. *J. Mol. Med. 1,* 325.
8. Pollow, K., Schmidt-Gollwitzer, H. and Nevinny-Stickel, J. (1977): Progesterone receptors in normal endometrium and endometrial carcinoma. In: *Progesterone Receptors in Normal and Neoplastic Tissues,* pp. 313–338. Eds: W.L. McGuire,

J.P. Raynaud and E.E. Beaulieu. Raven Press, New York.
9. Evans, L.H., Martin, J.D. and Hanel, R. (1974): Estrogen receptor concentration in normal and pathologic uterine tissues. *J. Clin. Endocrinol. Metab. 38,* 23.
10. Bayard, F., Damilano, S. and Robel, P. (1975): Les récepteurs de l'estradiol et de la progestérone dans l'endomètre humain au cours du cycle. *Comptes Rendus des Séances Acad. Sci. (Ser. D) 281,* 1341.
11. Limpaphayom, K., Lee, C., Jacobson, H.I. and King, T.M. (1971): Estrogen receptor in human endometrium during the menstrual cycle and early pregnancy. *Am. J. Obstet. Gynecol. 111,* 1064.
12. King, R.J.B., Townsend, P.T., Siddel, N. et al. (1981): Regulation of estrogen and progesterone receptor levels in epithelium and stroma from pre- and postmenopausal endometria. *J. Steroid Biochem.* 1845.
13. King, R.J.B., Whitehead, M.I., Campbell, S. and Minardi, J. (1979): Effect of estrogen and progestin treatments on endometria from postmenopausal women. *Cancer Res. 39,* 1094.
14. King, R.J.B. and Whitehead, M.I. (1980): Application of steroid receptor analyses to clinical and biological investigations of the postmenopausal endometrium. In: *Perspectives in Steroid Receptor Research,* pp. 259–272. Ed: F. Bresciani. Raven Press, New York.
15. King, R.J.B., Dyer, G., Collins, W.P. and Whitehead, M.I. (1980): Intracellular estradiol, estrone and estrogen receptor levels in endometria from postmenopausal women receiving estrogens and progestins. *J. Steroid Biochem. 13,* 377.
16. Broders, A.C. (1925): The grading of carcinoma. *Minn. Med. 8,* 726.
17. Broders, A.C. (1932): Practical point on the macroscopic grading of carcinoma. *N. Engl. J. Med. 32,* 667.
18. Novak, E.R. (1965): Endometrium histology. In: *Gynecologic and Obstetric Pathology,* pp. 160–187. Eds: E.R. Novak and J.D. Woodruff. W.B. Saunders Company, Philadelphia.
19. Sherman, B.H., West, J.H. and Korenman, S.G. (1976): The menopausal transition: analyses of LH, FSH, estradiol and progesterone concentrations during menstrual cycles of older women. *J. Clin. Endocrinol. Metab. 42,* 629.
20. Abraham, G.E., Odell, W.D. and Swerdloff, R.S. (1972): Simultaneous radioimmunoassays of plasma FSH, LH, progesterone, 17-OH-progesterone and estradiol during the menstrual cycle. *J. Clin. Endocrinol. Metab. 34,* 312.
21. Magdelenat, H. (1979): Simultaneous determination of estrogen and progestin receptors on small amount of breast tumor cytosol. *Cancer Treat. Rep. 63,* 1146.
22. Martin, P.M., Rolland, P.H., Jacquemier, J. et al. (1979): Multiple steroid receptors in human breast cancer. II. Estrogen and progestin receptors in 672 primary tumors. *Cancer Chemother. Pharmacol. 2,* 107.
23. Martin, P.M., Rolland, P.H., Jacquemier, J. et al. (1979): Multiple steroid receptors in human breast cancer. III. Relationships between steroid receptors and the state of differentiation and the activity of carcinomas throughout the pathologic features. *Cancer Chemother. Pharmacol. 2,* 115.
24. Martin, P.M., Rolland, P.H., Jacquemier, J. et al. (1978): Multiple steroid receptors in human breast cancer. I. Technological features. *Biomedicine 28*, 278.
25. McGuire, W.L., Horwitz, K.B., Pearson, O.H. and Segalogg, A. (1977): Current status of estrogen and progesterone receptors in breast cancer. *Cancer 39*, 2934.

26. Verga, A. and Henriksen, E. (1965): Histologic observations on the effect of 17-alpha-hydroxyprogesterone caproate on endometrial carcinoma. *Obstet. Gynecol. 26*, 656.
27. Hudson, C.N., Chu, M. and Stanfeld, A.G. (1966): The histological changes produced in untreated adenocarcinoma of the endometrium by a progestogen. *J. Obstet. Gynecol. Br. Commonwealth 74,* 442.
28. Kistner, R.W. (1959): Histological effects of progestins on hyperplasia and carcinoma in situ of endometrium. *Cancer 12*, 1106.
29. Gerschenson, L.E., Berliner, J. and Yang, J.J. (1974): Diethylstilbestrol and progesterone regulation of cultured rabbit endometrial cell growth. *Cancer Res. 34,* 2873.
30. Gerschenson, L.E., Conner, E. and Murai, J.T. (1977): Regulation of the cell cycle by diethylstilbestrol and progesterone in cultured endometrial cells. *Endocrinology 100,* 1468.
31. Hustin, J. (1975): Effect of protein hormones and steroids on tissue cultures of endometrial carcinoma. *Br. J. Obstet. Gynecol. 82,* 493.
32. Kimura, J. (1978): Effect of progesterone on cell division in chemically induced endometrial hyperplasia and adenocarcinoma in mice. *Cancer Res. 38*, 78.
33. Ishiwata, I., Nozawa, S. and Okumura, H. (1977): Effects of 17-beta-estradiol and progesterone on growth and morphology of human endometrial carcinoma cells in vitro. *Cancer Res. 37,* 4246.
34. John, A.M., Cornes, J.S., Jackson, W.D. and Bye, P. (1972): Effect of systemically administered progesterone on histopathology of endometrial carcinoma. *J. Obstet. Gynecol. Scand. 51*, 55.
35. Sekiya, S., Takayama, N. and Takamizawz, H. (1976): Effects of progesterone on rat uterine adenocarcinoma cells in vitro: an electron microscopic study. *Eur. J. Cancer 12,* 493.
36. Jensen, E.V., Suzuke, T., Kawashima, T. et al. (1968): A two-step mechanism for the interaction of estradiol with rat uterus. *Proc. Natl. Acad. Sci. U.S.A. 59,* 632.
37. Freifeld, M.L., Feil, R.D. and Bardini, C.W. (1974): The in vivo regulation of the progesterone receptor in guinea-pig uterus: dependence on estrogen and progesterone. *Steroids 23*, 93.
38. Bhakoo, H.S. and Katzenellenbogen, B.S. (1977): Progesterone modulation of estrogen stimulated uterine biosynthetic events and estrogen receptor levels. *Modern Cellular Endocrinol. 8,* 121.
39. Hsueh, A.J.W., Peck, E.J. and Clark, J.H. (1975): Progesterone antagonism of estrogen receptor and estradiol-induced uterine growth. *Nature (London) 254,* 337.
40. Hsueh, A.J.W., Peck. E.J. and Clark, J.H. (1976): Control of uterine estrogen receptor levels by progesterone. *Endocrinology 98*, 438.
41. Tseng, L. and Gurpide, E. (1975): Effects of progestins on estradiol receptor levels in human endometrium. *J. Clin. Endocrinol. Metab. 41*, 402.
42. Gerulath, A.H. and Borth, R. (1977): Effect of progesterone and estradiol-17-beta on nucleic acid synthesis in vitro in carcinoma of the endometrium. *Am. J. Obstet. Gynecol. 128,* 772.
43. West, N.B., Verhage, H.G. and Brenner, R.H. (1976): Suppression of the estradiol receptor system by progesterone in the oviduct and uterus of cat. *Endocrinology 99*, 1010.

44. Janne, O., Kontula, K., Luukainen, T. and Vihko, R. (1975): Estrogen-induced progesterone receptor in human uterus. *J. Steroid Biochem. 6,* 501.
45. Whitehead, M.I., Townsend, P.T., Pryse-Davies, J. et al. (1981): Effects of estrogens and progestins on the biochemistry and morphology of the postmenopausal endometrium. *N. Engl. J. Med. 27*, 1600.
46. Raynaud, J.P., Martin, P.M., Bouton, M.M. and Ojasoo, T. (1978): 11β-methoxy-17-ethynyl-1,3,5(10)-estratriene-3,17β-diol (Moxestrol). A tag for estrogen receptor binding sites in human tissues. *Cancer Res. 38*, 3044.
47. Sheridan, J.P., Buchanan, J.M., Anselmo, V.C. and Martin, P.M. (1979): Equilibrium: the intra-cellular distribution of steroid receptors. *Nature (London) 282*, 579.
48. Edwards, D., Martin, P.M., Horwitz, K. et al. (1980): Subcellular compartimentalization of estrogen receptors in human breast cancer cells. *Exp. Cell Res. 127*, 197.
49. Sheridan, P.J., Buchanan, J.M., Anselmo, V.C. and Martin, P.M. (1981): Unbound progesterone receptors are in equilibrium between the nucleus and cytoplasm in cells of the rat uterus. *Endocrinology 108*, 1533.
50. Martin, P.M. and Sheridan P.J. (1982): Toward a new model for mechanism of action of steroids. *J. Steroid Biochem. 16*, 215.

Clinical significance of female sex steroid hormone receptors in endometrial carcinoma treated with conventional methods and medroxyprogesterone acetate*

A.J.I. Kauppila[1], H. Isotalo[2], E. Kujansuu[1] and R. Vihko[1]
[1]Department of Obstetrics and Gynaecology; and [2]Department of Clinical Chemistry, University of Oulu, Oulu, Finland

Introduction

Data from epidemiological [1, 2] and biochemical [3, 4] studies clearly demonstrate that female sex steroid hormones are involved in the development and progression of endometrial carcinoma. It has been concluded that unopposed oestrogen activity helps promote malignant transformation of the endometrium [1]. Progesterone and progestins, on the other hand, may counteract this process [2, 5], and can often produce regressive changes in the malignant endometrial cells [6] or even total disappearance of endometrial malignancy [7], with objective remission in about one-third of patients with advanced malignancy [8, 9]. In addition, they reduce the number of cytosolic binding sites for oestrogens and progestins [4]. Our knowledge at present thus provides a rational foundation for progestin therapy in endometrial carcinoma, but calls for studies of the hormonal characteristics of endometrial carcinomas via assay of cytosol for oestrogen receptors (ER) and progestin receptors (PR). All patients in our hospital with endometrial carcinoma have been given supplementary treatment with medroxyprogesterone acetate (MPA) for 2 years, and, since 1976, concentrations of cytosolic ER and PR have been determined in 134 endometrial carcinoma specimens from 127 patients. In this paper we survey the clinical significance of the results of these receptor determinations in cases of endometrial carcinoma treated using conventional methods and prolonged administration of MPA.

* Supported by grants from The Finnish Foundation for Cancer Research and The National Research Council for Medical Sciences, Finland.

Materials and methods

Patients and therapy

Eighty-eight (69%) of the 127 patients had International Federation of Gynaecology and Obstetrics stage I disease. Twelve (9%) of patients had stage-II disease and 23 (18%) of patients had stage III to IV disease. A tissue specimen for receptor determination was taken from the distant primary malignant lesion in 4 cases (3%) before any therapy. In addition, 7 tissue samples from recurrent lesions were studied.

The principal treatment used in cases of stage I and II endometrial carcinoma consisted of pre-operative intracavitary irradiation with the Cathetron afterloading unit [10], and total abdominal hysterectomy and bilateral salpingo-oophorectomy. Postoperative external pelvic irradiation took place in cases in which one or more of the indicators of high risk (cervical, deep myometrial or lymph node involvement, histological anaplasia of the tumour) were present [11]. Otherwise, only the vagina was irradiated postoperatively. The treatment of patients with advanced primary malignancy was highly individual. In stage III disease, most cases were irradiated both internally and externally, and surgical therapy was undertaken, if possible. All patients with early or advanced primary malignancy were treated with oral MPA (100 mg a day) for 2 years. In cases of recurrence, or failure of primary therapy, cytotoxic combination chemotherapy, mostly involving cyclophosphamide, doxorubicin and 5-fluorouracil was initiated, as described previously, in detail [12].

Tissue samples and cytosolic ER and PR assay

Samples were taken from the primary endometrial carcinomas by curettage and from distant lesions at operation. Each specimen was divided into 2 parts, one for receptor assay, the other for histopathological examination, employing the criteria of the World Health Organization. The specimens for receptor assay were frozen immediately, and stored at $-70\,^{\circ}C$ until assayed. Tritiated oestradiol and a synthetic progestin, Org 2058 (16α-ethyl-21-hydroxy-19-nor-4-pregnene-3,20-dione), were used as labelled ligands. The assay methods have been described in detail elsewhere [4]. The detection limits for ER and PR were 3 and 6 femtomol ($= mol \times 10^{-15}$) (fmol)/mg of cytosolic protein, respectively.

Statistical analyses

Because there were substantial variations in the concentrations of cytosolic ER and PR, logarithmic transformations were performed before statistical analyses of the results, using Student's *t*-test.

Results

Cytosolic ER and PR and various indicators of risk

Clinical stage The concentrations of cytosolic ER and PR in stage III to IV

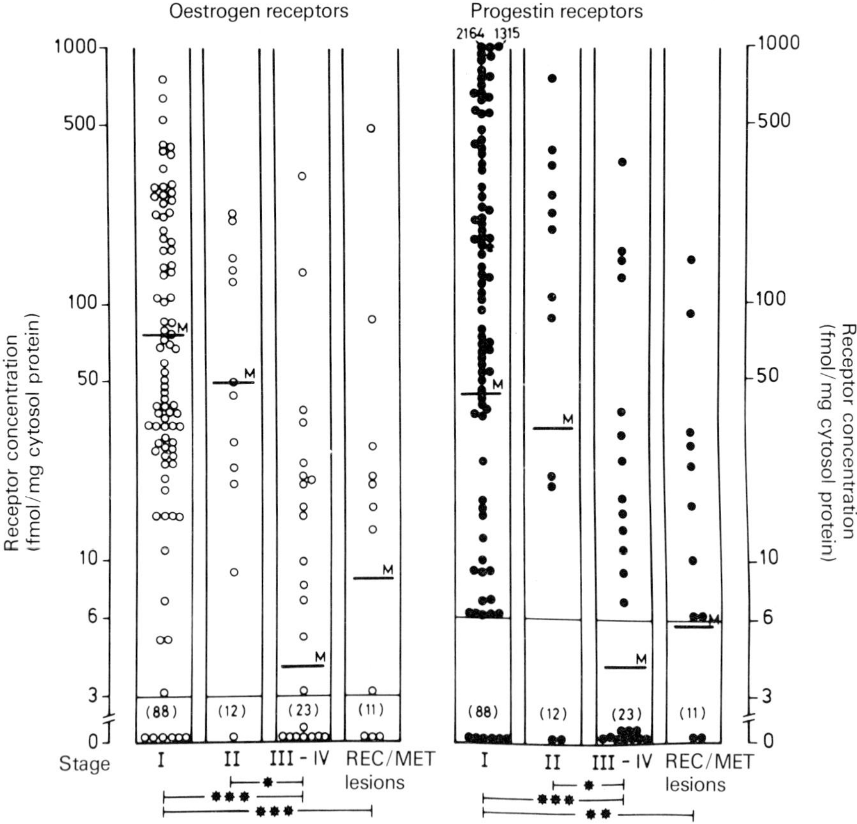

Fig. 1. Individual ER and PR concentrations in different clinical stages of endometrial carcinoma. M indicates geometric mean of values. Numbers in parentheses are numbers of cases. (= P<0.05, **= P<0.01, ***= P<0.001). (REC= recurrent, MET= metastatic).*

endometrial carcinomas and recurrent or metastatic lesions were lower than in stage I and II carcinomas (Fig. 1). The relative frequency of receptor-rich tumours (cytosolic ER and PR concentrations ≥30 fmol/mg protein) decreased markedly as the disease progressed (Table I).

Histological grade The concentrations of cytosolic ER and PR in anaplastic carcinomas (stage I subgroup G3) were lower than in well-differentiated (stage I subgroup G1) or moderately differentiated carcinomas (stage I subgroup G2) (Fig. 2). The relative frequency of receptor-rich tumours decreased as histopathological differentiation of the tumour decreased (Table II).

Myometrial invasion Approximately half of the stage I malignancies had infiltrated markedly into the myometria. The rest were superficial. Cytosolic PR concentrations in the infiltrating malignancies were lower than those in superficial tumours (Fig. 3).

Table I. Distribution of receptor-rich and receptor-poor endometrial carcinomas in relation to clinical stage.*

Clinical stage	No. of patients	Numbers (percentages) of tumours of receptor status shown			
		Receptor-rich		Receptor-poor	
I	88	57	(65)	31	(35)
II	12	6	(50)	6	(50)
III-IV	23	4	(17)	19	(83)
Recurrences/ metastases	11	0	(0)	11	(100)

* Receptor-rich indicates presence of cytosolic ER and PR in concentrations ≥30 fmol/mg protein.

Table II. Relative frequency of receptor-rich and receptor-poor tumours among stage I endometrial adenocarcinomas of different histological grades.

Grade	No. of cases	Numbers (percentages) of tumours of receptor status shown			
		Receptor-rich		Receptor-poor	
I	46	34	(74)	12	(26)
II	34	21	(62)	13	(38)
III	8	2	(25)	6	(75)

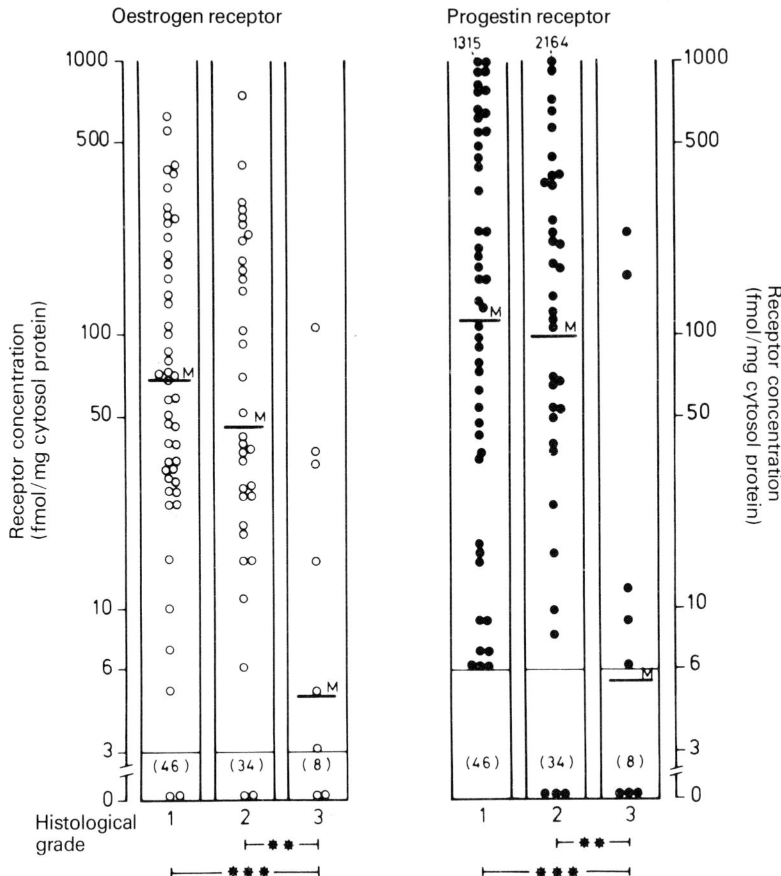

*Fig. 2. Individual cytosolic ER and PR concentrations in stage I endometrial carcinoma of different histological grades. M indicates geometric mean of values. Numbers in parentheses are numbers of cases. (** = P<0.01, *** = P<0.001).*

Cytosolic ER and PR and clinical outcome

Early disease Fifty-four patients with stage I disease were followed up for one year, 41 for 2 years and 25 for 3 years. About two-thirds of these endometrial malignancies were receptor-rich, the remainder receptor-poor (ER and/or PR ≤30 fmol/mg protein) (Table I). The corrected survival rate in patients with receptor-rich carcinomas tended to be better than that in patients with receptor-poor malignancies (Fig. 4). One patient in each group died of early postoperative complications (in one case pulmonary embolism, in the

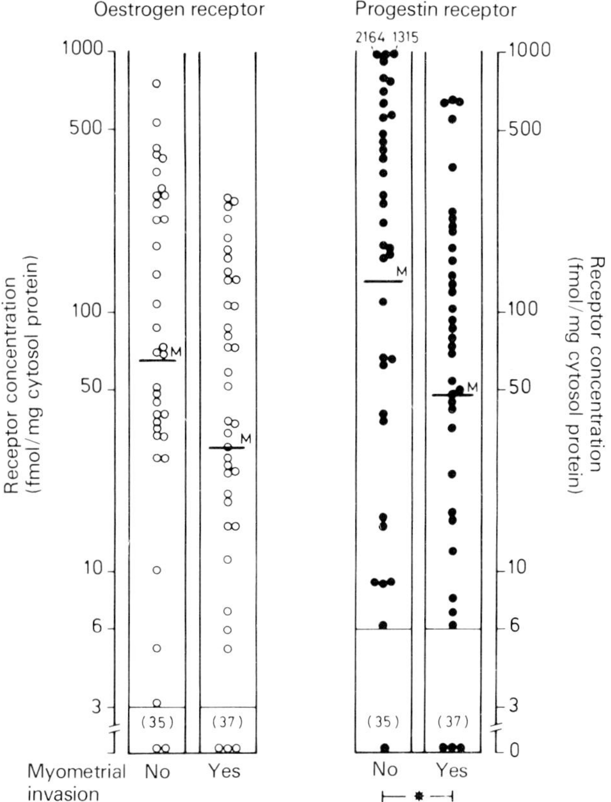

Fig. 3. Individual cytosolic ER and PR values in superficial and invasive stage I endometrial malignancies. M indicates geometric mean of values. Numbers in parentheses are numbers of cases. (= <0.05).*

other an anaphylactic reaction following a dextran infusion). In addition, one patient with a receptor-rich tumour died from a cardiac infarction during the third year of follow-up. All these patients have been excluded from analysis. A notable feature of these results is that there was no carcinoma-related death in any patient with a receptor-rich malignancy during the administration of MPA.

Advanced disease Twenty-one patients with clinical stage III or IV disease were followed-up for 2 years or more (Table III). Only 4 had a receptor-rich malignancy. Two died from endometrial carcinoma. Two are still alive. In contrast, only one of the 17 patients with a receptor-poor malignancy is still

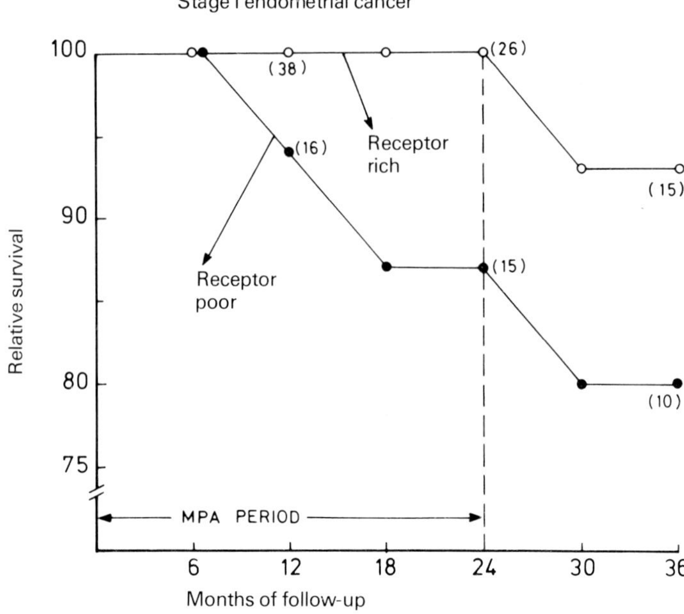

Fig. 4. Relative survival rate of patients with receptor-rich (○) or receptor-poor (•) carcinomas of clinical stage I. Numbers in parentheses are numbers of evaluable patients.

Table III. Survival of patients with stage III to IV receptor-rich or receptor-poor endometrial malignancy.

Receptor-status of tumour	No. of patients	Number (%) of survivors	Duration of survival (months)	Number (%) of deaths	Duration of survival (months)
Rich	4	2 (50)	45+ and 61+	2 (50)	12 and 23
Poor	17	1 (6)	25	16 (94)	2 to 19 (mean 9.6)

alive, and the duration of survival of those who died was mostly very short. Thus the presence of a receptor-poor carcinoma is a bad prognostic sign in both early and advanced malignancies.

In cases in which MPA therapy failed, the response to cytotoxic combination treatment of advanced or recurrent malignancies poor in receptors tended to be better than that of receptor-rich carcinomas (Table IV).

Table IV. Receptor status and response of advanced or recurrent endometrial malignancies to combined cytotoxic chemotherapy after failure of progestin therapy.

Receptor-status of tumour	No. of patients	Number (percentage) of responders		Number (percentage) of nonresponders	
Rich	6	1	(17)	5	(83)
Poor	14	8	(57)	6	(43)
Total	20	9	(45)	11	(55)

Discussion

We have previously detected the simultaneous occurrence of cytosolic ER and PR in about 80% of endometrial carcinoma specimens [4, 13]. This percentage is higher than the percentages recorded by other investigators [14, 15], possibly as a result of differences in methodology and detection limits applied [16]. It is not only the presence but also the concentrations of female sex steroid hormone receptors which are clinically important, as in breast carcinoma [17, 18]. In this, as in an earlier study [12], we therefore set a limit of 30 fmol/mg protein for cytosolic ER and PR, for division of tumours into receptor-rich and receptor-poor types, and found that about two-thirds of early malignancies but only 17% of advanced malignancies were receptor-rich. A similar reduction in the incidence of receptor-rich malignancies also took place as histopathological differentiation of the tumour decreased, a phenomenon also reported elsewhere [19]. In addition, the concentrations of cytosolic ER and PR in invasive malignancies tended to be lower than those in superficial tumours. The data presented here, showing a significant correlation between cytosolic ER and PR concentrations and such clinically important indicators of risk as clinical stage, degree of histopathological differentiation, and myometrial invasion by the endometrial malignancy, clearly indicate the prognostic significance of cytosolic ER and PR concentrations. Because the concentrations of cytosolic ER and PR varied greatly within each subgroup studied (Tables I and II, Figs 1–3), the information obtainable from results of receptor determinations seems likely to be unique, and capable of complementing information given by other risk indicators.

There is also evidence of the direct clinical importance of cytosolic ER and PR in endometrial carcinoma. We observed that the prognosis in cases of receptor-poor malignancies tended to be worse than in cases of receptor-rich malignancies, regardless of whether the malignancies were at an early stage, or advanced. A similar tendency has been observed in other clinical studies [20]. Determinations of cytosolic ER and, more particularly, PR, have been shown to be important for selection of the most appropriate chemotherapy for patients with advanced or recurrent endometrial carcinoma, as discussed elsewhere [19, 21].

The data arising from the present study, and recorded in the literature, clearly indicate the value of cytosolic ER and PR determinations in endometrial carcinoma. Concentrations of cytosolic ER and PR appear to be predictive of the clinical behaviour of tumours and their sensitivity to various forms of chemotherapy. Determinations of ER and PR might, therefore, be of help in deciding the extent of primary surgical and/or radiological therapy, and, in cases of advanced or recurrent malignancies, in selecting the most appropriate chemotherapy.

References

1. Gusberg, S.B. (1980): Current concepts in cancer. The changing nature of endometrial cancer. *N. Engl. J. Med. 302*, 729.
2. Gambrell, R.D. (1979): The role of hormones in the etiology of breast and endometrial cancer. *Acta Obstet. Gynecol. Scand. 88*, 73.
3. Nisker, J.A., Hammond, G.L., Davidson, B.J. et al. (1980): Serum sex hormone-binding globulin capacity and the percentage of free estradiol in postmenopausal women with and without endometrial carcinoma. *Am. J. Obstet. Gynecol. 138*, 637.
4. Jänne, O., Kauppila, A., Kontula, K. et al. (1979): Female sex steroid receptors in normal, hyperplastic and carcinomatous endometrium. The relationship to serum steroid hormones and gonadotropins and changes during medroxyprogesterone acetate administration. *Int. J. Cancer 24*, 545.
5. Whitehead, M.I., Townsend, P.T., Pryse-Davies, J. et al. (1981): Effects of estrogens and progestins on the biochemistry and morphology of the postmenopausal endometrium. *N. Engl. J. Med. 305*, 1599.
6. Nordqvist, S.R.B. (1973): Endometrial cancer. Facts and theories. *Path. Annu. 8*, 283.
7. Wentz, W.B. (1964): Effect of progestational agent on endometrial hyperplasia and endometrial carcinoma. *Obstet. Gynecol. 24*, 370.
8. Briggs, M.H., Caldwell, A.D.S. and Pitchford, A.G. (1967): The treatment of cancer by progestogens. *Hospital Medicine* (October), 63.
9. Bonte, J., Decoster, J.M., Ide, P. and Billiet, G. (1978): Hormono-prophylaxis and hormonotherapy in the treatment of endometrial adenocarcinoma by means of medroxyprogesterone acetate. *Gynecol. Oncol. 6*, 60.
10. O'Connell, K.M., Joslin, C.A., Howard, N. et al. (1967): The treatment of uterine carcinoma using the Cathetron. *Br. J. Radiol. 40*, 882.
11. Kauppila, A. and Kiviniitty, K. (1980): High dose-rate intracavitary irradiation in the treatment of cervical and endometrial carcinomas: Preliminary observations. In: *High Dose-Rate Afterloading in the Treatment of Cancer of the Uterus*, pp.

59–64. Eds: T.D. Bates and R.J. Berry. (Br. J. Radiol. Special Report No. 17).

12. Kauppila, A., Jänne, O., Kujansuu, E. and Vihko, R. (1980): Treatment of advanced endometrial adenocarcinoma with a combined cytotoxic chemotherapy; predictive value of cytosol estrogen and progestin receptor levels. *Cancer 46*, 2162.
13. Kauppila, A., Kujansuu, E. and Vihko, R. (1982): Cytosol estrogen and progestin receptors in endometrial carcinoma of patients treated with surgery, radiotherapy and progestin. Clinical correlates. *Cancer* (In press.)
14. Ehrlich, C.E., Young, P.C.M. and Einhorn, L.H. (1978): Progesterone and estrogen receptors in cancer treatment. In: *Estrogens and Cancer*, pp. 179–192. Eds: S.G. Silverberg and F.J. Major. John Wiley & Sons, New York.
15. McCarty, Jr., K.S., Barton, T.K., Fetter, B.F. et al. (1979): Correlation of estrogen and progesterone receptors with histological differentiation in endometrial adenocarcinoma. *Am. J. Pathol. 96*, 171.
16. Vihko, R., Jänne, O. and Kauppila, A. (1980): Steroid receptors in normal, hyperplastic and malignant human endometria. *Ann. Clin. Res. 12*, 208.
17. Knight III, W.A., Osborne, C.K., Yochomowitz, M.G. and McGuire, W.L. (1980): Steroid receptors in the management of human breast cancer. *Ann. Clin. Res. 12*, 202.
18. Vihko, R., Jänne, O., Kontula, K. and Syrjälä, P. (1980): Female sex steroid receptor status in primary and metastatic breast carcinoma and its relationship to serum steroid and peptide hormone levels. *Int. J. Cancer 26*, 13.
19. Ehrlich, C.E., Young, P.C.M. and Cleary, R.E. (1981): Cytoplasmic progesterone and estradiol receptors in normal, hyperplastic and carcinomatous endometria: Therapeutic implications. *Am. J. Obstet. Gynecol. 141*, 539.
20. Creasman, W.T., McCarty, Sr., K.S., Barton, T.K. and McCarty, Jr., K.S. (1980): Clinical correlates of estrogen- and progesterone-binding proteins in human endometrial adenocarcinoma. *Obst. Gynecol. 55*, 363.
21. Kauppila, A. and Friberg, L.-G. (1981): Hormonal and cytotoxic chemotherapy for endometrial carcinoma. Steroid receptors in the selection of appropriate therapy. *Acta Obstet. Gynecol. Scand. Suppl. 101*, 59.

Discussion

P. Robel (Bicetre, France): I have been very interested in both presentations. With regard to the measurement of oestradiol and progesterone receptors, we all agree that most endometrial cancer cases contain oestradiol receptors. In our experience, we have had slightly less progesterone receptor-positive cases (about 3 or 4).

Secondly, we have observed that after giving an anti-oestrogen to the patients, several progesterone receptor-negative patients became progesterone receptor-positive. Therefore, progesterone receptor-negative patients can be made eligible for progestogen therapy by inducing the progesterone receptor with anti-oestrogens or oestrogens.

Thirdly, we have also observed that by giving an anti-oestrogen for some days, about two-thirds of the oestradiol receptor-positive patients respond with a large increase in progesterone receptors.

Is it possible, in the opinion of Dr Martin and Dr Kauppila, to have a better selection of patients who are able to respond to hormone therapy, by comparing biopsies taken from their tumour before and after a hormone challenge test?

P.M. Martin: During this afternoon's Round Table I shall give the answer about the hormone challenge test. The problem is that the so-called 'anti-oestrogen' therapy with tamoxifen is not an antihormonal therapy for the endometrium. At the moment we have 7 patients treated for breast carcinoma by anti-oestrogens who have developed endometrial carcinoma which is hormone-dependent and which has developed under anti-oestrogen therapy. I think that the challenge test, stimulation by tamoxifen for a short period, is a very important test for screening the patients. Probably, the determination of the progesterone receptor is the most important parameter for prognosis and therapy, and the stimulation by anti-oestrogen is also very important.

A.J.I. Kauppila: I agree with Dr Martin, but I would like to add that there are still many practical difficulties in performing such tests. After the first or second curettage there is not much carcinomatous tissue left in the uterine cavity. Therefore, in many cases, there will be considerable difficulty in performing this kind of test. Theoretically, and in suitable cases, it is of clinical value and complements the information obtained from poor single receptor determinations.

C. Mangioni (Milan, Italy): Firstly, all the cases presented by Dr Kauppila are treated in the stage-I disease with internal radiotherapy, bilateral salpingo-oöphorectomy, hysterectomy and external radiotherapy. The experience in the United States and in Europe (Italy, Finland, etc.) is that more than 80–90% of endometrial cancer limited to the uterine cavity is cured by simple hysterectomy, bilateral salpingo-oöphorectomy and excision of the vaginal collar. It seems to me that Dr Kauppila's series have been greatly overtreated.

Secondly, how is it possible to determine and correlate the receptor and the myometrial infiltration in a surgical specimen that has previously been treated with internal radiotherapy? Myometrial infiltration can be determined only in fresh specimens, not in those previously treated with radiotherapy.

Thirdly, it is impossible to be sure about the histological grade on the curettage specimen alone. Serial sections are required from fresh specimens to be able to determine the true histological grade in endometrial cancer. Many papers on the international experience prove that there is at least 20 or 30% difference in the histological grades when determined on the curettage specimen as compared with those determined on serial section of the fresh uterine specimens.

A.J.I. Kauppila: As an answer to the first question I would like to say that intracavitary pre-operative irradiation was given in every case, and hysterectomy with salpingo-oöphorectomy was performed. However, the target for postoperative radiotherapy was either only the vagina or the whole pelvis. The extended form of postoperative radiotherapy was used only in those cases in which one or more of the following risk factors existed: anaplasia of the tumour, deep myometrial infiltration, or occult cervical or lymph node involvement. I think, therefore, that our treatment was not too extensive. We have tried to standardize our treatments as much as possible, following the principles described.

With regard to the second and third questions about myometrial infiltration and histological grading, I would like to say that it is possible to determine the depth of tumour invasion after radiotherapy if the surgical intervention is made immediately after radiotherapy. Serial sections of the specimens have been taken, and our pathologists were able to determine the depth of the infiltration without any difficulty.

I agree that histological differentiation is often difficult to determine and is not so accurate when done on the endometrial curettage specimen, but this is one way of dividing up the patients into different risk groups – and no better method is available for us to use. I admit that there may be some weaknesses in this method.

A. Fuchs: Dr Kauppila did sucrose density gradient centrifugation. Was any influence observed from the appearance of 4S or 8S oestrogen receptor on the response rate to MPA treatment? According to Whitcliffe and others, it is suggested that the appearance of 4S alone would not predict a hormonal response.

A.J.I. Kauppila: We have not correlated the response to MPA therapy. Our treatment in the early stages of therapy included so many different kinds of therapy – radiotherapy for different tumours and surgical intervention – that it was not very easy to make reliable comparisons. In the literature, there is a lot of evidence showing that progesterone determination and progesterone status are very important in the prediction of the response to hormonal therapy, and that they are better predictors than histological differentiation.

A. Fuchs: Sucrose density gradients were done, and 4S and 8S may be observed. In breast cancer it is under discussion whether there may be a response to hormonal treatment, when only the 4S form of oestrogen receptor is observed in sucrose density gradients. I wonder whether Dr Kauppila observed differences in response, depending on whether there was only the 8S oestrogen receptor or only the 4S in the sucrose density gradient. Perhaps I misunderstood.

A.J.I. Kauppila: In our study group, I am responsible for the clinical part of the trial. I am sorry, but I can not speculate about the methodological aspects.

A controlled clinical study on stage-I endometrial carcinoma: methodological approach and preliminary results*

G. De Palo[1], M. Merson[1], P. Periti[2], C. Mangioni[3], M. Del Vecchio[1] and study participants

[1]National Cancer Institute, Milan; [2]Department of Pharmacology, University of Florence; and [3]Department of Obstetrics and Gynaecology, University of Milan, Italy

Introduction

Survival rates in patients with Fédération Internationale de Gynécologie et d'Obstétrique (FIGO) stage I endometrial carcinoma, the stage most frequently diagnosed, vary widely. They depend on the precise clinical or pathological state, type of treatment pursued, and a number of other factors.

Many such factors have been identified. The degree of histological differentiation and the occurrence of myometrial invasion or retroperitoneal lymph node metastases are of unquestionable significance in relation to prognosis. Positive peritoneal cytology, the histological type of carcinoma, and invasion of the intramural tract of the fallopian tube are probably significant. The significance of the only factor taken into consideration by FIGO, the length of the uterine cavity (stage IA and IB), is negligible [1–4].

Review of factors affecting survival rates

The degree of histological differentiation is one of the most reliable prog-

*This study is being organized by the Subproject Group 'Clinical Multimodality Therapy' of the applications-oriented project Group 'Control of Neoplastic Growth', and is supported by a grant from the National Research Council of Italy. Reproduced in part from the 'International Symposium on the Role of Medroxyprogesterone Acetate (MPA) in Endocrine-Related Tumors' by kind permission of the editors L. Campio, G. Robustelli Della Cuna and R.W. Taylor, and the publisher Raven Press, New York.

nostic factors. The survival rate decreases as the histopathological tumour grading increases [1–3, 5, 6].

The histopathological grade of the tumour correlates with the extent of myometrial invasion. As the tumour becomes less differentiated, the degree of myometrial invasion increases [7, 8].

The depth of myometrial invasion and the proximity of the invading tumour to the uterine tunica serosa is another factor affecting survival. As myometrial invasion increases [9] and the nearer the tumour approaches to the uterine tunica serosa [10], the lower the 5-year survival rate.

The presence of retroperitoneal lymph node metastases is the major factor affecting survival. The 5-year survival rate in patients with stage I disease and histologically or lymphographically positive findings in retroperitoneal lymph nodes is markedly inferior to that in patients without retroperitoneal involvement [11–13].

Nevertheless, in published reports of lymphographic and surgical studies, data on the incidence and sites of lymph node metastases, whether limited to the pelvic chains, contemporaneously involving the pelvic and aortic nodes, or limited to the para-aortic region are confusing. In addition, there is not much information on prognosis in patients with para-aortic node involvement [14].

The incidence of abnormal lymphograms in cases reported in the literature [12, 15, 16] ranges between 8 and 12.8% in stage I pathological endometrial carcinoma, and between 10.9 and 20% in clinically diagnosed stage I disease. The incidence of histologically positive lymph node metastases ranges from 5% [17, 18] to 23% [19], with a mean of 9.9% [20].

In the lymphographic series of the Italian National Cancer Institute and the Mangiagalli, First Department of Obstetrics and Gynaecology of the University of Milan [12], metastases occurred most often in the pelvic nodes alone, and next most often in the pelvic nodes and the para-aortic nodes (in 56.2% and 34.3% of cases, respectively). The percentage of cases with metastases limited to the para-aortic area was 9.5.

These results do not confirm that the ovarian pedicle which drains along the gonadal vessels to the para-aortic nodes is of primary importance as a route for spread of the disease. Lymphatic drainage through the anatomically secondary parametrial channels which drains into the external and common iliac nodes seems to be most important in this connection.

In a series of 140 patients, Creasman et al. [21] found that 10 out of 102 patients (9.8%) in whom the para-aortic chains were histopathologically examined had metastases. On analysis of data gathered by the Gynaecological Oncology Group (GOG), 23 out of 206 patients with FIGO stage I endometrial carcinoma had pelvic node metastases. Seventy-five per cent of 23 patients underwent para-aortic node biopsies, and 16 of these were found to have metastases in the para-aortic nodes [22]. It is not clear if the metastases were para-aortic only, or para-aortic and pelvic.

Positive peritoneal cytological findings as regards malignant cells occur in approximately 15% of patients with stage I carcinoma of the endometrium [22]. There are 2 routes of spread, via the fallopian tubes, which, in a large number of elderly patients, are not patent, or via the uterine wall. The prognostic significance of positive peritoneal cytological findings in cancer of the endometrium is not at present known. Theoretically, these patients are at risk of developing metastases in the peritoneal cavity.

There is no clear evidence in the literature concerning the prognostic value of the histological type of tumour or invasion of the intramural tract of the fallopian tube.

Clinical and pathological staging of carcinoma

The current classification of carcinoma of the uterine corpus used by FIGO is based on clinical findings. Nevertheless it is common practice to use the data found at operation for classification. The results of classification may be different as between patients undergoing surgery and those primarily treated with radiotherapy.

Intensive surgical-pathological staging of the disease is essential. Clinical classification understates pathological classification by about 15–20%.

Treatment of endometrial carcinoma

Total abdominal hysterectomy with bilateral salpingo-oophorectomy and excision of the superior third of the vagina is the surgical treatment of choice, with simultaneous pelvic and para-aortic node biopsy.

With adequate attention to irradiation of the vaginal vault, using intracavitary radium techniques, or external high voltage therapy, the incidence of vaginal persistence after surgery can be diminished significantly as compared to that after surgery alone [23]. The incidence of vaginal recurrences after hysterectomy for carcinoma of the corpus uteri of FIGO stage I was between 9% [24] and 20% [25], whereas recurrences essentially did not occur if partial colpectomy, with or without irradiation of the vaginal vault, was performed [4, 26]. The incidence of pelvic recurrences (central and/or nodal) was significantly diminished by external high voltage radiotherapy of the pelvis after surgery [23].

The effectiveness of progestogens as adjuvant hormonal therapy is still unknown. A controlled clinical trial in 574 cases treated with medroxy-progesterone acetate (MPA) intramuscularly (i.m.) or placebo for 14 weeks did not suggest that MPA contributed significantly to survival [27]. In contrast, a pilot study conducted by the Italian National Cancer Institute in Milan (unpublished) seems to suggest that prolonged adjuvant hormone treatment (200 mg of gestonorone caproate a week, i.m., for one year) may extend survival time and the percentage of tumour-free survivors, in stage I endometrial carcinoma with deep myometrial invasion. For various reasons, neither study allows firm conclusions to be drawn.

Aims and design of controlled study on stage I endometrial carcinoma

In the light of the facts outlined above, in 1980 the Subproject Group 'Clinical Multimodality Therapy', of the Project Group 'Control of Neoplastic Growth' of the National Research Council of Italy, undertook a controlled study on endometrial carcinoma stage I.

The study has 3 aims:

1. To undertake complete presurgical and surgical staging in patients with FIGO stage I endometrial carcinoma, and to establish the rate of conversion from clinical to pathological stage.
2. To establish a treatment plan (surgery alone, surgery plus external high voltage therapy) on the basis of the degree of pathological extent of the disease.
3. To establish the effectiveness of adjuvant hormone therapy.

All patients in participating institutions with FIGO stage I endometrial carcinoma (diagnosed after dilatation and curettage (D & C)) are being enrolled.

Presurgical examinations consist of chest X-ray, intravenous urography, lymphography, X-ray of pelvic bones, and rectosigmoidoscopy and/or double contrast enema with, in some cases a liver scan.

Surgical examinations consist of peritoneal cytology (fluid of peritoneal cavity and peritoneal washing), performed as the first step during laparotomy, inspection of omentum and abdominal viscera, with biopsy of suspected lesions, and selective lymphadenectomy on pelvic and para-aortic nodes, in cases of pathological lymphographic findings, or enlarged lymph nodes found during surgery.

Surgical treatment consists of total abdominal hysterectomy with bilateral salpingo-oophorectomy and excision of the superior third of the vagina.

On the basis of histopathological grading, degree of myometrial invasion and histologically positive findings in pelvic or para-aortic nodes, patients are divided into 3 groups with different levels of risk. Other factors, namely, histological type of tumour and peritoneal cytology will subsequently be evaluated as regards their possible prognostic significance.

The histopathological grading is carried out on the basis of the classification which subdivides carcinomas into 3 types:
Grade I (GI), high degree of differentiation.
Grade II (GII), moderate degree of differentiation.
Grade III (GIII), low degree of differentiation, or no differentiation.

The maximum depth of tumour infiltration in the myometrium is used as a criterion to divide cases into 4 other groups:
M0, neoplasm confined to endometrium, no myometrial invasion.
M1, tumour involving as much as one-third of myometrium.
M2, tumour involving as much as two-thirds of myometrium.
M3, tumour involving the whole thickness of the myometrium, and reaching the tunica serosa.

All definitive histological specimens and peritoneal cytological slides are to be reviewed by the consultant pathologists and all lymphangiograms by the consultant radiologists.

The risk groups formed within the study are:
R1, GI-GII-M1 categories.
R2, GI-GII-M2-M3 or GIII-M1-M2-M3 categories.
R3, any G and M category with lymph node involvement.

The following groups of patients are not admitted to the study:
Age over 75 years. (In the course of the study the admission of patients was limited to the age of ≤ 75 years.)
Geographic inaccessibility.
Previous treatment.
Previous or synchronous neoplastic disease, with the exception of cutaneous epithelioma.
Patients who refuse full diagnostic procedure or postsurgical treatment.
Patients with mixed mesodermal tumour.
Patients with severe diseases, such as cardiovascular disorders, or neuropsychiatric difficulties.
Patients not recommended for surgery because of high operative risk, or who refuse surgical treatment.
Patients recommended for vaginal hysterectomy because of high operative risk.

The following categories of patients are also not eligible for inclusion in this comparative study:
RO, patients without myometrial invasion, any G.
RE, patients who subsequently are found to have pathological stage II disease

(occult involvement of cervix), stage III disease (involvement of ovaries, patent tract of fallopian tubes, pelvic peritoneum, parametrium), or stage IV disease (extension beyond the true pelvis).

The patients in the risk categories (R1, R2, R3) eligible for inclusion in the therapeutic study are divided at random into 2 groups, one of which receives adjuvant hormone treatment with MPA, 100 mg twice a day, per os, for 12 months, the other of which does not. The treatment schedule is as follows:
R1 patients, surgery alone versus surgery plus MPA.
R2 patients, surgery plus radiotherapy of the pelvis (50 Gray (Gy) in 5–7 weeks) versus the same plus MPA.
R3 patients, surgery plus radiotherapy of the pelvis, as in R2 patients, and on para-aortic chains (45 Gy in 5–7 weeks plus boost of 10 Gy on involved lymph nodes) versus the same plus MPA.

The patients are followed up (clinical and pelvic examination) every 2 months during the first year, every 3 months during the second year, every 4 months during the third year, every 6 months in the fourth year and at the end of the fifth year. Chest X-ray, X-ray of the pelvic bone, vaginal smear and blood chemistry investigations are to be performed every 6 months during the first year, and thereafter every 12 months. Intravenous urography is to be performed one month after surgery and, together with a double contrast enema, 6 months after radiotherapy.

Patients enrolled

The study began in February 1980. Twenty-one institutions are involved. From February 1st 1980 to May 31st 1981, a total of 530 patients have been enrolled. One hundred and sixteen were regarded as ineligible and 414 as eligible by the investigators concerned. Eighteen were subsequently excluded because of protocol violations. Three hundred and ninety six patients were, therefore, eligible for inclusion in the study. Of these, 270 (R1, 144; R2, 120; R3, 6) were allocated at random whether or not to receive adjuvant hormone treatment with MPA (Table I). The balance of 126 patients were excluded because there was no myometrial involvement, or because the disease turned out to be stage II, III or IV.

Findings in patients eligible for inclusion

Ages of patients, types of tumour and histopathological grade

The majority of the patients were aged between 51 and 70 years (Table II). Of

Table I. Patients enrolled.

Number of cases enrolled in study				530
Cases ineligible for inclusion in study				116
Reasons for ineligibility (numbers of cases)				
Age > 75 years				17
Refused diagnostic procedures				1
Previous neoplastic disease				11
Synchronous neoplastic disease				8
Previous treatment				1
Mixed mesodermal tumour				5
Died before surgery				1
No surgery because of high operative risk				10
Vaginal hysterectomy because of high operative risk				16
Geographic inaccessibility				5
Severe disease				4
Died after surgery				2
Radiotherapy not feasible				3
Incomplete radiological procedure				5
Incomplete surgical staging and/or radiological procedure				4
Other reasons				2
Multiple reasons				21
Cases considered eligible				414
Protocol violations				18
Cases with no myometrial invasion, or stage II, III or IV disease				126
Patients enrolled in controlled study				270
R1:	144	MPA	69	
		No MPA	75	
R2:	120	MPA	61	
		No MPA	59	
R3:	6	MPA	2	
		No MPA	4	

the 270 cases assigned to the different treatment groups, the majority (81.1%) had an adenocarcinoma and a minority (0.7%) a clear cell carcinoma. Adenoacanthoma accounted for 9.3% of cases, adenosquamous tumours for 6.7% of cases, and undifferentiated carcinoma for 1.5%; information is still lacking in 2 cases. Following surgery, there was a change in histological diagnosis, as compared with that following D & C, in 33 patients. The

Table II. Age distribution of patients.

Age (years)	Numbers of patients
≤ 40	4
41–50	15
51–60	118
61–70	102
71–75	25
> 75*	6
Totals	270

* In the course of the study the admission of patients was limited to the age of ≤ 75 years.

histopathological grade of the tumour was I in 55.9% of cases, II in 31.9% of cases, and III in 11.1%; information is still lacking in 3 cases.

Lymphography and lymph node biopsies

For the diagnosis of metastatic involvement the criteria described by Douglas et al. [28], Wallace et al. [29], and Musumeci et al. [30] are being used. At the time of writing, the lymphangiograms have yet to be re-interpreted by the consultant radiologists.

Of the 270 cases allocated to treatment groups, lymphography gave negative results in 206 patients, and positive results in 9 (external iliac 5, para-aortic and external iliac 3, external and internal iliac 1). Bilaterality was found in 3 case (para-aortic plus external iliac). In 55 patients the lymphangiographic findings were equivocal.

Retroperitoneal node biopsies were performed in a total of 133 out of the 270 cases allocated to treatment groups. Histological findings in retroperitoneal nodes were negative in 127 patients and positive in 6 (para-aortic 1, common iliac 1, external iliac 2, internal iliac 1, common and external iliac 1 (no bilaterality)).

Correlation of histological and radiological findings has, up to now, indicated that there are high percentages of false positive or false negative results of lymphography.

Peritoneal cytology

Once the peritoneal cavity has been opened, an assessment of the amount of free fluid in the Douglas cul-de-sac and the paracolic gutter is made. The free fluid is withdrawn and sent for cytological examination. Thereafter, 300 ml of normal saline is injected into the Douglas cul-de-sac, pelvis, and right and left paracolic gutters, using an aseptic syringe. The saline solution, withdrawn via the syringe, is sent within 30 minutes for cytological examination by the Pathology Departments. The cellular material of the fluid samples is examined after centrifugation at 1,500 revolutions per minute for 20 minutes, and spreading of the sample on glass slides. The preparations are fixed in 95% methanol and stained using the Papanicolaou method. The findings are classified as negative (normal mesothelial cells, histiocytes and blood elements), inadequate (no cell present), or positive (presence of cancer cells or cells suggestive of malignancy).

Out of a total of 396 patients, peritoneal cytology has been performed in 361 cases. Positive peritoneal cytology was found in 6.6% of the patients (Table III). At the time of writing, the slides have yet to be re-interpreted by the consultant pathologists.

Table III. Peritoneal cytology; numbers of cases (% of cases).

Negative	302 (83.7)
Positive	24 (6.6)
No cells present	35 (9.7)
Not performed	35 (9.7)
Total	396

Pathological stage

Out of 396 patients who were recommended for total abdominal hysterectomy, bilateral salpingo-oophorectomy, excision of the superior third of the vagina, and selective or systematic pelvic and/or para-aortic node biopsies, 329 patients were found to have stage I disease (83%). Forty-five patients (11.4%) were classified as having stage II disease, 43 with endocervical and 2 with exocervical involvement (Table IV). Twenty-one patients (5.3%) were classified as having stage III disease (Table V). In this group, there were 6 cases who had been placed in the R3 group (primary tumour limited to the uterus, with regional lymph node involvement). One patient (0.2%) was categorized as stage IV on the basis of omental involvement. Sixty-seven out of 396 patients (16.9%) had other than stage I disease, therefore, on the basis of surgical findings.

Table IV. Stage II disease discovered on surgery.

Endocervical involvement	Superficial extension over:		Totals
	<50% of cervix length	>50% of cervix length	
Invasion of mucosa only	21	–	21
Invasion of muscularis	16	6	22
Totals	37	6	43
Exocervix			2
Total number of stage II cases			45

Table V. Stage III disease discovered on surgery.

Extension of tumour to:	Numbers of cases
Ovary and/or fallopian tube (free tract)	8
Parametrium	3
Pelvic peritoneum	2
Ovary and retroperitoneal nodes	1
Retroperitoneal nodes and cervix	1
Retroperitoneal nodes alone	6*
Total	21

* All allocated to R3 group.

Adjuvant hormone therapy

A pilot pharmacokinetic study showed that plasma MPA, as determined by radioimmunoassay following a single dose of 100 mg, reached a mean peak concentration of 12.4 ng/ml after 2 hours, and declined with a half life of 8.6 hours, reaching a concentration of 5.17 ng/ml after 12 hours. The mean peak value increased in the first 6 months of treatment from 10 to 20 ng/ml. This level was then maintained until treatment came to an end. Oral MPA at a dose of 100 mg every 12 hours can, therefore, assure plasma concentrations of between 10^{-8} and 10^{-7} M in all patients [31].

Of 132 patients assigned to receive treatment with MPA, 33 have at present completed the planned 12 months of treatment without interruption, and 8 have started treatment but have had to interrupt it (range of duration of interruptions 5–95 days). Seven patients did not complete treatment, 3 because of toxicity, 3 because of refusal of treatment, and one because of complications. Among the total number of patients evaluable (48), toxicity was evident in 4 (8.3%) (Table VI).

Future plans

Apart from the comparative study, it should be possible to carry out a prospective study of the natural history of the disease and its spread, in a large number of cases not eligible for inclusion in the comparative study. Patients will be enrolled in the comparative study up to December 1983.

Study participants

C. Belloni, 1st Department of Obstetrics and Gynaecology, University of Milan; S. Bettocchi, 1st Department of Obstetrics and Gynaecology, University of Bari; U. Bianchi, 3rd Department of Obstetrics and Gynaecology, University of Milan; G. Cagnazzo, 2nd Department of Obstetrics and

Table VI. Treatment with MPA.

One year of treatment completed without interruption		33
One year of treatment completed with interruptions		8
One year of treatment not completed		7
Reasons for lack of completion of treatment:		
Refusal of therapy		3
		(after 9, 6 and 2 months)
Toxicity within 30 days of start of treatment:		2
Asthenia	1	
Allergy	1	
Toxicity after 30 days of start of treatment:		2
Tachycardia (?)		
(after 9 months)	1	
Overweight		
(after 6 months*)	1	
Complications		1
Hemiparesis		
(after 3 months)		

* Treatment not interrupted.

Gynaecology, University of Bari; L. Carenza, 2nd Department of Obstetrics and Gynaecology, University of Rome; V. Danesino, Department of Obstetrics and Gynaecology, University of Pavia; S. Dell'Acqua, Department of Obstetrics and Gynaecology, Sacro Cuore University, Rome; S. Di Leo, Department of Obstetrics and Gynaecology, University of Catania; P. Fioretti, Department of Obstetrics and Gynaecology, University of Pisa; F. Gasparri, Department of Obstetrics and Gynaecology, University of Florence; P. Marziale, Department of Gynaecological Oncology, Cancer Institute, Rome; G. Mollica, Department of Obstetrics and Gynaecology, University of Ferrara; R. Monti, 2nd Department of Obstetrics and Gynaecology, University of Turin; A. Onnis, Department of Obstetrics and Gynaecology, University of Padua; C. Orlandi, 2nd Department of Obstetrics and Gynaecology, University of Bologna; G. Pescetto, Department of Obstetrics and Gynaecology, University of Genoa; G. Sani, 1st Department of Obstetrics and Gynaecology, University of Bologna; E. Saraceno, 4th Department of Obstetrics and Gynaecology, University of Milan; P. Sismondi, 1st Department of Obstetrics and Gynaecology, University of Turin; M. Vignali, 5th Department of Obstetrics and Gynaecology, University of Milan.

References

1. Malkasian Jr., G.D. (1978): Carcinoma of the endometrium: effect of stage and grade on survival. *Cancer 41*, 996.
2. Berman, M.L. and Ballon, S.C. (1979): Treatment of endometrial cancer. *Cancer Treat. Rev. 6*, 165.
3. Aalders, J., Abeler, B., Kolstad, P. and Onsrud, M. (1980): Postoperative external irradiation and prognostic parameters in stage I endometrial carcinoma. Clinical and histopathologic study of 540 patients. *Obstet. Gynecol. 56*, 419.
4. De Palo, G., Kenda, R., Andreola, S. et al. (1982): Endometrial carcinoma: pathologic Stage I. A retrospective analysis of 262 patients. *Obstet. Gynecol.* (In press.)
5. Salazar, O.M., Feldstein, M.L., Depapp, E.W. et al. (1978): The management of clinical stage I endometrial carcinoma. *Cancer 41*, 1016.
6. Malkasian Jr., G.D., Annegers, J.F. and Fountain, K.S. (1980): Carcinoma of the endometrium: stage I. *Am. J. Obstet. Gynecol. 136*, 872.
7. Cheon, H.K. (1969): Prognosis of endometrial carcinoma. *Obstet. Gynecol. 34*, 680.
8. Ng, A.B. and Reagan, J.W. (1970): Incidence and prognosis of endometrial carcinoma by histologic grade and extent. *Obstet. Gynecol. 35*, 437.
9. Jones III, H.W. (1975): Treatment of adenocarcinoma of the endometrium. *Obstet. Gynecol. Surv. 30*, 147.
10. Lutz, M.H., Underwood Jr., P.B., Kreutner Jr., A. and Miller, M. (1978): Endometrial carcinoma: a new method of classification of therapeutic and prognostic significance. *Gynecol. Oncol. 6*, 83.

11. Morrow, C.P., Di Saia, P.J. and Townsend, D.E. (1973): Current management of endometrial carcinoma. *Obstet. Gynecol. 42*, 399.
12. Musumeci, R., De Palo, G., Conti, U. et al. (1980): Are retroperitoneal lymph node metastases a major problem in endometrial adenocarcinoma? Diagnostic and prognostic assessment with lymphography. *Cancer 46*, 1887.
13. Musumeci, R., Kenda, R., Volterrani, F. et al. (1979): Diagnostic and prognostic value of lymphography in patients with cancer of the endometrium. *Tumori 65*, 77.
14. Leibel, S.A. and Wharam, M.D. (1980): Vaginal and paraaortic lymph node metastases in carcinoma of the endometrium. *Int. J. Radiat. Oncol. Biol. Phys. 6*, 893.
15. Gerteis, W. (1967): The frequency of metastases in carcinoma of the cervix and corpus. In: *Progress in Lymphology*, pp. 209–212. Ed: A. Ruttiman. George Thieme Verlag, Stuttgart.
16. Kademian, M.T., Buchler, T.A. and Wirtanen, G.W. (1977): Bipedal lymphangiography in malignancies of the uterine corpus: *Am. J. Roentgenol. 129*, 903.
17. Rickford, R.B.K. (1968): Involvement of pelvic lymph nodes in carcinoma of the endometrium. *J. Obstet. Gynaecol. Br. Commonw. 75*, 580.
18. Lees, D.H. (1969): An evaluation of the treatment of carcinoma of the body of the uterus. *J. Obstet. Gynaecol. Br. Commonw. 76*, 615.
19. Roberts, D.W.T. (1961): Carcinoma of the body of the uterus at Chelsea Hospital for women, 1943–1953. *J. Obstet. Gynaecol. Br. Commonw. 68*, 132.
20. De Palo, G., Mangioni, C., Periti, P. et al. (1981): A controlled clinical trial on Stage I endometrial carcinoma: rationale and methodological approach. Paper read at: Second International Symposium on Role of Medroxyprogesterone Acetate (MPA) in Endocrine-related Tumors, Rome, 1981.
21. Creasman, W.T., Boronow, R.C., Morrow, C.P. et al. (1976): Adenocarcinoma of the endometrium; its metastatic lymph node potential. A preliminary report. *Gynecol. Oncol. 4*, 239.
22. Di Saia, P.J. and Creasman, W.T. (1981): *Clinical Gynecologic Oncology,* pp. 128–152. C.V. Mosby Co., St. Louis-Toronto-London.
23. Brady, L.W. (1975): Combined modality therapy of gynecologic cancer. *Cancer 35*, 76.
24. Salazar, O.M., Feldstein, M.L., Depapp, E.W. et al. (1977): Endometrial carcinoma: analysis of failures with special emphasis on the use of initial preoperative external pelvic irradiation. *Int. J. Radiat. Oncol. Biol. Phys. 2*, 1101.
25. Rutledge, F.H., Tan, S.K. and Fletchier, G.H. (1958): Vaginal metastases from adenocarcinoma of the corpus uteri. *Am. J. Obstet. Gynecol. 75*, 167.
26. Graham, J. (1971): The value of preoperative or postoperative treatment by radium for carcinoma of the uterine body. *Surg. Gynecol. Obstet. 132*, 855.
27. Lewis Jr., G.C., Slack, N.H., Mortel, R. and Bross, I.D.J. (1974): Adjuvant progestogen therapy in the primary definitive treatment of endometrial cancer. *Gynecol. Oncol. 2*, 368.
28. Douglas, G., Macdonald, J.S. and Baker, J.W. (1972): Lymphography in carcinoma of the uterus. *Clin. Radiol. 23*, 286.
29. Wallace, S., Jing, B.S. and Medellin, H. (1974): Endometrial carcinoma: radiologic assistance in diagnosis, staging and management. *Gynecol. Oncol. 2*, 287.

30. Musumeci, R., Banfi, A., Bolis, G. et al. (1977): Lymphangiography in patients with ovarian epithelial cancer. An evaluation of 289 consecutive cases. *Cancer 40*, 1444.
31. Periti, P., Mazzei, T., Ciuffi, M. and Savino, L. (1982): Pharmacokinetics of oral medroxyprogesterone acetate at moderate doses. Personal communication.

A preliminary report of a controlled study of the effectiveness of medroxyprogesterone acetate therapy in endometrial carcinoma

F. Calero Cuerda[1], E. Alonso Briz[2], E. Asins Codoñer[3], R. Diaz Castellanos[4], J.M. Garzón Sánchez[5], P. Gonzáles Gancedo[6], A. Herruzo Nalda[7], F.J. Rodriguez-Escudero[8], J.M. Rubio Martinez[9], F. Ugalde Bonilla[10] and A. Varela Nuñez[11]

[1]Maternidad, Ciudad Sanitaria La Paz, Madrid; [2]Servicio de Obstetricia y Ginecología, Residencia Sanitaria General Yagüe, Burgos; [3]Maternidad, Ciudad Sanitaria La Fe, Valencia; [4]Maternidad, Ciudad Sanitaria Reina Sofía, Córdoba; [5]Servicio de Obstetricia y Ginecología, Residencia Sanitaria Manuel Lois García, Huelva; [6]Laboratorio de Hormonas, Ciudad Sanitaria La Paz, Madrid; [7]Maternidad, Ciudad Sanitaria Virgen de Las Nieves, Granada; [8]Maternidad, Ciudad Sanitaria Enrique Sotomayor, Bilbao; [9]Servicio de Obstetricia y Ginecología, Centro Especial Ramón y Cajal, Madrid; [10]Servicio de Obstetricia y Ginecología, Residencia Sanitaria Virgen de Aránzazu, San Sebastián; and [11]Maternidad, Ciudad Sanitaria Juan Canalejo, La Coruña, Spain

Introduction

The incidence of endometrial cancer is increasing and has now reached a point where it almost equals that of cervical cancer [1].

Numerous factors favour the hormone dependency of endometrial cancer, both directly and indirectly [2], but it is not clear if all endometrial adenocarcinomas are hormone-dependent [3, 4], nor is their exact nature known.

The prognosis in this type of cancer is usually good if diagnosis is made in the early stages. However, once the myometrium or the endocervix is invaded, endometrial cancer behaves very aggressively [5].

The most appropriate treatment is still far from established: on reading the literature it is evident that there are numerous types of treatment in existence which depend upon the use of available methods such as surgery, radiation therapy, hormone therapy and chemotherapy on their own or in combination.

The beneficial action of progestins in advanced metastatic disease has been adequately demonstrated [6]. There are publications which describe the use of progestins as adjuvant therapy, and the improved results obtained with such therapy. Bonte et al. have achieved a 100% survival rate over a 5-year period in stage I disease using adjuvant progestin therapy [7].

The administration of medroxyprogesterone acetate (MPA) before surgery and radiotherapy is advantageous. The benefits of progestins for facilitating surgery and increasing the biological activity of ionizing radiation have been demonstrated [8].

This preliminary publication records the results of a prospective, randomized, multicentre clinical study in which results in a control group were compared with those in a group treated with MPA.

Patients and methods

The patients taking part in the study were drawn from the Gynaecological and Obstetrics Departments of 10 Spanish hospitals, namely, La Fe Hospital, Valencia, the Juan Canalejo Hospital, La Coruña, La Paz Hospital, Madrid, the Enrique Sotomayor Hospital, Bilbao, the Ramón y Cajal Centre, Madrid, the Reina Sofia Hospital, Córdoba, the Manuel Lois Hospital, Huelva, the General Yagüe Hospital, Burgos, the Virgen de Aránzazu Hospital, San Sebastián, and the Virgen de las Nieves Hospital, Granada. These hospitals make up the Spanish Group for the Study of Oncological Treatment.

Selection of patients

All the patients had an endometrial adenocarcinoma, diagnosed via fractional curettage of the uterus. All were 70 years of age or less. None had received previous treatment for their illness. Histological demonstration of other types of adenocarcinoma excluded participation from this study.

Experimental design

The stage of evolution of the disease was established in accordance with the International Federation of Gynaecology and Obstetrics (FIGO) classification by means of palpation, inspection, colposcopy, fractional endometrial and endocervical curettage, hysteroscopy, cystoscopy, proctoscopy, intravenous urography, and X-ray examinations of the lungs and skeleton. The general state of the patient, the degree of her obesity, the results of cardiopulmonary examination, and the results of clinical chemical investigations formed the basis of assessment of the risks of surgery.

The patients were distributed between 3 groups, each forming a therapeutic category. These 3 categories were:

1. Patients with stage I disease, surgically treated.
2. Patients with stage II disease, surgically treated.
3. Patients with stages III or IV disease, and those with stage I or II disease in whom surgical risk factors precluded operation.

After being allocated to one or other category, patients were allocated at random to the control group or to the group to be treated with MPA. The randomization procedure was carried out in each hospital using a list of random numbers. The patients in the first category were further subdivided according to histological findings in the uterus, on hysterectomy. In patients of one subdivision, the myometrium had been invaded. In patients in the other subdivision the disease was limited to the endometrium.

Hormones (oestradiol, LH and FSH) were determined in plasma by radioimmunoassay, and histological investigations and determinations of oestrogen receptors in cytosols using dextran-coated-charcoal assays were carried out before operation or radiotherapy, and after 4 weeks of MPA administration.

Therapy

The patients in the MPA group received 1 g of MPA per week, as 2 intramuscular injections of 500 mg. Four weeks later, the other treatment involved (see below) was initiated, and the administration of MPA maintained for one year. The treatment given to patients in the 3 categories was as follows:

Stage I The normal treatment for stage I adenocarcinoma was surgical. The technique followed consisted of total hysterectomy with double adnexectomy and extirpation of the vaginal cupula. If the myometrium was invaded, one of 2 types of radiotherapy was administered, either external pelvic cobalt therapy, (dose 5,000 rads) or external pelvic cobalt therapy with, in addition, insertion of radium into the vagina. Use of this second procedure depended upon the availability of radium in each hospital. Radium therapy was used after surgery in the present study, because of the requirement for a second sample of tumorous tissue for histological study and assay of oestrogen receptors.

Stage II With stage II patients, abdominal surgery was practised, consisting of extended total hysterectomy and pelvic lymphadenectomy. This was followed by external pelvic cobalt therapy using a dose of 5,000 rads. Radium was inserted into the vagina in those hospitals in which facilities were available.

Stage III or IV disease, or stage I or II disease with high surgical risk factors This heterogenous group was treated by means of intracavitary administration of radium at a dose of 6,000 rads, and external pelvic therapy using a dose of 5,000 rads. Patients with ovarian metastases are not treated in this way, but undergo operation. Results relating to these patients will be reported separately.

Patient numbers and distribution

The first patient was enrolled in this study on 23rd March, 1979. From then up to 26th October 1981, a total of 162 patients was enrolled. Sixty-five patients formed the control group, and 97 the group treated with MPA. A total of 40 patients was considered ineligible for analysis. Twelve of these were in the control group, 28 in the treated group. The reasons for exclusion from analyses are shown in Table I. A total of 122 patients thus remained for evaluation, 53 in the control group and 69 in the group treated with MPA.

Table I. Patients excluded from analysis.

	Control group	MPA-treated group	Totals
Numbers of patients	65	97	162
Excluded from analysis (%)	18.4	28.8	24.6
Reasons for exclusion from analysis:			
treatment not as assigned (%)	9.2	13.4	11.7
no presurgical MPA (%)	–	9.2	5.5
disease too advanced (%)	1.5	–	0.6
histological considerations (adenosquamous, clear cells, papillary) (%)	4.6	5.1	4.9
Too recently enrolled for follow-up (patients)	2	1	3
Numbers of patients included in analysis	53	69	122

The distribution of patients according to categories and sub-categories was as follows:
Stage I, myometrium not invaded, 9 patients in control group, 11 in treated group.
Stage I, myometrium invaded, patients treated both surgically and with cobalt therapy, 14 patients in control group, 19 in the treated group.
Stage I, myometrium invaded, patients treated by surgery, cobalt therapy and radium therapy, 9 patients in control group, 14 in treated group.
Stage II, 9 patients in control group, 10 in treated group.
Stage III or IV, or stage I or stage II with high degree of surgical risk, 12 patients in control group, 15 in treated group.

Patient characteristics

Patients in the control group and in the group treated with MPA had, in general, similar characteristics (Table II). The average age of the patients was 56.2 years in the control group and 57.7 years in the treated group.

Table II. Characteristics of the patients.

	Control group	MPA-treated group
Numbers of patients	53	69
Average age (years)	56.2	57.7
Associated pathology (% of cases):	37.7	47.8
hypertension	15.0	28.9
diabetes mellitus	5.6	10.1
obesity	15.0	18.8
other illnesses	5.6	4.3
High surgical risk factor (% of cases)	9.4	11.5
Premenopausal (% of cases)	13.2	14.4
Postmenopausal (% of cases)	86.8	85.6

Table III. Distribution of patients according to FIGO classification.

FIGO stage of disease	Control group	MPA-treated group	Totals
I	38	45	83
II	9	16	25
III	6	6	12
IV	–	2	2

Premenopausal patients in both groups were a minority, similar in numbers in each group. Associated pathology, frequently found in this form of tumour, occurred slightly more often in the treated group. Five patients in the control group and 8 patients in the treated group were considered to have high surgical risk factors. In the control group, the patients concerned all had stage I disease. In the treated group, there were 2 patients with stage I disease and 6 with stage II disease.

On the basis of the initial examination, patients were categorized according to the clinical stages of their disease as shown in Table III. The distribution of the different disease stages between groups was largely similar.

Histological and other findings

The length of the uterine cavity was measured during curettage. It was found to be 8 cm or less in 39 patients, and more than 8 cm in 44 patients. The distribution of lengths of uterine cavity was similar in both groups (Table IV).

The grade of histological differentiation of stage I disease was ascertained, as recommended in FIGO guidelines. The findings are also shown in Table IV. The most common finding (67 patients) was of a highly differentiated adenocarcinoma, followed by moderately differentiated adenocarcinoma (11 patients), and, finally, by poorly differentiated adenocarcinoma (5 patients). The differences between groups were not significant. Among the other patients, there were 28 highly differentiated adenocarcinomas, and 11 moderately differentiated tumours.

Table IV. Histological and other findings.

	Control group	MPA-treated group
Numbers of stage I cases	38	45
Uterine length		
≤8 cm (% of cases)	50.0	44.4
>8 cm (% of cases)	50.0	55.6
Degree of tumour differentiation		
Grade 1 (% of cases)	71.0	88.9
Grade 2 (% of cases)	21.0	6.7
Grade 3 (% of cases)	8.0	4.4
Myometrium invaded (% of cases)	74.2	75.0
Numbers of stage II, III and IV cases	15	24
Grade 1 (% of cases)	73.3	70.8
Grade 2 (% of cases)	26.7	29.2
Ovarian metastases (% of cases)	9.4	1.4

Histological study of the uterus in the 76 stage I patients operated on showed invasion of the myometrium in 56 cases. The number of cases of invasion was higher for the treated group, but the difference was not significant.

Ovarian metastases were found in 6 patients, 5 in the control group and 1 in the treated group.

Objectives of trial

The basic objectives of the trial were to obtain answers to the following questions:
How many adenocarcinomas are hormone-dependent?
What is the action of MPA upon:
a. hormones
b. cells and
c. molecules?
Is MPA beneficial to patients with endometrial adenocarcinoma?

Follow-up

The follow-up procedure for control-group patients was slightly different from that for patients in the treated group.

The first follow-up in control group patients took place 3 months after initiation of treatment.

The patients in the MPA-treated group underwent their first follow-up 2 weeks after the start of MPA administration. The check consisted of an evaluation of side-effects and a repetition of hormone analysis. In a second follow-up at 4 weeks, the side-effects were again evaluated. Hormone analysis and surgery were carried out when indicated. A sample was also taken at this time for quantification of oestrogen-receptors. During histological study of the uterus, the changes produced by the administration of the hormone were examined.

Subsequent checks were carried out with the same frequency in both groups, namely, every 3 months in the first year and every 6 months during the following 4 years.

At each check-up, in addition to a general examination, the Karnofsky index was evaluated, genital exploration was carried out, vaginal cytology was examined and blood and urine analyses undertaken. An X-ray was taken of the lungs and skeleton every 6 months. In patients of the MPA-treated group there was, in addition, an evaluation of side-effects and a hormone analysis every 3 months during the year of treatment.

Up to the present, the average follow-up period has been 15.5 months (range 3–32 months). The control group had an average follow-up period of 13.3 months, and the MPA-treated group a period of 17.1 months.

Statistical methods

The statistical methods used were Student's *t*-test, the chi-squared test, and the Wilcoxon test modified by Gehan [9].

Results

Tumours with oestrogen receptors

The measurement of oestrogen receptors was carried out in the Hormone Laboratory at the La Paz Hospital. Samples were taken from 33 patients. Measurement was possible in 28 patients. In 23 of these patients (82.1%) oestrogen receptors were detected, in an average amount of 65.66 femtomol (=mol $\times$ 10^{-15})(fmol)/mg of protein (range 13.7 to 190 fmol/mg protein). These 23 patients were considered to have a hormone-dependent endometrial adenocarcinoma. In 5 patients (17.9%) findings were considered negative, since in 3 patients oestrogen receptors were not detected, and in 2 the amount detected was less than 10 fmol/mg of protein. In 5 patients the sample obtained was not adequate for measurement of receptors.

Among the 18 patients in whom oestrogen receptors were found, and who were treated with MPA, oestrogen receptor measurement has been repeated in 5. The average amount found was 26.82 fmol/mg of protein (range 12 to 50 fmol/mg of protein).

Hormone analysis

Oestradiol was determined in 10 patients, and LH and FSH in 12 patients. The analyses were carried out before and after the first 4 weeks of MPA administration, but only in patients in whom oestrogen receptors had been found. A significant drop in LH levels was observed in 10 out of 12 patients (83.3%) after MPA. A fall in FSH levels occurred in 9 out of 12 patients (75%). Plasma oestradiol levels declined in 6 out of the 10 patients studied. This fall is also significant.

Histological changes

Microscopic study of the tumour after 4 weeks of MPA treatment revealed alterations in 23 out of 95 patients (24.2%) with highly differentiated adenocarcinomas, but in only one of the patients with moderately differentiated adenocarcinomas. The most common findings, relating to the effect of MPA on tumorous endometrial tissue, were stromal decidualization, increase of stroma between glands, appearance of glandular secretion, formation of one layer of glandular epithelium, and an increase in amount of cellular cytoplasm.

Disease free patients

The numbers of disease-free patients in each category are shown in Table V.

Table V. Disease-free patients.

Category of patient	Numbers of disease-free patients cf. total numbers of patients (%)		Average duration of follow-up (months)	Percentage of disease-free patients per month of follow-up
Stage I disease:				
myometrium not invaded				
control group	9	(100)	14.6	6.8
MPA-treated group	11	(100)	16.4	6.9
myometrium invaded				
S + Co, control group	13	(92.8)	11.5	8.0
S + Co, MPA-treated group	18	(94.7)	18	5.2
S + Co + Ra control group	8	(88.8)	15.6	5.6
S + Co + Ra MPA-treated group	14	(100)	18	5.5
Stage II disease:				
control group	9	(100)	13.7	7.2
MPA-treated group	8	(80)	14.7	5.4
Stage III or IV disease; stage I or II patients where surgery risky:				
control group	9	(75)	12.2	6.1
MPA-treated group	10	(66.6)	17.6	3.7
Control group overall	48	(90.5)	13.3	6.8
MPA-treated group overall	61	(88.4)	17.1	5.1

S = surgery, Co = cobalt therapy, Ra = radium therapy.

In patients with stage I disease, in whom the myometrium was not invaded, all 9 patients in the control group as well as all 11 patients in the MPA-treated group were disease-free.

In patients with stage I disease in whom the myometrium was invaded, the MPA-treated group overall fared slightly better than the untreated group, but the difference was not significant. The average follow-up period was slightly longer in MPA-treated patients.

Among patients with stage II disease all 9 patients of the control group were disease-free, and, in the MPA-treated group, 8 out of 10 patients were free of disease.

In patients with stage III or IV disease, or with stage I or II disease and high surgical risk factors, 9 out of 12 patients in the control group were disease-free, and 10 out of 15 patients in the MPA-treated group were disease-free.

Taking the patients as a whole, 48 out of 53 patients (90.5%) in the control group were disease-free, as compared with 61 out of 69 patients (88.4%) in the MPA-treated group. It should, again, be borne in mind that the follow-up period was longer in the case of the MPA-treated group.

Survival rate

Survival rates for the various groups of patients are shown in Table VI.

In stage I patients in whom the myometrium was not invaded, all patients in control and MPA-treated groups remained alive.

When the myometrium was invaded in cases of stage I disease in which treatment consisted of surgery plus cobalt therapy, 13 out of 14 patients (92.8%) in the control group remained alive, as compared with 18 out of 19 patients (94.7%) in the MPA-treated group. When treatment consisted of surgery, cobalt therapy and radium therapy, all patients in the control and MPA-treated groups remained alive.

In stage II cases all 9 patients in the control group remained alive, as compared with 9 out of 10 patients in the MPA-treated group.

In stage III and IV cases, and stage I and II cases associated with high surgical risk 10 out of 12 patients (83.3%) in the control group survived, as against 11 out of 15 (73.3%) in the MPA-treated group.

The survival rate overall was 50 out of 53 patients (94.3%) in the control group as compared with 63 out of 69 patients (91.3%) in the MPA-treated group.

Side-effects of MPA

MPA has generally been well tolerated. The side-effects at the dosage level

Table VI. Survival among patients with endometrial adenocarcinoma.

Category of patient	Numbers of patients surviving cf. total numbers of patients (%)		Average duration of follow-up (months)	Percentage of patients surviving per month of follow-up
Stage I disease:				
myometrium not invaded				
control group	9	(100)	14.6	6.8
MPA-treated group	11	(100)	16.4	6.9
myometrium invaded				
S + Co, control group	13	(92.8)	11.5	8.0
S + Co, MPA-treated group	18	(94.7)	18	5.2
S + Co + Ra control group	9	(100)	15.6	6.4
S + Co + Ra MPA-treated group	14	(100)	18	5.5
Stage II disease:				
control group	9	(100)	13.7	7.2
MPA-treated group	9	(90)	14.7	6.1
Stage III or IV disease; stage I or II patients where surgery risky:				
control group	10	(83.3)	12.2	6.8
MPA-treated group	11	(73.3)	17.6	4.1
Control group overall	50	(94.3)	13.3	7.0
MPA-treated group overall	63	(91.3)	17.1	5.3

S = surgery, Co = cobalt therapy, Ra = radium therapy.

used were hot flushes (4 patients), muscular aches and pains (2 patients), and headaches (2 patients). In one patient with hypertension treatment was discontinued because of an aggravation of this condition. Finally, 2 patients had gluteal abscesses which needed draining.

Comments

Our results are only preliminary. More patients will have to be enrolled in the trial and the follow-up period prolonged to 5 years before definite conclusions can be reached. Nevertheless, on the basis of the information currently available, it is clear that measurement of oestrogen receptors will show which endometrial adenocarcinomas are hormone-dependent. In patients selected in this way, the administration of MPA caused a significant fall in plasma LH levels in 83.3% of patients, in FSH levels in 75% of patients, and in oestradiol levels in 60% of patients. It therefore seems probable that, as in the case of breast cancer [9], a high percentage of cases of hormone-dependent endometrial adenocarcinoma, will respond favourably to hormone treatment, either with MPA or with anti-oestrogens [10]. Tumours which are not hormone-dependent would appear to be totally unaffected, or affected in only very few cases, by hormone therapy.

After an average of 15.5 months of follow-up, MPA appeared to increase both the number of disease-free patients and the survival rate in patients with stage I disease. On the other hand, in the other patients results were better in control group patients. The differences were not statistically significant.

References

1. Cramer, D.W. and Cutler, S.J. (1974): Incidence in histopathology of malignancies of the female genital organs in the United States. *Am. J. Obstet. Gynecol. 118*, 443.
2. Bjersing, L. (1977): Endometrial hyperplasia and carcinoma: histopathology and hormonal factors. *Acta Obstet. Gynecol. Scand. 65*, 83.
3. Pollow, K., Lubbert, H., Boquoi, E. et al. (1975): Characterization and comparison of receptor for 17 beta-estradiol and progesterone in human proliferative endometrium and endometrial cancer. *Endocrinology 96*, 319.
4. Young, P.C.M., Ehrlich, C.E. and Cleary, R.E. (1976): Progesterone binding in human endometrial carcinomas. *Am. J. Obstet. Gynecol. 125*, 353.
5. Kottmeier, H.L. and Kolstad, P. (1975): Classification and staging of malignant tumours in the female pelvis. In: *Annual Report on the Results of Treatment in Carcinoma of the Uterus, Vagina and Ovary*, Vol. 16, p. 8. Radium Clinic, Stockholm.
6. Kohorn, E.I. (1976): Gestagens and endometrial carcinoma. *Gynecol. Oncol. 4*, 398.
7. Bonte, J., Decoster, J.M., Ide, P. and Billiet, G. (1978): Hormonoprophylaxis and hormonotherapy in the treatment of endometrial adenocarcinoma by means of medroxyprogesterone acetate. *Gynecol. Oncol. 6*, 60.
8. Bonte, J., Decoster, J.M., Ide, P. et al. (1974): Progestagens in endometrial cancer. In: *Proceedings of the VII World Congress on Obstetrics and Gynaecology*, p. 285. Eds: L.S. Persianinov, T.V. Chervakova and J. Presl. Excerpta Medica, Amsterdam.
9. Gehan, E.A. (1965): A generalized Wilcoxon test for comparing arbitrarily single-censored samples. *Biometrika 52,* 203.
10. McGuire, W.L., Horowitz, K.B., Pearson, O.H. et al. (1977): Current status of estrogen and progesterone receptors in breast cancer. *Cancer 39*, 2934.
11. Swenerton, K.D. (1980): Treatment of advanced endometrial adenocarcinoma with tamoxifen. *Cancer Treat. Rep. 64*, 805.

Treatment of advanced or recurrent endometrial adenocarcinoma with progestins, including medroxyprogesterone acetate

H. Caffier, G. Horner and R.-J. Baum
University Hospital for Obstetrics and Gynaecology, Würzburg, Federal Republic of Germany

Introduction

It has frequently been stated that adenocarcinoma of the endometrium is a so-called 'good' cancer with regard to prognosis when compared with other cancers in women. Fortunately, in the majority of patients the disease is diagnosed at an early stage when it is limited to the endometrium or uterus. Conventional treatments, such as ablative surgery, radiation, or a combination of both, is fairly well standardized, and efficacies, as measured by 5-year survival rates, are about 80%. When the disease has spread to other organs of the pelvis, to distant sites, or has recurred after primary therapy, successful management is extremely difficult, and there is a role for systemic treatment.

That advanced endometrial adenocarcinoma may be amenable to control by means of progestational agents was first demonstrated by Kelly and Baker in 1960 [1]. Several other authors [for reviews see references 2, 3 and 4] have since described their experiences with progestin therapy, using a variety of drugs. According to the data of these authors, the response rate to progestin therapy in patients with advanced or recurrent endometrial adenocarcinoma is 30–40%. In the following paper, we report on our studies with progestin therapy in 54 patients with recurrent or advanced endometrial carcinoma.

Materials and methods

The records of 54 patients with advanced (stage III or IV) or recurrent endometrial adenocarcinoma who had been treated with progestins were analysed in detail. All patients had undergone as many surgical procedures as appropriate, or been subjected to as much radiation as possible, or both, either as primary treatment, or as treatment for recurrent disease, prior to progestin therapy. The drug initially employed was gestonorone caproate (GC), administered to 37 patients. More recently, 17 patients have been treated with medroxyprogesterone acetate (MPA). GC was administered intramuscularly (i.m.) at a dose of 3 × 200 mg weekly for 3 months. Maintenance therapy was 2 × 200 mg weekly in patients who showed either stable disease or partial response. MPA was administered at a dosage of 3 × 100 mg daily, by mouth, for 6 weeks. Maintenance therapy was 2 × 100 mg daily.

Response was defined as complete remission (no evidence of disease for 3 months or more), partial remission (50% or greater reduction in size of tumour for 3 months or more), no change (less than 50% reduction in size of tumour, or stable disease) and progression. Complete and partial remission for 3 months were considered as objective responses. Correlation of response to treatment with age, length of disease-free interval (for recurrent carcinomas only), status of disease (primary advanced or recurrent), site of lesion, degree of histological differentiation of the tumour, and type of treatment was investigated.

Results

As shown in Table I, 17 out of the 54 patients (31.5%) treated with progestins had objective responses. Six showed complete remission, 11 partial remission. No response was noted in 37 patients (68.5%) (no change in 19 patients, marked progression in 18). The median period of survival was 27 months for objective responders (range 3+ to 61+ months) and 7 months (range one to 26 months) for nonresponders.

Table I. Advanced or recurrent endometrial adenocarcinoma. Progestin treatment and response; numbers of patients (%).

Complete remission	6 (11.1)	Responders (31.5)
Partial remission	11 (20.4)	
No change	19 (35.2)	Nonresponders (68.5)
Progression	18 (33.3)	
Total	54	

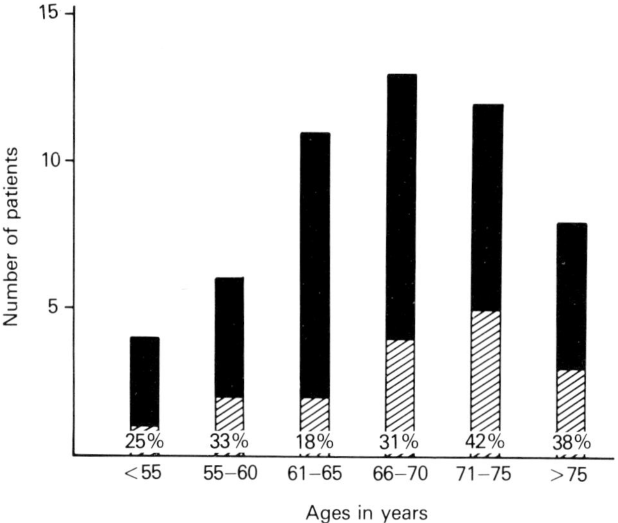

Fig. 1. Relationship between age of patient and response to progestin therapy. ■ *nonresponders;* ▨ *responders.*

Age of patient was not a factor markedly influencing the responses of the tumours to progestins. There was a slight tendency to higher response rates in older patients (Fig. 1), but the differences were small. The mean age of patients with responsive tumours was 68.9. The mean age of patients with nonresponsive lesions was 66.8.

Responses to progestin therapy in relation to disease status and site of lesion are shown in Table II. There were no substantial differences between response rates in patients with primary advanced, or recurrent tumours. Patients with local pelvic lesions responded better than those with distant metastases. The objective response rates were 39.4 and 19.1%, respectively. Further evaluation of the group with distant metastases, categorizing patients by predominant site of metastases, revealed that 2 out of 13 cases with pulmonary metastases, one out of 2 cases with hepatic metastases and one out of 2 cases with bony metastases showed objective responses. No nodal lesion or abdominal mass responded to progestin therapy.

Patients in whom long periods had elapsed between initial therapy and the onset of recurrent or metastatic disease, or both, responded better than these with a short disease-free interval. Table III shows the disease-free intervals in the 36 patients with recurrent disease. This interval was shorter in the group of nonresponders than in responsive patients.

Table II. Disease status and site of lesion in patients with endometrial adenocarcinoma, and response to progestin therapy (numbers of patients, and percentage response rates).

	Responders	Nonresponders	Response rate (%)
Totals	17	37	31.5
Disease status			
Primary advanced	5	13	27.8
Recurrent	12	24	33.3
Site of lesion			
Local	13	20	39.4
Distant	4	17	19.1
Lung	2	11	
Liver	1	1	
Bone	1	1	
Node	0	2	
Abdomen outside pelvis	0	2	

Table III. Disease-free interval and response to progestin therapy in patients with recurrent endometrial adenocarcinoma.

	Responders	Nonresponders
Numbers of patients	12	24
Disease-free interval (months)		
Range	6–126	4–120
Mean	40.1	25.2
Median	31	19

Table IV. Histological grade and response to progestin therapy in advanced or recurrent endometrial adenocarcinoma.

Grade	Total number of patients with grade of tumour shown	Numbers (percentages) of patients responding
I	15	8 (53)
II	20	6 (30)
III	13	1 (8)
Totals	48	15 (31)

Table V. Responses in patients with endometrial adenocarcinoma treated with GC or MPA; numbers of patients (percentages).

	Treatment				Totals	
	GC		MPA			
Complete remission	3 (8)	(24)	3 (18)	(47)	6 (11)	(32)
Partial remission	6 (16)		5 (29)		11 (21)	
No change	14 (38)	(76)	5 (29)	(53)	19 (35)	(68)
Progression	14 (38)		4 (24)		18 (33)	
	37 (100)		17 (100)		54 (100)	

Response rates in relation to degree of histological differentiation are shown in Table IV. Three grades of differentiation were defined, corresponding to the grade I (well-differentiated), grade II (moderately differentiated) and grade III (undifferentiated) categories in the Fédération Internationale de Gynécologie et d'Obstétrique (FIGO) staging of endometrial cancer. The response rate was highest (53%) in grade I tumours. Six out of 20 grade II tumours (30%) responded to progestin treatment, and only one out of 13 patients (8%) with grade III tumours.

A higher rate of objective response was obtained in MPA-treated patients than in those treated with GC (Table V). The objective response rate in the

Table VI. Clinical characteristics of patients with endometrial adenocarcinoma treated with GG or MPA.

	Treatment	
	GC	MPA
Total numbers of patients	37	17
Mean ages (years)	67.3	67.9
Mean disease-free interval (months)	29.1	35.3
Numbers (%) of patients with primary advanced disease	11 (30)	7 (41)
Numbers (%) of patients with distant metastases	12 (32)	9 (53)
Numbers (%) of patients with tumours of histological grade		
I	9/31 (29)	6/16 (37)
III	9/31 (29)	4/16 (25)

MPA group was 47% (3 complete responses, 5 partial), as compared with 24% (3 complete responses, 6 partial) in the GC group. No change was observed in 29% of MPA-treated patients and 38% of GC-treated patients. In the remaining 24% of MPA-treated patients and 38% of GC-treated patients, there was progression.

The distribution of host and tumour characteristics was not markedly different between the 2 treatment groups overall (Table VI). The mean ages and the distribution of histological grades were almost identical for both treatment groups. The mean disease-free interval was slightly longer in MPA-treated patients, leading to better prognoses in these patients. On the other hand, a higher percentage of patients in the MPA group had distant metastases which would worsen prognosis in these cases.

Survival curves, plotted according to the actuarial method, and analysed in terms of type of treatment, are shown in Figure 2. For the patients as a whole, the overall survival period ranged from one month to more than 61 months, with a median survival period of 13 months. Subdivision by type of treatment revealed better results for the MPA group (median survival period 25 months) than for the GC group (median survival period 9 months). This difference was not only attributable to the higher objective response rate obtained with MPA but also to survival for longer periods in patients not responding to MPA (Fig. 3). Figures showing survival periods in patients responding to MPA and GC are not shown, because, except for one, who died after 14 months, all of the

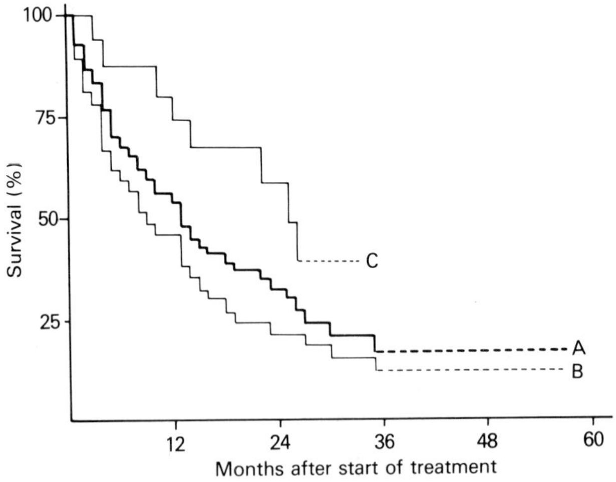

Fig. 2. Survival in relation to type of treatment. A = total (n = 54); B = GC (n = 37); and C = MPA (n = 17).

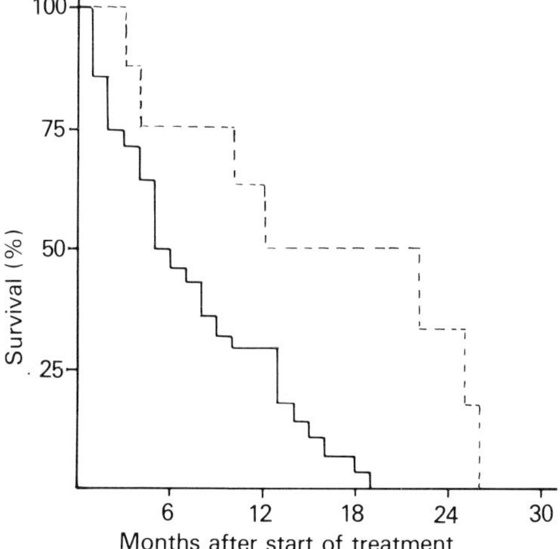

Fig. 3. Survival of patients not responding to progestin therapy. ---- = *nonresponders MPA (n = 9); and* —— *nonresponders GC (n = 29).*

MPA-treated patients are still alive. Among the 9 patients showing no response to MPA, the median duration of survival was 12 months, with no patient surviving more than 26 months, whereas the median survival period among the 29 nonresponders to GC was only 5 months, with no patient surviving more than 19 months.

Comments and conclusions

The overall objective response rate of 31.5% in patients with advanced or recurrent endometrial adenocarcinoma treated with GC or MPA is in general agreement with that reported by other authors [2–4]. Differences between responders and nonresponders in respect of host and tumour characteristics can be identified, but it does not appear possible to predict with great accuracy which individual patient is likely to respond. According to our data slow growing, recurrent tumours, well-differentiated tumours, and local pelvic masses, either as recurrent or primary disease, as opposed to metastatic lesions, responded best. The histological grade of the tumour and duration of disease-free interval have already been shown by other authors [2, 5, 6] to be correlated with response rates. Contrary to Smith and coworkers [7], in our study age was not a factor important in determining response.

MPA is probably more effective than GC. The response and survival rate of MPA-treated patients was higher than that of GC-treated patients, with major prognostic factors almost equally distributed among the 2 treatment groups. Our series is, however, too small to allow any more definite assertion that MPA is better than GC.

Side-effects were less pronounced in patients treated with MPA. No patient on MPA had severe side-effects, but 3 patients in the group treated with GC died of pulmonary embolism, which could have been attributable to medication. Five patients with distant metastases treated with GC, and one such patient treated with MPA, developed vaginal bleeding not attributable to the disease, as shown by curettage. A favourable side-effect of both drugs was improvement in appetite and sense of well-being. This side-effect was more frequent in MPA-treated patients, even in the presence of progressive disease.

Because patients were kept on medication until subjective progression occurred, this may serve to explain why nonresponders to MPA showed longer survival periods than GC-nonresponders.

References

1. Kelly, R.M. and Baker, W.H. (1961): Progestational agents in the treatment of carcinoma of the endometrium. *N. Engl. J. Med. 264,* 216.
2. Wait, R.B. (1973): Megestrol acetate in the management of advanced endometrial carcinoma. *Obstet. Gynecol. 41*, 129.
3. Reifenstein, E.C., Jr. (1974): The treatment of advanced endometrial cancer with hydroxyprogesterone caproate. *Gynecol. Oncol. 2,* 377.
4. Kohorn, E.I., (1976): Gestagens and endometrial carcinoma. *Gynecol. Oncol. 4,* 398.
5. Geisler, H.E., (1973): The use of megestrol acetate in the treatment of advanced malignant lesions of the endometrium. *Gynecol. Oncol. 1,* 340.
6. Malkasian, G.D., Jr., Decker, D.G., Mussey, E. and Johnson, C.E. (1971): Progestogen treatment of recurrent endometrial carcinoma. *Am. J. Obstet. Gynecol. 110,* 15.
7. Smith, J.P., Rutledge, F. and Soffar, S.W. (1966): Progestins in the treatment of patients with endometrial adenocarcinoma. *Am. J. Obstet. Gynecol. 94*, 977.

Hormonal therapy associated with combination chemotherapy in the treatment of advanced endometrial cancer

T. Battelli[1], F. Saccani[2], G. Saccani Jotti[3], P. Manocchi[1], L. Giustini[1], R. Mattioci[1] and A. Ginnetti[1]

[1]F. Angelini Oncological Centre for Nuclear Medicine, Ancona; [2]Associated Hospitals of Reggio Emilia; and [3]Pathological Anatomy Institute, University of Parma, Italy

Introduction

After the first studies of hormone therapy using progestins, described by Kelley and Baker [1], there have been many others, both clinical and experimental, which have confirmed that progestin therapy has favourable results in the treatment of endometrial cancer (Table I).

The cells of the endometrium undergo continuous endocrine stimulation during the premenopausal life of a woman. When, during the menopause, hormonal stimuli are reduced, the endometrial cells cease their monthly fluctuations in activity and transformation, and the endometrium becomes atrophic.

A most interesting fact is that neoplastic cells of the endometrium also become modified under hormonal stimulus. This happens in highly differentiated tumours, in particular. With progestin therapy, there is a cessation of mitotic activity, a tendency to normalization of the nucleocytoplasmic ratio, through reduction in nuclear size and increase in cytoplasm of finely vacuolated appearance. The stroma increases in size and separates the glandulae, which, being more regular, are covered with only one cellular layer.

Macroscopically, the uterine cavity shows neoplasms, sometimes separated by an apparently normal mucous membrane, sometimes covered by such a membrane, coating the entire uterine cavity. The colour of the mucous membrane is yellowish, similar to the colour during the normal secretory phase of the endometrium. Abundant mucous material coats necrotic and haemor-

Table I. Results of hormone therapy of endometrial cancer.

Investigators	Drug	No. of cases	Percentage of partial and complete response
Kistner et al. [2]	Hydroxyprogesterone caproate	---	33
Kistner et al. [2]	Medroxyprogesterone acetate (MPA)	---	50
Anderson [3]	Hydroxyprogesterone caproate	431	30
Anderson [3]	MPA	20	40
Briggs et al. [4]	MPA	822	31
Kennedy [5]	Hydroxyprogesterone caproate	596	30
Peck and Boyes [6]	MPA	23	34
Hreschchyshyn and Graham [7]	Hydroxyprogesterone caproate	83	20
Malkasian et al. [8]	Hydroxyprogesterone caproate	20	25
Malkasian [8]	Medrogestone	30	23
Malkasian [8]	MPA	25	24
Reifenstein [9]	Hydroxyprogesterone caproate	314	30
Lewis [10]	MPA	16	62
Bonte [11]	Hydroxyprogesterone caproate	327	33
Bonte [11]	MPA	234	45
Rozier [12]	MPA	34	38
Bonte et al. [13]	MPA	106	53
Battelli and Saccani [14]	MPA	55	40

rhagic areas, which are residues of neoplasms which have partly regressed following progestin therapy. The classic theory of the aetiology of endometrial carcinomas postulates their origin in an increase of oestrogens, which may be responsible for the proliferative processes of the endometrium.

However, it has been observed that the urinary excretion of oestrogens in women with endometrial cancer is similar to that in normal women.

Sherman found hyperplasia in the cells of the hilus ovarii in 80% of cases of adenocarcinoma of the endometrium [15]. These cells are stimulated by the hypophysis through secretion of luteinizing hormone (LH), and can be inhibited by progesterone through its blocking action of the production of LH.

This might explain why the endometrial cancer is distinctly more common in postmenopausal women. In such women, the physiological decrease in progesterone means that production of LH is no longer reduced. The hilus cells, stimulated by LH, might thus initiate endometrial hyperplasia.

Hypophyseal block could also be achieved through the use of oestroprogestins with anti-ovulatory properties, and Pincus has, in fact, recorded that there is a low percentage of endometrial tumours in women who have been on contraceptive pills for a long time [16].

Other authors, such as Novak, trace endometrial cancer back to increased production of androgens by the ovary [17].

It is not yet evident whether the action of progestins is direct or indirect.

It has been shown that addition of progesterone to a culture of endometrial cells results in a decrease in synthesis of nucleic acids, together with a slowing of the rate of cell multiplication. Oestrogens have the opposite effect. Nordquist has shown that by adding high doses of progestins to cultures of cells of endometrial cancer cell death can be provoked [18]. This is not observed with either low-dose progestins or androgens.

The discovery of steroid receptors in the cytoplasm of the cells reacting to hormonal therapy has undoubtedly explained the direct mechanism of action of progestins, which block receptor sites. The presence of hormonal receptors in the cells of the body of the uterus has been demonstrated.

Flickinger has demonstrated the presence of receptors for oestrogens in about 60% of cases [19]. In various samples taken from the uterine cavity the authors have, however, found different concentrations of receptors.

Oestrogen receptors are also present, though in reduced amount, in postmenopausal women. In premenopausal women it has been shown that the largest concentration of oestrogen (oestradiol) receptors is present during the proliferative phase. In some endometrial neoplasms, particularly those most highly differentiated histologically, receptors for both oestrogen (oestradiol) and androgen (androstanolone) are present. Such tumours react best to hormonal therapy.

The sensitivity of a tumour to endocrine therapy is very likely to be proportional to the concentration of progesterone receptors. On the other hand, we are very doubtful about the use of oestrogens in cases not sensitive to progestogen therapy to induce the neoplastic cells to produce progesterone receptors. It would appear that a response has been obtained in 20% of cases using this approach.

According to Young the most highly differentiated tumours contain higher quantities of progesterone receptors [20]. The number of progesterone receptors decreases with age.

Metastic tumours are often lacking in hormone receptors. In different metastatic areas in any given patient, variable numbers of receptors may be found, with the consequence that a metastasis may respond to endocrine therapy in one area, while in another location therapy is ineffective.

This can be explained on the basis of metastatic colonization by different types of cell. Metastases composed of cells with hormonal receptors will respond to hormone therapy, those without will not.

If, in the primary tumour, hormonal receptors cannot be found even after repeated biopsy, metastases are also very likely to be lacking in receptors. On the other hand, the presence of receptors in the primary tumour does not signify that they will necessarily be present in the metastatic cells also.

From a practical point of view, to test the responsiveness of an endometrial carcinoma to hormones, progestins are administered to the patient (via the usual routes, or even directly within the uterine cavity). Histological examination of the endometrium on re-inspection of the cavity after some days' treatment allows determination of whether response has occurred.

Progestational therapy

We believe that progestins are always useful in the treatment of patients suffering from endometrial cancer, both in the pre-operative phase, to test the patient's response to hormone therapy, and to reduce the size of the neoplastic masses and the danger of their dissemination during surgery, and in the immediate postoperative phase, as therapy complementary to surgery and to any radiotherapy which may be undertaken.

It has been shown experimentally with, e.g., MPA added to a culture of endometrial cancer cells, that progestins increase the effect of ionizing radiation.

In cases of advanced endometrial cancer, not capable of being treated by radical surgery because of local diffusion of the neoplasm, or because of the poor state of health of the patient, and in cases of recurrence of neoplasms, progestin therapy is, in practice, the only available therapy, if the use of the radiotherapy is not possible. We have no experience of preventative treatment with progestins in endometrial hyperplasias, or of cancer therapy in situ in young patients who refuse surgery. However, investigators of these approaches have obtained satisfactory results.

The patients upon whom we can report include only patients with advanced cancer, usually having recurred following previous treatments.

We observed no significant differences in results as between different progestin products. In contrast, there is a marked dependence of outcome on dose.

In a previous paper, we have described results obtained with high doses of MPA [14]. There was a favourable response in 18 out of 41 patients who received 500 mg intramuscularly (i.m.) per day for a month, then 500 mg i.m. every other day for another month, and then 500 mg i.m. twice per week continuously. In contrast, favourable responses occurred in 4 out of 14 patients treated with 500 mg i.m. per week continuously. On the basis of our experience, results are more satisfactory in patients over 60, are dependent upon the degree of differentiation of cells, and on the principal site of metastases, those in the lungs being more responsive than bony or vaginal metastases. Response to hormone therapy is distinctly better, in our opinion, in obese, diabetic patients, and in those suffering from hypertension.

The average period of remission in our patients was 11 months. The average period of survival was 17 months in patients responding to treatment, and 6 months in those not responding. We did not observe any significant toxicity, even on prolonged treatment with high doses of progestins. We never once saw a gluteal abscess, even though many patients were diabetic. This contrasts with what has been observed in the treatment of mammary neoplasms with MPA.

The results of treatment with high-dose i.m. MPA are satisfactory, in relation to remission of symptomatology also. The latter can be achieved in more than 50% of cases treated with low or high doses, but occurs more quickly with higher doses.

Cytotoxic chemotherapy

Experience with chemotherapy in the treatment of endometrial neoplasms is fairly limited. The belief is, in fact, widely held that these neoplasms are made up of well-differentiated cells, not very sensitive to antiproliferative drugs (Table II). In addition, the favourable responses seen in many cases treated with hormones, without any major side-effects, have usually led to the latter treatment being preferred. However, in advanced stages of the illness, it is often necessary for patients to undergo chemotherapy, since the tumour is no longer hormone-responsive.

Chemotherapy and hormone therapy combined

Chemotherapy and hormone therapy act on different types of cell. In hormone-responsive tumours, hormone-dependent and hormone-independent cells co-exist. It is, therefore, evident that hormone treatment alone will favour the development of a predominance of hormone-independent cells, i.e.

Table II. Chemotherapy of advanced endometrial cancer.

Investigators	Drug	No. of cases	Complete and partial remissions
Bruckner and Deppe [21]	Doxorubicin (ADR) + cyclophosphamide (CTX) + 5-fluorouracil (5FU) (+MPA)	7	6
De Vita et al. [22]	5FU	43	10
De Vita et al. [22]	ADR	18	7
De Vita et al. [22]	CTX	33	7
Cohen et al. [23]	5FU + melphalan (+ MPA)	7	6
Thipgen et al. [24]	ADR	49	17
Muggia et al. [25]	CTX + ADR	8	5
Koretz et al. [26]	Platinum + ADR + CTX	7	4
Piver et al. [27]	MPL + 5FU (+ MPA)	11	6

the most undifferentiated and malignant cells. The object of combined chemotherapy and hormone therapy is to obtain the sum of the effects of the 2 types of treatment, to limit recurrence of the tumour, and to improve the general and haematological condition of the patient, in many cases, as a result of the anabolic activity of the hormone. The 2 treatments do not show any additive toxic effects, and have different mechanisms of action.

In 1979, we began a study in patients suffering from advanced endometrial cancer which was either inoperable, or had recurred after previous surgery and/or radiation treatment, and which had never before been the subject of high-dose progestin therapy. Patients received high doses of MPA or high doses of MPA together with chemotherapy with ADR, 5FU and CTX. The doses of MPA used were 1 g i.m. daily for 7 days, followed by 500 mg i.m. daily for a month, followed by 500 mg twice a week. In patients receiving chemotherapy in addition, the doses were 600 mg CTX/mq on day 1, 600 mg 5FU/mq on days 1 and 8 and 50 mg ADR/mq on day 1, with repetition of dosage every 28 days thereafter.

The criteria for admission of patients to the study were:

- no previous treatment with high-dose MPA,
- postmenopausal patients,
- age less than 65,
- Karnofsky status greater than 50,
- no cardiopathies or grave metabolic problems.

Up to December 1981, 53 patients had been admitted to the study. Twenty-seven received MPA alone, 26 MPA and chemotherapy. Thirty-one (15 MPA, 16 MPA and chemotherapy) have undergone at least 2 months' treatment, or more than one year has passed from the beginning of treatment. The other patients began treatment in 1981. In these cases the objective and subjective response can be assessed, but not the duration of response or survival period.

Table III summarizes the results in the 31 patients defined above. The mean duration of remission was of 11 months in the group treated with MPA, and 13 months in the group treated with MPA and chemotherapy.

Of the 13 patients who started treatment in 1979, 4 patients in the group treated with MPA who did not respond to treatment survived for 3, 5, 6 and 7 months. In the group treated with MPA and chemotherapy, 4 patients who did not respond survived for 3, 4, 5 and 7 months. In 2 patients responding to MPA treatment, survival lasted 17 and 19 months. In 3 patients responding to MPA combined with chemotherapy, survival lasted 15, 16 and 20 months.

Table IV shows responses of metastases in different areas to the 2 treatments.

Table V shows the main side-effects and toxic effects observed after 2 and 6 months of treatment.

Table III. Results of treatment with MPA and MPA combined with chemotherapy.

MPA	No. of cases	Complete or partial remission	Stationary	Progressing
MPA	15	5	6	4
MPA combined with chemotherapy	16	8	5	3

Table IV. Response of metastases in various areas to treatment (numbers of patients).

Site of metastases	MPA	MPA combined with chemotherapy
Pelvis	1/4	1/2
Vagina	1/3	1/2
Lung	1/2	2/3
Bones	1/2	1/2
Liver	0/1	0/1
Peritoneum	– – –	1/1

Table V. Side-effects and toxic effects (percentage incidence).

Side-effect	MPA	MPA combined with chemotherapy	MPA	MPA combined with chemotherapy
	(After 2 months)		(After 6 months)	
Leukopenia	–	20	–	50
Low platelet count	–	10	–	30
Anaemia	–	10	–	20
Liver cell damage	–	–	10	15
Liver congestion	5	10	10	15
ECG changes	–	–	5	30
Cardiac insufficiency	–	–	–	–
Water and electrolyte retention	15	10	20	20
Arterial hypertension	15	15	25	25
Hyperglycaemia	20	10	20	20
Thrombophlebitis	5	5	5	10
Cramps and tremors	15	20	20	25
Asthenia	20	30	30	30
Gluteal abscess	–	–	5	10
Gluteal seepage	25	30	40	60

In the group receiving MPA, it has never been necessary to interrupt therapy. In the other group, 20% of patients had to reduce the doses of the cytostatic agents after 2 months, and 75% after 6 months. Cessation of treatment after 6 months was necessary in 20% of patients on cytostatics.

Subjective responses, such as reduction of pain symptoms, increase in appetite, improved well-being, and reduction in dyspnoea and metrorrhagia are shown in Table VI.

Table VI. Subjective response.

	MPA	MPA combined with chemotherapy
Reduced pain	3/6	4/6
Increased appetite	4/4	3/4
Improved well-being	2/4	1/3
Reduced dyspnoea	0/1	2/3
Reduced metrorrhagia	0/1	1/2

Discussion

The investigation reported here is still in progress, and it is not yet possible to draw conclusions. The numbers are relatively small. However, chemotherapy combined with MPA therapy has tended to give better results, both subjectively and objectively. Pulmonary, pelvic and bone metastases responded more promptly than metastases elsewhere.

Side-effects and toxic effects were more marked in patients undergoing therapy with cytostatic agents, as would be expected. In many cases we have been compelled to reduce the doses of the cytostatics, and sometimes even to discontinue treatment with them.

References

1. Kelley, R.H. and Baker, W.H. (1961): Progestational agents in the treatment of carcinoma of the endometrium. *N. Engl. J. Med. 264*, 216.
2. Kistner, R.W., Griffiths, G.T. and Craig, J.M. (1965): Use of progestational agents in the management of the endometrium. *Cancer 18*, 1563.
3. Anderson, D.G. (1965): Management of advanced endometrial adenocarcinoma with medroxyprogesterone acetate. *Am. J. Obstet. Gynecol. 92*, 87.
4. Briggs, M.H., Caldwell, A.D.S. and Pitchford, A.G. (1967): The treatment of cancer by progestogens. *Hosp. Med. 2*, 63.
5. Kennedy, B.J. (1968): Progestogens in the treatment of carcinoma of endometrium. *Surg. Gynecol. Obstet. 127*, 103.
6. Peck, J.G. and Boyes, D.A. (1969): Treatment of advanced endometrial carcinoma with a progestational agent. *Am. J. Obstet. Gynecol. 103*, 90.
7. Hreschchyshyn, M.M. and Graham, R.M. (1969): 17-alpha-hydroxyprogesterone caproate treatment of gynecologic cancer. *Am. J. Obstet. Gynecol. 104*, 916.
8. Malkasian, G.D., Decker, D.G., Mussey, E. and Johnson, C.E. (1971): Progestogen treatment of recurrent endometrial carcinoma. *Am. J. Obstet. Gynecol. 110*, 15.
9. Reifenstein, E.C. (1971): Hydroxyprogesterone caproate therapy in advanced endometrial cancer. *Cancer 27*, 485.
10. Lewis, G.C. (1971): Progestin therapy for cancer of the uterine corpus. *Pennsyl. Med. 74*, 47.
11. Bonte, J. (1973): Radium therapy and medroxyprogesterone treatment in the management of primary and recurrent or metastatic uterine adenocarcinoma. In: *Endometrial Cancer*. Eds: M.G. Brush, R.W. Taylor and D.C. Williams, William Heinemann Medical Books, London.
12. Rozier, J.C. and Underwood, P.B. (1974): Use of progestational agents in endometrial adenocarcinoma. *Obstet. Gynecol. 44*, 60.
13. Bonte, J., Decoster, M.J., Ide, P. and Billiet, G. (1978): Hormonoprophylaxis and hormonotherapy in the treatment of endometrial adenocarcinoma by means of medroxyprogesterone acetate. *Gynecol. Oncol. 6*, 60.

14. Battelli, T. and Saccani. F. (1979): Il tumore dell'utero: il trattamento della fase avanzata. In: *Chemioterapia dei Tumori Solidi Vol. II*, Ed: Pàtron, Bologna.
15. Sherman, W. (1959): An endocrine basis for endometrial carcinoma. *Am. J. Obstet. Gynecol. 77*, 233.
16. Pincus, G. (1961): Les médicaments anticonceptionnels ont-ils une action anticancéreuse? *Med. Hyg. 29*, 238.
17. Novak, E. (1962): Come influiva l'influenza delle nostre esperienze e osservazioni sulla scelta dell'operazione nel cancro del corpo dell'utero. *Proceedings of the International Symposium on Therapy of Cancer of the Uterine Body*, Florence.
18. Nordquist, S. (1972): Effect of progesterone on human endometrial carcinoma in different experimental systems. *Acta Obstet. Gynecol. Scand. 19*, 25.
19. Flickinger, G.L., Muechler, E.K. and Mikhail, G. (1974): Estradiol receptors in the human fallopian tube. *Fertil. Steril. 25*, 900.
20. Young, P.C.M. and Cleary, R.E. (1974): Characterization and properties of progesterone-binding components in human endometrium. *J. Clin. Endocrinol. 425.*
21. Bruckner, H.W. and Deppe, G. (1977): Combination chemotherapy of advanced endometrial adenocarcinoma with adriamycin, cyclophosphamide, 5-fluorouracil and medroxyprogesterone acetate. *Obstet. Gynecol. 50*, suppl. 10.
22. De Vita, V.T., Wasserman, T.H., Young, R.C. and Carter, S.K. (1976): Perspectives on research in gynecologic oncology. Treatment protocols. *Cancer 38*, suppl. 509.
23. Cohen, C.J., Deppe, G. and Bruckner, H.W. (1977): Treatment of advanced adenocarcinoma of the endometrium with melphalan, 5-fluorouracil and medroxyprogesterone acetate. A preliminary study. *Obstet. Gynecol. 50*, 415.
24. Thipgen, T., Torres, J. and Buchsbaum, H. (1977): Phase II trial of adriamycin in the treatment of advanced endometrial adenocarcinoma. *Proc. Am. Assoc. Cancer Res. 18.*
25. Muggia, F.M., Chia, G., Reed, L.J. and Romney, S.L. (1977): Doxorubicin-cyclophosphamide. Effective chemotherapy for advanced endometrial adenocarcinoma. *Am. J. Obstet. Gynecol. 128*, 314.
26. Koretz, M.M., Ballon, S., Friedman, M.A. and Donaldson, S. (1980): Platinum, adriamycin and cyclophosphamide (PAC) chemotherapy in advanced endometrial carcinoma. *Proc. Am. Assoc. Cancer Res. 65.*
27. Piver, M.S., Lele, S. and Barlow, J.J. (1980): Melphalan, 5-fluorouracil and medroxyprogesterone acetate in metastatic endometrial carcinoma. *Proc. Am. Assoc. Cancer Res. 66.*

Discussion

E. Bercovich: With regard to the MPA doses, Professor De Palo used 100 mg twice a day, orally, and Dr Caffier spoke about 300 mg a day, orally. Are these doses sufficient to induce pharmacologically effective levels of MPA?

G. De Palo: I do not know whether it is sufficient to achieve an efficient pharmacological level. The protocol was designed some time ago and the study began in February, 1980. At the time of protocol preparation, we did not have any data to show whether 200 mg administered twice daily was a fully sufficient dose.

H. Caffier: We preferred to use a higher dose, 100 mg 3 times a day for a period of 6 weeks, because we did not have the possibility of measuring the levels in the patients. All patients had advanced or metastatic disease, and this was the reason for using the higher MPA dose.

Session V: Kidney – prostate – ovarian cancer

Chairmen: M. Pavone-Macaluso – Palermo, Italy
C. Tropé – Lund, Sweden

Progestational therapy for human renal cell carcinoma*

G. Concolino[1] and F. Di Silverio[2]
[1]Istituto di Clinica Medica Generale e Terapia Medica V; and [2]Cattedra di Patologia Urologica, Università di Roma, Rome, Italy

Introduction

During the last 15 years we have been investigating the possibilities of influencing the growth of human renal cell carcinoma (RCC) through hormonal manipulation [1].

It is well known that the kidney is a target organ for many hormones, and both the normal kidney and RCC are able to synthesize erythropoietin [2], plasma renin precursor [2] and chorionic gonadotropin [3]. Steroid hormones are of particular interest, since they have been shown in a number of experimental animals to induce various effects, e.g., androgenic or oestrogenic, depending on the type of hormone considered [4, 5].

The likelihood that human RCC is hormone-sensitive is strengthened by the higher incidence of RCC in men than in women [5], its higher incidence in obese than in slim women [7], the adrenal tumours found in cases of regressing RCC [8], the greater frequency of spontaneous regression in men than in women [9], and the greater 10-year survival rate in women [10].

On analysing data from to 74 RCC patients studied between 1975 and 1981, we found the death rate in both sexes to be similar, regardless of histological stage of the tumour (pT), histological tumour grade (G), or the presence of steroid receptors. However, in 50 male and 20 female patients eligible for follow-up studies, there was a higher percentage mortality rate (61.1 vs 16.7%) in male than in female N_0M_0 (tumour nodes metastases staging system) patients, and 83.3% of female N_1M_1 patients died vs 38.9% of male N_1M_1 patients (Table I).

*This work was supported, in part, by a grant from the Italian Research Council (Special Project on Control of Neoplastic Growth).

Table I. Patient characteristics, TNM status and mortality rates in 70 RCC patients.

	Males	Females
Numbers of patients	50	20
Numbers of deaths	18	6
Percentage of deaths	36.0	30.0
Number of deaths in N_0M_0 patients	11	1
Number of deaths in N_1M_1 patients	7	5
Percentage of N_0M_0 patients among those dying	61.1	16.7
Percentage of N_1M_1 patients among those dying	38.9	83.3

In previous reports, we have always regarded extended disease-free intervals [11] and extended survival periods as positive hormonal effects on tumour growth [12]. Although such extensions cannot be regarded as rigorous oncological criteria for assessment of the effects of endocrine treatment on tumours, and although we were aware of the unsuccessful results reported with androgen therapy (3.8% response rate) and with low-dose progestin therapy (9.02% response rate) [13] in RCC, investigations were carried out on patients with N_0M_0 disease, in order to offer an explanation for the differences in mortality rates observed between the 2 sexes to establish whether patients with less aggressive cancers had prolonged periods of stable disease, and whether high-dose progestin therapy had a beneficial effect. It would be particularly useful to be able to predict, on the basis of histopathological and biochemical data, which patients were likely to suffer rapid progression, and to attempt to improve the prognosis by means of high-dose progestational therapy.

Forty-eight N_0M_0 RCC patients have been studied. The ratio of males to females was 2.2 : 1. The mean age of the patients was 57.5 years. All had been submitted to radical nephrectomy, and all were treated with medroxyprogesterone acetate (MPA) [14]. As in the group of patients described above, there was a higher death rate in male than in female patients (27.3% vs 6.7%) (Table II). The histological stage was pT_2 in 36 patients, and pT_3 in 12 patients, and the histological grades (data available for 40 patients) were G_1 in 30.0% of the patients, G_2 in 60.0%, and G_3 in 10.0%. No correlation was found between histological stage and histological grade. The overall death rate in the 48 patients examined could be related to the histological stage

Table II. Death rates in $pT_{2-3}N_0M_0$ RCC patients.

	Males		Females
Numbers of patients	33		15
Mean age of patients (years)		57.5	
Overall number of deaths		10	
Percentage of deaths overall		20.8	
Number of deaths according to sex	9		1
Percentage of deaths according to sex	27.3		6.7

Table III. Histopathological stage, grade and death rates in patients with RCC.

	Stage		Grade		
	pT_2	pT_3	G_1	G_2	G_3
Numbers of patients	36	12	12	24	4
Numbers of deaths	5	5	1	5	2
Percentage of deaths	13.9	41.6	8.3	20.8	50.0

(Table III). Too few patients with G_3 tumour were available to allow any definite conclusions to be drawn regarding the relationship between tumour grade and mortality rate.

The present observations did not explain the difference in death rates between male and female patients. Studies on the risk factors relating to death, and the statistical significance of these factors, and of the results obtained relating death rates to the histological stage or grade, and to steroid receptor status, were therefore also carried out.

Risk factors were studied using the Walker-Duncan method [15]. Data on 36 patients were analysed. These patients were all N_0M_0 RCC patients for whom data covering a 2-year follow-up period were available. The factors studied were histological stage of tumour, sex, tumour grade, and progesterone receptor (PR), androgen receptor (AR) and oestrogen receptor (ER) status. It was possible to give coefficients to these risk factors, with different degrees of significance when correlated with death. Histological stage was found to be the most significant risk factor, followed by sex, tumour grade, PR status and ER status, in that order (Table IV). Only histological stage was, however, significantly correlated with the incidence of death. Combining all

Table IV. Application of Walker-Duncan method to data from 36 N_0M_0 RCC patients.

Variable	Risk coefficient	Standard error of coefficient	T	Statistical significance of variable as risk factor
pT	2.19	1.11	1.98	significant
Sex	1.21	1.23	0.98	not significant
G	0.80	1.32	0.60	not significant
PR status	0.46	1.16	0.40	not significant
ER status	0.20	0.97	0.21	not significant

these factors for each patient it was possible to group all RCC patients in 10 deciles, according to overall risk coefficient. Most deaths occurred in the top 2 deciles. When quantitative, statistical calculations were performed relating to individual variables (using censored data and the Breslow or Mantel-Cox tests [16–18]) significant differences were found only between pT_2 and pT_3 patients, not between males and females.

Further statistical analysis of data on all 48 male and female N_0M_0 patients was then performed, taking into account histological stage and grade, and survival period, using Student's *t*-test and lamda (λ) values. The latter allow assessment of the statistical significance (*P*) obtained between the 2 groups of patients, higher values of *P* being related to a greater significance.

The difference in death rates between pT_2 and pT_3 patients is more significant for men than for women ($P=0.95$ vs 0.29) (Table V), and the difference in death rates between G_1 and G_2 patients is more significant for women than for men ($P=0.68$ vs 0.07). These findings should, however, be regarded with caution, since only one female patient died. A larger series of patients needs to be examined before definite conclusions can be drawn.

Table V. Statistical analysis of death rates in pT_2 vs pT_3 and in G_1 vs G_2 RCC patients.

Sex	Risk factor	t	λ	P
Male	pT	1.99	1.41	0.95
Female	pT	0.38	0.27	0.29
Male	G	0.11	7.20	0.07
Female	G	1.09	0.77	0.68

Table VI. Distribution of oestrogen (ER), progesterone (PR) and androgen (AR) receptors in 48 pT_2 and pT_3 patients with RCC. (Numbers of patients (percentages).)

Receptor status	Histological stage	
	pT_2	pT_3
ER^+	22 (61.1)	7 (58.3)
ER^-	14 (38.9)	5 (41.7)
PR^+	19 (52.8)	9 (75.0)
PR^-	17 (47.2)	3 (25.0)
AR^+	14 (66.7)	6 (66.7)
AR^-	7 (33.3)	3 (33.3)

As far as receptor studies are concerned, it should be noted, firstly, that receptors were more frequently found in male than in female patients, secondly, that there was a slight predominance of ER-, PR- and AR-positive tumours in both the pT_2 and pT_3 groups (Table VI), and, thirdly, that when histological grade and steroid receptor status in pT_2-pT_3 RCC patients were correlated, receptor-positive tumours were predominantly G_2, for all 3 receptors studied. It is, however, known that grading has little prognostic value in RCC.

On the question of whether the presence of receptors allows prediction of the clinical course of the disease, and explains the observed differences in mortality rates between male and female patients, data from the present study show that the death rate was slightly higher in patients with receptor-negative cancers than in those with receptor-positive cancers. On the question of whether the presence of receptors improves prognosis regardless of endocrine treatment, or whether receptor status can help to differentiate hormone-responsive from hormone-nonresponsive tumours, as previously reported hormonal treatment improves the survival rate in nephrectomized patients (Fig. 1) [12]. Survival rates for patients treated with MPA and for patients not treated with MPA coincide in the first 2 years, and decrease only thereafter. This finding could be explained on the basis that radical nephrectomy affects mainly tumour stage, but not other factors such as sex, grade and receptor status. Hormonal therapy, in contrast, can hardly affect tumour stage, but can modify risk factors which, though less important than stage, may contribute to prolonging the survival period. More recently, an attempt has been made to determine whether the life expectancy in nephrectomized, MPA-treated patients differed between ER-positive and ER-negative patients, or between PR-positive and PR-negative patients [19]. The overall life expectan-

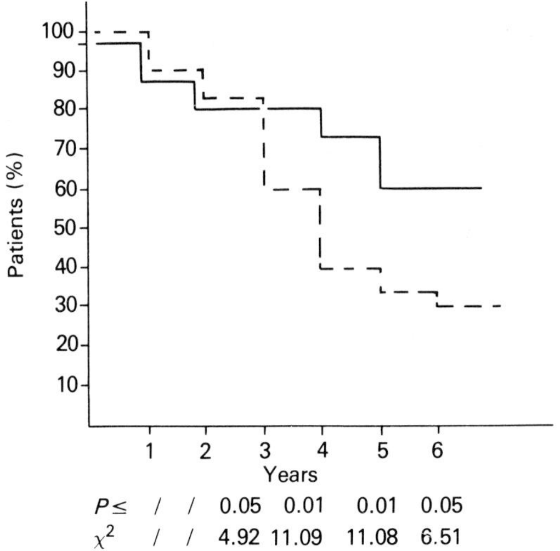

Fig. 1. Survival rates in 2 groups of patients nephrectomized for RCC and treated (solid line) or not treated (broken line) with hormonal therapy.

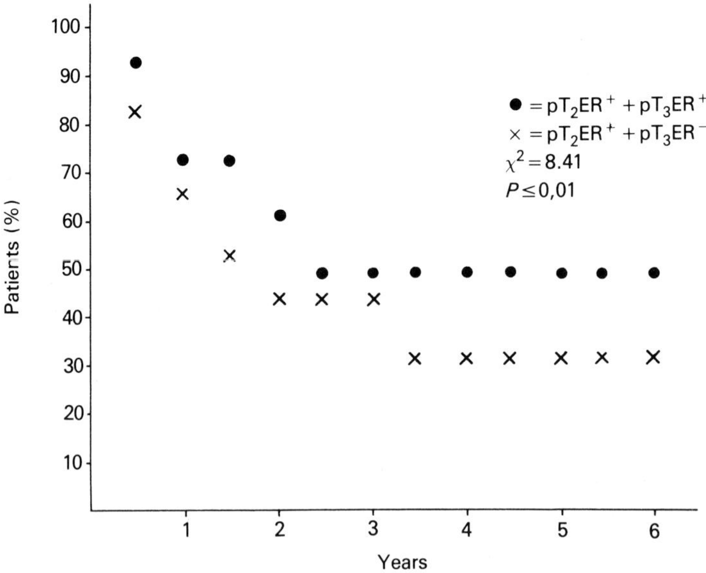

Fig. 2. Overall life expectancy in 2 groups of patients nephrectomized for RCC, and treated with MPA, with ER-positive (●) and ER-negative (x) tumours.

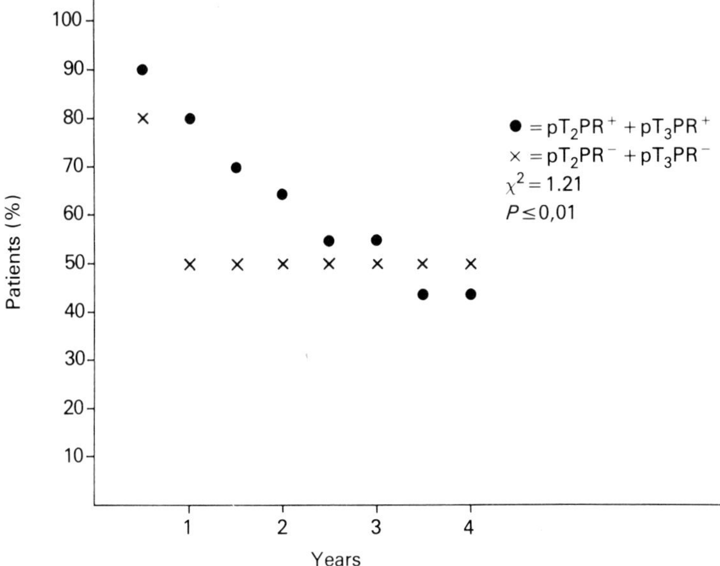

Fig. 3. Overall life expectancy in 2 groups of patients nephrectomized for RCC, and treated with MPA, with PR-positive (●) and PR-negative (x) tumours.

cy was found to be higher in ER-positive than in ER-negative patients after the third year of follow-up (Fig. 2), but was higher in PR-positive than in PR-negative patients only during the first 2 years of follow-up (Fig. 3).

Recent data on the value of determination of nuclear AR status has led us to investigate whether the favourable action of MPA on RCC patients could be particularly related to the presence of the nuclear AR, which are responsible for the androgenic activity of MPA. Progestins could, in fact, counteract the tumour growth-promoting effect of oestrogens via nuclear AR. The clinical response to MPA treatment is, therefore, at present being evaluated mainly in patients with RCC in which nuclear AR can be demonstrated, allowing the relationship between nuclear AR and hormone-responsiveness to be studied. ER and PR status have been shown to be related to hormone dependence in renal tumours [20].

In addition, recognizing that the 'positive' hormonal effect sought is only prolonged survival, not an effect conforming to current rigorous oncological criteria, a controlled study in 2 homogeneous groups of RCC patients is in progress, in an attempt to establish the predictive value of steroid receptor status, and confirm the efficacy of high dose progestin treatment in RCC patients.

Acknowledgement

Thanks are extended to Drs Antonietta Marocchi and Giuseppina Margiotta of the Istituto di Clinica Medica Generale e Terapia Medica V for their work on receptor analyses, and to Drs Raffaele Tenaglia, Ermanno Pannunzio and Giuseppe La Pera of the Cattedra di Patologia Urologica for their help with follow-up studies and statistical analyses.

References

1. Concolino, G., Di Silverio, F., Marocchi, A. et al. (1978): Human renal cell carcinoma as a hormonedependent tumor. *Cancer Res. 34*, 4340.
2. Sufrin, G., Mirand, E.A., Moore, R.H. et al. (1977): Hormones in renal cancer. *J. Urol. 117,* 433.
3. Gibbons, R.P., Montie, J.E., Correa, R.J. and Mason, J.T. (1976): Manifestations of renal cell carcinoma. *Urology 8*, 201.
4. Terada, M. (1927): Changes in ovaries and other organs in animals injected with various substances. *Jpn. Med. World 7,* 233.
5. Bullock, L.P. and Bardin, C.W. (1977): Androgenic, synandrogenic and antiandrogenic actions of progestins. *Ann. N.Y. Acad. Sci. USA, 286*, 321.
6. Matsuda, M., Osafune, M., Kotake, T. and Sonoda, T. (1976): A clinical study on renal cell carcinoma. *Jpn. J. Urol. 67*, 635.
7. Wynder, E.L., Mabuchi, C.H. and Whitmore, W.F., Jr. (1974): Epidemiology of adenocarcinoma of the kidney. *J. Natl. Cancer Inst. 53,* 1619.
8. Bartley, O. and Hultquist, G.T. (1950): Spontaneous regression of hypernephromas. *Acta Pathol. Microbiol. Scand. 27*, 448.
9. Bloom, H.J.G. (1973): Hormone-induced and spontaneous regression of metastatic renal cancer. *Cancer (Philadelphia) 32*, 1066.
10. Mostofi, F.K. (1967): Pathology and spread of renal cell carcinoma. In: *Renal Neoplasia,* p. 63. Ed: J.S. King Jr. Little Brown and Company, Inc., Boston.
11. Di Silverio, F., Concolino, G., Giacobini, S. et al. (1977): Significato ed importanza dei recettori steroidei nella terapia dei tumori ormono-dipendenti delle vie urinarie. *Prog. Med. 33,* 249.
12. Concolino, G., Marocchi, A., Conti, C. et al. (1980): Endocrine treatment and steroid receptors in urological malignancies. In: *Hormones and Cancer,* p. 403. Eds: S. Iacobelli, R.J.B. King, H.R. Lindner and M.E. Kippman. Raven Press, New York.
13. Hogan, T.F. (1979): Hormonal therapy of renal cell carcinoma. In: *Endocrinological Cancers,* vol. II, p. 69. Ed: G. Rose. CRC Press Inc. Boca Raton.
14. Bracci, U. and Di Silverio, F. (1976): Attuali orientamenti nella diagnosi e terapia dei carcinomi del rene: l'ormonodipendenza. In: *Atti della Società Italiana di Urologia,* Vol. I, p. 167. Ed: C. Corbi. Tripi De Maria, Rome.
15. Walker, S. and Duncan, D.B. (1967): Estimation of the probability of events as a function of several independent variables. *Biometrika 54,* 167.
16. Breslow, N. (1970): A generalized Kruskal-Wallis test for comparing sample subjects to unequal patterns of censorship. *Biometrika 57,* 579.

17. Mantel, N. (1966): Evaluation of survival data and two new rank order statistics arising in its consideration. *Cancer Chemother. Rep. 50,* 163.
18. Mantel, N. and Haenszel, W. (1959): Statistical aspects of the analysis of data from retrospective studies of diseases. *J. Natl. Cancer Inst. 22,* 719.
19. Bracci, U., Di Silverio, F. and Concolino, G. (1981): Hormonal therapy of renal cell carcinoma. In: *Proceedings of the First International Symposium on Kidney Tumor, Paris, November 9–11, 1981.* Eds: R. Küss, G.P. Murphy, S. Khoury and J.P. Karr. Alan R. Liss, Inc., New York. (In press.)
20. Concolino, G., Marocchi, A., Toscano, V. and Di Silverio, F. (1981): Nuclear androgen receptor as marker of responsiveness to medroxyprogesterone acetate in human renal cell carcinoma. *J. Steroid Biochem. 15,* 397.

High-dose medroxyprogesterone acetate in patients with advanced renal cell carcinoma

H. Wicklund
Department of Oncology, University Hospital, Uppsala, Sweden

Introduction

Metastatic renal cell carcinoma has been highly resistant to most therapeutic approaches, and has an extremely poor prognosis [1–3]. Hormonal treatment has been reported to induce subjective and objective improvement [2, 4–10]. Some evidence of regression in metastatic tumours treated with medroxyprogesterone acetate (MPA) at various dosages has been observed [2, 6, 8, 9, 11–15]. The aim of this pilot study, which has been in progress from September 1980 to December 1981, was to assess the clinical effect of high-dose MPA in patients with advanced renal cell carcinoma, and how well treatment was tolerated.

Material and methods

The material consisted of 12 patients, 9 males and 3 females, with histologically-proven renal cell carcinoma and metastases. The mean age of the patients was 59 years (range 30–75 years). Ten of the 12 patients had undergone nephrectomy, and 2 patients had previously been treated with tamoxifen and 1 patient with MPA, orally. Seven patients had been subjected to palliative irradiation. At the time of MPA treatment, 2 patients had bone metastases, 1 had lymph node metastases, 2 had pulmonary and bone metastases, and all the others had very disseminated disease, with metastases in 3 or more organs. In 6 patients the disease first became evident via metastases. Nine patients died from the disease within 1.5–10 months of the beginning of MPA treatment. The median Karnofsky performance index was 40 (range 20–70).

The patients were treated with 500 mg of MPA administered intramuscularly (i.m.) daily for 5 days a week, for a period of 6 weeks and then with a maintenance dose of 1 g a week until progression of disease was detected. Before MPA therapy was started a physical examination was carried out, haemoglobin, leucocyte count, platelet count, liver function, serum creatinine, serum glucose, and serum electrolyte status determined the urinary sediment examined microscopically, chest radiography, isotope-scanning of the liver, skeleton and brain, and ultrasonic and computed tomography examinations of the abdominal and pelvic cavities were performed. These examinations were repeated regularly during MPA treatment.

During treatment, plasma concentrations of MPA were measured every week. Blood samples were taken immediately prior to each MPA injection. MPA was determined by radioimmunoassay using an antiserum prepared by Cornetti et al. [16]. The method used has been described by Hesselius and Johansson [17].

The criteria for evaluation of response were:

Complete remission (CR): complete disappearance of all lesions for a period of at least 3 months.

Partial remission (PR): 50% reduction in the area of all measurable lesions.

Minimal remission (MR): 25–50% decrease in the area of one measurable lesion, with no change in the others, for at least one month.

No change (NC): no marked change in size of measurable lesions, or less than 25% decrease in area.

Progression (P): a 25% increase, in the area of at least one measurable lesion, or appearance of new lesions.

Subjective response: increase in appetite and sensations of well being. The subjective response was also correlated with the Karnofsky performance index.

Results

The therapeutic outcome is summarized in Table I.

Three patients responded with minimal objective remissions lasting for a median period of 3 months (range 2–4 months). One of these patients, who relapsed after 4 months, is still alive 10 months after the start of MPA treatment, and in very good subjective condition. This patient had lymph node metastases in the left supraclavicular fossa and in the left axilla. These nodes decreased in size but, after 4 months, there was progression in the retroperitoneal nodes. For a period of 2 months, one patient exhibited a decrease of 25% in the size of one metastasis located in the left iliac fossa. During the same period there was no progression of his pulmonary metastases. A regression in size of about 30% occurred in a metastasis located

Table I. Results of MPA therapy in 12 patients.

Therapeutic outcome	Numbers of patients	Duration of remission (months)		Alive but relapsed
		Median	Range	
Complete remission	0			
Partial remission	0			
Minimal remission	3	3	(2–4)	1
No change	0			
Progression	9			
Subjective improvement	9	4	(2–10)	3

Table II. Side-effects of treatment with MPA in 12 patients.

Side-effect	Numbers of patients
Hypercalcaemia	2
Thrombosis	1
Alopecia	1
Sweating	1

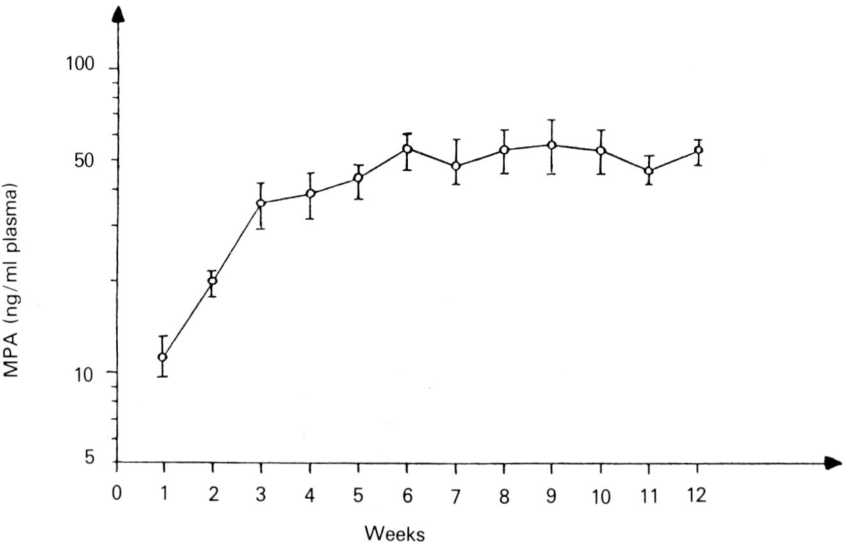

Figure. Plasma concentrations of MPA in 9 patients treated with 500 mg of MPA administered i.m. daily for 5 days a week for 6 weeks, followed by 1 g weekly. (Mean ± SEM.)

in the thyroid gland of one patient but, after 3 months, progression of his pulmonary metastases was observed. Subjective improvement was seen in 9 of the 12 patients. As measured by the Karnofsky performance index, there were subjective improvements of 10–20 points (mean 15). The mean duration of subjective improvement was 4 months (range 2–10 months).

The therapy was well tolerated, and no severe side-effects were seen (Table II). In 2 patients who had exhibited slight increases in serum calcium levels before MPA treatment, levels increased still further during treatment. One patient, who was confined to bed with paraparesis, developed a thrombosis in her right leg. One patient developed partial alopecia and one patient complained of sweating. No side-effects were seen at the injection sites.

Although plasma levels of MPA showed great interindividual variation, mean plasma concentration curves all had similar shapes. During the loading phase, when MPA was being administered at the rate of 500 mg once a day, i.m., MPA plasma levels increased steadily from a mean of 11 ng/ml to a mean of 53 ng/ml. During the maintenance phase, however, when MPA was being administered at a dose of 1 g once a week, i.m., the plasma levels remained fairly constant at 50–55 ng/ml (Figure).

Discussion

High-dose MPA treatment, when used alone, seems in this pilot study to have an extremely low objective response rate in advanced renal cell carcinoma. The percentage of cases showing subjective improvement is relatively high, and the degree of palliation seems to be fairly good, with no severe side-effects. Subjective improvement is, however, difficult to evaluate and can depend on many other factors, for example better general medical care.

No definite conclusions can be made from this pilot study, but MPA, when used alone, can not be considered effective in the treatment of advanced renal cell carcinoma. The next step could be a trial of a combination of high-dose MPA and chemotherapy.

The MPA concentration level studies show that the dosage schedule used, with daily i.m. loading doses followed by weekly i.m. maintenance doses, produces a rapid increase in MPA levels, which is important for achieving an effect as quickly as possible in these patients with advanced renal carcinoma.

References

1. Middleton, R.G. (1967): Surgery for metastatic renal cell carcinoma. *J. Urol. 97,* 973.

2. Morales, A., Kiruluta, G. and Lott, S. (1975): Hormones in the treatment of metastatic renal cancer. *J. Urol. 114,* 692.
3. Bellinger, M.F., Koontz, Jr. W.W. and Smith, M.J.V. (1979): Renal cell carcinoma: Twenty Years of Experience. *Virginia Med. Monthly 106,* 819.
4. Bloom, H.J.G., Dukes, C.E. and Mitchley, B.C.V. (1963): Hormone-dependent tumours of the kidney, I. *Br. J. Cancer 17,* 611.
5. Bloom, H.J.G., Baker, W.H., Dukes, C.E. and Mitchley, B.C.V. (1963): Hormone-dependent tumours of the kidney, II. *Br. J. Cancer 17,* 646.
6. Samuels, M.L., Sullivan, P. and Howe, C.D. (1968): Medroxyprogesterone acetate in the treatment of renal cell carcinoma (hypernephroma). *Cancer 22,* 525.
7. Talley, R.W., Moorhead, E.L.II., Tucker, W.G. et al. (1969): Treatment of metastatic hypernephroma. *J.Am.Med.Assoc. 207,* 322.
8. Paine, C.H., Wright, F.W. and Ellis, F. (1970): The use of progesterone in the treatment of metastatic carcinoma of kidney and uterine body. *Br. J. Cancer 24,* 277.
9. Wagle, D.G. and Murphy, G.P. (1971): Hormonal therapy in advanced renal cell carcinoma. *Cancer 28,* 318.
10. Van der Werf-Messing, B. and van Gilse, H.A. (1971): Hormonal treatment of metastases of renal carcinoma. *Br. J. Cancer 25,* 423.
11. Bloom, H.J.G. (1971): Medroxyprogesterone acetate (Provera) in the treatment of metastatic renal cancer. *Br. J. Cancer 25,* 250.
12. Von Lieven, H. and Hahn, D. (1977): Die Behandlung des metastasierenden hypernephroiden Nieren Karzinoms mit Medroxyprogesteroneazetat (Clinovir). *Münch. Med. Wochenschr. 119,* 1089.
13. Pannuti, F., Martoni, A. and Cricca, A. (1978): Pilot study of treatment of renal clear-cell carcinoma by high doses of medroxyprogesterone acetate (MAP). *IRCS Med. Sci. Cancer 6,* 177.
14. Bono, A.V., Benvenuti, C., Gianneo, E. et al. (1979): Progesterone in renal cell carcinoma. *Eur. Urol. 5,* 94.
15. Rao, M.K. and Soloway, M.S. (1980): Medroxyprogesterone in metastatic renal cell carcinoma. *South. Med. J. 73,* 247.
16. Cornette, J.C., Kirton, K.T. and Duncan, G.W. (1971): Measurement of medroxyprogesterone acetate (Provera) by radioimmunoassay. *J. Clin. Endocrinol. Metab. 33,* 459.
17. Hesselius, I. and Johansson, E.D.B. (1980): Medroxyprogesterone acetate (MPA) plasma levels after oral and intramuscular administration in a long-term study. *Acta Obstet. Gynecol. Scand. Suppl. 101,* 65.

Combined chemotherapy and hormonal therapy in metastatic renal adenocarcinoma. A controlled trial

S.A. Engelholm, M. Kjaer, S. Walbom-Jørgensen and H.H. Hansen
The Radiumstation, The Finsen Institute, Copenhagen, Denmark

Introduction

The prognosis in metastatic renal adenocarcinoma is extremely poor. Many antineoplastic agents and hormones have been employed in the treatment of this disease. Response rates following single agent chemotherapy vary from 5–16%. Following progestational agents the response rate is 8%, and following androgens it is 3% [1]. In view of the toxicity of chemotherapy, coupled with the low expectation of objective response to such therapy, we conducted a pilot study on a relatively atoxic therapeutic regimen consisting of vinblastine (VLB) and medroxyprogesterone acetate (MPA). Objective response was demonstrated in 6 out of 16 patients (37%). Encouraged by these results, we therefore designed a controlled trial to compare this regimen with a combination of cytotoxic agents which have shown some activity in metastatic renal carcinoma, namely, cyclophosphamide (CTX), lomustine (CCNU), and hydroxycarbamide (HDU). The purpose of the study was to compare response rates, durations of response, durations of survival, and toxicity of the 2 regimens.

Material

Fifty-two patients (29 male, 23 female) of mean age 58.5 years (range 32–69), took part in the trial. All patients had histologically proven renal adenocarcinoma, and all patients had been nephrectomized. No patients had previously received chemotherapy or hormonal therapy.

Methods

All patients had metastatic disease meeting the following criteria:

Lung metastases Demonstrated by chest X-ray but not proven histologically.

Bone metastases Demonstrated by a Tc^{99} radioisotope scintigram, followed by roentgenographic evaluation of suspected foci, together with bone marrow biopsy and aspiration according to Radner [2], in all patients. Bone metastases not demonstrated by X-ray or biopsy were disregarded.

Liver metastases Demonstrated, in cases of abnormal liver function tests or liver enlargement, by ultrasonic scanogram and fine needle biopsy, or peritoneoscopy with liver biopsy. Liver metastases not verified by biopsy were disregarded.

Other locations Demonstrated by biopsy or fine needle aspiration of lymph nodes, skin, and laparotomy scars. Only histological evidence of metastases was accepted. One case of contralateral renal metastases was demonstrated by angiography and ultrasonic fine needle aspiration.

Treatment

Patients were allocated at random (using the sealed envelope procedure) to one of the following treatments, after informed consent had been obtained:

Regimen 1 VLB, 6 mg/m^2 intravenously (i.v.), weekly. MPA 500 mg intramuscularly (i.m.), weekly.

This regimen was continued for 10 weeks, after which the patients were re-evaluated. In cases of progression of disease, cross-over to regimen 2 (see below) was performed. In cases of response or no change treatment continued with administration of VLB every 4 weeks, and MPA weekly.

Regimen 2 CCNU, 70 mg/m^2 per os (p.o.), on day 1, CTX, 700 mg/m^2, i.v., on day 1, and HDU, 2 g/m^2, p.o., on days 15, 18 and 21.

Treatment was repeated every 4 weeks. This treatment continued until progression occurred, when cross-over to regimen 1 was undertaken.

Dose reduction MPA was given in the doses stated, throughout the study. In the case of the cytotoxic agents, the doses mentioned were reduced by 50% if the white blood cell count (WBC) was 2,500 to 2,900/mm^3 and/or the thrombocyte count was 50,000 to 99,000/mm^3. If the WBC was 2,500/mm^3 or less, and/or the thrombocyte count was 50,000/mm^3 or less, treatment was discontinued until the heamatological values regained their original levels.

Other forms of therapy Radiotherapy was allowed only in cases of brain metastases or symptomatic bone metastases. Corticosteroids were administered in cases in which there was increased intracranial pressure, or hypercalcaemia.

Evaluation of response

The following criteria were used to evaluate response:

Partial response (PR) A regression of a measurable/evaluable parameter of more than 50% in the absence of progression elsewhere, or occurrence of fresh lesions.

Complete response (CR) Complete disappearance of all evidence of disease.

Statistical evaluation

Survival rates were calculated as described in references 3 and 4. Comparisons were performed using the log-rank test. Findings were regarded as statistically significant at the 5% level.

Results

Three patients were excluded from evaluation because of major protocol violations. Of the remaining 49 patients, 24 had received regimen 1, and 25 patients regimen 2. The characteristics of patients in the 2 groups with regard to sex, age and metastatic foci are shown in Table I. No significant differences existed between the groups.

Response

Four out of 24 patients (16%) responded objectively (2 CR, 2 PR) to regimen 1, and 2 out of 25 (8%) (1 CR, 1 PR) to regimen 2. Under regimen 1, one patient with lung metastases and one patient with bone metastases experienced CR, and 2 patients with bone metastases experienced PR. Under regimen 2, one patient with a soft tissue lesion on the chest wall, and bone metastases, experienced CR, and one patient with lung metastases experienced PR. Three males and 3 females responded to treatment.

The median duration of response was 267 days (range 125–1,100 days), with no significant differences between the 2 regimens.

Table I. Characteristics of patients.

	Regimen	
	1	2
Number of patients evaluable	24	25
Sex		
Female (%)	45	45
Male (%)	55	55
Ages (years)		
Median	60.6	58.2
Range	50–69	32–69
Number of patients with metastatic foci in locations indicated		
Bone	10	5
Bone marrow	1	1
Liver	2	2
Renal (contralateral)	0	1
Distant lymph nodes	1	2
Skin	2	1
Lung	16	17

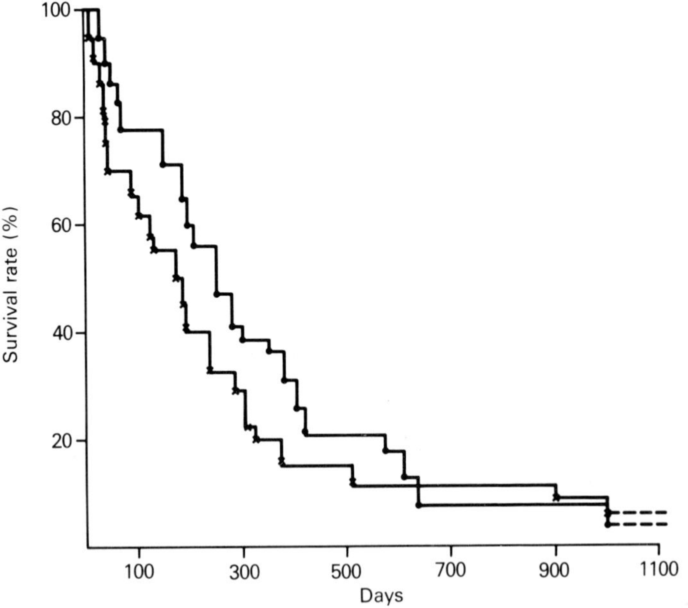

Fig. 1. Survival rates in relation to treatment in 49 patients with renal adenocarcinoma. •———• = VLB + MPA, ×———× = CTX + CCNU + HDU.

Survival rates in relation to treatment are shown in Figure 1. Patients receiving regimen 1 had a significantly longer median survival period (250 days) than patients receiving regimen 2 (129 days) ($P<0.05$). No difference in long-term survival rates could be demonstrated.

In Figure 2, the survival rates of the patients according to response are shown. The 6 patients who experienced CR or PR survived significantly longer than the 43 patients who did not respond ($P<0.05$).

Cross-over between the 2 treatment regimens was undertaken in 20 patients (10 from each regimen). Two patients, one from each regimen, experienced a PR or less than 2 months' duration after cross-over.

Toxicity

Regimen 2 was significantly more toxic than regimen 1 with regard to median number of blood transfusions, and median leucocyte and thrombocyte nadir during treatment. ($P<0.01$ for each comparison (Table II).)

Chemotherapy was discontinued in 2 patients on regimen 2 because of toxicity. Discontinuance of therapy was not necessary in any patient on regimen 1.

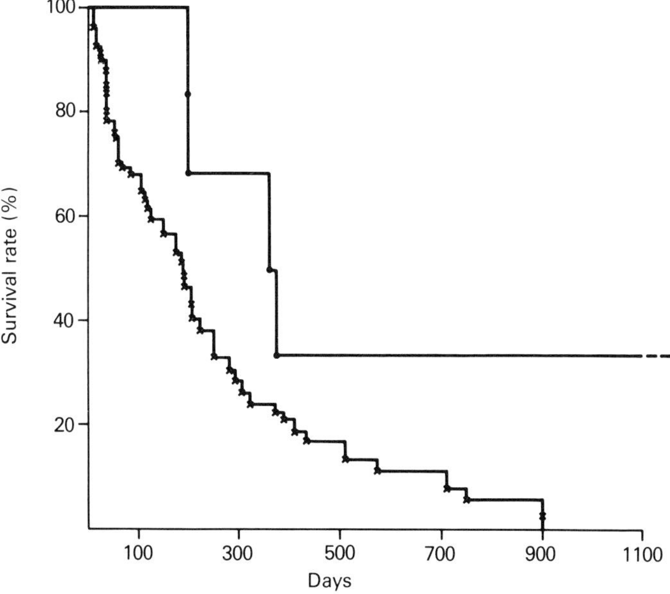

Fig. 2. Survival rates in relation to response in 49 patients with renal adenocarcinoma. •——• = responders, ×——× = non-responders.

Table II. Median minimal WBC and platelet count values, and median numbers of blood transfusions in patients on the 2 regimens.

	Regimen	
	1	2
Leukocytes × 10^3	2.9	1.1
Platelets × 10^3	282	144
Median numbers of blood transfusions	14	17

Discussion

The overall response rate in the trial (6 out of 49 patients, 12%) was disappointingly low, but confirmed the results of earlier studies [1]. We were unable to achieve the 37% response rate seen in our pilot study with VLB + MPA.

Metastatic renal adenocarcinoma is a condition with a wide range of clinical courses, extending over a few months, or up to 50 years [4]. The disease is, on the whole, unaffected by treatment. One finding from the present study is noteworthy. Patients treated with VLB + MPA had a significantly longer median survival period than patients treated with combination chemotherapy. The response rate with VLB + MPA, 16%, equals response rates with the most active single agents in this disease [1]. In view of the lack of toxicity of VLB + MPA, it would seem justified to treat patients with VLB + MPA until new and more potent agents can be identified.

Acknowledgement

The authors would like to thank J. Nyboe, Department of Medical Statistics, Rigshospitalet, for help and advice concerning the statistical evaluation of the data.

References

1. Luderer, R.C., Opipari, M.I. and Perrotta, A.L. (1978): Treatment of metastatic renal cell carcinoma: Review of experience and world literature. *J. Am. Osteopath. Assoc. 77*, 590.
2. Hansen, H.H. (1974): *Bone Metastases in Lung Cancer. A Clinical Study of 200 Consecutive Patients with Bronchogenic Carcinoma and its Therapeutic Implications for Small Cell Carcinoma*. Munksgaard, Copenhagen.

3. Peto, R., Pike, M.C., Armitage, P. et al. (1976): Design and analysis of randomized clinical trials requiring prolonged observation of each patient. I. Introduction and design. *Br. J. Cancer 34,* 585.
4. Peto, R., Pike, M.C., Armitage, P. et al. (1977): Design and analysis of randomized clinical trials requiring prolonged observation of each patient. II. Analysis and examples. *Br. J. Cancer 35,* 1.
5. Walter, C.W. and Gillespie, D.R. (1960): Metastatic hypernephroma of fifty years' duration. *Minn. Med. 43,* 123.

Discussion

M. Pavone-Macaluso: With regard to the treatment of renal cell carcinoma, there are several controversial points. Many people may know that some papers published before 1975 showed a very high response rate of between 15 and 25%. On the other hand, papers that have appeared since 1975 reported only 2–5% response rate – and even lower. There must be something unusual; either patients have changed or perhaps the response criteria are different. Of course, this difference has created much discussion about whether or not MPA is an effective treatment in this particular tumour. I think that our discussion will probably bring to light some new data and new ideas.

Another controversial point: if we have an agent such as MPA, which, according to the latest resuls, is not very effective in metastatic disease or in the primary tumour in renal cell carcinoma, can this agent reasonably be employed as an adjuvant treatment following nephrectomy? In other cancers, if we have a combination of chemotherapeutic agents which does not lead to complete regression or leads to partial regression at a rate less than 40%, this drug or combination of drugs is very unlikely to be used in the adjuvant situation. Yet, Dr Concolino reported that the survival of patients after radical nephrectomy for renal carcinoma is much better with the addition of MPA than without anything at all. Again, this is controversial.

A third controversial point is the presence of receptors. Dr Concolino works in Rome with a very competent team. If they say that they have found receptors in a high percentage of their tumours, we must believe them. On the other hand, however, other workers, in Germany and the U.S.A. for example, have been unable to compare their results with those from the group in Rome. There are, therefore, many topics to discuss.

A. Beni (Rome, Italy): Apart from my congratulations concerning the design of the study and the statistical elaboration of the data, I would like to ask Dr Concolino a question relative to the 60% survival achieved if I am not mistaken, in 5 years. I would like to know whether this is a 'disease-free' survival time or not?

Furthermore, I would like to ask Dr Wicklund why she has not considered controlling the glycaemia also, as, in our experience, often a preclinical diabetic becomes clinically evident during MPA treatment?

G. Concolino (Rome, Italy): The 5-year survival was related to the disease-free interval of the patients. At the beginning of our studies, we considered a tumour-free interval to be a positive effect of therapy. As I said in my presentation, that may not be such a rigorous oncological criterion as is now being used in considering complete or partial remission. But if one wants to get an answer about the effect of this type of treatment in mainly patients with no other metastatic disease, taking only that event into consideration, it provides an answer – which, up to now, seems to be 'yes' in the patients who are receptor-positive.

In answer to Professor Pavone-Macaluso's remarks about our receptor findings in Rome, I would like to say that other workers in Paris and the U.S.A. recently published data comparable with ours. Initially, in Milan, they were unable to measure oestradiol, progesterone and androgen receptors, but they are doing that now and are approaching our present stage.

I would also like to make it clear that the receptor mechanisms are effective in the kidney, as is shown with the tamoxifen challenge test.

H. Wicklund: In answer to Dr Beni's questions, I would first like to say that we have measured serum glucose values weekly, and they appeared to be normal. Secondly, we do not know why the patient developed alopecia; she had received no other drugs that might have explained its occurrence.

S. Fosså (Oslo, Norway): We must be very cautious in claiming anything about a response to MPA if there are no more than 3 out of 12 patients responding and this is only a minimal response. This result might be within the limits of spontaneous regression. Professor van der Werf-Messing, in Sicily, showed a 22% spontaneous regression rate. Other people have not observed such a high rate – but nobody looks carefully at spontaneous regression. Usually, the patients stay at home until they die – they do not come back to the doctor, 3-weekly x-rays of the chest are not performed (as they are in patients receiving therapy). I think that what is needed is a comparative phase-II or a phase-III study comparing MPA – or anything else – with no treatment, but the control arm should have x-rays and other examinations as often as the treatment arm.

G. Concolino: I agree with Dr Fosså, but may I remind her that on this topic of spontaneous regression, other workers only found a 0.8% spontaneous regression rate.

S. Fosså: That is because no one ever looks at the patients who do not get any treatment. X-rays are not taken at 3-weekly intervals – these patients just stay at home. Spontaneous regression will not be found if it is not looked for.

M. Pavone-Macaluso: The spontaneous regressions were only in the lungs; there were no regressions in bone or in other organs. Even in patients treated with MPA I do not know of any regression demonstrated elsewhere than in the lungs.

H. Bojar (Düsseldorf, Federal Republic of Germany): I think Dr Concolino will agree with me that receptor analysis in human renal cell carcinoma, as performed in the past, did not represent the state of the art. We have a lot of experience with receptor analysis in over 100 human renal cell carcinomas. This work was published some years ago. We did not agree with Dr Concolino's group that there are progesterone receptors in the tissue. It is very dangerous, when measuring a specific binding by dextran-coated charcoal, to jump to the conclusion that progesterone receptors are present. With R-5020, for example, used as a relatively specific ligand, we were able to demonstrate that there is some specific binding. However, the binding components sediment only in the 4S region of the gradients. The experiments failed to induce the progesterone-binding components in the human renal cell carcinomas by oestrogens.

In addition, experiments were done in intact cells. These were binding studies, and they failed to demonstrate significant amounts of progesterone binding. However, a low concentration of glucocorticoid receptors and also a very low concentration of androgen-binding components could be demonstrated. By a variety of techniques it was possible to demonstrate that the androgen-binding components, although present in a low concentration, seem to be hormone receptors. I think it can not be concluded from specific binding experiments that progesterone receptors are present in the tissue.

M. Kjaer: Dr Wicklund showed 3 (what she called) 'minimal' responses in her presentation. First, in what organs were these lesions located? Were they present in lung or in bone?

Secondly, does she think it is possible, both objectively and reproducibly, to measure a 25% regression? People have worked with blind studies for such evaluations, and I think that 25% regression is within the interpersonal variation of such measurements. Nothing can be said about a 25% regression.

H. Wicklund: The measurable lesions were in the lymph nodes and the thyroid gland. I agree that it is rather difficult to measure a 25% regression.

J.G.M. Klijn: With regard to hypercalcaemia, in her abstract Dr Wicklund mentioned 2 patients with increasing plasma calcium levels. It was demonstrated earlier in this meeting that the main effect of MPA is a corticosteroid-like effect. It is known that corticosteroids are useful in the treatment of malignant hypercalcaemia because of the decreasing prostaglandin levels and of other osteoclast-stimulating factors that result from their use. In those 2 patients, were parathyroid hormone (PTH) levels measured? It is known that corticosteroids have no effect on hypersecretion of PTH, and therefore on hypercalcaemia.

H. Wicklund: Both patients had disseminated bone metastases, and were changed to corticosteroid treatment, but we have not measured PTH.

M. Pavone-Macaluso: The message that we are left with is that we must demonstrate the efficacy of MPA in renal cell carcinoma. It still remains doubtful and, of course, the story of receptors is an extremely interesting avenue for research. When there is another meeting on MPA, we will probably hear some more definitive comments on this particular topic.

Medroxyprogesterone acetate, diethylstilboestrol and cyproterone acetate in the treatment of prostatic cancer. Interim report of a prospective study of the European Organization for Research on the Treatment of Cancer (EORTC) Genito-urinary Tract Co-operative Group*

M. Pavone-Macaluso[1], M. De Pauw[2], S. Suciu[2], R. Sylvester[2], H. de Voogt[3], B. Lardennois[4], A. Nasta[5], R. Zolfanelli[6], E. Barasolo[6] and the EORTC Urological Group**

[1]Polyclinic Hospital, School of Medicine, University of Palermo, Palermo, Italy; [2]EORTC Data Centre, Brussels, Belgium; [3]Free University of Amsterdam, Amsterdam, The Netherlands; [4]Maison Blanche Hospital, Reims, France; [5]Ospedale Civile Umberto I, Mestre; and [6]S. Andrea Hospital, Vercelli, Italy

Introduction

New forms of drug treatment are presently under investigation as alternatives to conventional oestrogenic therapy in advanced prostatic cancer, particularly since the cardiovascular toxicity of high doses of oestrogens is now clear.

The value of orchidectomy or hormonal treatment of prostatic cancer still remains controversial, as do the indication for these measures. In our present state of knowledge, it is not possible to lay down any firm rules as to the best treatment at the various stages of the disease. This is especially true in situations such as poorly differentiated carcinomas, or cancers unresponsive to hormonal treatment as a result of either primary resistance or relapse [1].

*Reproduced in part from the Proceedings of the International Symposium on the Role of Medroxyprogesterone Acetate (MPA) in Endocrine-related Tumors (1982), by kind permission of the editors (L. Campio, G. Robustelli Della Cuna and R.W. Taylor) and the publishers (Raven Press, New York).
**A list of the other participants in this study is given at the end of this paper.

Although oestrogen therapy is an effective form of treatment, the enthusiasm for it has been decreased by the discovery of its cardiovascular side-effects, and it is well known that oestrogen treatment does not lead to permanent cure. Objective regression can be demonstrated in less than half the treated cases. Oestrogen treatment is, therefore, basically a palliative measure, but may have a fairly prolonged effect, and lead to stabilization in a relatively large number of cases. There is obviously a need to investigate new kinds of hormonal treatment for prostatic cancer in the hope of discovering new therapies displaying higher efficacy and lower incidences of side-effects. Unfortunately, the majority of published papers on hormonal therapy deal with small series of patients, and are lacking in control groups, and variable criteria of response have been used.

The Genito-urinary Tract Co-operative Group of the EORTC has begun a series of prospective, controlled clinical trials in recent years, in the hope of obtaining at least some answers to as yet unresolved questions. Medroxy-progesterone acetate (MPA) was one therapeutic component in trial number 30761, the results of which have been submitted to preliminary analysis. The study was begun in February 1977, and enrolment stopped in April 1981 after 295 patients had been enrolled. The results of the most recent analysis are reported here.

Aim of the study

The aim of this study, the coordinator of which was M. Pavone-Macaluso, was to compare diethylstilboestrol (DES), MPA and cyproterone acetate (CPA) in a controlled manner with regard to objective response, duration of remission, toxicity and survival in patients with advanced prostatic cancer.

Drugs employed

DES is the oestrogen conventionally used in the U.S.A., U.K., and some other European countries. It is no longer commercially available in Italy or in Germany.

MPA, like other progestational agents, inhibits release of luteinizing hormone (LH), and decreases plasma testosterone levels and testosterone synthesis. As shown by Massa and Martin, it also acts directly upon prostatic tissue by inhibiting 5-α-reductase, thereby reducing the formation of androstanolone (DHT) in normal and neoplastic prostatic cells [2]. A few pilot studies demonstrated MPA to be active in prostatic cancer. In 1972, Ferulano et al. described a number of palliative and objective responses [3]. In 1976,

Denis and Leclerq [4] and Bouffioux [5] obtained similar results. A co-operative study in Italian urological institutions showed that, in 62 evaluable patients, an objective response was obtained in 38.7% of patients, and stabilization in another 37% of patients [6]. It is of interest that responses were obtained even in patients in a state of relapse after initially favourable responses to orchidectomy and/or oestrogenic treatment. In the controlled Veterans' Administration Co-operative Urological Research Group (VACURG) study III [7], 30 mg of MPA daily was not significantly inferior to 1 mg of DES per day. Better results were not obtained by combining DES and MPA.

CPA, apart from inhibiting LH release, acts by competitive inhibition of androgen receptors in target tissues. Since the reports published by Bracci and Di Silverio [8] and Giuliani [9], it has gained considerable popularity in Italy, where it is usually employed in conjunction with orchidectomy. It has not yet been accepted in the United States as a treatment for prostatic cancer.

Admission criteria

Only patients who had not undergone hormonal treatment or orchidectomy previously were eligible for this study. All patients had histologically confirmed, locally advanced, prostatic carcinoma (categories T3 and T4), with or without distant metastases. Patients with a life expectancy of less than 90 days, and those with severe cardiovascular disease contra-indicating oestrogenic treatment were not eligible for the study.

Dosage and administration of hormonal therapy

Patients were allotted at random to one of 3 groups. The treatment given to patients in the 3 groups consisted of 3 mg of DES daily, (1 mg every 8 hours, per os (p.o.)), 500 mg of MPA intramuscularly (i.m.), 3 times a week, for 8 weeks, followed by 100 mg of MPA twice daily, p.o., or 250 mg of CPA daily, p.o.

Patients received a minimum of 2 months' treatment, followed by initial evaluation of response to therapy. In cases in which response had occurred, treatment was continued until progression, with follow-up evaluations 6 months after the start of treatment, and every 6 months thereafter. In the case of patients with stable disease at 2 months, further treatment was at the investigator's discretion. However, the majority of such patients continued with their initial treatment.

Table I. Response criteria.

Complete remission:
1. Absence of any clinically detectable soft tissue tumour mass.
2. Recalcification of any osteolytic lesions present.
3. No evidence of progression of any osteoblastic lesions present.

Partial remission:
1. Significant decrease in size of at least 50% in all soft tissue lesions.
   - measurable lesions: decrease of 50% in the product of the 2 largest tumour dimensions.
   - nonmeasurable lesions: reduction of at least three-quarters in the estimated volume.
2. Recalcification of some osteolytic lesions, if present.

(Complete and partial remission:)
No increase in any other lesion, and no new areas of malignant disease.
No significant (>10%) deterioration in weight, no significant deterioration in symptoms or performance status (one score level).
Return of elevated acid phosphatase values to normal levels.
If hepatomegaly was taken a significant indicator, there had to be a reduction in liver size and a 30% improvement, at least, in all abnormal pretreatment liver function values.

No change:
No new lesions, and no increases in size of any lesion.
No significant deterioration in weight, symptoms or performance status.

Progression:
Any increase in size of any lesion, or appearance of any new lesion, regardless of response of other lesions.
Significant deterioration in symptoms, decrease in weight, or decrease in performance status.
(Increases in acid or alkaline phosphatase values alone were not considered as indication of progression).

Response criteria

Response to treatment, classified as CR (complete remission), PR (partial remission), NC (no change) or PD (progressive disease) was assessed by each participating investigator in accordance with the criteria in Table I.

Preliminary results

A total of 295 patients were enrolled in urological institutions in Austria, Belgium, France, Italy, The Netherlands, Portugal, Spain and the U.K.

Table II. Reasons for withdrawal from study (numbers of patients).

Reason	Therapy			
	CPA	MPA	DES	Totals
Progression (including deaths resulting from prostatic cancer)	26	35	24	85
Lost to follow-up	16	8	6	30
Ineligibility*	4	9	6	19
Treatment refused	6	5	3	14
Death (not due to cancer)	4	2	4	10
Excessive toxicity	1	3	2	6
Protocol violations	1	1	1	3
Other reasons	3	4	8	15
Patients remaining in study	42	34	37	113
Totals	103	101	91	295

*Ineligibility was mainly due to previous hormonal treatment, which was one of the criteria for exclusion according to the protocol.

Table III. Overall response rates (numbers of patients).

Treatment	CR	PR	NC	Progression	Totals	Percentage of CR + PR
CPA	2	15	14	21	52	33
MPA	—	10	23	23	56	18
DES	7	18	18	14	57	44
Totals	9	43	55	58	165	32

Significances of differences in overall response rates: MPA vs DES, $P<0.005$; CPA vs DES, $P<0.32$; CPA vs MPA, $P<0.12$.

About half the patients were treated in urological centres in Italy.

The current status of the study is shown in Table II. Of the patients enrolled, 29% have left the study because of progression, or death resulting from malignant disease. A preliminary analysis of objective response to treatment and of toxicity has been undertaken.

The overall objective response rates (CR + PR) observed were 44% for DES, 33% for CPA and 18% for MPA. Only the difference between the response rates for DES and MPA is statistically significant ($P<0.005$). No cases of CR were noted with MPA (Table III).

Table IV. Severity of cardiovascular side-effects reported during treatment (numbers of patients (percentages)).

Severity of cardiovascular side-effects	Treatment			Totals
	CPA	MPA	DES	
None	49	49	36	134 (75)
Not affecting treatment	4	11	18	33 (18)
Requiring cessation of treatment	— (14)	3 (23)	2 (38)	5 (3) (25)
Fatal	4	1	2	7 (4)
Total	57	64	58	179

Significance of difference between 14% incidence of cardiovascular side-effects with CPA and 38% incidence of cardiovascular side-effects with DES: $P<0.01$.

Table V. Incidence of cardiovascular side-effects in relation to previous history of cardiovascular disease (numbers of patients (percentages)).

Previous cardio-vascular disease	Treatment			Totals
	CPA	MPA	DES	
Yes	5/17 (29)	5/26 (19)	10/21 (48)	20/64 (31)
No	3/40 (8)	10/38 (26)	12/37 (32)	25/115 (22)
Totals	8/57 (14)	15/64 (23)	22/58 (38)	45/179 (25)

Significance of difference between 8% incidence of cardiovascular side effects in patients with no previous history of cardiovascular disease treated with CPA and 32% incidence of cardiovascular side-effects in patients with no previous history of cardiovascular disease treated with DES: $P<0.02$.

The overall incidence of cardiovascular side-effects was 25%. The incidences on therapy with CPA, MPA and DES were 14, 23 and 38% respectively (Table IV). The difference between the incidences of cardiovascular side-effects with CPA and DES is significant at $P<0.01$. Patients treated with DES have a significantly higher chance of developing cardiovascular side-effects than patients treated with CPA.

If patients without any cardiovascular history on entry to the study are considered separately (Table V), the frequencies of cardiovascular side-effects reported during treatment are found to be 8, 26 and 32% for CPA, MPA and DES, respectively. The difference between CPA and DES is, again, significant

Table VI. Types of cardiovascular complications (numbers of patients (percentages)).

Types of cardiovascular complications	Treatment			Totals
	CPA	MPA	DES	
Ischaemic cardiopathy	2	4	6	12 (27)
Thromboembolic disease	2	4	6	12 (27)
Fluid retention	4	4	10	18 (40)
Other	—	1	—	1
Not specified	—	2	—	2
Totals	8/57	15/64	22/58	45/179

Table VII. Painful gynaecomastia (numbers of patients).

Treatment	Total number of patients	Painful gynaecomastia
CPA	52	3
MPA	52	3
DES	52	21 (40%)
Totals	156	27

($P<0.02$). The figures in the table suggest that only patients with no previous history of cardiovascular disease develop significantly fewer cardiovascular side-effects when treated with CPA than with DES. In the patients with a history of cardiovascular disease, no statistically significant difference was observed in incidence of cardiovascular side-effects between the 3 treatments, although the data indicate that this group of patients tended to develop fewer cardiovascular side-effects when treated with MPA than with DES ($P<0.11$). No other significant differences between the treatments were observed.

The cardiovascular side-effects reported during treatment involved mainly fluid retention (40% of instances) in the form of heart failure, hypertension, oedema and dyspnoea. Ischaemic heart disease (infarct, right bundle branch block, ventricular ectopic beats) and venous thromboembolism (thrombophlebitis, deep venous thromboembolism, cerebrovascular accidents, pulmonary embolism) were reported in 27% of the patients (Table VI).

As regards other side-effects, painful gynaecomastia was more frequent in DES-treated patients than in patients treated with either MPA or CPA (Table VII).

Conclusions

In previously untreated patients with advanced prostatic cancer, DES appears to be no worse than the newer hormonal compounds. It is certainly cheaper, and shows a statistically significant superiority over MPA. However, 3 mg of DES per day is accompanied by cardiovascular toxicity in an appreciable proportion of patients.

The present data from the EORTC Genito-urinary Tract Co-operative Group appear to indicate, therefore, that MPA is not a treatment to be employed as first choice in the majority of patients with previously untreated adenocarcinoma of the prostate, at the dosage employed in this trial, at least. However, our own pilot studies, as well as those of other investigators, indicate that MPA may be of value in inducing a response in about one-third of patients in relapse after initial response to oestrogens. It may be a useful alternative in patients with a history of cardiovascular disease.

CPA does not appear to be superior to DES in previously untreated patients, but it is active and its relatively low incidence of cardiovascular side-effects is noteworthy. Its value in association with orchidectomy is currently being evaluated by the EORTC Genito-urinary Tract Co-operative Group in a study in which orchidectomy alone is being compared with orchidectomy plus CPA, and with 1 mg of DES per day.

Investigators participating

J. Frick (Austria), C. Bouffioux, C. Schulman (Belgium), B. Lardennois, J. Guerrin (France), M. Pavone-Macaluso, C. Bondavalli, M. Laudi, F. Merlo, V. Nadalini, A. Nasta, M. Porena, C. Viggiano, E. Visentini, R. Zolfanelli, E. Barasolo (Italy), H. de Voogt, J. Alexieva-Figusch (The Netherlands), F. Calais da Silva (Portugal), J.A. Martinez-Pineiro, E.A. Barrilero, L. Resell-Esteve (Spain), P.H. Smith, D. Newling, B. Richards, M.R.G. Robinson (United Kingdom).

References

1. Chisholm, G.D. and Pavone-Macaluso, M. (1980): Cancer of the prostate; advances in diagnosis and treatment. Report of a round table discussion held at the Third Congress of the European Association of Urology, Monte Carlo, June 16, 1978. *Eur. Urol. 6,* 197.
2. Massa, R. and Martini, L. (1971–72): Interference with the 5 alpha-reductase system. A new approach for developing antiandrogens. Hormones and antagonists. *Gynecol. Invest. 2,* 253.

3. Ferulano, O., Petrarola, F. and Castaldo, A. (1972): Trattamento del cancro della prostata con il controllo ormonico dell'arco diencefalo-ipofisario. *Minerva Urol. 24,* 274.
4. Denis, L. and Leclerq, G. (1978): Progestogens in prostatic cancer. *Eur. Urol. 4,* 162.
5. Bouffioux, C. (1976): Traitement du cancer de la prostate par les agents progestatifs. *Acta Urol. Belg. 44,* 336.
6. Pavone-Macaluso, M., Melloni, D., La Piana, E. et al. (1978): La terapia del carcinoma prostatico con medrossiprogesterone acetato. Dati bibliografici e risultati preliminari. *Urologia 45*, 595.
7. Byar, D. (1977): Preliminary experience with 30 mg daily of medroxyprogesterone (abstract). In: *The Tumours of the Genito-urinary Apparatus*, p. 275. Ed: M. Pavone-Macaluso. Cofese, Palermo.
8. Bracci, U. and Di Silverio, F. (1979): Terapia chirurgica ed ormonale del carcinoma prostatico, In: *Terapia dei Tumori Ormonodipendenti,* pp. 173–201. Eds: U. Bracci and F. Di Silverio. Acta Medica Ciarrapico, Rome.

High-dose medroxyprogesterone acetate in the treatment of advanced prostatic carcinoma. A preliminary report

T. Nilsson
Department of Urology, Helsingborg Hospital, Helsingborg, Sweden

Introduction

The hormonal treatment of prostatic carcinoma has aroused increasing interest ever since Huggins demonstrated the hormonal responsiveness of the tumour in 1941 [1]. In 1967, the Veterans' Administration Cooperative Urological Research Group report appeared [2]. This questioned the use of oestrogens and aroused further interest. Today, it seems to be accepted that prostatic carcinoma at the localized stages, not giving rise to symptoms, should not be treated with oestrogens. The side-effects of oestrogen treatment are considered to be worse than any palliative effect in such cases. In the course of the search for therapeutic compounds with fewer side-effects, interest has focused on progestogens [3, 4]. In previous studies, an effect comparable to that of conventional oestrogen therapy has been proven. In this small scale preliminary study, a possible cytotoxic effect of 1-g doses of medroxyprogesterone acetate (MPA) was investigated in patients who were no longer responding to previous therapy. These patients had advanced, progressing prostatic carcinoma.

Methods and results

Between July 1980 and December 1981 successive patients who no longer responded to estramustine phosphate therapy (280 mg twice daily, by mouth), and in whom progression of the disease was clinically evident, were switched to MPA treatment. A daily dose of 1 g of MPA was given intramuscularly for at least 2 weeks. If the patient responded well subjectively or objectively, injections were continued until the patients died. The longest period of treatment was 9 months.

Table I. Diagnosis and treatment.

Patient	Degree of differentiation/ year of diagnosis	Previous treatment and its duration		Duration of MPA treatment	Side-effects of MPA treatment
		Oestrogen	Estramustine phosphate		
1	Poor/1980	—	8 months	5 weeks	None
2	Poor/1979	—	—	4 weeks	None
3	Moderate/1978	3 weeks	12 months	8 months	None
4	Moderate/1972	6 years	18 months	6 months	None
5	Anaplastic/1975	—	3 months (in 1980)	9 months	None
6	Moderate/1978	—	13 months	3 weeks	None
7	Anaplastic/1980	—	1 month	3 months	None
8	Good/1977	—	48 months	4 months	None
9	Moderate/1980	—	6 months	6 weeks	None
10	Unknown/1977	—	40 months	2 months	None
11	Good/1977	6 years	30 months	8 months	Weight gain
12	Good/1974	6 years	1 month	5 months	None
13	Good/1979	—	24 months	4 weeks	None
14	Unknown/1974	6 years	6 months	8 months	Weight gain Symptoms like Cushing's disease
15	Poor/1977	18 months	2 months	7 weeks	None

All patients were categorized as T_4M+ according to the tumour-nodes-metastases staging system. Some of the patients had been treated from the beginning with conventional oestrogen therapy. When this therapy failed they were switched to estramustine phosphate, and, on further progression, MPA was given (Table I).

The number of patients in the trial was 15. Fourteen had failed to respond to estramustine phosphate treatment. The criteria for objective response used were those agreed by EORTC and NPCP. Subjective response was assessed on the basis of clinical judgement, arrived at from the patient's own account of how he felt.

The clinical results are summarized in Tables I and II. Three patients (patients 4, 11 and 14) showed objective signs of regression. In addition, 4 patients (patients 1, 3, 10 and 15) showed normalization of serum acid phosphatase (SAP) levels. Five out of these 7 patients also exhibited subjective responses, mostly in the form of pain relief and improved well-being. All reported increased appetite. Apart from these 5 patients, 3 (patients 5, 8 and 12) reported subjective response, mostly in the form of pain relief.

Side-effects were recorded in 2 patients (patients 11 and 14). The most obvious effects were substantial weight gain and moon face, as occurs after prolonged corticosteroid therapy. Two complications recorded as pulmonary emboli at autopsy might be mentioned under this heading (patients 4 and 10).

Discussion

Once treated hormonally, prostatic carcinoma will always progress and become a therapeutic problem. Estramustine phosphate and cytotoxic compounds are sometimes of value when conventional oestrogen therapy has failed. It could theoretically be worthwhile trying progestogens in these instances. The progestogens should be used in very high dosages, in the expectation of profiting from the cytotoxic effects which have been postulated [5]. Very high doses of progestogens can be given with a very low incidence of side-effects.

The aim of this study was to find out if any objective response to 1 g doses of MPA could be registered clinically in cases of prostatic carcinoma. Fifteen consecutive patients who did not respond to estramustine phosphate therapy were offered this treatment. An objective response was demonstrated in 3 out of 15 patients. The numbers are too small to allow the statistical significance of this finding to be assessed.

Progestogens, apart from their suppressive action on the pituitary, have been postulated to have a direct cytotoxic effect, through inhibition of the binding of dihydrotestosterone to the nucleus. The effect is most pronounced

Table II. Results of MPA treatment.

Patient	Clinical response		Time of survival after MPA treatment	Cause of death	Over-all result
	Subjective	Objective			
1	—	SAP fell to normal level	5 weeks	Uraemia	Nil
2	Nil	Nil	8 weeks	Prostatic carcinoma	Nil
3	Nil	SAP fell to normal level	32 weeks	Prostatic carcinoma	Nil
4	Pain relief. Discharge from hospital	SAP fell to normal level. Serum creatinine level normalized	24 weeks	Pulmonary embolism	Good
5	Pain relief. Micturition normalized	—	32 weeks	Still alive	Good
6	—	—	6 weeks	Prostatic carcinoma	Nil
7	—	—	12 weeks	Prostatic carcinoma	Nil
8	Pain relief. Discharged	—	7 weeks	Prostatic carcinoma	Nil
9	Oedema disappeared	—	7 weeks	Prostatic carcinoma	Nil
10	Pain relief. Discharged	SAP fell to normal level	8 weeks	Pulmonary embolism	Good
11	Pain relief. Discharged	Renal function returned to normal. Rectal tumour disappeared. SAP fell to normal level	32 weeks	Prostatic carcinoma	Very good
12	Pain relief	—	20 weeks	Still alive	Good
13	—	—	9 weeks	Prostatic carcinoma	Nil
14	Pain relief. Epileptic seizure ended	Brain metastases regressed. Pulmonary metastases disappeared. SAP fell to normal level	36 weeks	Still alive	Very good
15	Pain relief	SAP fell to normal level	13 weeks	Still alive	Good

in the case of cyproterone acetate. Our decision to use 1-g doses of MPA in the treatment of advanced prostatic carcinoma was intended as a test of this hypothesis. We knew, from clinical experience with this treatment in other cancerous conditions (ovarian cancer, renal carcinoma) that high doses of this kind have an effect on tumour tissue. Only minor side-effects have been recorded with such therapy. The results obtained in this study so far are interesting, and suggest that a 1-g dose of MPA may have a cytotoxic effect similar to or exceeding that of estramustine phosphate. Apart from the objective response recorded in 3 out of the 15 patients involved, 8 patients felt the treatment had helped them.

Side-effects were negligible. However, in one patient there were striae, substantial weight gain, a moon face and hump like those seen in Cushing's syndrome. In another patient there was weight gain. No cardiovascular side-effects were recorded clinically. However, 2 patients showed pulmonary emboli at autopsy.

The results in this report indicate that MPA may have a cytotoxic effect in 1-g doses. These results require verification by a prospective randomized study. A study using MPA as initial treatment in patients with advanced prostatic carcinoma is in progress.

References

1. Huggins, C. and Hodges, C.V. (1941): Studies on prostatic cancer: effect of castration, of estrogens and of androgen injection on serum phosphatases in metastatic carcinoma of the prostate. *Cancer Res. 1,* 293.
2. Veterans' Administration Cooperative Urological Research Group (1967): Carcinoma of the Prostate. Treatment comparison. *J. Urol. 98,* 516.
3. Bouffioux, C. (1976): Traitement de cancer de la prostate par les agents progestatifs. *Acta Urol. Belg. 44,* 336.
4. Geller, J., Fruchtman, B., Newman, H. et al. (1967): Effect of progestional agents on carcinoma of the prostate. *Cancer Chemother. Rep. 51*, 41.
5. Anderson, D.G. (1972): The possible mechanisms of action of progestins on endometrial adenocarcinoma. *Am. J. Obstet. Gynecol. 113,* 195.

Medroxyprogesterone acetate in prostatic cancer. Five-year results in advanced untreated and oestrogen-resistant cases

C.R. Bouffioux
Urological Department, University of Liège, Liège, Belgium

Introduction

Gutierrez (1949) [1] and Trunnel and Duffy [2] were the first to report favourable results with progestational compounds in prostatic cancer. However, as a result of the success of oestrogens, and because the progestins available were weaker than the oestrogens available, natural progestins did not come to be widely used in the treatment of prostatic cancer.

More recently, the synthesis of new compounds such as medroxyprogesterone acetate (MPA) [3, 4] with high progestational activity, active by the oral route, and well tolerated, has led to the wider use of progestins in the treatment of endocrine-related tumours [5]. Our preliminary studies [6], and pilot trials by other investigators [7–9] have demonstrated objective and subjective responses to MPA in some cases of advanced prostatic cancer, and have prompted controlled trials on a larger scale.

Pavone-Macaluso has reported the preliminary results of trial number 30761, performed by the European Organization for Research on Treatment of Cancer (EORTC) Genitourinary Group [10]. We have reported elsewhere preliminary results arising from a personal study conducted between 1974 and 1976, in which MPA was compared with diethylstilboestrol (DES) in the treatment of advanced, previously untreated prostatic cancer, and with estramustine phosphate (Estracyt®) in the treatment of oestrogen-resistant cancer [11, 12]. The 5-year results of this study are presented here.

Methods

Forty previously untreated patients with advanced prostatic cancer of stage C (tumour-nodes-metastases classification T_{3-4} N_xM_0) or stage D (T_{0-4}, N_x, M_1) were treated randomly with either MPA or DES. The treatment schedule used for MPA consisted of loading doses of 500 mg intramuscularly, 2–4 times weekly, for 2 weeks, followed by maintenance doses of 100 mg per os (p.o.), daily. DES was given in doses of 3–5 mg, p.o., daily. Equal numbers of patients received the 2 drugs.

Thirty patients in a state of relapse during oestrogen therapy were given MPA or estramustine phosphate. The treatment schedule used for MPA was as described above. In the case of estramustine phosphate, a loading dose of 560–840 mg was given daily, p.o., for 2 weeks, followed by a maintenance dose of 280 mg, daily, p.o.

The response criteria were very similar to those used subsequently in EORTC trial number 30761. The patients were followed up every 3 months until progression and/or death. The side-effects of treatment were recorded.

In both the MPA/DES comparison and the MPA/estramustine phosphate comparison, the distribution of tumours of different stages and grades was essentially the same between treatment groups.

Results

Results were assessed in terms of subjective and objective response, duration of response (time until progression) and survival. In connection with results relating to survival, it must be remembered that there was a switch to various treatments (cyproterone acetate, estramustine phosphate, chemotherapy, corticotherapy), with varying degrees of success, if patients showed progression under the treatment first used.

Untreated cases – MPA vs DES

The subjective response takes into account general status, degree of pain (if present) and ease of micturition. Seventeen patients out of the 20 in each group exhibited subjective improvement. In patients showing subjective response, the mean duration of response was 18 months in the MPA group, and 24 months in the DES group.

For assessment of objective response, we used parameters similar to those proposed in EORTC studies 30761 and 30762 [10]. Objective responses were classified as complete remission (CR), partial remission (PR), no change (NC) or progressive disease (PD). We observed an immediate 40% objective response rate with MPA, and an immediate 60% objective response rate with DES (Table I).

Table I. Objective response (numbers of patients).

	MPA	DES
CR	0/20	1/20
PR	8/20	11/20
NC	9/20	6/20
PD	3/20	2/20

Table II. Survival periods (numbers of patients).

Duration of survival (years)	MPA			DES		
	Numbers of survivors out of original 20 patients	Causes of death		Number of survivors out of original 20 patients	Causes of death	
		Cancer	Other		Cancer	Other
1	19	1	0	16	2	2
2	15	3	2	14	3	3
3	8	9	3	11	5	4
4	4	12	4	8	7	4
5	2	14	4	5	10	5

After 5 years, 4 patients in the MPA group had died from a cause other than cancer (2 cardiovascular disease, one respiratory disease, one unknown cause). Fifteen patients had shown progression of disease during treatment. Fourteen of these had died of cancer. Among these 15 patients, the mean duration of objective remission was 14.5 months. In the DES group, 5 patients had died of a cause other than cancer (4 cardiovascular disease, one liver disease). Thirteen patients had shown progression of disease under treatment. Ten had died of cancer. Among these 13 patients, the mean duration of objective remission was 19.8 months.

The duration of survival is illustrated in Table II and in the Figure.

Of the 2 patients alive in the MPA group after 5 years, one showed no signs of progression of disease. In the DES group, 5 patients were alive after 5 years, 2 without signs of progression of disease.

As regards side-effects, one patient in the MPA group complained of mild gynaecomastia, with tenderness of the nipples. Nine patients in the DES group had painful gynaecomastia. No significant gastro-intestinal disturbances

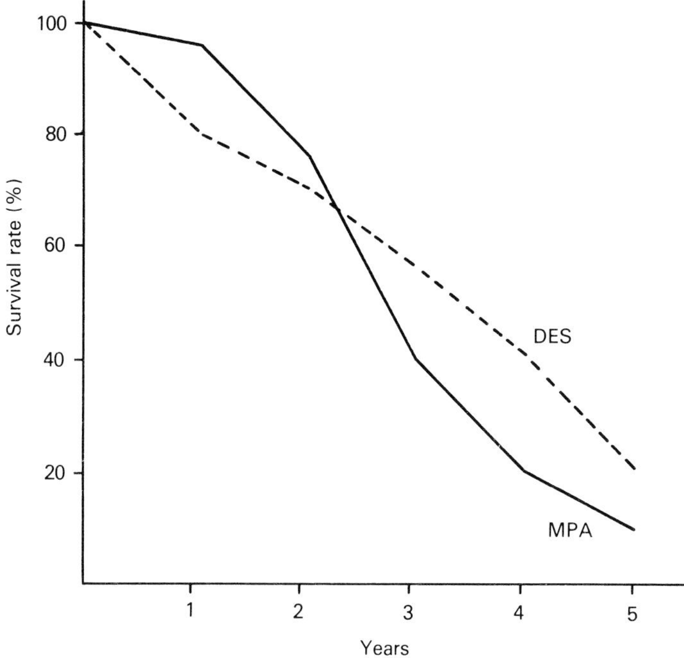

Figure. Percentage survival rates over a 5-year period in prostatic cancer patients treated with MPA or DES.

necessitating discontinuance of treatment were observed. The incidence of deaths from cardiovascular disease is recorded above. No conclusions can be drawn from these statistics.

Oestrogen-resistant cases – MPA vs estramustine

The 30 patients in this study had relapsed on oestrogen therapy. Most had widespread distant metastases. Fourteen received MPA. A. Of these, 6 did not show any response to treatment. Their disease continued to progress, and 2 died shortly after. In 4 patients, treatment was changed to estramustine. Two did not show any response. The other 2 showed significant subjective improvement, for 7 and 9 months, respectively. These 2 patients died 12 and 15 months after therapy had been begun. B. Six patients showed a subjective response to MPA, lasting for periods of 3–9 months (mean 5.5 months). Four of these then received estramustine. One patient did not respond and one showed subjective remission for a period of 8 months. In the remaining 2 pa-

Table III. Results of treatment of oestrogen-resistant prostate cancer cases with MPA or estramustine (numbers of patients).

Response to therapy	MPA	Estramustine
None	6	5
Transient subjective response	6	6
Partial objective remission	2	5
Totals	14	16

tients, objective remissions were observed for periods of 8 and 15 months. C. Two patients showed partial objective remission on MPA, lasting for 6 and 12 months, respectively.

Of the 16 cases who received estramustine; A. 5 did not show any response. Four of these were then treated with MPA, which resulted in a short-lasting, mild, subjective improvement in 2 cases, for periods of 2 and 4 months, respectively. B. Six patients showed subjective responses only, lasting for 10 months on average. At the end of the period of subjective response, 5 patients were given MPA. No response was recorded in 3 patients, but 2 exhibited objective and subjective improvement for periods of 6 and 8 months. C. In 5 patients, estramustine therapy resulted in objective partial remission for periods of 4–17 months. In one of these patients, MPA had a pain-relieving effect for some months after estramustine therapy had ceased to be effective (Table III).

Conclusions

We would not presume to draw firm conclusions from our studies. The numbers of patients are too small to allow the statistical significance of differences to be assessed. Nevertheless, our clinical experience, the published data of Denis and others [7–13], and preliminary results in EORTC trial 30761 indicate that MPA, although not inactive, is less efficient than DES in the treatment of previously untreated advanced prostatic cancer. Objective remission is less frequent, and the periods of remission shorter.

In oestrogen-resistant cases, estramustine therapy results in a higher remission rate than MPA therapy, but the latter, in some cases, gave good results for some months, even in instances in which estramustine had proved ineffective.

One advantage of MPA therapy is that it is normally well tolerated. It does not result in gynaecomastia, or testicular atrophy. The risk of cardiovascular complications seems less than with DES, but this aspect still needs clarifying.

MPA should, in future, be considered for use as additional hormonal treatment, not as sole, primary therapy in the treatment of prostatic adenocarcinoma.

References

1. Gutierrez, R. (1949): New horizons in surgical management of carcinoma of the prostate gland. *Am. J. Surg. 78*, 147.
2. Trunnel, J. and Duffy, B. (1950): Influence of certain steroids on behaviour of human prostatic cancer. *Trans. N.Y. Acad. Sci. 12,* 238.
3. Sala, G., Camerino, B. and Cavallero, C. (1958): Progestational activity of 6-alpha-methyl-17-alpha-medroxyprogesterone acetate. *Acta Endocrinol. 29*, 508.
4. Babcock, Y., Gutsell, E., Heve, N., Hogg, Y., Stucky, Y., Barnes, W. and Dublin, W. (1958): 6-α-methyl-17-α-medroxyprogesterone-17-acylates: a new class of potent progestins. *J. Am. Chem. Soc. 80*, 2904.
5. Iacobelli, S. and Di Marco, A. (1980): *Role of Medroxyprogesterone in Endocrine-related Tumors,* p. 29. Raven Press, New York.
6. Bouffioux, C. (1976): Traitement du cancer de la prostate par les agents progestatifs. *Acta Urol. Belg. 44,* 336.
7. Denis, L. and Leclerq, G. (1978): Progestogens in prostatic cancer. *Eur. Urol. 4*, 162.
8. Ferulano, O., Petrarola, F. and Castaldo, A. (1972): Trattamento del cancro della prostata con il controllo ormonico dell'arco diencefalo-ipofisario. *Minerva Urol. 24,* 274.
9. Pavone-Macaluso, M., Melloni, D., La Piana, E. et al. (1978): La terapia del carcinoma prostatico con medrossiprogesterone acetato. *Urologia 45*, 595.
10. Pavone-Macaluso, M., De Pauw, M., Suciu, S. et al. (1982): Medroxyprogesterone acetate, diethylstilboestrol and cyproterone acetate in the treatment of prostatic cancer. Interim report of a prospective study of the European Organization for Research on the Treatment of Cancer (EORTC) Genito-urinary Tract Co-operative Group. In: *Proceedings of an International Symposium on Medroxyprogesterone Acetate*, pp. 436–444. Eds: F. Cavalli, W.L. McGuire, F. Pannuti, A. Pellegrini and G. Robustelli Della Cuna. Excerpta Medica, Amsterdam.
11. Bouffioux, C. (1979): Le cancer de la prostate. Rapport présenté au XLIVe Congrès de la S.B.U. *Acta Urol. Belg. 47*, 189.
12. Bouffioux, C. (1980): Treatment of prostatic cancer with medroxyprogesterone acetate (MPA). In: *Bladder Tumors and Other Topics in Urological Oncology,* p. 463. Eds: M. Pavone-Macaluso, M.A. Smith and F. Edsmyr. Plenum Publishing Corporation, New York-London.
13. Denis, L. and Bouffioux, C. (1982): *Progestins in Prostatic Cancer.* (In press.)

Discussion

M. Pavone-Macaluso: I think that the papers presented so far seem to be in some agreement that perhaps neither MPA nor estramustine phosphate is probably the drug of choice as an initial treatment in previously untreated patients. Not only are they more expensive but they are also not more efficacious than the conventional treatment with oestrogens. In the present ongoing study of the European Organization for Research on Treatment of Cancer (EORTC) orchidectomy is now being compared with low-dose oestrogens. Both MPA and estramustine phosphate, however, seem to be of interest in the relapsing patients. This has also been shown elsewhere. I think that Dr Andersson (who is present here) and the Swedish group have also confirmed in another randomized trial that there is no difference between oestrogens and estramustine phosphate in previously untreated patients. Again, they stress that perhaps a cheaper and more conventional method should remain the treatment of first choice, leaving MPA or estramustine phosphate as a second choice in relapsing patients.

It is of some interest to emphasize that many patients receiving MPA had some interesting degree of palliation, even if they showed no objective remission.

Another topic to discuss is whether the correct dose of MPA is being used. Our friends from Bologna said that we have used *low-dose* MPA. When breast cancer is being treated, much higher doses are used, so perhaps our results in prostatic cancer could be improved by using higher doses – but nobody knows because nobody has tried to do it.

I was very interested to hear Professor Nilsson's comments, which are again in agreement that MPA can be a valuable tool in patients who relapse, even after estramustine phosphate treatment. So, MPA is not something to forget about, but probably not something to use as a first-choice therapy.

We do not want to have a secondary prolactin rise in patients treated with hormones. Contrary to oestrogens or cyproterone acetate, MPA produces no increase in serum prolactin, so there is no need to add any antiprolactin agent in MPA-treated patients.

Finally, diethylstilboestrol given 3 times daily gives rise to some cardiovascular side-effects. This had not been known previously, although it was known that 5 mg was dangerous. It was thought that 1 mg a day was almost innocuous from the point of view of cardiovascular toxicity, and also that 3 mg 3 times a day produced a low level of plasma testosterone, which remains constant throughout the day. Certainly, some degree of cardiovascular toxicity has been observed with the latter regimen.

E. Bercovich: With regard to the dose, I think that both the EORTC and Dr Bouffioux's trials are a little unfair to MPA. This is because the other drugs are given in high doses – i.e., high doses of diethylstilboestrol and of cyproterone acetate – whereas MPA is given in very low doses which, I believe, are below the pharmacologically effective level of this drug.

S. Fosså: From the VACURG studies it is known that no hormonal treatment prolongs or reduces cancer-related survival in patients. Even no treatment gives the same survival rate. Therefore, the design of any trial in which survival is compared between 2 hormonal treatments is wrongly designed. At best, hormonal therapy only leads to palliation in these patients, so the question to be asked is much more whether the palliation effect is as good in the 2 or 3 treatment arms. It is not really very important to know what the local response is if the patient is asymptomatic, but in symptomatic patients we want to know whether the palliative effect of the hormonal treatment is as good. In the treatment regimens for the primary hormonal treatment of prostatic cancer, these aspects must be much more seriously considered. I have seen a partial response in 5 patients when MPA has been used as a second-line treatment, but I have never seen an objective remission among 80 patients treated with estramustine phosphate. I think, therefore, that MPA is a drug which should be considered more as a secondary treatment.

M. Pavone-Macaluso: I think that Dr Fosså is in agreement with our point of view. With regard to palliation and response criteria, the present EORTC trial considers time to progression as the sole criterion for response. We believe it is more critical than survival – as Dr Fosså pointed out. We now treat only metastatic patients.

E. Robinson: I think that stage-III patients were also included in the trials. Would the same be done now? Following the results from the Stanford group, and also from our own group, which show a 70% 5-year disease-free survival in prostatic carcinoma using radiotherapy, is there now any justification for giving hormone therapy, bearing in mind both the complications and Dr Fosså's comments?

M. Pavone-Macaluso: I think Dr Robinson is probably right – and perhaps I have already answered in replying to Dr Fosså. The present EORTC study considers only patients who have distant metastases, not the T3 and T4 patients without distant metastases. Of course, irradiation is known to be a very valuable tool in the treatment of those patients. The one difficult point with regard to the value of irradiation is that the T3 and T4 patients have about 40–50% and 70–80% metastatic involvement of the lymph nodes, respectively. No radiologist has so far been able to answer the question whether the lymph nodes are really cured by irradiation. It is known that the primary tumour shows a high response rate after irradiation, but how effective is radiotherapy on the lymph node metastases? To say the least, this has not yet been clearly established. Nevertheless, we believe that irradiation is a very valuable tool for the treatment of the T3 patients in particular. The EORTC is not treating patients without metastases in any hormonal trial.

V.E. Hofmann: When does cardiovascular toxicity occur with the 3 different drugs used?

M. Pavone-Macaluso: Cardiovascular toxicity is a complication that occurs at a relatively early stage, usually within the first year. This is very much in agreement with the data from the Veterans Administration Co-operative Research Group. David Byar showed at the last meeting in Erice (Sicily), that most of the cardiovascular complications due to oestrogens occurred within the first 6 months after starting the treatment.

All I can say about the other 2 substances is that the cardiovascular toxicity occurred within the first year. I do not think it was analysed in the first 6 months – but I hope to be able to answer that question after having visited the Data Centre in Brussels to find out other data about the 2 studies that I have just presented.

G. Concolino: As we have heard yesterday from Professor McGuire, when we are dealing with hormone-dependent tumours, receptor studies ought to be done. I am slightly surprised that none of the 3 speakers has carried out this type of study and, in particular, that no one has tried to compare the effects of the various treatments with their action upon the receptors, which are known to be present in prostatic cancer.

M. Pavone-Macaluso: That is a pertinent remark. However, it should be remembered, first, that these were large co-operative studies involving many centres and, secondly, that our studies were started in 1976 and 1977, respectively. I think that Dr Concolino might agree that the technical aspects of proper receptor determination then, were not as advanced as they are nowadays. But, of course, Dr Concolino is the king of receptors, and if he carries out a similar study he will certainly determine them. It should be done by each laboratory that has the facilities. However, it is difficult to include it in a large co-operative trial involving many hospitals.

L. Beex (Nijmegen, The Netherlands): It is of interest that in one of Professor Nilsson's patients with brain metastases, there was a response on MPA treatment, possibly due to an anti-inflammatory effect of the drug. Has Professor Nilsson (or anybody else) further experience with brain metastases and MPA treatment?

T. Nilsson: My results should be looked upon as more or less anecdotal. I do not know the kind of brain metastases that were present in that patient. We do not know if it *was* a metastasis in his brain – it was a lesion which was visualized on a computed-tomography scan and then disappeared. We have no histologically-proven diagnosis. I have not seen any other brain metastases disappear on MPA treatment.

J.L. Misset (Villejuif, France): With regard to the 2 cases of pulmonary embolism Professor Nilsson reported, was that the main cause of death in those patients, or were they coincidental events in terminal patients? If they were the main cause of death, can pulmonary embolism be considered as a side-effect of the drug?

T. Nilsson: I apologize for not having pointed that out. The 2 pulmonary emboli were detected at autopsy and had nothing to do with the cause of death – but I thought that they should be reported.

L. Andersson (Stockholm, Sweden): It would be interesting to know the extent to which pituitary and testicular function are inhibited by the various forms of treatment. I could not discover from any of the 3 presentations whether the plasma testosterone values are known and whether they decrease to the castration levels. Is the dosage of MPA that is required to have a complete abolition of testosterone production known? Until that is known, it is impossible to discuss what would be an adequate dosage.

M. Pavone-Macaluso: In the EORTC study, all the plasma testosterone levels have been recorded although they have not yet been evaluated. I can say, however, that the MPA-treated patients usually had a plasma testosterone value between 30 and 50 ng/ml (which is more or less the castrate range) on the dose used. It will be interesting to find out whether there is a correlation between the clinical response and the decrease in the plasma testosterone level. We believe that it is of course an important factor, but probably not the only one that is responsible for the clinical response. It is known that an oestrogen, chlorotrianisene, is supposed to be clinically effective in spite of the extremely small reduction in the plasma testosterone levels that it causes. From our preliminary experience we are to believe that 1 mg of diethylstilboestrol is probably as effective as 3 mg – in spite of the fact that, while giving only 1 mg a day, there are wide fluctuations in the plasma testosterone levels, whereas the levels remain stable if the same amount is given every 8 hours.

But are we really treating the patient or the hormonal levels? And how important are the latter? Only when our final evaluation is available, comparing the hormonal levels with the clinical response, will it be possible to answer Dr Andersson's question.

High-dose progestin therapy for advanced ovarian cancer. An updated report

C. Mangioni[1], S. Franceschi[2], F. Landoni[1], C. La Vecchia[2], E. Colombo[1] and P. Molina
[1]Obstetrics and Gynaecological Department, San Gerardo Hospital, Monza, and [2]the Mario Negri Institute of Pharmacological Research, Milan, Italy

Introduction

In spite of a large number of reports claiming effectiveness for various chemotherapeutic regimens in advanced ovarian cancer, survival rates have not changed appreciably in the last 3 decades [1]. The benefits of second line treatment with either single chemotherapeutic agents or very aggressive polychemotherapeutic regimens appear fairly minimal in comparison with their toxic side-effects. Progestins have low toxicity and are reportedly efficacious in malignancies in hormone-dependent tissues (e.g. breast or endometrial cancer), but few studies have yet been conducted allowing evaluation of their activity in epithelial ovarian cancer. A prospective, controlled phase-II study of these agents in a substantial number of ovarian cancer patients, using standardized criteria to define response, has been urged [2]. The reported presence of oestrogen and progestin receptor in 40–70% of ovarian cancers [3, 4], gives further support to the biological rationale for such a study. In the First Obstetric and Gynaecological Clinic of the University of Milan, and in the Obstetric and Gynecological Department of the San Gerardo Hospital in Monza, high-dose medroxyprogesterone acetate (MPA) has been given since July 1978 to all patients with advanced ovarian cancer no longer responding to surgery, radiation therapy or conventional cytotoxic chemotherapy. The present paper is an up-to-date report of findings, which have been previously published, in part [5].

Patients and methods

From July 1st 1978 to December 31st 1981, a total of 103 patients, aged from

28 to 76 (median age 59) with advanced epithelial ovarian cancer were given high-dose MPA, orally (p.o.) or intramuscularly (i.m.).

Patients without measurable disease were ineligible. All patients enrolled had received at least one course of polychemotherapy. Seventy-three had received 2 or more courses. Two patients had received only cyclophosphamide, because old age and low performance status precluded their being treated with other cytotoxic drugs. Sixteen patients were not evaluable because they died within one month of starting therapy. In all, 87 patients were evaluable.

The main characteristics of the 2 groups of patients are listed in Table I.

Patients were categorized according to histological grade of tumour (Broders grades 1 and 2, 30 patients; Broders grades 3 and 4, 57 patients).

Table I. Patient characteristics.

	Route of administration	
	P.o.	I.m.
Age		
Median	58	59
Range	33–76	28–75
Karnofsky index (numbers of patients (%))		
≤50	5 (13)	11 (23)
60–80	21 (54)	28 (58)
90–100	13 (33)	9 (19)
Histological category (numbers of patients (%))		
Serous	21 (54)	30 (43)
Endometrioid	8 (20)	10 (21)
Clear cell	4 (10)	— —
Mucinous	3 (8)	3 (6)
Undifferentiated	3 (8)	5 (10)
Histological grade (numbers of patients (%))		
1–2	15 (38)	14 (29)
3–4	24 (62)	34 (71)
Totals	39 (100)	48 (100)

From July 1978 to September 1980 patients in each category were allocated at random to one of the following 2 MPA regimens:
1. 800 mg daily, p.o. for at least 12 weeks (33 patients)
2. 500 mg daily, i.m., for the first 4 weeks; 500 mg twice weekly, i.m., for the second 4 weeks and 500 mg once weekly i.m. for the next 4 or more weeks (33 patients).

Since October 1980, when the first analysis of results revealed a significantly higher response rate in the group treated i.m., the 800-mg p.o. regimen has been withdrawn. The maintenance dose in the i.m. schedule was increased to 500 mg twice weekly (15 patients). Recently, a higher dose p.o. regimen (2000 mg daily) has begun to be tested.

Response was classified according to the following criteria:
Partial response: ≥ 50% decrease in size of measurable lesions (for at least 3 months);
Minimal response: < 50% but ≥ 25% decrease in size of measurable lesions (for at least 3 months);
Stable disease: < 25% decrease or < 25% increase in size of measurable lesions (for at least 3 months);
Progression: ≥ 25% increase in size of measurable lesions, or appearance of lesions at new sites.

Karnofsky's index was used to evaluate subjective status at the beginning of therapy. Sixteen patients (18.4%) had an index of ≤ 50; 49 patients (56.3%) an index between 60 and 80, and 22 patients (25.3%) an index ≥ 90. Subjective improvement was defined as a Karnofsky index improvement of at least 20 points.

Results

As reported in Table II, there were 7 partial or minimal responses in the 48 patients of the group treated i.m. (15%). The durations of these responses were 5, 5, 6, 8, 11.5 + and 9 + months. No partial or minimal response was obtained in patients treated p.o. (χ_1^2 with continuity correction = 4,32; $P < 0.04$). Seven patients had stable disease (2 p.o., 5 i.m.; durations 3, 3, 4, 3, 3, 5 and 7 + months). The mean duration of survival of partial and minimal responders (10.7 months) and of patients with stable disease (7.6 months) was longer than that for patients in progression (3.3 months).

Among the 58 less differentiated tumours, there were 4 cases of partial or minimal response, and 5 cases of stable disease. Three partial and minimal responses were observed among the 29 better differentiated tumours. The histological findings shown in Table II reveal a slightly better responsiveness

Table II. Response in relation to histotype and route of administration.

Histological category of tumour	Partial and minimal responses	Stable disease	Progression
I.m. administration (numbers of patients)			
Serous	4	2	24
Endometrioid	2	1	7
Clear cell	—	—	—
Mucinous	—	1	2
Undifferentiated	1	1	3
Totals (%)	7 (15)	5 (10)	36 (75)
P.o. administration (800 mg dose) (numbers of patients)			
Serous	—	1	16
Endometrioid	—	1	7
Clear cell	—	—	4
Mucinous	—	—	2
Undifferentiated	—	—	2
Totals (%)	—	2 (6)	31 (94)
P.o. administration (2,000 mg dose) (numbers of patients)			
Serous	—	3	1
Endometrioid	—	—	—
Clear cell	—	—	—
Mucinous	—	—	1
Undifferentiated	—	—	1
Totals (%)	—	3 (50)	3 (50)

among endometrioid tumours (2 partial or minimal responses and 2 cases of stable disease among 18 patients), but the difference is not statistically significant. Overall, subjective improvement was noted in 25% of patients.

MPA treatment was well tolerated by both the i.m. and p.o. routes. No haematological toxicity and no significant alterations in serum electrolyte values or liver enzyme levels were observed during monthly checks. Only one patient suffered from a gluteal abscess. Administration was changed from the parenteral to the oral route, as a result.

Discussion

Our findings to date confirm our previous observation that high-dose MPA, given i.m., can induce objective response in about one out of 7 ovarian cancers refractory to other treatments. Such a result, though hardly exciting in absolute terms, can be considered to have some clinical implications, having regard to the fact that the patients in this study had already been extensively treated with other chemotherapeutic regimens, and the likelihood of their benefiting from any conventional chemotherapeutic agent was poor. Except for the performance status index which was slightly better in the p.o.-treated group, the characteristics of the groups of patients receiving MPA by the 2 routes (Table I) were very similar, but no patient receiving MPA p.o. responded to treatment, suggesting that systemic bio-availability after administration of 800 mg p.o. daily is not sufficient to achieve or maintain drug levels [6]. Even with a very high p.o. dosage (2,000 mg daily) no objective responses have been observed. However, the number of patients enrolled (6) is too low to permit conclusions to be drawn. Studies by Malkasian, though also relating to a very small number of patients, also suggested that the efficacy of MPA when given p.o. is low [7].

Earlier studies had indicated that high-dose i.m. progestin therapy might be effective in ovarian cancer, but the results of these studies were difficult to assess, since patient numbers were limited [4, 7–11], or because the progestins were combined with other hormones or cytotoxic drugs [4, 12].

Recently, Ehrlich treated 24 patients with advanced or recurrent endometrial adenocarcinoma with progestin, having previously determined oestrogen and progestin receptor levels. He recorded one complete response, and 6 partial responses in 8 patients who were progestin receptor-positive, but only one complete response of 16 patients who were progestin receptor negative [13]. Two recent phase-II studies have shown only a minimal effect of MPA in refractory ovarian cancer [14, 15]. Our slightly better results, in which the response rate was 15% are, however, not statistically significantly different from those in other studies.

The results obtained justify further studies, with a view to determining more precisely the efficacy of MPA, not only in endometrioid ovarian cancer, where some activity is to be expected on the basis of its structural similarity to endometrial cancer, but also in the other histotype, where some effect has been observed. Determination of the progestin receptor status of ovarian cancer cells, together with MPA plasma levels, may help to define those tumours likely to be susceptible to endocrine therapy, and the most efficacious therapeutic schedules.

References

1. Editorial (1980): *The Lancet II,* 1010.
2. Tobias, J.S. and Griffiths, C.T. (1976): Management of ovarian carcinoma (second of 2 parts). *N. Engl. J. Med. 294,* 877.
3. Holt, J.A., Caputo, T.A., Kelly, K.M. et al. (1979): Estrogen and progestin binding in cytosol of ovarian adenocarcinoma. *Obstet. Gynecol. 53,* 50.
4. Bergquist, A., Kullander, S. and Thorell, J. (1981): A study of estrogen and progesterone cytosol receptor concentration in benign and malignant ovarian tumors and a review of ovarian tumors treated with medroxyprogesterone acetate. *Acta Obstet. Gynecol. Scand. Suppl. 101,* 75.
5. Mangioni, C., Franceschi, S., La Vecchia, C. and D'Incalci, M. (1981): High-dose medroxyprogesterone acetate (MPA) in advanced epithelial ovarian cancer resistant to first or second-line chemotherapy. *Gynecol. Oncol. 12,* 314.
6. Hesselius, H. and Johansson, E.D.B. (1981): Medroxyprogesterone acetate (MPA) plasma levels after oral and intramuscular administration in a long-term study. *Acta Obstet. Gynecol. Scand. Suppl. 101,* 65.
7. Malkasian Jr., G.D., Decker, D.G., Jorgensen, E.O. and Webb, M.J. (1973): 6-dehydro-6, 17 alpha-dimethylprogesterone (NSC-123018) for the treatment of metastatic and recurrent ovarian carcinoma. *Cancer Chemother. Rep. 57*, 241.
8. Ward, H.W. (1972): Progesterone therapy for ovarian carcinoma. *J. Obstet. Gynaecol. Br. Commonw. 79,* 555.
9. Malkasian Jr., G.D., Decker, D.G., Jorgensen, E.O. and Edmonson, J.H. (1977): Medroxyprogesterone acetate for the treatment of metastatic and recurrent ovarian carcinoma. *Cancer Treat. Rep. 61*, 913.
10. Jolles, B. (1962): Progesterone in the treatment of advanced malignant tumors of breast, ovary and uterus. *Br. J. Cancer 16,* 209.
11. Varga, A. and Heriksen, E. (1964): Effect of 17-alpha-hydroxyprogesterone 17-n-caproate on various pelvic malignancies. *Obstet Gynecol. 23,* 51.
12. Guthrie D. (1979): The treatment of advanced cystoadenocarcinoma of the ovary with gestronol and continuous oral cyclophosphamide. *Br. J. Obstet. Gynecol. 86,* 497.
13. Ehrlich, C.E., Young, P.C.M. and Clear, R.E. (1981): Cytoplasmic progesterone and estradiol receptors in normal, hyperplastic, and carcinomatous endometria: therapeutic implications. *Am. J. Obstet. Gynecol. 141,* 539.
14. Slyton, R.E., Pagano, M. and Creech, R.H. (1981): Progesterone therapy for advanced ovarian cancer: a phase II Eastern Cooperative Oncology Group trial. *Cancer Treat. Rep. 65*, 895.
15. Aabo, K., Pedersen, A.G., Hald, I. and Dombernowsky, P. (1982): High-dose MPA in advanced chemotherapy-resistant ovarian carcinoma: a phase II study. *Cancer Treat. Rep. 66,* 407.

Discussion

C. Tropé: There are only 3 good phase-II studies on chemoresistant ovarian cancer. Slayton's study was one which showed no response, and Professor Mangioni's showed a 15% response. The third is the study from Lund with more than 25 patients participating.

In the Lund study the so-called high-dose MPA was used, given in a dose of 500 mg a day, intramuscularly, for a period of 3 weeks, followed by 500 mg weekly, intramuscularly, for at least 2 months.

The results in the first 25 patients showed that there was no complete remission and one partial remission, with a median duration of 5-plus months, and a median survival of 6-plus months. Fifteen patients had progressive disease.

I think that we could discuss the above results after Dr Maskens' presentation.

Role of medroxyprogesterone acetate in the management of ovarian carcinoma. Programme of the European Organization for Research on the Treatment of Cancer (EORTC) Gynaecological Cancer Co-operative Group (GCCG)

A.P. Maskens[1], J.V. Hamerlynck[2], V.N. Kozyreff[3], I.R. Hesselius[4] and E.E. Johansson[4]

[1]EORTC GCCG, Brussels, Belgium; [2]Antoni van Leeuwenhoek House, Amsterdam, The Netherlands; [3]Clinical Biology Laboratory, St. Etienne Clinic, Brussels, Belgium; and [4]The Academic Hospital, Uppsala, Sweden

Introduction

Progress in the treatment of ovarian carcinoma is taking place in 2 main directions. The first, and probably most promising, direction is concerned with early diagnosis, extensive surgery, and adjuvant therapy.

Unfortunately, however, the majority of cases are first diagnosed after disease has spread beyond the pelvis (stages III and IV of the Fédération Internationale de Gynécologie et d'Obstétrique classification). In most instances of this kind, primary surgery will be limited to partial debulking, at best, leaving significant residual tumour masses.

What is the effect of chemotherapy in this category of patients? A large number of chemotherapeutic regimens have recently been under investigation. They are summarized in Table I, which is based on reports presented at 2 of the major cancer meetings in 1981, the Union Internationale contre le Cancer meeting in Lausanne, and the American Society for Clinical Oncology meeting in Washington [1–11]. The overall response rates obtained with these various treatments range from 29–83% (Table II), with an apparent correlation between the number of drugs used in the combination, and the antitumour effect. This correlation is also evident when complete clinical response rates are taken into consideration (Table III). The latter range from 7–60%. It should, however, be remembered that ovarian cancer is a disease character-

Table I. Ovarian carcinoma stages III/IV (summary, ASCO and UICC meetings, 1981). Chemotherapy regimens.

L-PAM										
L-PAM	+	ADM								
CPM	+	ADM								
CPM	+	ADM	+	CDDP						
CPM	+	ADM	+	CDDP	+	HMM				
L-PAM	+					HMM				
		ADM	+	CDDP						
CPM	+	ADM					+	5-FU		
CPM	+	ADM	+	CDDP	+			5-FU		
CPM	+					HMM	+	5-FU	+	MTX
CPM	+			CDDP	+	HMM	+	5-FU		

Abbreviations: CPM, cyclophosphamide; CDDP, cis-diamminedichloroplatinum; ADM, adriamycin; HMM, hexamethylmelamine; MTX, methotrexate; FU, fluorouracil; L-PAM, melphalan.

Table II. Ovarian carcinoma stages III/IV (summary, ASCO and UICC meetings, 1981). Overall response rates.

Number of drugs in combination	Mean response rate (%)	Range (%)
1	36.5	(29–43)
2	48.1	(44–52)
3	64.2	(57–80)
4	66.9	(52–83)

Table III. Ovarian carcinoma stages III/IV (summary, ASCO and UICC meetings, 1981). Complete response rates.

Number of drugs in combination	Mean response rate (%)	Range (%)
1	15.3	(7–20)
2	27.0	(21–32)
≥ 3	45.8	(39–60)

ized by predominantly intraperitoneal spread, or by extension to the para-aortic nodes; only laparotomy can reliably demonstrate complete remission. Five recent studies give figures for surgically-verified complete response. These range from 12–29%, with durations of response probably in excess of 2 years (Table IV).

Table IV. Ovarian carcinoma stages III/IV (summary, ASCO and UICC meetings, 1981). Surgically-verified complete response rates.

Numbers of patients	Regimen	Complete responders (%)	Duration (months)	Reference
43	CPM + ADM + CDDP	19	18^{+}	[1]
(47)	CPM + ADM + CDDP + HMM	26	$25^{(*)}$	[3]
(47)	CPM + MTX + 5FU + HMM	12	$9^{(*)}$	[3]
51	CPM + CDDP + 5FU + HMM	20	$24^{+(\diamond)}$	[11]
21	CPM + MTX + 5FU + HMM/ ADM + CDDP	29	21^{+}	[8]
34	CPM + ADM + 5FU	16		[6]
18	CPM + ADM + 5FU + CDDP	17		[6]

(*) : progression-free survival of all responders.
(◇): median survival time of responders.
For explanation of other abbreviations see Table I.

Although such findings certainly reflect a significant improvement in the management of ovarian cancer, the majority of patients will continue to receive little or no benefit from treatments which are unpleasant, and at the limit of acceptable toxicity.

New therapeutic approaches therefore require investigation. Attempts are being made, inter alia, to optimize the use of existing drugs. Examples of this approach are the intraperitoneal administration of medication, and the in-vitro testing of chemosensitivity. Immunotherapy is another new field deserving investigation. A third approach consists of seeking new drugs devoid of marrow or kidney toxicity, which might supplement current regimens.

This latter category includes hormones, or, more specifically, progestins. Their activity in the treatment of ovarian carcinoma has been reported to be rather low in a review of the studies conducted before 1977 [12]. The recent introduction of preparations containing high doses of medroxyprogesterone acetate (MPA), and indications that such high dosages give good results in the treatment of breast cancer [13], with a possible dose/response relationship [14], have revived interest in this class of agents for the management of ovarian carcinoma, a tumour which can contain hormone receptors [15].

Recent phase II studies using MPA in this disease [16–18] are listed in Table V. Although the results may seem disappointing, it is of interest that the study in which greatest activity was found [17] is the study in which the dosage and route of administration likely to give the highest serum levels, based on cur-

Table V. Ovarian carcinoma stages III/IV. Previous studies with MPA.

Number of patients	Dose (mg) and frequency of dosage	Route	Response rate (%)	Reference
19	100 to 400, daily	oral	5	[16]
19	1000, weekly	intramuscular	0	[18]
30	800, daily	oral	0	[17]
33	500, daily	intramuscular	15	[17]

rent knowledge of MPA pharmacokinetics [19, 20] were used. The 15% response rate is also significant within the context of such phase-II studies, in which the medication tested is given after failure of 1 or 2 chemotherapeutic regimens. It has, in fact, been reported that second-line chemotherapy in ovarian cancer usually produces very low response rates, even when primarily active agents such as melphalan [21], 5-fluorouracil [21], doxorubicin [21, 22], or hexamethylmelamine [21] are used.

Having regard to the above considerations, the EORTC GCCG decided to test whether the results reported by Mangioni [17] could be confirmed, and whether the antitumour activity of MPA is, in fact, dose-dependent. A phase-II protocol was devised towards the end of 1981 (Protocol Committee: Drs J. Hamerlynck, Amsterdam; C. Mangioni, Milan; I. Hesselius, Uppsala; F. Cheix, Lyon; P.F. Conte, Genoa; V. Kozyreff, Brussels; A. Maskens, Brussels; and Ms N. Rotmensz, Brussels).

The study was designed to cover patients with epithelial ovarian carcinoma progressing after conventional therapy. The treatment plan involved a 4-week loading phase, during which MPA was given intramuscularly at a daily dose of 500 mg, and a maintenance phase during which the dose was reduced to 1,000 mg weekly, given as 1 or 2 injections. In all patients, the serum level of MPA was determined at regular intervals, using both gas liquid chromatography (GLC) and radio-immunoassay (RIA) techniques.

Although it is too early to present our results, preliminary information on the serum levels of MPA observed in the first 11 patients enrolled is presented in Figure 1. The observation that large individual variations can occur in this category of patients is interesting. In the 6 cases in which the loading phase has been completed, serum levels have been found to vary more than tenfold. If any dose/response effect in fact exists, this study would be expected to reveal it, unambiguously.

In Figure 2, levels obtained using the 2 analytical techniques are compared, for 4 patients. The data indicate that both methods appear reliable. The levels

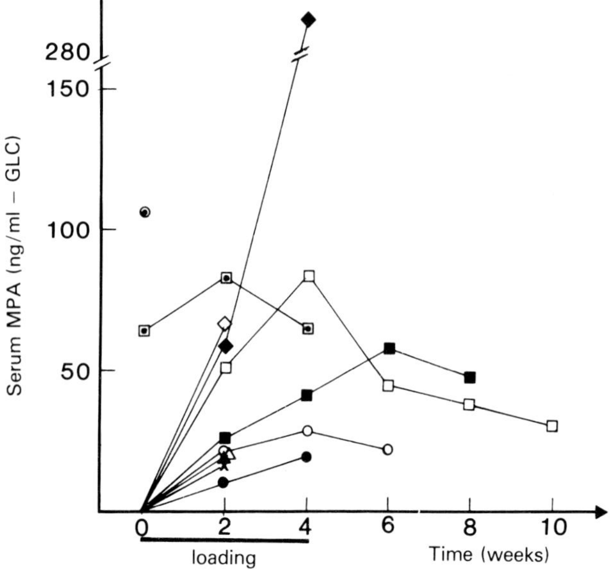

Fig. 1. Serum levels of MPA determined at various intervals using GLC in 11 patients with ovarian carcinoma. Two patients had apparently already received the drug before the study.

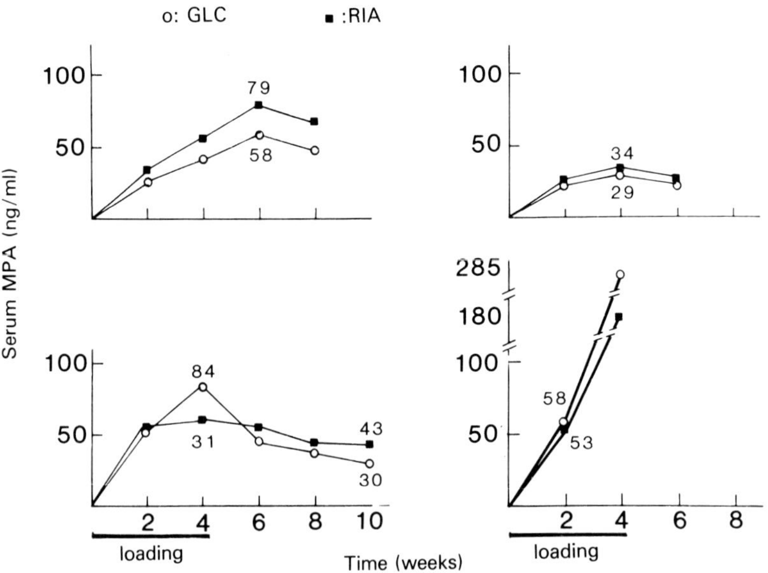

Fig. 2. Comparison between serum levels of MPA obtained using GLC and RIA techniques, in 4 patients taken from the same series as in Figure 1.

vary in parallel, with only minor deviations. The RIA values are usually slightly higher than those observed using GLC.

In conclusion, recent data have indicated that high dose MPA may have antitumour activity in ovarian carcinoma. A large scale study is now under way in an attempt to study this possibility definitively. Care will be taken to analyse the relationship between serum levels of MPA in treated patients, and possible therapeutic benefits.

References

1. Bolis, G., Sessa, C., Molina, P. et al. (1981): Cisplatinum (P), adriamycin (A) and cyclophosphamide (C) in combination for previously untreated advanced ovarian cancer. Paper read at: UICC Conference on Clinical Oncology, Lausanne, 1981
2. Griffin, J.P., Belinson, J., Lynn, J. et al. (1981): Combination chemotherapy of ovarian carcinoma with CAP. *Proc. Am. Assoc. Cancer Res. and ASCO 22,* 468.
3. Neijt, J.P., ten Bokkel Huinink, W.W., van den Burg, M.E.L. et al. (1981): Combination chemotherapy with HEXA-CAF and CHAP-5 for stage III and IV ovarian carcinoma. Paper read at: UICC Conference on Clinical Oncology, Lausanne, 1981.
4. Omura, G.A., Blessing, J.A., Morrow, C.P. et al. (1981): Follow up on a randomized trial of melphalan (M) vs. melphalan plus hexamethylmelamine (M + H) vs. adriamycin plus cyclophosphamide (A + C) in advanced ovarian adenocarcinoma. *Proc. Am. Assoc. Cancer Res. and ASCO 22,* 470.
5. Posada, J.G., Marantz, A.B., Yeung K.Y. et al. (1981): Hexamethylmelamine, cytoxan, and 5-fluorouracil (HEXA CF) in stages III and IV of ovarian carcinoma. *Proc. Am. Assoc. Cancer Res. and ASCO 22,* 466.
6. Pouillart, P., Palangie, T., Bretaudeau, B. et al. (1981): Role of CIS DDP in a combination of chemotherapy in patients with ovarian carcinoma, stage III and IV. Paper read at: UICC Conference on Clinical Oncology, Lausanne, 1981.
7. Tropé, C. (1981): A prospective and randomized trial comparison of melphalan vs. adriamycin-melphalan in advanced ovarian carcinoma by the Swedish Cooperative Ovarian Cancer Study Group (SCOCSG). *Proc. Am. Assoc. Cancer Res. and ASCO 22,* 469.
8. Varini, M., Geiger, U., Preitner, J. and Cavalli, F. (1981): HEXA-CAF (hexamethylmelamine, cyclophosphamide, methotrexate, 5-fluorouracil) alternating with DDP-ADM (cisdiammineplatinum, adriblastine) in the treatment of advanced ovarian cancer. Paper read at: UICC Conference on Clinical Oncology, Lausanne, 1981.
9. Vogl, S., Kaplan, B. and Pagano, M. (1981): CHAD (cyclophosphamide, hexamethylmelamine, adriamycin and diamminedichloroplatinum) is superior to melphalan in the therapy of bulky advanced ovarian cancer – an Eastern Cooperative Oncology Group randomized trial. Paper read at: UICC Conference on Clinical Oncology, Lausanne, 1981.
10. Williams, C., Mead, G., Arnold, A. et al. (1981): Platinum based chemotherapy (PACe) of advanced ovarian carcinoma. Paper read at: UICC Conference on Clinical Oncology, Lausanne, 1981.

11. Young, R.C., Howser, D.M., Myers, C.E. et al. (1981): Combination chemotherapy (Chex-UP) with intraperitoneal maintenance in advanced ovarian adenocarcinoma. *Proc. Am. Assoc. Cancer Res. and ASCO 22*, 465.
12. Young, R.C. (1979): Gynecologic malignancies. In: *Cancer Chemotherapy 1979*, Chapter 17, pp. 340–375. Ed: H.M. Pinedo. Excerpta Medica, Amsterdam.
13. Pannuti, F., Di Marco, A.R., Martoni, A. et al. (1980): Medroxyprogesterone acetate in treatment of metastatic breast cancer: seven years of experience. In: *Role of Medroxyprogesterone in Endocrine-related Tumors*, pp. 73–92. Eds: S. Iacobelli and A. Di Marco. Raven Press, New York.
14. Cavalli, F., Goldhirsch, A., Jungi, F. et al. (1982): Low versus high dose medroxyprogesterone acetate in the treatment of advanced breast cancer. In: *Proceedings of the International Symposium on Medroxyprogesterone Acetate*, pp. 224–233. Eds: F. Cavalli, W.L. McGuire, F. Pannuti, A. Pellegrini, and G. Robustelli Della Cuna. Excerpta Medica, Amsterdam.
15. Holt, J.A., Caputo, T.A., Kelly, K.M. et al. (1979): Estrogen and progestin binding in cytosols of ovarian adenocarcinoma. *Obstet. Gynecol. 53*, 50.
16. Malkasian, G.D., Decker, D.G., Jorgensen, E.O. and Edmonson, J.H. (1977): Medroxyprogesterone acetate for the treatment of metastatic and recurrent ovarian carcinoma. *Cancer Treat. Rep. 61*, 913.
17. Mangioni, C., Franceschi, S., La Vecchia, C. and D'Incalci, M. (1981): High dose medroxyprogesterone acetate (MPA) in advanced epithelial cancer resistant to first or second-line chemotherapy. *Gynecol. Oncol. 12*, 314.
18. Slayton, R.E., Pagano, M. and Creech, R.H. (1981): Progestin therapy for advanced ovarian cancer: a phase II Eastern Cooperative Oncology Group trial. *Cancer Treat. Rep. 65*, 895.
19. Hesselius, I.R. (1982): Pharmacokinetics and bioavailability of medroxyprogesterone acetate in cancer treatment. In: *Proceedings of the International Symposium on Medroxyprogesterone Acetate*, pp. 169–176. Eds: F. Cavalli, W.L. McGuire, F. Pannuti, A. Pellegrini, and G. Robustelli Della Cuna. Excerpta Medica, Amsterdam.
20. Maskens, A.P., Hap, B., Kozyreff, V.N. et al. (1980): Serum levels of medroxyprogesterone acetate under various treatment schedules. *Proc. Am. Assoc. Cancer Res. and ASCO 21*, 165.
21. Stanhope, C.R., Smith, J.P. and Rutledge, F. (1977): Second trial drugs in ovarian cancer. *Gynecol. Oncol. 5*, 52.
22. Bolis, G., D'Incalci, M., Gramellini, F. and Mangioni, C. (1978): Adriamycin in ovarian cancer patients resistant to cyclophosphamide. *Eur. J. Cancer 14*, 1401.

Discussion

C. Tropé: Professor Mangioni and we ourselves have shown that high-dose MPA has a moderate activity in chemoresistant ovarian cancer. We should concentrate on the endometrial type of ovarian cancer, and determine the receptor status before treating the patients. That is my opinion.

C. Mangioni: Since September 1981, another 10 patients have been treated in the GCCG of the European Organization for Research on Treatment of Cancer, and so far there have been 3 objective responses confirmed – although not any partial responses yet. The trends from the first analysis in September 1980 and the second analysis in September 1981 are the same. These data provide some help in this situation. Our experience in 180 patients who received second-line chemotherapy between 1975 and 1981 is that only platinum seems to be able to lead to 33% minimal or partial responses in well-treated patients with epithelial ovarian cancer. After mono- or polychemotherapies, when used as second-line treatment, we were unable to achieve any kind of result – any more than MPA alone.

All these data should be discussed because MPA gives at least a subjective or objective improvement. I know of no chemotherapy that is at least able to give a better quality of life.

C. Tropé: I agree with Professor Mangioni. In our study, 40% of the patients improved their performance status according to the Karnofsky index. Perhaps we are slightly unfair to MPA in testing it as a third-line therapy (as we have done). If chemotherapy is used, as Professor Mangioni said, as a third-line therapy, only about 2–5% of the patients respond. MPA must be tested with receptor status. In particular, the endometrial type of ovarian cancer is interesting because MPA may be good as a first-line therapy in that situation.

M. Kjaer: In many of the papers presented we have heard about objective improvement following MPA treatment, a better Karnofsky index, weight gain and so on. I would like to draw attention to the fact that (as everybody knows) all can be obtained with prednisone. The number of responses at present is very low – although that may be improved in the future – and MPA is rather expensive. If we are going for a subjective response, perhaps prednisone should be included in some of the trials because a subjective response could be obtained in that way, without spending enormous amounts of money on MPA.

Multi-agent chemotherapy with and without medroxyprogesterone acetate in the treatment of advanced ovarian cancer*

K.V. Kahanpää, J. Kärkkäinen and U. Nieminen
Obstetrics and Gynaecology Departments I and II, University Central Hospital, Helsinki, Finland

Introduction

Hormonal treatment with derivatives of progesterone, such as medroxyprogesterone acetate, (MPA), is widely used in gynaecological oncology, especially for the treatment of endometrial carcinoma. Initially, the hormone was mostly used in endometrial carcinomas which had reached an advanced stage, and in recurrent endometrial carcinoma. Subsequently, MPA was used in cases at earlier stages [1–3]. In most of the earlier studies, MPA was given at doses of 50–300 mg daily. In recent years, high-dose MPA treatment has frequently been used and advocated, especially for patients with recurrent tumours.

There are only a few reports in the literature on the use of MPA in the treatment of ovarian carcinoma, and these are to some extent contradictory [4–6]. It has been suggested that the best targets for MPA treatment may be serous papillary adenocarcinomas, together with endometrioid and mesonephric types of ovarian carcinoma. Highly differentiated tumours are believed to be more sensitive to therapy. Senn and his collaborators were unable to find evidence confirming the previously reported trend towards a beneficial effect of MPA as adjuvant treatment in advanced ovarian cancer [7]. Bumma and Bertetto were able to demonstrate a significantly longer postoperative duration of response in ovarian cancer patients receiving cytotoxic drugs together with MPA, as compared with patients receiving cytotoxic drugs only [8].

*The financial assistance of Farmitalia Carlo Erba is gratefully acknowledged.

However, the percentage remission rates were similar in the 2 groups. Tropé et al. were not able, in a recent study, to demonstrate any clear enhancement of response rate in late stage ovarian carcinoma with high-dose MPA treatment [9]. However, they drew attention to the beneficial effect of the hormone on the general condition of the patients, and recommended MPA as a component of palliative therapy, especially in cases of highly differentiated tumours.

In our clinics, 100 mg of MPA daily, per os (p.o.), for 2 years, has been used routinely as adjuvant treatment of endometrial carcinoma since 1965. During the last 2 years we have given MPA in high doses to patients with advanced or recurrent endometrial carcinoma, and also to patients with advanced endometrial stromal sarcoma. In the light of the encouraging results, we started a controlled study in 1980 to investigate the effects of high-dose MPA treatment in advanced or recurrent ovarian carcinoma.

Material and methods

At present, results relating to 20 patients are available for assessment. The patients had Fédération Internationale de Gynécologie et d'Obstétrique Stage III to IV ovarian carcinoma, or were relapsed ovarian carcinoma cases (5 patients). All patients had been operated upon, and as much of the tumour tissue as possible removed. Following surgery, all patients were treated using combination therapy with cytotoxic drugs (Cis Pt(II)diaminodichloride, 50 mg/m^2, doxorubicin, 40 mg/m^2, and cyclophosphamide, 500 mg/m^2, given intravenously (i.v.) as single doses at 4-weekly intervals). Patients were randomly divided into 2 groups. Group A (10 patients) received the combination mentioned above plus MPA, 500 mg daily, for 7 days, followed by 1 g once a week, intramuscularly (i.m.). Group B patients received no MPA.

In addition to the routine blood tests necessary for the follow-up of treatment with the cytotoxic drugs, concentrations of MPA in the sera of patients were regularly determined, using radioimmunoassay as previously described [10, 11].

The general condition of the patients (Karnofsky index) and side-effects possibly resulting from treatment were recorded. Remissions were mainly classified on the basis of the European Organization for Research on the Treatment of Cancer (EORTC) criteria. Clinically detectable and quantifiable neoplastic foci were sought and measured. Physical examination, ultrasound, and radiological methods were used. Laparotomy was repeated in only a few cases. Subjective criteria such as weight gain, regression of ascites and pain relief were also used.

Results

In all cases, the diagnosis of ovarian malignancy was confirmed histologically. The distribution of tumours by histological type is shown in Table I. Table II shows the degree of differentiation and clinical stages of tumours.

All 5 cases with recurrent malignancies fell in group A. Other prognostic factors such as histological classification, and degrees of differentiation, showed a fairly even distribution between the 2 treatment groups. Table III

Table I. Distribution of histological types of tumour. (Numbers of patients.)

	Group A	Group B
Serous-papillary adenocarcinoma	2	4
Pseudomucinous adenocarcinoma	2	1
Adenomatous carcinoma	1	4
Granulosa cell carcinoma	2	—
Mesonephric carcinoma	1	—
Anaplastic carcinoma	2	1

Table II. Degrees of differentiation and clinical stages of tumours. (Numbers of patients.)

	Group A	Group B
Well-differentiated (G1)	2	—
Intermediate degree of differentiation (G2)	1	2
Anaplastic (G3)	5	5
Undefined	2	3
Stage III	3	8
Stage IV	2	2
Recurrent carcinoma	5	—

Table III. Responses to therapy. (Numbers of cases, with durations of remission, in months, in parentheses.)

Treatment group	Number of cases	CR	PR	NC	Progression
A	10	—	—	6 (3–12)	4
B	10	2 (12,16)	1 (11)	3 (5–14)	4

shows the results of chemotherapy. Complete remission (CR) was obtained in only 2 cases (follow-up times 12 and 16 months). These 2 patients are still alive, without any evidence of disease. There was one case of partial remission (PR). All these patients were members of group B. No change (NC) was observed in 3 cases in group B and in 6 cases in group A. However, the significance of the above-mentioned differences cannot be assessed, as numbers of patients are too small. Follow-up continues in some cases. For the time being, at least, no marked differences between the 2 groups can be regarded as established.

At least 4 weeks of treatment were required before serum levels of MPA higher than 100 nmol/l were achieved. These levels were then maintained, except in one case. The mean maintenance level of MPA in the other 9 patients was 150 nmol/l (range 105–168 nmol/l).

Discussion

The role of hormones in the natural history and treatment of malignant tumours is well established. The relationships between ovarian hormones, breast cancer and endometrial cancer have been the subject of study for several years. Oestrogen and progesterone receptors have been found in 25–50% of malignant ovarian tumours [8, 12, 13].

The endometrioid type of ovarian carcinoma had previously been most often regarded as receptor-positive. Bumma and Bertetto have suggested that the natural history of epithelial ovarian carcinoma also indicates hormonal aetiology, in some cases at least [8].

The effects of MPA on malignant tumours could be mediated other than solely via oestrogen and progesterone receptors. Baulieu et al. have shown that progestins have great affinity for glucocorticoid receptors [14]. Other suggestions in the literature regarding the mediation of MPA effects have involved roles for prostaglandins, prolactin, or proteins other than receptor proteins.

The concentrations of MPA which need to be achieved in the sera of patients for a beneficial effect are still not established. In the present study, serum MPA levels greater than 100 nmol/l were achieved in all cases except one. According to Bonte, these levels are sufficiently high for therapeutic effects in endometrial carcinoma to be expected [6]. MPA concentrations in tumour tissue would, obviously, be the best indicator, but, for practical reasons, these cannot be determined in serial tissue preparations.

On the whole, durations of remission appeared fairly brief in both groups. This reflects the fact that our patients, in contrast to those in many other studies reported in the literature, formed a group with advanced disease, in which therapeutic and prognostic factors were unfavourable. More than half of the cases were poorly differentiated or anaplastic tumours.

A more careful selection of patients, based on determinations of oestrogen and progesterone receptor levels, needs to be undertaken in future clinical studies. At present, we are trying to find out whether patients with better differentiated tumours and/or higher receptor concentrations respond better to MPA. We are also trying to determine which histological types of tumours react better. According to a recent paper there may be areas within the same tumour differing in receptor concentrations, and these concentrations may, in addition, change during tumour growth [15]. The degree of differentiation may vary within the same tumour, and may also change during growth. Concentrations of receptors in the metasases may differ from receptor concentrations in the primary tumours. Heterogeneity of malignant tumours may explain why combination chemotherapy often succeeds in controlling or even curing cancers in situations where a single drug is ineffective. We agree with Tropé and his colleagues [9], that the lack of serious side-effects, and the frequent beneficial effects of MPA on the general condition of patients make high-dose MPA worth trying, as a palliative, if nothing else, in late stage or recurrent ovarian carcinomas.

References

1. Bonte, J. (1981): New perspectives in solid tumours: endometrial carcinoma. Paper read at: Second International Symposium on the Role of Medroxyprogesterone Acetate (MPA) in Endocrine-related Tumors, Rome, 1981.
2. Kauppila, A., Grönroos, M. and Nieminen, U. (1982): Clinical outcome in endometrial carcinoma. *Obstet. Gynecol.* (In press.)
3. Taylor, R.W. (1981): The treatment of endometrial carcinoma with medroxyprogesterone acetate. Paper read at: Second International Symposium on the Role of Medroxyprogesterone Acetate (MPA) in Endocrine-related Tumors, Rome, 1981.
4. Senn, H.J. (1973): Zur Therapie des fortgeschrittenen inoperablen Ovarialkarzinoms. *Ther. Umsch. 30*, 651.
5. Malkasian, G.D., Decker, D.G., Jorgensen, E.O. and Webb, M.J. (1973): 6-Dehydro-6,17-α-dimethylprogesterone (NSC-123018) for the treatment of metastatic and recurrent ovarian carcinoma. *Cancer Chemother. Rep. 57,* 241.
6. Bonte, J. (1979): Developments in endocrine therapy of endometrial and ovarian cancer. In: *Reviews on Endocrine-related Cancer, No. 3,* pp. 11–17. Ed: B.A. Stoll. I.C.I., Holmes Chapel.
7. Senn, H.J., Lei, D., Castaõ-Almendral, A. et al. (1980): Chemo-(Hormon)-Therapie fortgeschrittener Ovarialkarzinome der FIGO-Stadien III und IV. *Schweiz. Med. Wochenschr. 110,* 1202.
8. Bumma, C. and Bertetto, O. (1981): Treatment with chemotherapy versus treat-

ment with medroxyprogesterone acetate plus chemotherapy in advanced ovarian carcinoma. Paper read at: Second International Symposium on the Role of Medroxyprogesterone Acetate (MPA) in Endocrine-related Tumors, Rome, 1981.

9. Tropé, C., Johnsson, J.-E., Sigurdsson, K. and Simonsen, E. (1981): Högdos medroxyprogesteronacetat vid avancerad recidiverande ovarialcancer. *Acta Soc. Med. Suecanae Hygiea 90*, 337.
10. Martin, F. and Adlercreutz, H. (1977): Aspects of megestrol acetate and medroxyprogesterone acetate metabolism. In: *Symposium on the Pharmacology of Steroid Contraceptive Drugs,* p. 99. Ed: S. Garattini. Raven Press, New York.
11. Laatikainen, T., Nieminen, U. and Adlercreutz, H. (1979): Plasma medroxyprogesterone acetate levels following intramuscular or oral administration in patients with endometrial adenocarcinoma. *Acta Obstet. Gynecol. Scand. 58*, 95.
12. Holt, J.A., Caputo, T.A., Kelly, K.M. et al. (1979): Estrogen and progestin binding in cytosols of ovarian adenocarcinomas. *Obstet. Gynecol. 53,* 50.
13. Jänne, O., Kauppila, A., Syrjälä, P. and Vihko, R. (1980): Comparison of cytosol estrogen and progestin receptor status in malignant and benign tumors and tumorlike lesions of human ovary. *Int. J. Cancer 25,* 175.
14. Baulieu, E.-E. (1981): Combined effects of estradiol, progesterone and tamoxifen. 1. Studies in the chick oviduct model system. 2. A 'hormonal challenge test' in human breast and endometrium cancers. Paper read at: Second International Symposium on the Role of Medroxyprogesterone Acetate (MPA) in Endocrine-related Tumors, Rome, 1981.
15. Marx, J.L. (1982): Tumours: A mixed bag of cells. *Science 215,* 275.

Failure of low-dose medroxyprogesterone acetate to improve tumour response or to reduce haematological toxicity in ovarian cancer. A randomized, co-operative trial by the Swiss Study Group for Clinical Cancer Research*

W.F. Jungi, D. Lei and H.J. Senn
Medical Clinic C, Cantonal Hospital, St. Gallen, Switzerland

Introduction

The obvious contrast between the progress made in the treatment of many solid tumours with combination chemotherapy and the lack of progress in the management of ovarian cancer led the Swiss Study Group for Clinical Cancer Research (SAKK) to initiate, in 1971, a comparative trial of hormonal therapy and chemotherapy in patients with ovarian cancer of Fédération Internationale de Gynécologie et d'Obstétrique (FIGO) stages III to IV.

At the time, chemotherapy of ovarian cancer was normally monotherapy, mostly with alkylating agents. The goals of the SAKK-study (No. 20/71) were:
1. To investigate the contributions made by an antimetabolite, 5-fluorouracil (5-FU), and progestogenic hormone, medroxyprogesterone acetate (MPA), to the tumour response achievable with the alkylating agent cyclophosphamide (CYT), alone.
2. To assess whether haematological tolerance in chemotherapy could be improved by addition of a progestational hormone (MPA).

The study was terminated in 1973. The results have been reported orally several times, and have also recently been published [1].

*Supported by funds from the Swiss Cancer League and the Regional Cancer Research Programme of Eastern Switzerland.

Materials and methods

Between 1971 and 1973, 89 patients with histologically proven, advanced ovarian cancer (stage III or IV) were admitted to this prospective co-operative study. The patients were allocated at random to 3 different treatment schedules involving CYT alone (group A), CYT + MPA (group B), and CYT + 5-FU (group C). Table I shows drug doses and the schedule of administration.

All patients had either failed to respond to previous therapy, consisting of attempted curative surgery and/or radiotherapy, or were inoperable at the time of diagnosis. Patients who had previously had chemotherapy were excluded. Eighteen of the 89 patients who were enrolled were not evaluable, for the following reasons: no primary tumour in the ovaries (5 patients), too short a duration of treatment (5), faulty randomization (3), refusal of treatment (2), lost to follow-up (3). The distribution of tumour stages and histological subtypes in the 3 treatment regimes is shown in Table II. Radical surgery had been performed in 13 patients, non-radical surgery, or only excisional biopsy, in 53 patients. Nineteen patients had received radiotherapy after surgery. Only 5 patients were completely untreated.

After 6 months, the initial therapy was discontinued and a second laparotomy was recommended in all patients with objective clinical remission or stable disease. On day 189, maintenance therapy was started. This consisted of 4-week courses of the initial dosage regimes, followed by 4-week rest periods. Treatment was continued in this way until evidence of tumour progression or relapse was obtained. Survival data was recorded for all patients. Alterations in dose were undertaken in accordance with standard SAKK criteria.

The criteria used to evaluate the outcome of therapy were as follows:
Complete remission (CR): disappearance of all measurable tumours and tumour-related subjective symptoms.

Table I. Drug doses and schedule of administration.

Group	Drugs	Dosage, frequency of dosage and route of administration
A	CYT	100 mg/m^2/day, per os (p.o.)
B	CYT +	100 mg/m^2/day p.o.
	MPA	500 mg/week intramuscularly (i.m.)
C	CYT +	100 mg/m^2/day p.o.
	5-FU	500 mg/m^2/week, intravenously

Table II. Mean age of patients, distribution of tumour stages (FIGO) and histological types of tumour.

	Group		
	A	B	C
Mean age (years)	61.2	53.5	55.8
Tumour stage:			
III (numbers of patients)	10	7	10
IV (numbers of patients)	14	14	16
Histology (numbers of patients)			
Papillary serous	10	12	10
Pseudomucinous	2	2	4
Undifferentiated	2	—	2
Unclassified adenocarcinoma	3	3	4
Mixed adenocarcinomas	4	4	4
Granulosa cell tumour	2	—	2
Teratocarcinoma	1	—	—
Totals	24	21	26

Partial remission (PR): at least a 50% reduction in measurable tumour size (chest films, lymph node assessments, etc.), or at least 50% decrease in palpable (abdominal) tumour masses.
No change (NC): no significant change in tumour size (less than 50% decrease to less than 25% increase).
Progression (P): more than a 25% increase in tumour size, or appearance of new lesions after at least 4 weeks of treatment.
Duration of response (CR + PR + NC) was measured from the first signs of tumour regression up to the time of evidence of tumour progression.

Results

Table III summarizes the response rates in the 3 treatment regimes. The highest remission rate was observed in patients treated with the combination of CYT and 5-FU (group C). However, none of the differences between the 3 remission rates reached statistical significance. Only one complete remission was observed, in a patient of group C. This lasted for only 5.6 months. Overall, 34 out of 71 evaluable patients (47.8%) responded to one or other of the treatment regimes. Sixteen out of 71 patients (22.6%) showed stabilization

Table III. Remission rates; numbers of patients (%).

Group	Numbers of patients	PR		NC		P	
A (CYT)	24	10/24	(42)	5/24	(21)	9/24	(38)
B (CYT + MPA)	21	9/21	(43)	8/21	(43)	4/21	(19)
C (CYT + 5-FU)	26	16/26*	(58)	3/26	(12)	7/26	(27)
Totals	71	34/71	(48)	16/71	(23)	20/71	(28)

*Including 1 CR.

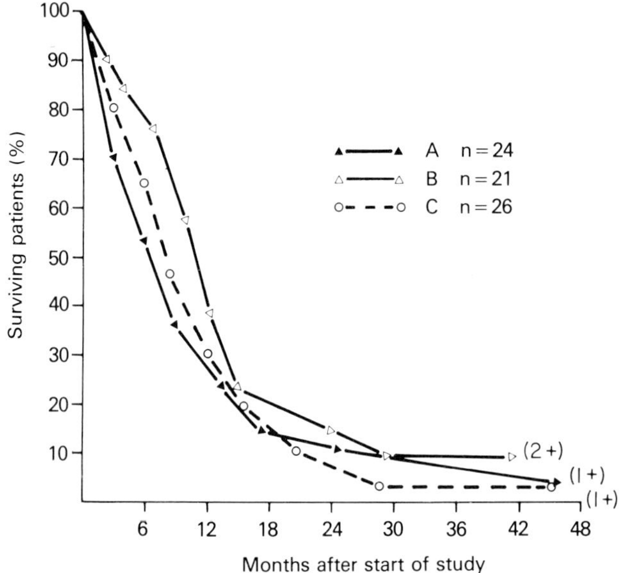

Figure. Survival from time of initiation of chemotherapy in SAKK study 20/71. (Ovarian cancer, FIGO stage III to IV).

of their disease (NC). The durations of remission were longest in patients of group C (median duration 5.8 months). The next longest durations of remission were in patients of group B (4.6 months), followed by patients of group A (3.0 months). The differences between these 3 durations are not statistically significant.

Survival curves calculated on an actuarial basis from the time of initiation of chemotherapy are shown in the Figure. The survival time in the 24 patients receiving CYT alone (group A) was 6.6 months or more. In those on CYT + MPA it was 10.3 months or more, and in those on CYT + 5-FU it was 8.2 months or more. In assessing these findings, the considerable differences in mean age between patients on the 3 regimes must be kept in mind. At present, there is still one long-term survivor from group B, in excellent health after more than 127 months. At second laparotomy she was found to have minimal residual disease. After radiotherapy to the entire abdomen complete remission persists.

When the durations of survival of responders (CR + PR + NC) are compared with those non-responders (P), a significant difference in median survival times (11 months or more versus 2.9 months or more, respectively) is found.

Toxicity

As recorded in Table IV, the haematological toxicity of the 3 dosage regimens was mild to moderate, and was easily managed by adjustment of the drug dosage. There was no difference between the 3 regimes in this respect. In particular, haematological toxicity was not ameliorated by the concomitant use of MPA.

Gastro-intestinal side-effects were somewhat more frequent in patients of group C. Alopecia to varying degrees was seen in patients on all 3 regimes. Haemorrhagic cystitis, attributable to CYT, was seen in 9 out of 71 patients, but was clinically relevant, leading to discontinuation of the drug in only 3 cases. In none of the 71 patients was the course complicated by significant treatment-related infections or bleeding.

Second laparotomy

Only 5 patients were considered suitable for this procedure by the in-

Table IV. Haematological toxicity.

Group	Lowest value/mm^3	
	White blood cells	Platelets
A	2,600	159,000
B	2,600	145,000
C	2,400	121,000

vestigators concerned. In 2 additional patients, therapeutic laparotomy was performed because of tumour-related bowel obstruction. Another 2 patients underwent laparoscopy for the purposes of reassessment.

In 2 out of the 5 patients in whom a second laparotomy was undertaken, the good partial remission assumed to have occurred on the basis of clinical evidence could not be confirmed, and disseminated peritoneal metastases were detected.

Discussion

The overall remission rate in our 71 patients with advanced ovarian cancer of stages III to IV was 48%. This value is very comparable to those found with other chemotherapeutic combinations currently in use, but is decidedly inferior to those achievable with the newer, more intensive chemotherapeutic combinations, including doxorubicin and cis-platinum. There was no statistically significant difference in remission rates between the 3 regimes. On the other hand, there was also no statistically significant difference in toxicity as between the 3 branches of the study. All 3 regimes were well tolerated, and must be regarded as mild according to 1982 criteria.

The addition of MPA at a dosage of 500 mg per week, i.m., had no effect on remission rate or haematological tolerance. We explain this result, firstly, by the relatively low doses of the suppressive agents in all 3 groups, and, secondly, because, in the light of more recent findings, the MPA dosage was insufficient [2, 3].

A prospective randomized study comparing the low dosage of MPA which we studied with the more recent high-dose MPA, in both cases in addition to standard chemotherapy, seems advisable.

Participating institutions in the study (No. SAKK 20/71)

Oncology Centre, Basel University Hospitals (Professor J. Obrecht, Professor A. Almendral), Oncology Department, Insel Hospital, Berne (Professor K.W. Brunner, Dr R. Sonntag), Specialized Oncology Section, Radiotherapy Department, Hanover Medical School (Professor Dr W. Rhomberg), Oncology Section, Department of Gynaecology and Obstetrics, University of Mainz (Professor Dr F. Melchert), Oncology Centre, Cantonal Hospital, St. Gallen (Professor H.J. Senn, Dr W.F. Jungi), Oncology Section, Department of Internal Medicine, Cantonal Hospital, Zürich (Professor G. Martz, Professor Dr Chr. Sauter).

References

1. Senn, H.J., Lei, D., Castaño-Almendral, A. et al. (1980): Results of chemo-(hormono)-therapy in advanced ovarian cancer with special reference to the randomized study SAKK 20/71. *Schweiz. Med. Wochenschr. 110,* 1202.
2. Robustelli della Cuna, G. et al. (1980): High dose medroxyprogesterone acetate (HDMPA) combined with chemotherapy for metastatic breast cancer. In: *Role of MPA in Endocrine-related Tumors,* pp. 53–64. Eds: S. Iacobelli and A. Di Marco. Raven Press, New York.
3. Pellegrini, A. et al. (1980): CAMF vs. CAMF + MPA nel carcinoma avanzato della mammella. Valutazione a 42 mesi. *Tumori* (suppl.) *66*, 99.

High-dose medroxyprogesterone acetate for the treatment of advanced ovarian carcinoma resistant to chemotherapy

C. Tropé, P. Buchhave and U. Stendahl
Gynaecological Section, Department of Oncology, University Hospital, Lund, Sweden

Introduction

Progestins of various kinds have been reported to have activity in patients with advanced ovarian adenocarcinomas, but there has been no uniform recording of objective response or histological type, and hormones and doses used have varied. The results have been conflicting, and response rates have varied from 5–65% [1–10] (Table I). Some of the differences in response rates may, however, be explained by differences in defining response. Jolles [1], Paraskevas [6] and Ward [3] did not use WHO criteria. If the response rates in Table I are reviewed according to WHO criteria, the mean response rate is 16.5% (range 0–38%) (Table II). Progestin treatment has usually been

Table I. Results of treatment of advanced ovarian cancer with progestins, using a variety of response criteria.

Investigators	Response rates (%)
Jolles [1]	40
Varga et al. [2]	50
Ward [3]	65
Malkasian et al. [4]	22
Tobias and Griffith [5]	38
Paraskevas et al. [6]	40
Malkasian et al. [7]	5
Mangioni et al. [8]	15
Slayton et al. [9]	0
Tropé et al. [10]	4

Table II. Results of progestin treatment in ovarian cancer patients using WHO response criteria.

Investigators	Response rates (%)
Jolles [1]	10
Varga [2]	30
Ward [3]	13
Malkasian et al. [4]	22
Tobias and Griffith [5]	38
Mangioni et al. [8]	15
Slayton et al. [9]	0
Tropé et al. [10]	4

employed when all other forms of treatment such as surgery, radiotherapy and chemotherapy have failed. If chemotherapy is used as second or third line treatment, the overall response rate is also very low (5–15%). The progestin most often used today is medroxyprogesterone acetate (MPA).

Material and methods

Twenty-eight patients with recurrent advanced (Fédération Internationale de Gynécologie et d'Obstétrique stage III or IV) ovarian carcinoma resistant to chemotherapy fulfilling the following criteria were enrolled: leukocyte count $\geq 3.0 \times 10^9/l$, platelet count $\geq 100 \times 10^9/l$, normal blood sugar levels, normal blood pressure, Karnofsky index ≥ 60, and measurable or evaluable lesions. All but 3 patients had previously had surgery. Five had undergone salpingo-oophorectomy-hysterectomy, 12 had undergone salpingo-oophorectomy and 8 had undergone explorative laparotomy. Prior to MPA treatment, one patient had received radiotherapy, 10 had received chemotherapy and 17 had received both types of therapy. Histological examination showed serous adenocarcinoma in 16 patients (8 highly or moderately well differentiated carcinomas, and 8 poorly differentiated), anaplastic cancer in 10 patients, and highly differentiated endometrioid cancer in 2 patients.

Before MPA treatment was started, the extent of the disease was assessed by physical and gynaecological examination, chest X-ray, isotope scanning of the liver, and fine-needle aspiration biopsy of accessible metastatic lesions in the small pelvis, lymph nodes, lungs, pleurae, and liver. When indicated, the examinations were supplemented by ultrasonic examination, computerized tomography of the abdomen, and various isotope scans. Routine blood examinations were regularly performed.

MPA (6-alpha-methyl-17-alpha-hydroxy-progesterone-acetate), a synthetic steroid derived from progesterone was given intramuscularly (i.m.) at a daily dosage of 500 mg for 3 weeks, and thereafter at a dosage of 500 mg, once a week, for at least 2 months. Patients showing objective response or stable disease continued treatment with 500 mg every week until progression of disease.

The responses to treatment were defined as follows: complete remission = complete disappearance of all measurable lesions for at least one month; partial remission = at least a 50% reduction in measurable tumour size, with no pleural or ascitic fluids persisting; stable disease = 0–49% decrease in measurable tumour volume, and no new lesions, or improvement in nonevaluable lesions such as ascitic and pleural fluids (ascitic and pleural fluids could persist, but could not increase, and an increase in time intervals between thoracocentesis and laparocentesis had to have occurred); progressive disease = increasing volume of tumour, or new lesions during treatment, without remission, or shortening of time intervals between paracenteses; relapse = a new lesion following remission, or recurrence in an area previously showing regression.

Results

Twenty-eight patients entered the study. Three patients were excluded from evaluation because of early death. Twenty-five patients, with a median age of 61 (range 43–81) were evaluable. Of these, 7 had stage III disease, and 18 had stage IV disease.

Of the 25 evaluable patients, one experienced partial response lasting for more than 3 months, and survived for over 4 months, 9 had stable disease for a median period of over 5.5 months, and a median survival period of over 6.5 months, and 15 had progressive disease, with a median survival period of 3 months. The partial remission occurred in a 73-year old woman with undifferentiated carcinoma, stage IV. This patient had a greater than 50% reduction of the central pelvic mass and inguinal nodes metastases. Eight of the 25 patients (32%) experienced an increase in their Karnofsky index (mean 20 points).

On examining response in relation to histology, 6 out of 8 patients with highly or moderately well differentiated serous adenocarcinoma were found to have had stable disease. In 66% of these patients, the Karnofsky index increased by a mean of 20 points. This compares with 1 partial remission and 2 cases of stable disease in 15 patients with poorly-differentiated adenocarcinomas. Disease in the 2 patients with endometrioid cancer was progressive. There were no changes during drug therapy in blood counts, serum levels of creatinine, bilirubin, alkaline phosphatase, or fasting blood sugar levels. One patient gained weight, as a result of fluid retention, and also developed high blood pressure. More severe complications (deep venous thrombosis) were seen in 2 patients, but both had large pelvic tumour masses and would perhaps, have developed deep venous thrombosis in any case.

Discussion

The overall response rate was 4%, which is about the same as that reported by Malkasian et al. [7], but far from the high response rate of 60% reported by Ward [3]. Since most of the epithelial ovarian carcinoma cell types were included in this study it is, therefore, reasonable to conclude that objective responses can only be obtained in a minority of patients with ovarian adenocarcinoma resistant to cytostatic drugs. However, we used MPA as third line therapy. When using chemotherapy as second or third line therapy, the overall response rate is also very low. Even although we saw no objective response, we believe that the patients with highly or moderately well-differentiated serous adenocarcinomas benefited from their treatment. Seventy-five per cent of them experienced stable disease, with a median survival period of over 6.5 months, and 66% had a better quality of life. Patients with progressive disease had a median survival period of 3 months.

Stable disease lasting for such periods, even though in only small numbers of patients, warrants further study, and we think it remains to be determined whether MPA at the dosages used can provide effective control in a large series of endometrioid carcinomas of the ovary. Recent studies in our laboratory indicate that many patients with ovarian adenocarcinoma have progesterone receptors. Such studies may be useful in defining patients particularly likely to be responsive to MPA.

Three studies have been published in which oral, high dose MPA has been used [7–9] (Table III). In the study of Mangioni et al. [8], either patients were allocated at random to high doses MPA orally, or high dose MPA intramuscularly. The conclusion from these 3 studies is that high dose MPA in-

Table III. Response to oral high dose MPA.

Investigators	Dosages	Numbers of patients	Objective response rates (%)
Malkasian et al. [7]	100 mg/day 200 mg/day 400 mg/day	19	4
Mangioni et al. [8]	800 mg daily for at least 4 weeks	30	0
Aabo [9]	500 mg/m^2 daily for at least 4 weeks	30	4

Table IV. MPA combined with chemotherapy in advanced ovarian cancer.

Investigators	Treatment	Objective response rate (%)	Period of survival (days)
Senn [13]	Cyclophosphamide	28	180
	Cyclophosphamide + 450 mg/week i.m. MPA	64	231 +
	Cyclophosphamide + 5	61	220 +
Bumma et al. [14]	CAF	55	—
	CAF + MPA 500 mg i.m. for 30 days then 500 mg twice weekly	59	Significantly longer than CAF
Curcio et al. [15]	MPA + melphalan	80	40% alive after 2 years
Guthrie [16]	Gestonorone + Cyclophosphamide	76	10% alive after 2 years
Bergkvist et al. [17]	MPA + melphalan	85	—

tramuscularly is superior to high dose MPA orally.

There are encouraging reports by Robustelli et al. [12] that a combination of chemotherapy and hormone therapy might prolong survival in breast cancer. There has recently been particular interest in evaluating hormonal therapy combined with chemotherapy in ovarian cancer. Results appear encouraging, with improvements in response rates. Five studies [13–17], 2 of which [13, 14] were controlled, have so far been published. In these, MPA was used together with cytostatic agents (Table IV). All 3 uncontrolled studies suggest that results were better than with cytostatic drugs alone, but without controls this cannot properly be judged. Curcio et al. reported an 80% objective response rate, with 40% of their patients alive after 2 years [15]. Guthrie reported a 76% objective response rate [16]. Ten per cent of his patients were still alive after 2 years. Bergkvist et al. reported an 85% objective response rate, but gave no survival data [17].

The investigators conducting controlled studies stressed that there were no significant differences in response rates, but that durations of response and survival times were longer, although not significantly, in the MPA-treated groups. The side-effects were also less in the MPA-treated groups. They conclude that MPA therapy combined with chemotherapy could possibly maintain the therapeutic results of chemotherapy.

Conclusions

1. High-dose MPA has some activity in ovarian epithelial cancer. 2. In unselected patients with advanced ovarian cancer refractory to conventional chemotherapy, high dose MPA is not an effective treatment. 3. High dose MPA intramuscularly is superior to high dose MPA orally. 4. Most patients experience an increase in their Karnofsky index when treated with high dose MPA. 5. Further trials of high dose MPA on its own in the therapy of ovarian cancer should be limited to patients for whom endometrial histology data is available, with special emphasis on the relationships between receptor activity and response. 6. High dose MPA combined with chemotherapy could reduce side effects, increase response rate and prolong survival. Prospective controlled investigations are, therefore, warranted, to check both the validity of this approach, and the optimal sequencing of the 2 treatments.

References

1. Jolles, B. (1962): Progesterone in the treatment of advanced malignant tumours of breast, ovary and uterus. *Br. J. Cancer 16,* 209.
2. Varga, A. and Henrikssen, E. (1964): Effect of 17-α-hydroxy-progesterone

17-n-caproate on various pelvic malignancies. *Obstet. Gynecol. 23,* 51.

3. Ward, H.W.C. (1972): Progesterone therapy for ovarian carcinoma. *J. Obstet. Gynecol. Br. Commonw. 79,* 555.
4. Malkasian Jr., G.D., Decker, D.G., Jorgensen, E.O. and Webb, M.J. (1973): 6-Dehydro-6; 17-α-dimethylprogesterone (NSC-123018) for the treatment of metastatic and recurrent ovarian carcinoma. *Cancer Chemother. Rep. 57,* 241.
5. Tobias, J.S. and Griffiths, C.T. (1976): Management of ovarian carcinoma. Current concepts and future prospects. *N. Engl. J. Med. 294,* 877.
6. Paraskevas, G.A., Angelakis, P.H. and Deligeorgi-Politi, H. (1976): Changes in clinical and histological patterns observed in patients with advanced carcinoma of the ovary treated with progesterone. In: *Chemotherapy,* Vol. 8. pp. 611–614. Cancer Chemotherapy II. Eds: Hellman and Connors. Plenum Press, New York and London.
7. Malkasian, G.D., Decker, D.G., Jorgensen, E.O. and Edmonson, J.H. (1977): Medroxyprogesterone acetate for the treatment of metastatic and recurrent ovarian carcinoma. *Cancer Treat. Rep. 61,* 913.
8. Mangioni, C., Franceschi, S., Vecchia, C. and D'Incaki, M. (1981): High dose medroxyprogesterone acetate (MPA) in advanced epithelial ovarian cancer resistant to first or second line chemotherapy. *Gynecol. Oncol. 12,* 314.
9. Aabo, K., Pedersen, A.G., Held, J. and Dombernowsky (1982): High dose medroxyprogesterone acetate (MPA) in advanced chemotherapy-resistant ovarian carcinoma: a phase II study. *Cancer Treat. Rep. 66,* 407.
10. Slayton, R.E., Pagano, M. and Creech, R.H. (1981): Progestin therapy for advanced ovarian cancer: a phase II Eastern Cooperative Oncology Group Trial. *Cancer Treat. Rep. 65,* 895.
11. Tropé, C., Johnsson, J.E., Sigurdsson, K. and Simonsen, E. (1982): High dose medroxyprogesterone acetate for the treatment of advanced ovarian carcinoma. *Cancer Treat. Rep.* (In press.)
12. Robustelli Della Cuna, G., Martinetti, L., Bernardo-Testa, M.R. and Pizzamiglio, D. (1978): FAC (5 Fu, Adm, CTX) versus FAC + HD MAP (high dose medroxyprogesterone acetate) in metastatic breast cancer. Paper read at: XIIth International Cancer Congress, Buenos Aires, October 1978.
13. Senn, H.J. (1973): Treatment of advanced inoperable ovarian carcinoma. *Ther. Umsch. 30,* 651.
14. Bumma, C. and Bertetto, O. (1981): Treatment with chemotherapy versus treatment with medroxyprogesterone acetate plus chemotherapy in advanced ovarian carcinoma. International Symposium on Role of Medroxyprogesterone acetate (MPA) in endocrine-related tumours, Rome, 1981. Abstract 18.
15. Curcio, C.G., Casati, A., Cianciotta, A. et al. (1978): Chemo-hormonotherapeutic management of twenty cases of metastatic ovarian carcinoma. *Clin. Ter. 90,* 137.
16. Guthrie, D. (1979): The treatment of advanced cystadenocarcinoma of the ovary with Gestonol and continuous oral cyclophosphamide. *Br. J. Obstet. Gynaecol. 86,* 497.
17. Bergkvist, A., Kullander, S. and Thorell, J. (1981): A study of estrogen and progesterone cytosol receptor concentration in benign and malignant ovarian tumours and a review of malignant ovarian tumours treated with medroxyprogesterone acetate. *Acta Obstet. Gynecol. Scand. 101 (Suppl.),* 75.

Discussion

C. Tropé: On the basis of the last 2 papers, obviously no definite beneficial effect of MPA combined with multi-agent chemotherapy has been shown in ovarian cancer. I think that Dr Jungi's suggestion to use high-dose MPA is right. Professor Nieminen's study included only 20 patients, so no conclusions can be drawn from that study.

M. Kjaer: We heard something about nadir values in Dr Jungi's presentation, but I think nothing was said about them in Professor Nieminen's paper. One of the interesting things in combining chemotherapy and MPA is that perhaps more chemotherapy could be given when MPA is given simultaneously, because MPA has a sort of protective effect. Probably it removes leucocytes to the peripheral blood*. That is why I do not think that the question about the possibility of giving more chemotherapy can be answered, unless we go for equivalent toxicity in the 2 regimens. We have to go for the same nadir values; the doses of chemotherapy have to be escalated if it is given in combination with MPA. I would like to hear from the Finnish group whether the total doses of chemotherapy given in the 2 arms, CDP (cyclophosphamide, doxorubicin, platinum) and CDP plus MPA, were equivalent, and what about the nadir values – the leucocytopenia?

U. Nieminen: The number of patients was so small that we have not done that.

C. Tropé: In Lund we are now going to use CDP plus or minus high-dose MPA. However, I can not give any results yet.

D.V. Razis: Both papers included granulose-cell ovarian tumours. This type of tumour should be studied separately; their natural history is different, their treatment and response to treatment are also very different. They respond nicely to radiation therapy. I do not think that this type of tumour should be

*Up to now, we do not know the mechanism(s) underlying the leucocytes' and platelets' protecting activity of MPA against chemotherapy toxicity.

included in the chemotherapeutic studies of all other sorts of ovarian tumours.

The dose schedule was possibly low in the Finnish study, which might explain the relatively low response rate for both partial and complete remissions. There are at least 2 reports from the United States, and another from Greece, saying that using the 3 drugs, cis-platinum, doxorubicin and cyclophosphamide, plus hexamethylmelamine, as a first-line therapy, gives a very high response rate. The problem is that the recurrence rate is also very high. Perhaps it is there that MPA may play a role in preventing recurrence in the cases of complete remission.

C. Mangioni: From September 1980 to December 1981, 47 patients with advanced epithelial ovarian cancer were treated with 3 different schedules of second-line chemotherapy at our Oncology Gynaecology Unit. All patients, whose age ranged from 20–70 years, were resistant or relapsed to previous first-line chemotherapy. The second-line chemotherapy consisted of the following 3 different schemes repeated every 4 weeks. 1. Doxorubicin + platinum + hexamethylmelamine in patients previously treated with alkylating agents and/or antimetabolites (20 patients). 2. Platinum + hexamethylmelamine in those previously treated with doxorubicin and alkylating agents (18 patients). 3. High doses of platinum alone in those previously treated with doxorubicin, hexamethylmelamine and alkylating agents (9 patients).

Randomly, 23 out of the 47 patients received also 500 mg of MPA, i.m., daily for the first 4 weeks and then 500 mg twice a week. Patients were evaluated at least after 3 months and the responses were classified as complete, partial, minimal, no change and progression. The bone marrow toxicity was evaluated according to ECOG criteria.

The responses obtained in the patients treated with MPA were: one complete response (4%), 6 partial (26%) and 5 minimal (22%). In the group of patients not treated with MPA, the responses were: one complete response (4%), 7 partial (29%) and one minimal (4%). Myelodepression was less marked in the patients treated with MPA: a statistically significant difference between the 2 groups was observed ($P < 0.01$). In fact, the number of patients with 3- and 4-grade bone marrow toxicity (according to ECOG) was lower in the group treated with MPA. Side-effects observed in the patients treated with MPA were: 4 Cushing-like syndromes, 2 indurations and abscesses in the site of injection.

In conclusion, the use of high-dose MPA in addition to the polychemotherapy regimens in second-line treatment of patients with advanced epithelial ovarian cancer does not seem to improve the clinical response rate. On the other hand, minimal response and subjective improvement were observed more frequently in the MPA-treated group, that is, a better quality of life normally not observed in second line-treated patients. In addition, a lower grade of bone marrow toxicity was observed in the group of patients treated with MPA.

C. Tropé: The conclusion about MPA and ovarian cancer may be that high-dose MPA has some activity in epithelial ovarian cancer (in fact, there is no doubt about that). In unselected patients with advanced ovarian cancer refractory to conventional chemotherapy, however, high-dose MPA is not an effective treatment. However, as has been said, there is no other treatment to give these patients – a third-line treatment with chemotherapy also gives response in only 5–10% of the patients. High-dose MPA, intramuscularly, is superior to high-dose MPA given orally. Professor Mangioni has beautifully demonstrated that.

Most patients increase their Karnofsky index rating when treated with high-dose MPA.

Further trials of high-dose MPA as a single drug for ovarian cancer therapy should be limited to patients with endometrial histology, with special emphasis on the relationship between receptor activity and response.

High-dose MPA combined with chemotherapy might reduce the side-effects, increase the response rate and prolong the survival. Prospective, controlled investigations are therefore warranted to check the validity of this new approach and the optimal ways of using the 2 treatments.

Round table: Hormone receptors

Chairman: W.L. McGuire, San Antonio, U.S.A.

Panelists:

F. Cavalli	(Bellinzona, Switzerland)
A. Di Marco	(Milan, Italy)
J.A. Gustafsson	(Huddinge, Sweden)
P.M. Martin	(Marseille, France)
E. Milgrom	(Le Kremlin Bicêtre, France)
Y. Nomura	(Fukuoka, Japan)
A. Pellegrini	(Cagliari, Italy)
K. Pollow	(Mainz, Federal Republic of Germany)
S. Saez	(Lyon, France)
N. Weigel	(Houston, U.S.A.)
D. Zava	(Bern, Switzerland)

Contents:

Introduction

We shall start with what will hopefully be some new (and I emphasize *new*) concepts in the mechanism of hormone action, proceeding to some other, more practical, aspects, such as developments in assay procedures. I hope that the panelists will not review older, traditional methods but will present only new and exciting innovations in receptor assays. Another topic will be receptors in adjuvant disease – again, not reviewing the literature but only presenting new, perhaps speculative but interesting data. Receptors in advanced disease is an old story – let us hope new information on that subject will be presented. The changing receptor status is also an old topic, but the literature on the subject is scant, so perhaps we can have some definitive numbers in terms of how many people switch from positive to negative receptors and vice versa. Finally, we have heard many reports of receptors being measured in non-classical tissues, and perhaps that can be put into perspective during this round table.

W.L. McGuire,
University of Texas,
Health Science Center
at San Antonio,
San Antonio
Texas
U.S.A.

The mechanism of hormone action

N. Weigel

For the last few years we have been using the chicken oviduct as a model system to study the mechanism of steroid hormone action. We have investigated the biochemistry of the progesterone receptor as one aspect of this study.

Some of the characteristics of this system are: progesterone can induce the synthesis of ovalbumin messenger ribonucleic acid in vivo. This action is mediated by an intracellular receptor protein. The receptor consists of 2 hormone-binding subunits with different molecular weights (MW): A, with a MW of 79,000, and a deoxyribonucleic acid (DNA)-binding activity; B, with a MW of 108,000, and a chromatin-binding activity. Both subunits have been purified to apparent homogeneity from chicken oviducts. Recent experiments done by Dr Kate Horowitz (University of Colorado School of Medicine, Denver, Colorado, U.S.A.) using human progesterone receptor suggest that it also has 2 subunits of these sizes.

The intact cytosol receptor exists as a complex of the A and B proteins which can bind to chromatin but not to DNA (Fig. 1). Warming or treatment with salt will dissociate the complex. Gel filtration and sucrose gradient studies have shown that both receptor proteins are highly asymmetric

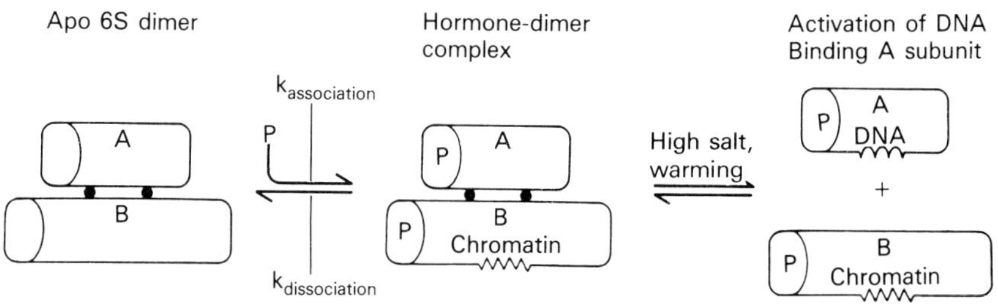

Fig. 1. Receptor activation by subunit dissociation.

molecules. In contrast, the hormone-binding portion (the meroreceptor) released by proteolysis appears to be globular. The A subunit has a high affinity for DNA in general. However, experiments done recently in our laboratory by Dr Compton demonstrate that the receptor binds preferentially to the DNA of the ovalbumin gene and of other hormonally-regulated genes.

We have been studying the structure and function of the receptor, and have also begun to isolate functional domains for further study of individual activities. I will describe the results of some of our more recent experiments, using techniques not commonly used to study receptors. We first looked at the structural relationship between A and B by peptide mapping. Since both subunits have hormone-binding sites, it was possible that the smaller subunit A was derived from the larger subunit B by proteolysis either as a biological processing mechanism or as an artifact of the isolation procedure. The purified proteins from hen oviduct were iodinated on the tyrosines, digested with trypsin, and mapped.

The peptides were separated in the first dimension by high-voltage electrophoresis followed by chromatography in the second dimension. Figure 2 shows a drawing of the map obtained from the analysis of A, B, and a mixture of both. If A were a proteolytic fragment of B, all the peptides in A would be

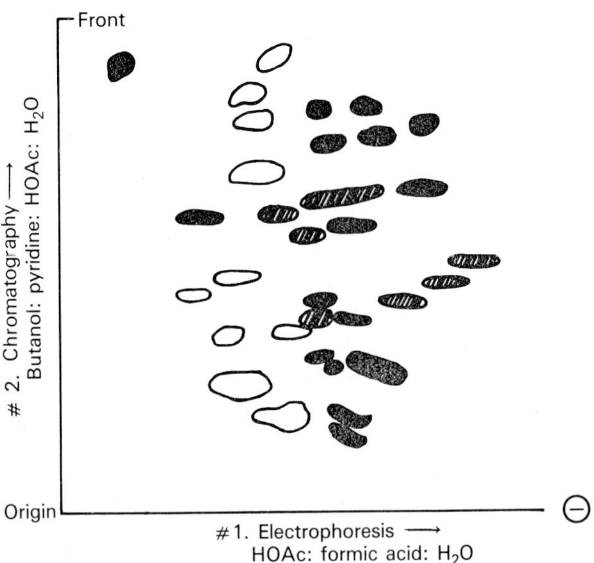

Fig. 2. Tryptic map of iodinated peptides in the hen receptors A and B (□ = peptides found only in A; ■ = peptides found only in B; ▨ = peptides found in both A and B).

found in B with the possible exception of 2: the amino terminal and carboxyl terminal peptides. Although there are a few overlapping peptides, most of the peptides are different. These results indicate that the 2 receptors are distinct molecules probably arising from separate genes.

We have also located the hormone-binding domain of the 2 proteins using a progesterone analogue, 17α-methylpromegestone (commonly known as R5020), as a photo-affinity label. These studies were done in our laboratory by Dr Birnbaumer. R5020 contains a conjugated double bond which absorbs at 320 nm, and can thus be activated without destroying amino acids.

Figure 3 shows a fluorograph of partially-purified, covalently-labelled A and B, analysed on a sodium dodecyl sulphate (SDS) gel. Cold progesterone completely blocks the reaction, as expected for a specific label.

The covalently-labelled proteins were then exhaustively digested with *Staphylococcus aureus* protease and analysed by 2-dimensional gel electrophoresis. The labelled peptides derived from A and B were indistinguishable by this method. Although a 9,500-MW fragment was obtained after exhaustive digestion, earlier experiments had shown that peptides of about 25,000 MW, depending upon the protease used, are the smallest that can retain noncovalently-bound hormone. The larger hormone-binding domains (or meroreceptors) derived from A and B by partial proteolysis are also indistinguishable by size. These experiments suggest that the hormone-binding

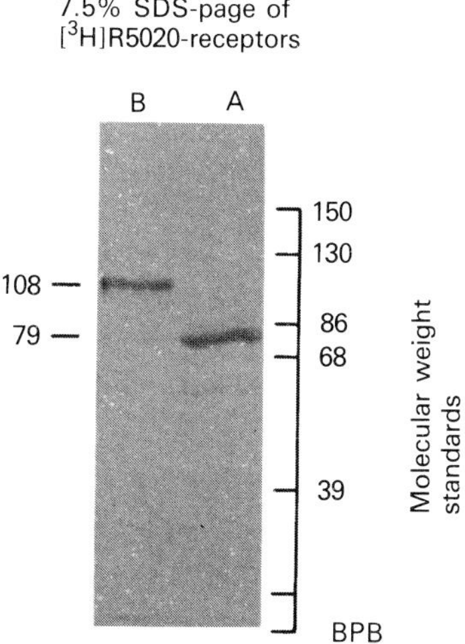

Fig. 3. Fluorograph of partially-purified, covalently labelled A and B, analysed on an SDS gel.

receptor sites are very similar, if not identical, although other portions are clearly different, based on peptide mapping.

We have also localized the DNA-binding site of the A protein. Earlier experiments with crude receptor suggested that proteolytic fragments of A with a MW $\geq$ 40,000, containing the hormone-binding site, also contained the DNA-binding site. We have now used the protein blotting method of Bowen et al. to look for smaller peptides containing a DNA-binding activity [1]. Proteins or peptides are separated by SDS gel electrophoresis, transferred to nitrocellulose paper by diffusion, and the paper containing the partially-renatured proteins is incubated with ^{32}P-DNA to detect the DNA binders. Because of the high specific activity of DNA, less than 1% of the protein needs to renature in order to see a band.

Figure 4 shows the results of a typical experiment with the A protein. Purified A was digested with *S. aureus* protease, either for a brief time or overnight, and the peptides were separated by SDS gel electrophoresis. The autoradiograph of the blotted lane containing purified A is shown. The left lane shows that the A protein binds DNA under these conditions. Also shown (centre lane) are the results of a 5-minute incubation with an enzyme and (right lane) the results of an overnight digestion. As digestion proceeds, the DNA-binding activity progressively decreases in size until a limited size of

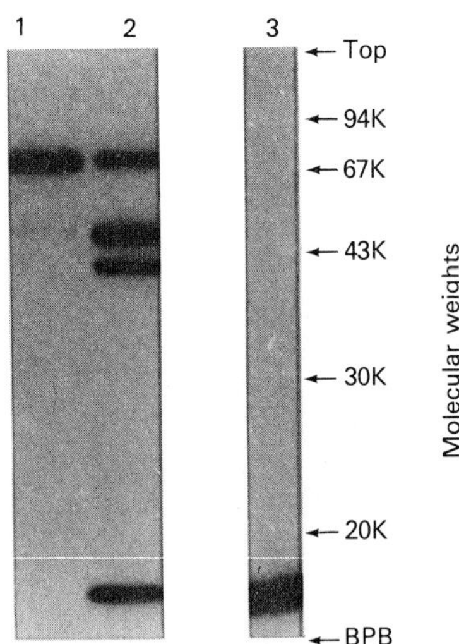

Fig. 4. Typical experiment with the A protein. Lane 1 shows the binding of DNA, lane 2 the result of a 5-minute incubation with an enzyme, and lane 3 the result of an overnight digestion.

15,000 is seen. The intermediate fragments also contain hormone-binding activity, based on R5020 experiments as well as experiments using DNA cellulose. The smallest fragment contains only the DNA-binding site (data not shown).

These and other studies have resulted in a partial map of the receptor subunits, as shown in Figure 5. The hormone-binding domain resides in a proteolytically-resistant region of the protein, of about 23,000 MW, depending upon the enzyme used. Sequence analysis of the receptors reveals that the amino terminal ends are blocked. The 23,000-MW hormone-binding domain (or meroreceptor) is also blocked, and thus is apparently the amino terminal end of the protein. Digestion of a covalently-labelled receptor with *S. aureus* protease produces a smaller peptide with a MW of 9,500 (the H fragment) which contains the covalently-attached R5020. Since peptides (called from IV) containing both hormone- and DNA-binding activity can be isolated, the DNA-binding domain must be adjacent to the hormone-binding domain. This domain is resistant to *S. aureus* protease digestion (as has been shown in

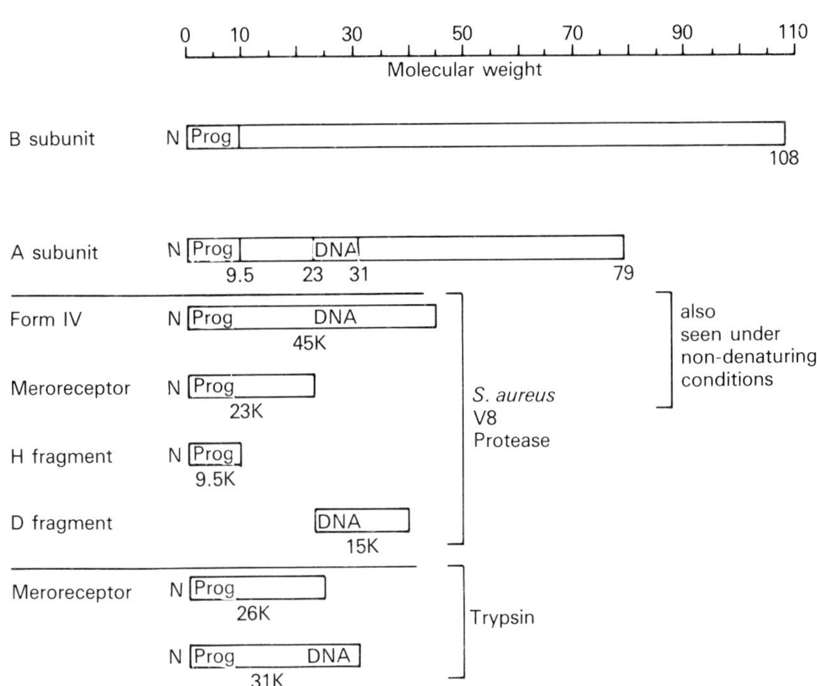

Fig. 5. Protease digestion maps of receptor subunits.

Figure 4). The 26,000-MW meroreceptor from the tryptic digest contains no DNA-binding activity, yet the 31,000-MW tryptic fragment contains at least a portion of the DNA-binding activity. Thus, the DNA-binding portion begins between 26,000 and 31,000, and extends towards the carboxyl end of the molecule. Using column chromatography, we are now isolating these domains to study the DNA- and hormone-binding activities of these fragments.

We have also started to look for post-translational modification of the receptor proteins. When the purified proteins were analysed by 2-dimensional gel electrophoresis charge heterogeneity was found suggesting that the proteins may be phosphorylated.

In Figure 6, lane 1 is the Coomassie blue-stained gel of B. Lane 2 is the phosphorylation autoradiograph of B by the catalytic subunit of the cyclic adenosine monophosphate-dependent protein kinase, showing that B is phosphorylated by the protein kinase. Lanes 3 and 4 are the results of the control incubation lacking protein kinase showing that the reaction is dependent upon added kinase. Lanes 5 and 6 show the autophosphorylation of the protein kinase.

Two-dimensional gel electrophoresis of the A and B subunits is shown in Figure 7. Panel 1 on the left shows the Coomassie blue-stained gel of a partially-phosphorylated B preparation and panel 2 below it, the correspond-

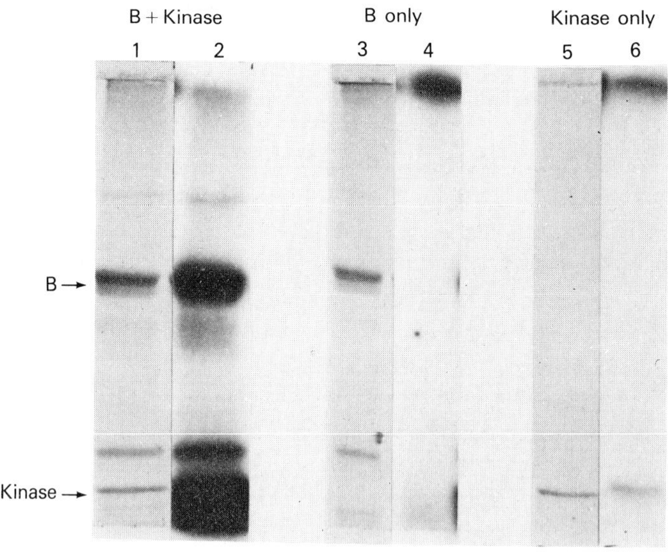

Fig. 6. Phosphorylation of hen receptor B using bovine heart protein kinase.

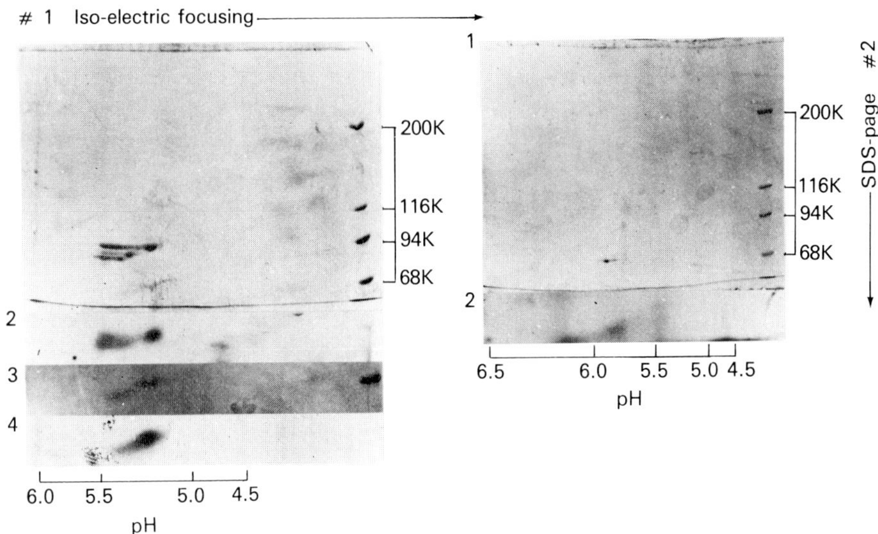

Fig. 7. Two-dimensional gel electrophoresis of phosphorylated receptors.

ing autoradiograph. Panel 3 shows the stained gel of extensively-phosphorylated B, showing a shift of the protein to the more acidic positions and panel 4 the corresponding autoradiograph. The right-hand panels show the stained A preparation (panel 1) and the corresponding autoradiograph (panel 2). Other experiments have demonstrated that both receptor subunits are phosphorylated rapidly, and apparently quantitatively. The 2-dimensional gel analysis suggests that the heterogeneity is caused by phosphorylation. If the in-vivo modification were something other than phosphorylation, the entire pattern should shift to more acidic positions and a new, more acidic spot should appear. Although the receptor was extensively phosphorylated, no new, more acidic spots were seen. Phospho-amino acid analysis of the ^{32}P-labelled receptor shows that it is phosphorylated on serine.

These experiments suggest that the receptors are phosphoproteins. We are also studying the effect of phosphorylation on the function of the receptor. I will briefly describe the one alteration we have found so far.

Dr Maggi, from our laboratory, has found that the chick progesterone receptor has a second, weaker hormone-binding site. This site is affected by alkaline phosphatase treatment, although the stronger site is not so affected.

Scatchard plots of the treated and untreated receptor are shown in Figure 8, with (on the left) the untreated receptor showing both sites and (on the right) the Scatchard plot after treatment. The second site is greatly diminished after

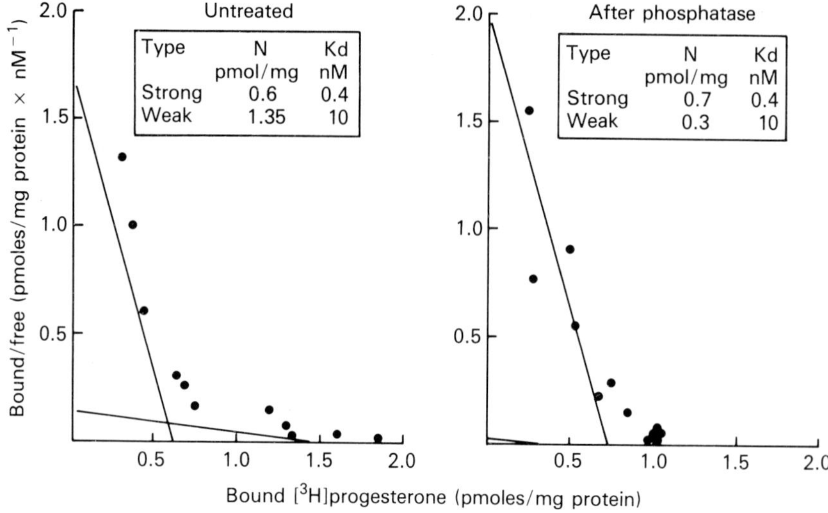

Fig. 8. Effect of alkaline phosphate treatment on receptor hormone-binding sites.

treatment, but the strong site remains unaffected. Phosphatase inhibitors, such as glucose 1-phosphate, prevent loss of the second site. Thus, this loss appears to be a result of dephosphorylation.

In conclusion, we can say that the 2 receptor subunits are distinctly different and can not share a precursor-product relationship; they have closely-related or identical hormone-binding sites; the DNA-binding site is present on a separate domain, adjacent to the hormone-binding domain; and both proteins appear to be phosphoproteins.

Reference

1. Bowen et al. (1980): *Nucleic Acids Res.*

W.L. McGuire: Those people who do not work with receptors should take my word for it that this work is really at the cutting edge of the attempts to understand the biochemical nature of the receptor as a protein, studying its binding site both to hormone and nuclear components.

The mechanism of hormone action

E. Milgrom

I would briefly like to introduce 2 types of studies in which we are interested and which are pursued on other models or other systems in many laboratories throughout the world. These studies will probably provide new tools for studying the various practical aspects of hormonotherapy described at this symposium.

The first problem is the study of the receptors. As we have heard, there are many problems with the present methods for measuring receptors: problems due to the compartmentalization of the receptors; the fact that measurement has to be made in the cytosol or the nuclei; problems due to endogenous hormone which necessitates the use of complicated exchange assays; and the problems due to the lability (the fragility) of the hormone-binding receptor site.

An important possible way of trying to solve these problems and to have more easily-handled receptor assays is, of course, to try not to use the hormone-binding properties of the receptor but obtain receptor antibodies and use these to measure the receptor. Although I think that Professor Gustafsson has some results, this has not yet been widely achieved. I would like to present some characteristics of an antibody obtained against the progesterone receptor, which may perhaps be used in such a way in the future.

The existence of this antibody is demonstrated in Figure 1. A sucrose gradient will be recognized with a rabbit progesterone receptor, prepared from the uterus, which is migrating at 4S. With increasing amounts of the antiserum, there is precipitation at the bottom of the receptor tube. The specificity of this antibody is interesting.

Figure 2 shows one of the elements of this specificity. The receptor prepared from human breast cancer runs as 4S, because it is in high ionic strength and again precipitated by the antibody.

Similar studies have been performed on various receptors and proteins, and the specificity is summarized in the Table.

The general picture given here is very close to the picture which has been

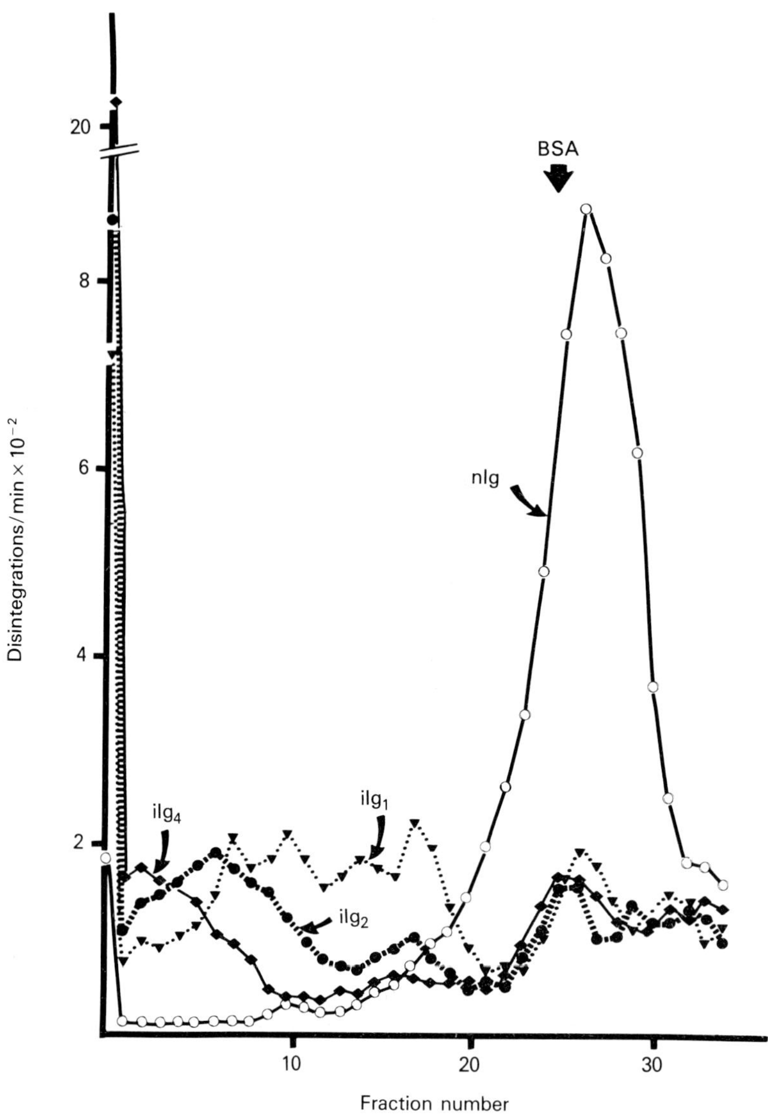

Fig. 1. Detection of antibodies against the cytosolic progesterone receptor from rabbit uterus (iIg = immunoglobulins from immunized goat; nIg = immunoglobulins from non-immunized goat; BSA = sulisobenzone).

given previously, for instance, by Dr Jensen, with the antibodies against the oestrogen receptor. There is the fact that these antibodies recognize the receptors from various tissues, and there is also a great similarity inter-species. This type of antibody, and perhaps even better monoclonal antibodies against

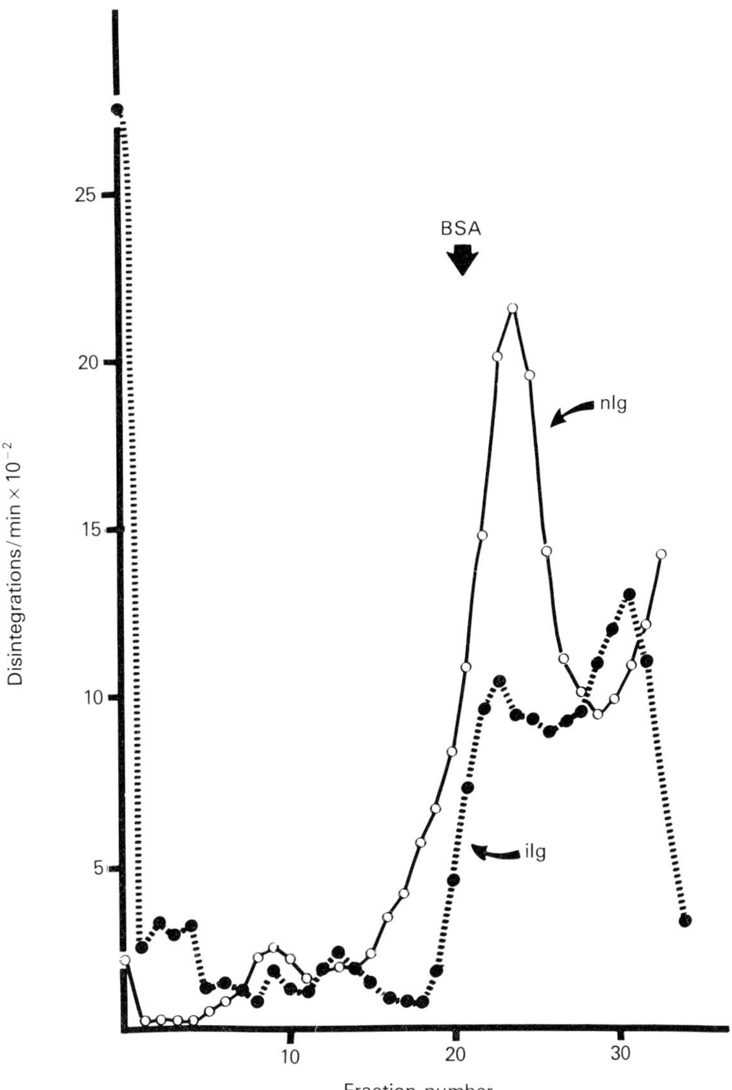

Fig. 2. Immunoprecipitation of progesterone receptor from human breast cancer (iIg = immunoglobulins from immunized goat; nIg = immunoglobulins from non-immunized goat).

these receptors which are now being prepared in various laboratories, will probably allow easier and more reproducible methods of progesterone receptor assay in the future.

The second problem which I shall briefly try to introduce is the response to

Table. Cross reactivity of antibodies elicited against progesterone receptor from rabbit uterine cytosol.

	Cross reactivity
Nuclear progesterone receptor from rabbit uterus	+
Cytosolic progesterone receptor from rabbit vagina	+
Cytosolic progesterone receptor from rabbit pituitary	+
Cytosolic progesterone receptor from human breast cancer	+
Cytosolic progesterone receptor from human endometrium	+
Nuclear progesterone receptor from human endometrium	+
Cytosolic progesterone receptor from guinea-pig uterus	+
Cytosolic progesterone receptor from rat uterus	+
Cytosolic progesterone receptor from chick oviduct	–
Rabbit corticosteroid-binding globulin (progesterone- and cortisol-binding plasma protein)	–
Rabbit uteroglobin (progesterone-binding protein from uterine fluid)	–
Cytosolic oestradiol receptor from rabbit uterus	–
Cytosolic glucocorticoid receptor from rabbit liver	–

the hormone and the possibility of using specific nucleic acids as tools for following this response. Since we were interested in the response of the rabbit endometrium to progesterone, we have focused on a protein, uteroglobin. The mRNA for uteroglobin which is induced by progesterone can be translated and also purified from this source. From the purified messenger it is of course possible to prepare a radioactive complementary DNA (cDNA). I would like to emphasize that such a cDNA is a very powerful tool with which to measure the hormone effect.

For instance, Figure 3 shows the time course of the effect of progesterone in prepubertal rabbit endometrium. The control experiment involves the measurements of less than 10 molecules of messenger per endometrial cell, and it is perfectly specific and very easily measured. The time course (which represents here rather short intervals of some hours) can be seen very easily by these hybridization methods with the specific cDNA. This kind of methodology is developed for very many systems and will probably be used in clinical situations in the future – that is, to measure the actual effect of hormones, and not simply the possibility of an effect (which is the receptor).

The other part of such studies is the possibility of bacterial cloning of cDNA. Once cDNA is cloned, it is a perfect tool. First, because it is perfectly homogeneous and reproducible and can be spread through many laboratories, and secondly, because it may then be used to assay the messenger without any problems or specificity difficulties.

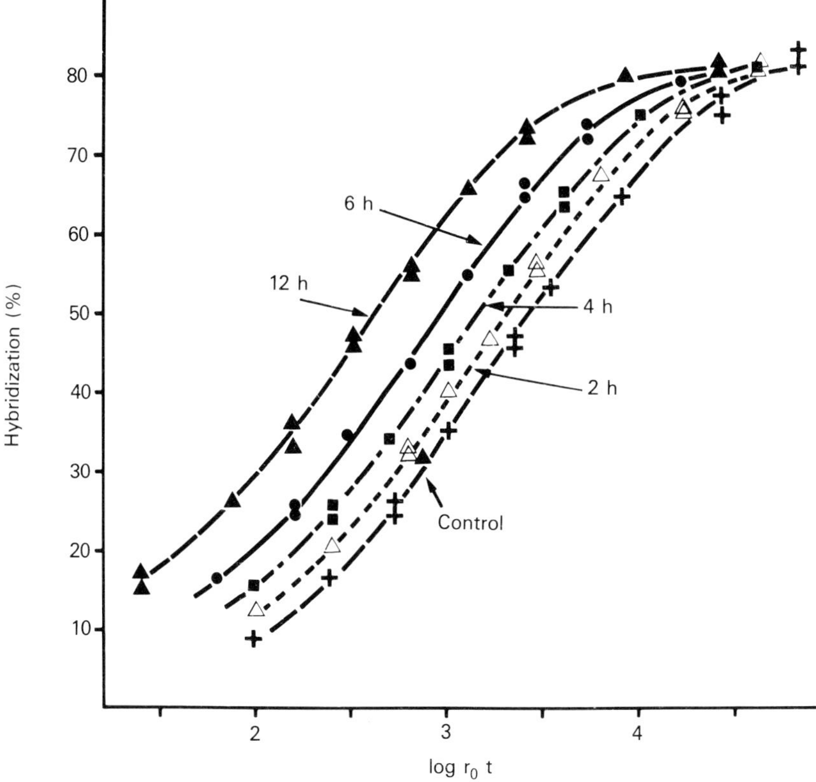

Fig. 3. Time course of induction by progesterone of uteroglobin mRNA.

Figure 4 shows a gel electrophoresis in which the DNA from a recombinant plasmid – in which uteroglobin cDNA has been cloned into the PST_1 site – has been excised by PST_1. There are 2 fragments, the bigger one which corresponds to the 3′ end of the messenger, and the other to the 5′ end (the opposite end) of the messenger. Those DNA fragments may then be used as very specific homogeneous probes, if we want to measure the messenger and also if we want to go up in the system and try to isolate the chromosomal gene for this hormone-responsive protein.

We have been screening a gene library prepared by Tom Maniatis which comprises the entire genome of the rabbit contained in about 850,000 different phages. We have screened about 200,000 of these phages. There are 10,000 of them on the Petri dish – and there is one positive spot which is recloned. After recloning, there are more spots which give a positive response with the cloned DNA used as a probe.

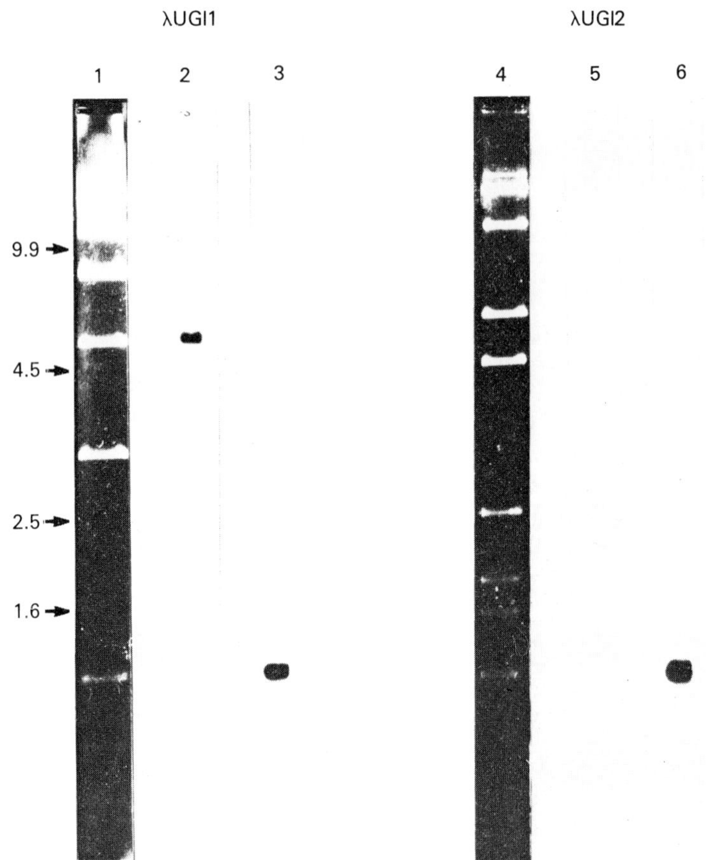

Fig. 4. Hybridization of λ-uteroglobin (UGL)$_1$ and λUGL$_2$ EcoRI DNA fragments with 5′ and 3′ fragments of cloned cDNA. Lanes 1 and 4: ethidium bromide fluorescence; lanes 2 and 5: autoradiography after hybridization with 5′ end probe; and lanes 3 and 6: autoradiography after hybridization with 3′ end probe. The size of markers is given in kilobase pairs.

With this method, therefore, we have obtained 2 different phages (Fig. 5). Shown are polyacrylamide gels after action of an enzyme – a restriction enzyme, EcoRI – on the DNA, and the different DNA fragments which have been isolated from the 2 phages. There is hybridization to the 5′ end as well as to the 3′ end of the gene. One of the phages contains the totality of the gene. Both ends are present in that phage, whereas the other phage contains only part of the gene, the 3′ end. We have now sequenced most of this gene and

Fig. 5. Comparison of uteroglobin gene sequence in phage λUGL_l and rabbit liver DNA, which were digested by EcoRI. 5′ and 3′ specific probes were used.

know exactly its structure. In one of the phages there is the totality of the gene and a lot of 5′-adjacent DNA; in the other phage there is half the gene and a lot of 3′-adjacent DNA.

This type of study enables us to do experiments in an attempt to understand what effect the progesterone has on the gene. We have also shown a comparison of what has been cloned in the phage with what is present in the cell, using DNA prepared from rabbit liver which has been treated by various enzymes. After hybridization there is the same disposition of the DNA; there have been no changes during recloning. Also, there is only a single gene present in the DNA for this protein.

In conclusion, I would like to say that this information is now far from the practical aspects on which this symposium has focused in the earlier sessions. However, I think that practical points will result rather rapidly from this kind of study with regard not only to the measurement of steroid hormone receptors but also with regard to the fact that the hormone response may also probably be measured by rather simple methods (an aspect which is currently not greatly developed).

W.L. McGuire: It is apparent that, for those of us who will be attending the meetings involving receptors in the 1980's, we will have to be able to understand the language of recombinant DNA, hybridomas and so on.

The mechanism of hormone action

J.A. Gustafsson

I would like to address 2 issues with regard to steroid receptors, in particular, the glucocorticoid receptor. 1. Some research we have performed recently, in collaboration with Dr Keith Yamamoto's laboratory in San Francisco, concerning specific binding of the glucocorticoid receptor to DNA. 2. During the new assays' section, I shall discuss our studies on an antiserum against the glucocorticoid receptor, and an enzyme-linked immunosorbent assay (ELISA) method based on this antiserum.

We have purified the glucocorticoid receptor to near homogeneity using a procedure, which is now used on a routine basis in our laboratory (Fig. 1). We start with the livers from 15 rats (which contain about 400 μg of glucocorticoid receptor). The receptor is labelled with [^{3}H]-triamcinolone acetonide and is then chromatographed on phosphocellulose and DNA-cellulose. Since the receptor is not activated, it will not stick to the gel but goes through the columns. Following that, the receptor is activated using incubation for 30 minutes at 25° C. It will then stick to the DNA in the second step. Using this

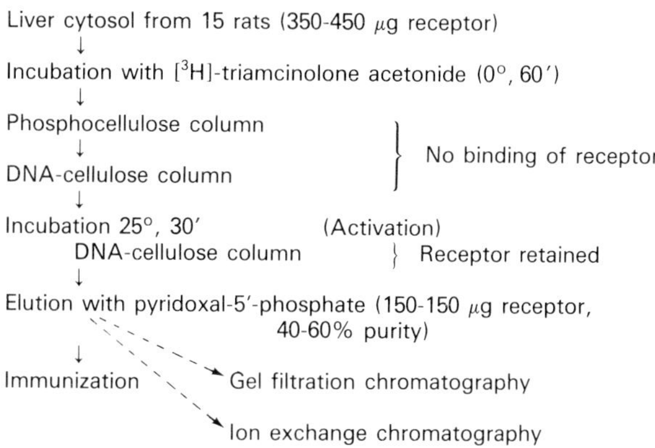

Fig. 1. Purification of the glucocorticoid receptors.

differential chromatography, and affinity-eluting the receptor from the second DNA-cellulose with pyridoxal-5′-phosphate, it is possible to rapidly obtain a 50% homogeneous preparation of the receptor in quite good yield.

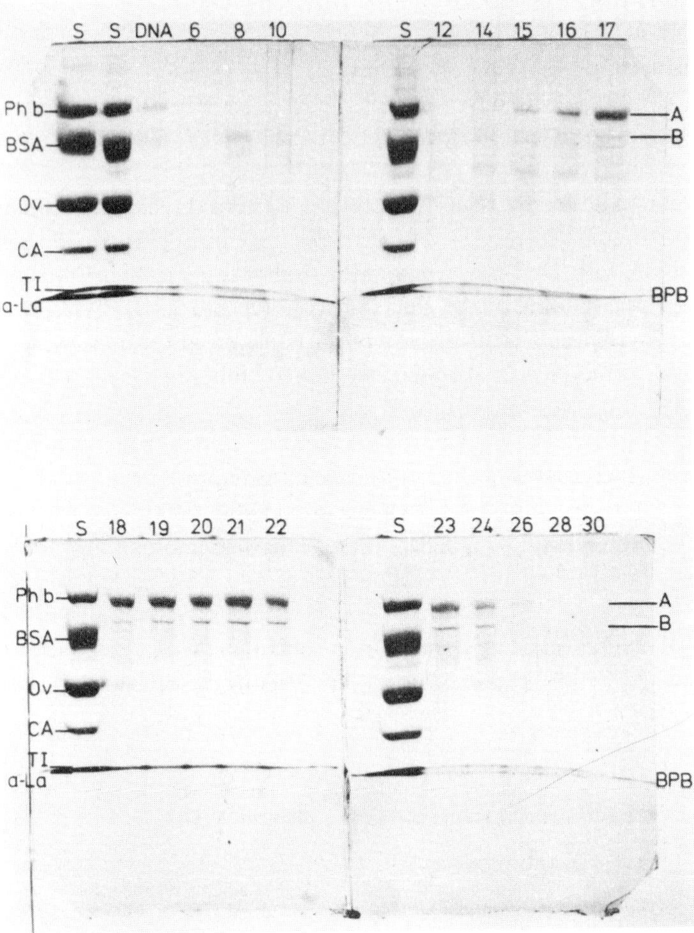

Fig. 2. SDS-polyacrylamide gel electrophoresis of fractions from DEAE-sepharose chromatography of the glucocorticoid receptor. All samples except the first standard on the top left gel were acid precipitated. The samples from the DEAE-sepharose chromatogram contained 0–15 μg of receptor. The fraction numbers of the samples are shown at the top of each gel. A portion from the pool from the second DNA-cellulose column was analysed simultaneously (DNA). S, standard proteins; Ph b, phosphorylase b; BSA, bovine serum albumin; Ov, ovalbumin; CA, carbonic anhydrase; TI, soybean trypsin inhibitor; a-La, α-lactalbumin; BPB, bromophenol blue.

When greater purification is required it is possible to further the receptor in a third and last step, with gel filtration or ion-exchange chromatography.

Figure 2 shows SDS-gel electrophoresis from consecutive fractions of the cross-linked dextran G-150 column, showing the glucocorticoid receptor and also a component with a slightly smaller MW. We do not know what this second component is; it may be a proteolytic fragment of the receptor. In any case, the receptor is about 90% pure [1]. This is the receptor preparation which is continuously and reproducibly being produced in our laboratory, and we have used it in our collaboration with the San Francisco laboratory.

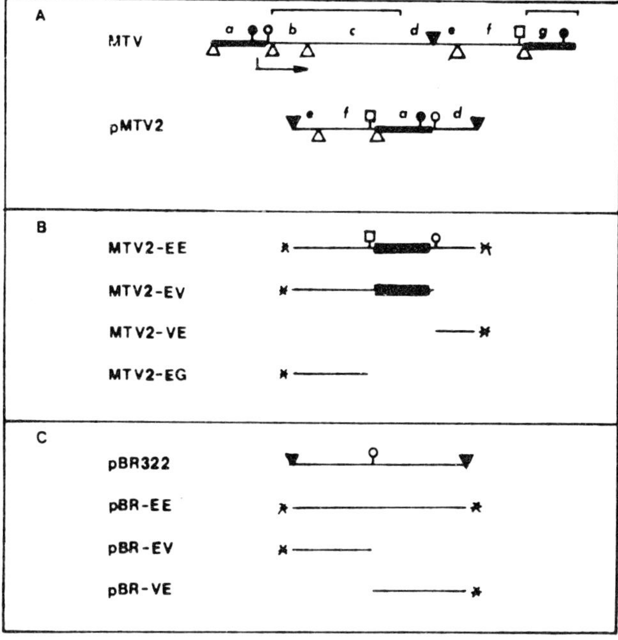

Fig. 3. *Restriction endonuclease map of pMTV2 and end-labeled fragments used for receptor binding experiments. (Top, row 1) Map of intact MTV DNA arranged as found in the integrated proviral state. Heavy lines denote the 1.3-kbp long terminal repeat sequence; the arrow marks the apparent start site for MTV DNA transcription; brackets delineate the regions deleted in pMTV2; lower case letters are to facilitate orienting the permutation seen in pMTV2. (Top, row 2) Map of the MTV insert in pMTV2; note that it is permuted to the single EcoRI site in the MTV sequence. ▼, EcoRI; △, Pst I; •, Sac I; ○, Pvu II; □, Bgl II. (Middle and Bottom) MTV and pBR322 fragments, respectively, ^{32}P end-labeled (*) at the EcoRI sites in the absence of further cleavage (MTV2-EE and pBR-EE) and after cleavage by Pvu II (MTV2-VE) and by Pvu II/Bgl-II (MTV2-EG, pBR-EV, and pBR-VE).*

One of the big problems in steroid receptor research has been to show whether there is a specific binding of the glucocorticoid receptor to DNA or whether the binding only represents nonspecific binding.

Figure 3 shows the genome of the mammary tumour virus (MTV), which is used a lot in glucocorticoid receptor research. Shown here is the 5′ end with the long terminal repeat of bases, which is supposed to be the site where the glucocorticoid receptor sticks. When this viral genome is introduced into a eukaryotic cell it can respond to glucocorticoid hormones. Following exposure of the infected cells to glucocorticoid hormones, viral RNA is produced. Keith Yamamoto has cloned certain segments of this genome – he calls it pMTV2 – and it contains about half the genome of the full virus. It also contains the long terminal repeat region, believed to bind the glucocorticoid receptor.

The way in which the experiment has been performed is simply to incubate receptor from Stockholm with DNA from San Francisco. If there is a binding of DNA to the receptor, it will stick to a nitrocellulose filter; if there is no protein binding, the DNA will go right through the filter. The DNA that is stuck

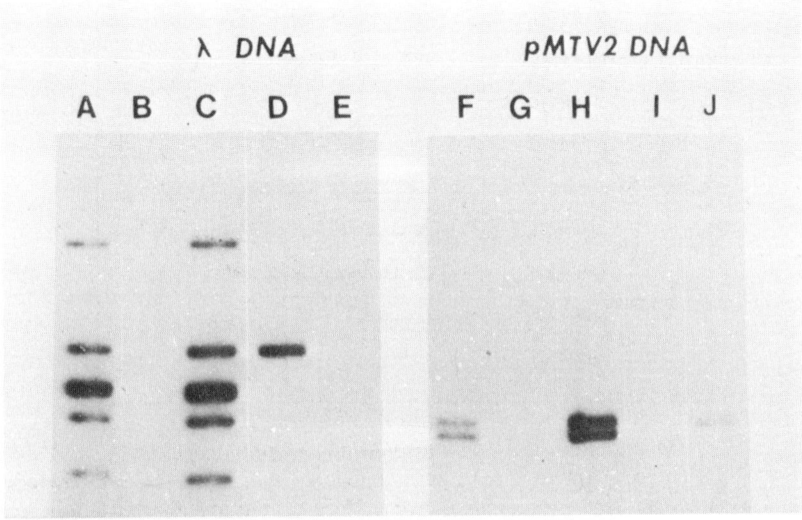

Fig. 4. Agarose gel electrophoresis of end-labeled EcoRI fragments of phage λ (Left) and pMTV2 (Right) DNA before and after nitrocellulose filter binding. Lanes: A-E, phage λ DNA; F-J, pMTV2 DNA; A and F, DNA prior to filter binding; B and G, DNA bound to filters in the absence of added proteins; C and H, DNA bound to filters in the presence of calf thymus histones; D and I, DNA bound to filters in the presence of phage λ repressor protein; E and J, DNA bound to filters in the presence of glucocorticoid receptor protein.

to the filter can then be eluted and chromatographed on an agarose gel. We work with radioactive DNA so the DNA can be visualized using autoradiography.

In Figure 4 a control experiment with phage λ DNA (which is not sensitive to glucocorticoid hormones) is shown. If this DNA is cleaved using so-called

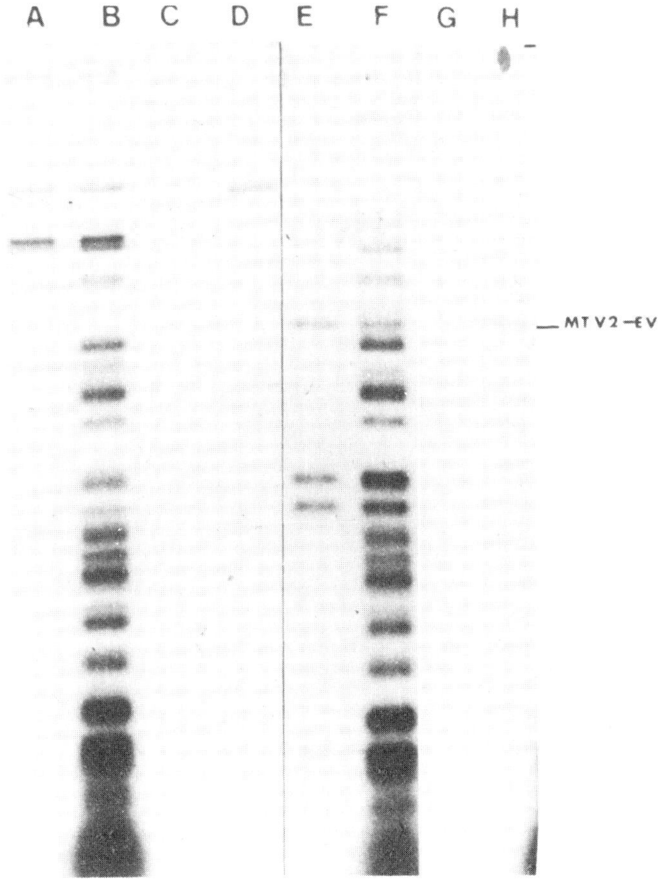

Fig. 5. Selectivity of DNA binding in the presence of ^{32}P end-labeled EcoRI fragments from bacteriophage T4 DNA. T4 DNA fragments (250 ng) were mixed with 100 ng of labeled EcoRI fragments of phage λ DNA (lanes A and B) or with labeled EcoRI fragments of pMTV2 DNA that had then been digested with Pvu II (lanes E and F). DNA fragments were then bound to nitrocellulose in the absence of added protein (lanes C and G), in the presence of phage λ repressor protein (lane D), or in the presence of glucocorticoid receptor protein (lane H).

restriction enzymes, there will be 5 fragments of DNA. If no incubation with protein is performed, no DNA will stick to the nitrocellulose filter. If calf thymus histones are added to the DNA, all the DNA fragments will stick. There is no selection; all DNA fragments stick to the filter.

If purified phage λ-repressor protein is added, it will selectively pick out one of the 5 DNA fragments and bind it. This fragment contains the operator region of the phage. If our glucocorticoid receptor is added, nothing is retained on the filter of these phage λDNA fragments.

Turning now to the pMTV2 DNA, no DNA will stick to the filter, if no protein is added. If calf thymus histones are added, both pMTV2 DNA and vector DNA will stick to the filter. If phage λ-repressor protein is added, no DNA sticks to the filter, but if our glucocorticoid receptor is added it will specifically bind the viral genome but not the vector. This is the first indication of a specific binding of the glucocorticoid receptor to a selective DNA region.

We can make it more difficult now for the receptor. Thirty-eight different DNA fragments from various sources, including DNA from the viral genome, can be mixed to see whether the glucocorticoid receptor can 'extract' the DNA fragment from this mixture. This is indeed what happens. The only fragment that is bound on the nitrocellulose filter is the viral DNA region containing the assumed glucocorticoid-sensitive region (Fig. 5).

This is the first evidence of a specific interaction of a steroid receptor with a selective DNA region [2]. We have recently been able to confirm this finding with electron microscopy, showing very neatly that the glucocorticoid receptor (presumably in the form of a tetramer) seems to stick to the long terminal repeat region of the virus (Payvar, F. et al., unpublished observations).

References

1. Wrange, Ö., Carlstedt-Duke, J. and Gustafsson, J.-A. (1979): Purification of the glucocorticoid receptor from rat liver cytosol. *J. Biol. Chem. 254,* 9284.
2. Payvar, F., Wrange, Ö., Carlstedt-Duke, J. et al. (1981): Purified glucocorticoid receptors bind selectively in vitro to a cloned DNA fragment whose transcription is regulated by glucocorticoids in vivo. *Proc. Natl. Acad. Sci. U.S.A. 78,* 6628.

The mechanism of hormone action

A. Di Marco

To elucidate the mode by which MPA exerts its action, we felt it opportune to examine the effects of oestrogen and MPA on a hormone-responsive human breast cancer cell line (MCF-7) derived from a pleural effusion [1]. This cell line has been demonstrated to have high levels of cell receptors for oestrogens, androgens, progestins, glucocorticoids, insulin and other hormones [2–5]. In this study we were primarily concerned with the antagonistic effect of MPA on oestradiol-stimulated cellular functions and on the cellular levels of oestrogen receptors (ER) and progesterone receptors (PgR).

In our experiments we used a cloned MCF-7, provided by Dr Jørgen Fogh (Sloan-Kettering Memorial Institute, Rye, New York). The human and mammary nature of this line was substantiated by chromosomal analysis and morphologic features. Chromosomal analysis revealed heteroploidy with a median chromosomal number of 81. These cells were also checked to see if they contained ER of PgR and if they were oestrogen-responsive.

For the experiments described in this work, cells were plated in Falcon plastic tissue culture dishes and grown at 37 °C in a humidified incubator supplied with a constant flow of 5% CO_2 in air.

Growth medium consisted of Eagle's MEM supplemented with nonessential amino acids, 60 ng/ml bovine insulin, and 10% calf serum. Cells from passage 63 through 78 were used. They were free of Mycoplasma contamination during the period of this study.

Cells growing in log phase were changed to serum-free medium (Eagle's MEM supplemented with 60 ng/ml insulin) 18 hours before treatment with hormones. Hormones were added at time zero; 1 hour before the cells were harvested, 0.5 μCi of (^{3}H) thymidine or 2.5 μCi of (^{3}H) leucine were added to each dish (Fig. 1). Cells were harvested by washing the dishes with ice-cold 0.9% BaCl buffered solution, suspending the cells in trypsin-EDTA, and collecting cell pellets by centrifugation.

Cell pellets were suspended in ice water and sonically dispersed for 4 seconds, at the lowest setting, with an ultrasonic probe (Biosonik III, Bron-

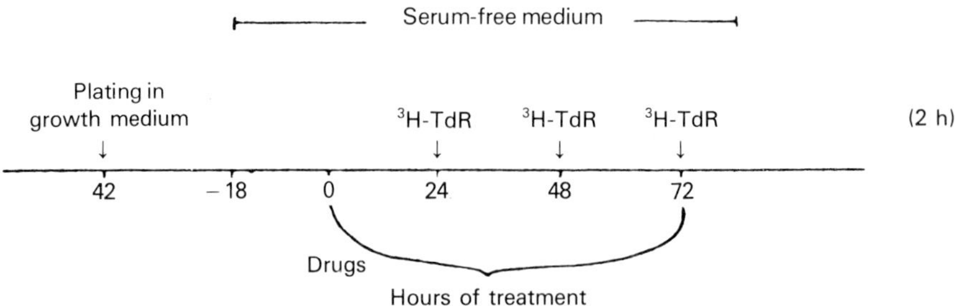

Fig. 1. Drug and labelled-precursor administration scheme.

will, Rochester, N.Y). Aliquots were then used for the determination of protein content, according to the method of Oyama and Eagle [6], and using BSA as protein standard, or for precipitation in 10% trichloro-acetil acid. Acid-insoluble counts were collected and washed on 0.45 μm Millipore filters. After drying, the filters were solubilized in 5 ml of a Filter Count Cocktail (Packard). The scintillation vials were shaken by hand and left in a refrigerator (4° C) for 1–2 hours before radioactivity counting.

Whole-cell binding studies

Cells growing logarithmically were changed to serum-free medium (Eagle's MEM supplemented with 60 ng/ml insulin) 24 hours before treatment with 10^{-8} M MPA dissolved in ethanol. The final concentration of ethanol in the growth medium was always less than 0.1% (v/v) and did not influence cell growth or hormone synthesis.

After 48 hours cells were harvested with trypsin-EDTA, washed twice with ice-cold physiological 0.9% NaCl solution to eliminate the endogenous hormone unbound before the saturation kinetics by radioactive ^{3}H steroids, and then suspended in 0.9% buffered NaCl solution at a density of 10^6 cells/ml. Solutions (0.2 ml) at decreasing concentrations of ^{3}H-E_2 (5.0–0.5 nM) or ^{3}H-R5020 (11.0–1.0 nM), with or without 100-fold molar excess of unlabeled binding competitor DES or R5020, respectively, were added to the 0.8-ml cell suspension tubes and incubated at 37° C for one hour. Cells were collected by centrifugation and washed 5 times in 0.9% buffered NaCl solution at 0° C to eliminate the unbound radioactivity.

The sediment was suspended in ice-cold water and sonically dispersed for 4 seconds at the lowest setting with an ultrasonic probe. Aliquots were then collected for the determination of protein content or for radioactivity counting.

The total number of cells arrested in metaphase was evaluated after treatment of the cells with 1μg/ml colchicine for 150 minutes before fixation.

In these conditions MCF-7 cells were able to synthesize DNA and enter in mitotic activity even when pre-incubated in synthetic medium without oestradiol. This was also previously observed [7] and was considered due to the persistance in the cells of an amount of oestradiol sufficient to permit one or more reproductive cycles.

Effect on macromolecular synthesis and mitotic activity

As indicated in Figure 2, oestradiol significantly speeds up and enhances (^{3}H)

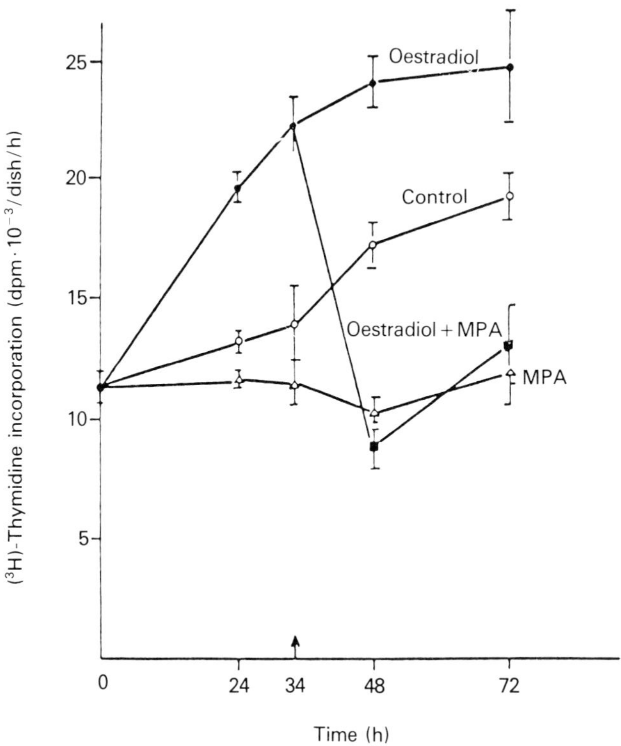

Fig. 2. Effects of 17-oestradiol and MPA on (^{3}H) thymidine incorporation into the precipitable acid material. Experiments were performed in serum-free medium. MPA or oestradiol were added at time 0: (○) = control; (●) = 10^{-8} M oestradiol; (△) = 10^{-8} M MPA; (■) = 10^{-8}M oestradiol with 10^{-8}M MPA added at 34 h as indicated by the arrow. (^{3}H) thymidine was added to each dish one h before harvesting. The values shown are averages of triplicate determinations ± SE.

thymidine incorporation into DNA with respect to the control, whereas MPA inhibited almost 50% of the (^{3}H) thymidine incorporation after 48 or 72 hours' exposure to a 10^{-7} M concentration. There was no significant inhibition by MPA of (^{3}H) leucine incorporation when protein synthesis was measured at 48 hours.

The MPA-inhibiting effect on (^{3}H) thymidine incorporation could be reversed by the addition of oestradiol to the cells. The kinetic of the response is shown in Figure 3. In these experiments, 10^{-8} M oestradiol or 10^{-8} M MPA was added to the cells at time zero. After 24 hours oestradiol-stimulated cells incorporated (^{3}H) thymidine at a rate greater than that of control cells. MPA-treated cells showed inhibition at the same time. After 34 hours oestradiol was added to half of the cells incubated in 10^{-8}M MPA. After 3/48 hours a sharp

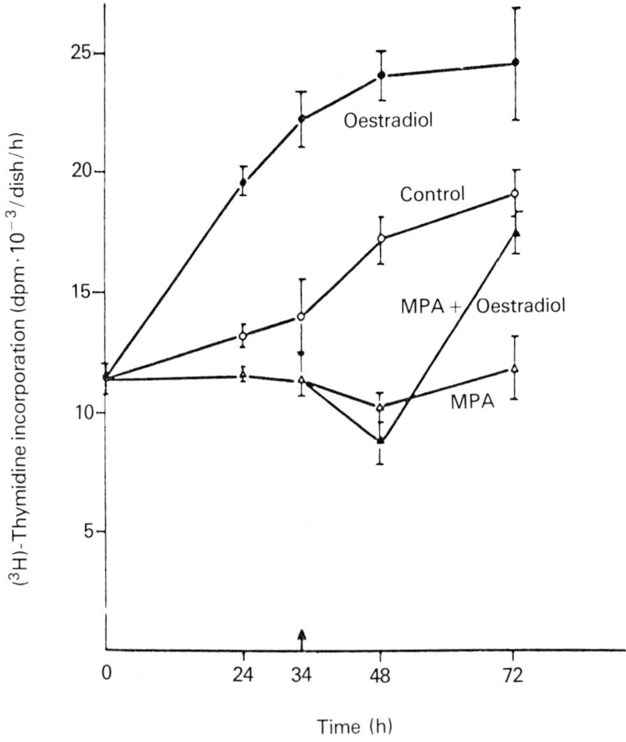

Fig. 3. Effects of 17-oestradiol and MPA on (^{3}H) thymidine incorporation into the precipitable acid material. MPA or oestradiol were added at time 0 (for explanation of the symbols, see Figure 2). (^{3}H) thymidine was added to each dish one h before harvesting. The values shown are averages of triplicate determinations ± SE.

Table. Effects of MPA, cortisol, progesterone and 21-acetoxy-17-hydroxy-6α-methylprogesterone on (^3H) thymidine incorporation in MCF-7 cells after 48 hours treatment.

Concentration of steroid (M)	MPA	Cortisol	Progesterone	21-Acetoxy-17-hydroxy-6α-methyl-progesterone
0	189.12 ± 18.89	—	—	—
10^{-9}	122.84 ± 22.63	288.85 ± 57.00	—	182.66 ± 16.36
10^{-8}	97.27 ± 8.31*	152.84 ± 29.29	92.08 ± 0.02**	127.12 ± 20.60
10^{-7}	84.10 ± 10.22**	147.79 ± 6.53	89.88 ± 2.64**	106.63 ± 8.22*
10^{-6}	85.20 ± 4.00**	113.73 ± 11.12*	58.92 ± 5.34**	58.41 ± 9.70**
10^{-5}	—	—	15.92 ± 2.24**	—

Values are dpm [^{3}H] thymidine $\cdot 10^{-3}$ per mg of protein per h ± SE.
*$P < 5\%$.
**$P < 1\%$.

rise in nucleoside precursor incorporation was observed in these MCF-8 cells. The antagonistic effect when 10^{-8} M MPA was added to the cells, stimulated (^{3}H) thymidine incorporation decreased to the level of MPA-treated cells. Since the inhibitory effect of MPA with (^{3}H) thymidine incorporation may not be due to the introduced molecular species but a possible metabolic product of the glucocorticoid series, we compared the effect of MPA with cortisol, progesterone and the possible metabolic product of MPA, i.e., 21-acetoxy-17-hydroxy-6-methylprogesterone [8]. MPA appeared to be the most active drug, but the dose-response line leveled at 10^{-7} M (Table). Progesterone, as well as 21-acetoxy-17-hydroxy-6-methylprogesterone, had a comparable activity, which was more dose-dependent (linear correlation coefficients respectively, $r = 0.7$ and 0.98). Cortisol was less effective and showed a nonlinear response curve ($r = 0.58$). The inhibiting effect of MPA on (^{3}H) thymidine incorporation was paralleled by a decreased mitotic activity. It appears from Figure 4 that the number of cumulated metaphase during 150-minute periods of incubation with colchicine at each experimental point

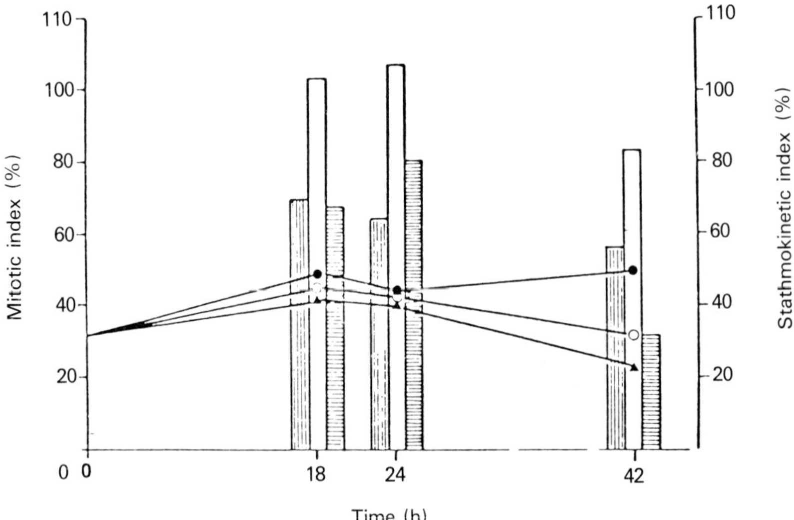

Fig. 4. Interference of oestradiol and MPA with mitotic activity. Oestradiol or MPA were added at time 0. Mitotic index: control (○——○); 10^{-8} M oestradiol (●——●); 10^{-8} M MPA (▲——▲). Stathmokinetic index was obtained from the accumulation of the mitosis in the presence of colchicine 4 h before fixation: control (▥); oestradiol (□); MPA (▤).

(stathmokinetic index), was increased by oestradiol and remained significantly higher than the control values up to 24 and 42 hours. This may indicate that in oestradiol-treated cultures there is a higher number of cells entering into the mitotic cycle than there is in the control cultures.

MPA did not influence the stathmokinetic index at 18 and 24 hours, and it was only at 42 hours that an evident reduction in the number of cumulated mitotic cells and the mitotic index appeared with respect to the control cultures.

Effect on oestradiol and progesterone binding

The results shown in Figure 5 clearly establish that MPA, after the long incubation time of 48 hours reduced both ^{3}H-E_2 and ^{3}H-5020 total (cytoplasmatic and nuclear) receptor binding in whole cells. The ER (432.12 fmol/mg) and PgR (135.11 fmol/ml) sites were reduced in MPA-pretreated cells (113.14 and 61.17 fmol/mg, respectively), both also with respect to the apparent affinity constant (K_a) (3.88×10^9 versus 1.65×10^9 M^{-1} for ER and $3.59 \cdot 10^9$ M^{-1} versus $1.54 \cdot 10^9$ M^{-1} for PgR).

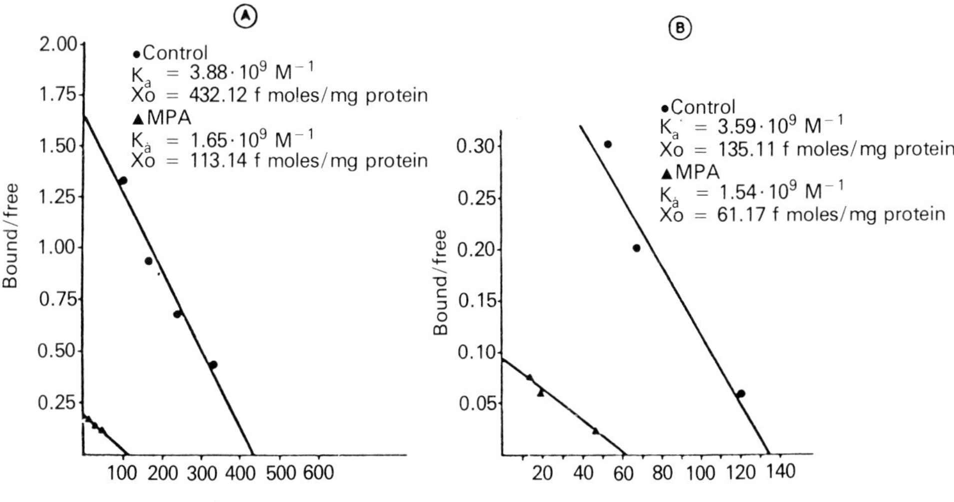

Fig. 5. Binding of (^{3}H) oestradiol (A) and ^{3}H-5020 (B) to intact MCF-7 human breast cancer cells. Cells growing logarithmically were changed to serum-free medium 24 h before the start of the experiment and incubated for 48 h with MPA. The binding data (A) are plotted according to the Scatchard analysis.

Conclusions

The experiments performed in 'vitro' on hormone-responsive MCF-7 breast cancer cells show that MPA inhibits (^{3}H) thymidine incorporation and proliferative activity (as expressed by the stathmokinetics index) of these cells. As previously shown, oestradiol added to the culture medium of MCF-7 cells greatly speeds up both these processes [9].

MPA specifically antagonizes these oestradiol effects on thymidine incorporation, whether given before or after oestradiol. From this antagonism it may be speculated that MPA like Pg interferes with an oestrogen-stimulated process related to the ability of the hormone-responsive cells to enter in the proliferative cycle. According to O.I. Epifanova, oestrogens regulate the number of hormone-dependent cells leaving G_0 status and entering in a shortened G_1 phase [10].

The interference of MPA with oestrogen-stimulated processes could, in agreement with the previous observation of K.B. Horwitz and W.L. McGuire, with progesterone [2], be exerted at the level of the oestrogen-induced activation of specific genes. An antagonistic effect of progesterone on oestrogen-stimulated growth has been observed in CAMA-1 cells by B.S. Leung [11]. The expression of these genes may induce a differentiation stage of the cells which is no more responsive to oestrogen effect on the entering of the hormone-responsive cells into the proliferation cycle.

Due to the long incubation time required for the observed effects, the possibility that MPA does not act by itself but through an active metabolite should be considered. The inhibitory effect on DNA synthesis of 21-acetoxy-17-hydroxy-6-methylprogesterone (a MPA metabolite of the glucocorticoid family) is compatible with this hypothesis.

At variance with MPA, the dose-response curve for Pg is linear in the range 10^{-5}–10^{-7} M, and this may indicate that the effect does not require previous metabolic modification from an inactive to an active metabolic form with the corticosteroid structure. However, this point is complicated by the recent demonstration of the broad receptor specificity of MPA for androgen, progesterone and glucocorticoid receptors [12, 13]. Since all these receptors are present in relatively high amounts in MCF-7 cells [4, 14], it cannot be excluded that the inhibitory effects on cell proliferation could be modulated by the binding to these receptors.

References

1. Soule, H.D., Vazquez, J., Long, A., Albert, S. and Brennam, M. (1973): A

human cell line from a pleural effusion derived from a breast carcinoma. *J. Natl. Cancer Inst. 51,* 1409.
2. Horwitz, K.B. and McGuire, W.L. (1977): Induction of progesterone receptor in a human breast cancer cell line. *Clin. Res. 25,* 295A.
3. Lippman, M., Bolan, G. and Huff, K. (1976): The effects of androgens and antiandrogens on hormone-responsive human breast cancer in long-term tissue culture. *Cancer Res. 36,* 4610.
4. Monaco, M.E. and Lippman, M.E. (1978): Interaction between hormones and human breast cancer in long-term tissue culture. In: *Endocrine Control in Neoplasia,* pp. 209–301. Eds: R.K. Sharma and W.E. Criss. Raven Press, New York.
5. Strobl, J.S. and Lippman, M.E. (1978): Studies of steroid hormone effects on human breast cancer cells in long-term tissue culture. In: *Hormones, Receptors and Breast Cancer,* pp. 85–106. Ed: W.L. McGuire. Raven Press, New York.
6. Oyama, V.I. and Eagle, H. (1956): Measurement of cell growth in tissue culture with a phenol reagent (Folin-Ciocalteau). *Proc. Soc. Exp. Biol. Med. 91,* 305.
7. Clark, J.H., Hardin, J.W., Padikula, H.A. and Cardesin, C.A. (1978): Role of estrogen receptor binding and transcriptional activity in the stimulation of hyperestrogism and nuclear bodies. *Proc. Natl. Acad. Sci. N.Y. 75*, 2781.
8. Glenn, E.M., Richardson, S.L. and Bowman, B.J. (1959): Biologic activity of 6-alpha-methyl compounds corresponding to progesterone, 17-alpha-hydroxyprogesterone acetate and compound S. *Metabolism 8,* 265.
9. Lippman, M. (1976): Hormone-responsive human breast cancer in continuous tissue culture. In: *Breast Cancer: Trends in Research and Treatment,* pp. 111–139. Eds: J.C. Heuson, W.H. Mattheiem and M. Rozencweig. Raven Press, New York.
10. Epifanova, O.I. (1971): Effects of hormones on the cell cycle. In: *The Cell Cycle and Cancer,* pp. 145–182. Ed: R. Baserga. Marcel Dekker, New York.
11. Leung, B.S. (1978): Hormonal dependency of experimental breast cancer. In: *Hormones, Receptors and Breast Cancer,* pp. 219–261. Ed: W.L. McGuire. Raven Press, New York.
12. McLaughlin, D.T. and Richardson, G.S. (1979): Specificity of medroxyprogesterone acetate binding in human endometrium. Interaction with testosterone and progesterone binding sites. *J. Steroid Biochem. 10,* 371.
13. Teuling, F.A., van Gilse, H.A., Henkelman, M.S., Portengen, H. and Alexeva-Figusch, J. (1980): Estrogen, androgen, glucocorticoid, and progesterone receptors in progestin-induced regression of human breast cancer. *Cancer Res. 40,* 2557.
14. Lippman, M., Bolan, G. and Huff, K. (1976): The effects of glucocorticoids and progesterone on hormone-responsive human breast cancer in long-term tissue culture. *Cancer Res. 36,* 4602.

The mechanism of hormone action: one-step procedure for progestin receptor purification

K. Pollow

To more clearly define the role of progestin receptors in gene transcription it is necessary to isolate this receptor from target tissue and purify this protein to homogeneity. Affinity chromatography is a technique of proven value and widespread application which has been exploited with varying degrees of success for the isolation of steroid receptors.

One of the major problems in purification of intact progestin receptors is the instability of these proteins. Earlier reports indicated that the presence of thiols in the buffer used for receptor preparation significantly stabilized the relatively labile protein [1]. Therefore, we prepared a biospecific adsorbent in which the specific ligand is bound to the stationary matrix through a disulphide linkage: addition of a thiol to the elution buffer would release the receptor protein by reduction of the disulphide linkages, and also stabilize it.

A further problem of progestin receptor purification is the presence of other high affinity binders for progesterone, such as corticosteroid binding globulin (CBG) in the cytosolic preparation. This problem can be solved by the choice of a synthetic steroid with high affinity for the progestin receptor, negligible interference with other steroid receptors, and a lack of tight serum binding.

We would like to report the isolation and purification of the progestin receptor from human uterine tissue by a single step method using a highly effective biospecific adsorbent that was prepared by attaching a derivative of the synthetic progestin Org2058 via a spacer, containing a disulphide bound to cross-linked sepharose. The advantages of our affinity chromatography system are the very specific interaction of the matrix-bound Org2058 with the progestin receptor and the easy elution of the matrix-bound progestin receptor by reducing the disulphide bond.

In order to select the most efficient Org2058 derivative modified in the side-chain at position 17 of the steroid molecule the binding affinity of these compounds to the progestin receptor was measured by competition with ^{3}H-R5020 and ^{3}H-Org2058, respectively.

Figure 1 shows that Org2058 is a clearly better competitor than progesterone itself. Its affinity resembles that of the synthetic gestagen R5020. Periodic acid oxidation of the side-chain to the corresponding 17β-carboxylic acid decreases the binding affinity nearly 3 orders of magnitude, whereas esterification or amidation of the 17β-carboxylic acid derivative of Org2058 partly restores the binding affinity (e.g., the affinity of the methylester is

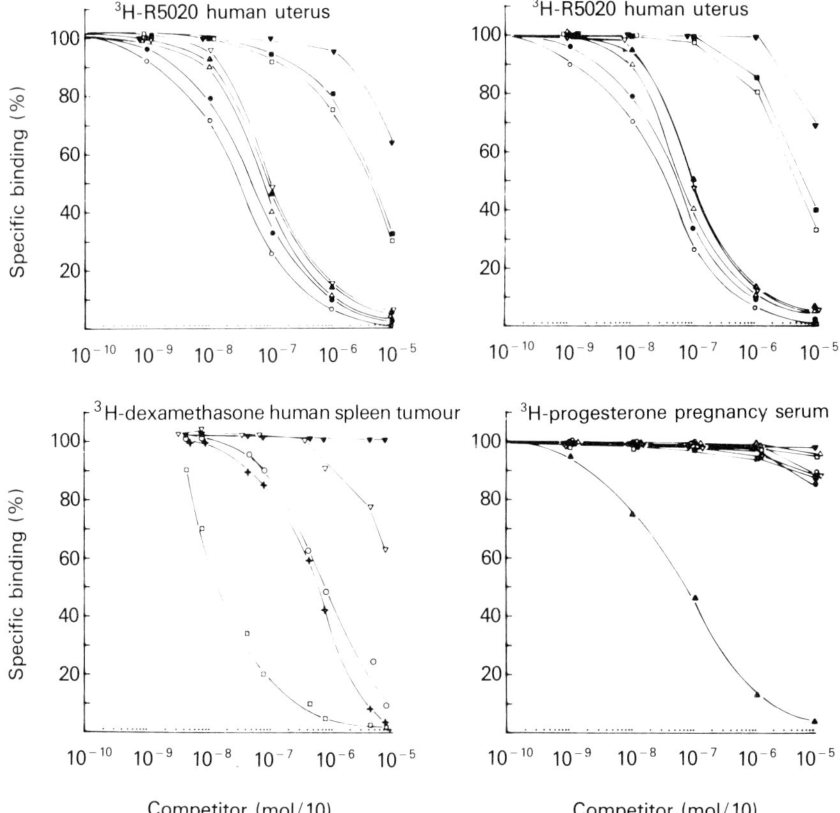

Fig. 1. Specificity of the binding of ^{3}H-R5020 and ^{3}H-Org2058 to the cytoplasmic progestin receptor of human uterine tissue, of ^{3}H-dexamethasone to the cytoplasmic glucocorticoid receptor of human spleen tumor, and of ^{3}H-progesterone to corticosteroid binding globulin of diluted pregnancy serum. R5020 (•), Org2058 (○), progesterone (▲), DHT (■), Org2058-17β-COOH (▼), Org2058-17β-COOH$_3$ (△), Org2058-17β-CONH (CH$_2$)$_2$-SH (▽), deoxycorticosterone (+).

similar to that of progesterone). Furthermore, this Figure also demonstrates that Org2058 and its derivatives compete for ^{3}H-dexamethasone binding to human spleen tumour cytosol. The affinity of Org2058 is even lower than that of progesterone. Side-chain modification of Org2058 additionally decreases the affinity. Neither Org2058 nor one of its side-chain modified descendants compete with ^{3}H-progesterone for binding to CBG in diluted human pregnancy serum.

Figure 2 shows the structure of the Org2058 affinity resin. The gel was synthesized by coupling the Org2058 17β-carboxylic acid through a spacer containing a disulphide linkage to Affigel 10 (obtained from BioRad), a N-hydroxysuccinimide active ester derivative of cross-linked agarose beads.

For coupling the progestin receptor to the affinity gel 200 ml of human uterine cytosol were incubated with 5 ml of the gel for 60 minutes at room temperature. After intensive washing of the incubation mixture the progestin receptor was eluted from the matrix with a buffer containing 100 mmol/l of β-mercaptoethanol.

The purification of the progestin receptor was greater than 24,000-fold over the starting material after only one step. The recovery of the receptor protein was 40% (Table).

The SDS-polyacrylamide gel electrophoresis of the final purified receptor preparation (affinity eluate II) exhibits 2 major bands of protein, which correspond to molecular weights of 108,000 and 43,000, respectively. But there

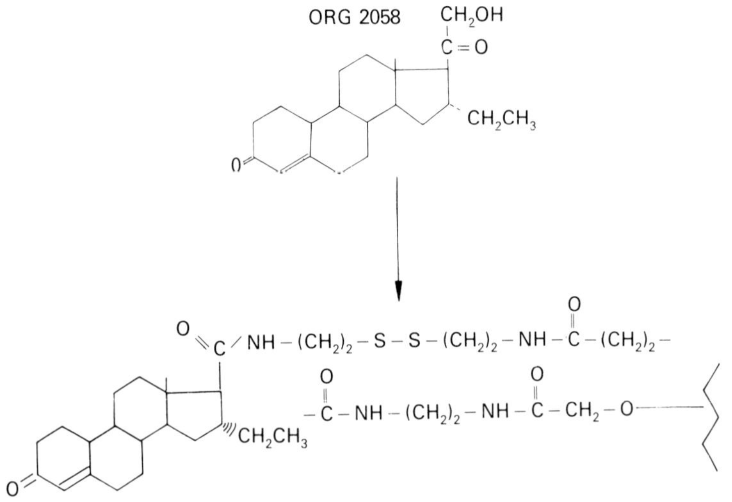

ORG 2058

CH_2OH
$C=O$
CH_2CH_3

$-C(=O)-NH-(CH_2)_2-S-S-(CH_2)_2-NH-C(=O)-(CH_2)_2-C(=O)-NH-(CH_2)_2-NH-C(=O)-CH_2-O-$

CH_2CH_3

Fig. 2. Structure of Org2058-agarose derivative synthesized for progestin receptor purification.

are also a few barely visible minor bands (Fig. 3). The 43,000 d band is also predominant in experiments using the precursor gel which contains only free amino groups. Whether these 2 43,000 d bands are really identical or peptides of similar molecular weight remains open. The molecular weight of the 108,000 d peptide is similar to the previously described chick oviduct progesterone receptor [2]. Specific antibodies raised against both, the 108,000 d and 43,000 d peptide should help to clarify this point.

Table. Purification scheme of human uterine progestin receptor.

Fraction	Total protein (mg)	Total labeled receptor hormone complexes (10^{-6} × dpm)	Specific activity (10^{-6} × dpm/mg protein)	Yield (%)	Purification (n-fold)
Cytosol	1186	152.7	0.128	100	1
Affinity chromatography eluate	0.0196	61.1	3113	40	24322

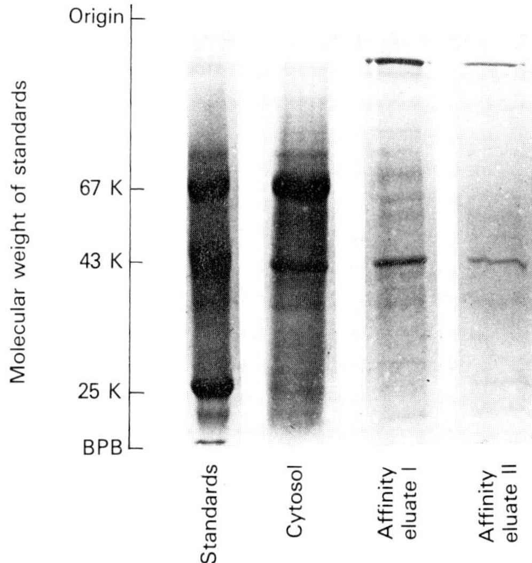

Fig. 3. Sodium dodecyl sulphate-polyacrylamide gel electrophoresis of the purified progestin receptor.

The following measurements of the physical and chemical properties of the purified receptor were carried out to determine whether any modifications of the receptor occurred during the purification procedure.

Determination of K_d-value: The affinity eluant was stripped off released steroid with dextran-coated charcoal and aliquots were incubated with increasing concentrations of ^{3}H-R5020 ± R5020 for 2 hours at 25° C (exchange conditions; Fig. 4). The K_d-values, calculated according to Scatchard, were 2.4×10^{-9}M/l for progestin receptor in native cytosol compared to 1.22×10^{-8}M/l in the affinity eluant.

Sucrose density gradient analysis was performed on linear 5–20% low salt sucrose gradients. Native cytosol, incubated with ^{3}H-R5020 ± R5020 at 4° C showed specific binding in the 4–5 S and 8 S region. After temperature activation (i.e. 4 hours at 4° C and 1 hour at 25° C) specific binding was exclusively found in the 4–5 S area. The isolated progestin receptor of the affinity eluant (incubated with ^{3}H-R5020 under exchange conditions) migrated as a single 4–5 S entity. The ^{3}H-R5020 bound to the purified progestin receptor could be almost completely displaced by R5020 and progesterone, whereas testosterone or cortisol did not show any competition (Fig. 5).

Finally, the above evidence leads to the conclusion that the affinity com-

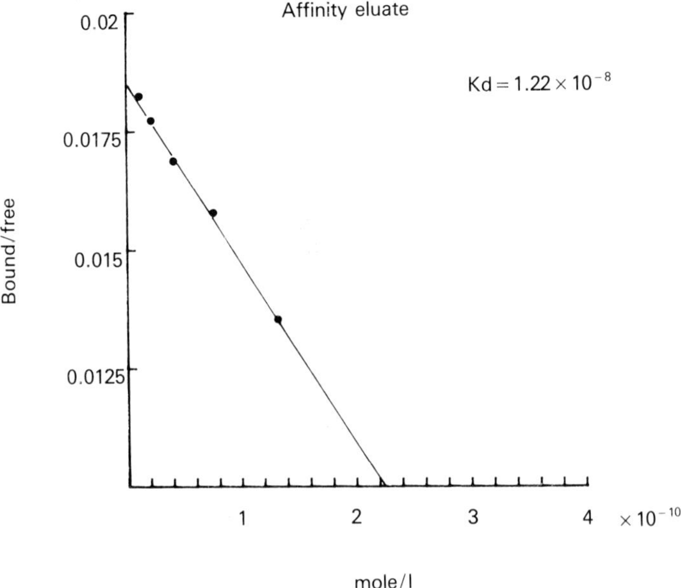

Fig. 4. Scatchard analysis of specific ^{3}H-R5020 binding protein in affinity eluate.

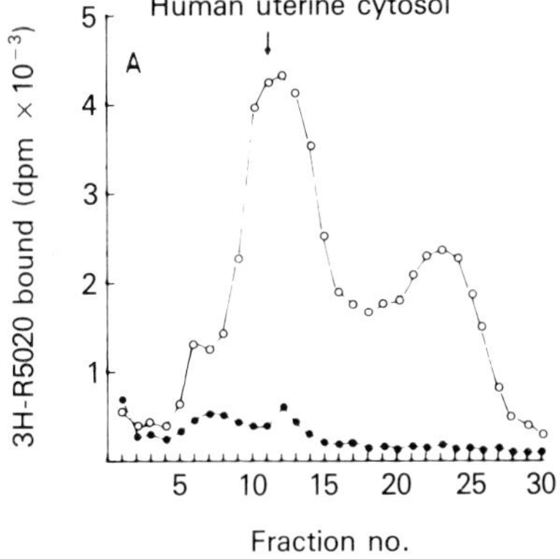

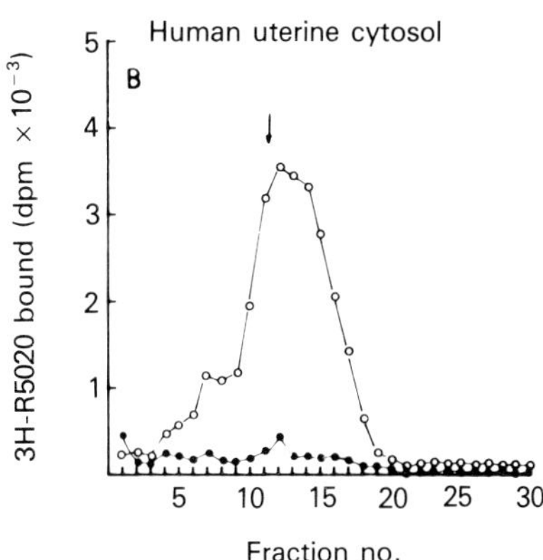

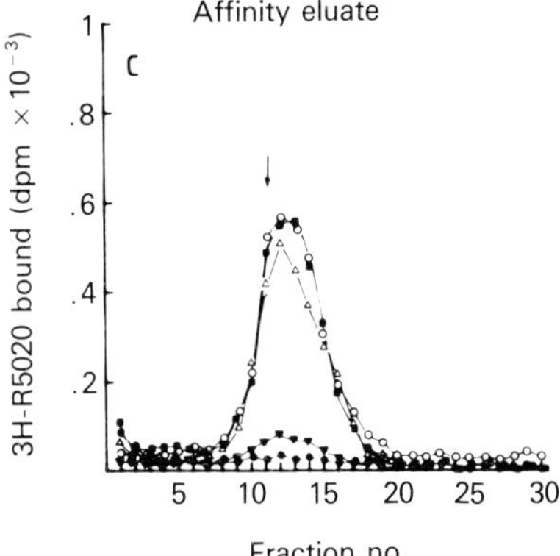

Fig. 5. Sedimentation analysis of the progestin receptor in human uterine cytosol after incubation at 4 °C (A) and 25 °C (B) and in the purified receptor preparation (affinity eluate II) at 25 °C (C) with or without a 100-fold excess of various competitor steroids (^{3}H-R5020 ○, R5020 •, progesterone ▼, cortisol ■, testosterone △). Arrow indicates the position of BSA.

pound described here resulted in a significant purification within a short time and with the minimum number of steps. The optimization of the conditions for this procedure is currently under investigation.

References

1. Sweet, F. and Adair, N.K. (1975): *Biochem. Biophys. Res. Commun. 63,* 99.
2. Kuhn, R.W., Schrader, W.T., Smith, R.G. and O'Malley, B.W. (1975): *J. Biol. Chem. 250,* 4220.

Discussion

W.L. McGuire: There must be at least a minimum of 10 different fundamental ways of measuring receptors. For each of those 10 fundamental ways there must be probably at least 10 modifications that people have employed for their own purposes. In all, we must have 100 different ways to measure receptors. The problem for clinicians or people who use the assays, who would like to trust the laboratory assays, is that they have difficulty in sorting out the 10 different ways or the 10 different modifications. I think that what Dr. Gustafsson referred to, and what Drs. Green and Jensen, in Chicago, are already well on the way to achieving, is to have a monoclonal antibody (or 2 or 3 monoclonal antibodies) where the supply is almost unlimited so that it can be distributed to any laboratory that wants to measure a receptor – so that, in effect, the quality control could be *almost* perfect. That is where the real progress will be made in receptor assays over the next year or two.

G. Concolino (Rome, Italy): Professor Pollow's 'gimmick' is good, and I like it. Has he any suggestions about the incubation time for oestradiol and progesterone receptors because for exchange condition the incubation time and temperature might be different?

K. Pollow: In the double-labelling assay the incubation time at 4° C is overnight, like the standard assay which is used worldwide.

G. Beretta: Can Dr Martin tell us if, with his micro samples he obtained the same results from many samples taken from the same tissue?

P.M. Martin: The problem in the follow-up of patients during therapy is that we use very small samples, and with some patients one, 2 or 3 needle aspirations are needed to obtain sufficient cells to make the measurement, and to determine the heterogeneity of the tumours. The assay is performed with 10 mg of tissue.

G. Beretta: If you take different samples within the same bulk of tumour (perhaps 2 or 3 cm in size), do you get the same results?

P.M. Martin: Using the fine-needle aspiration there is now some evidence that a subpopulation is extracted from the tumour, but it is not yet known whether this subpopulation is the high-risk metastatic population or another one.

W.L. McGuire: A number of people have taken a piece of tumour and subdivided it, measuring receptor levels in those subdivisions. Receptor levels do vary; there is clear-cut heterogeneity.

S. Parboo (London, UK): Can Dr Martin give us a quantitative result from his microsamples as well as a qualitative result?

P.M. Martin: Per mg of DNA.

J.A. Gustafsson: Perhaps I should mention that there are also alternative methods with which the oestrogen receptor may be measured in fine-needle aspiration biopsies. For several years now in Sweden we have used a method based on isoelectric focusing in polyacrylamide gel [1]. In fact, it is now the standard method used in several places in Sweden. With this method it is possible to measure the oestrogen receptor in fine-needle aspiration biopsies [2].

References

1. Wrange, Ö., Nordenskjöld, B. and Gustafsson, J.-A. (1978): Cytosol estradiol receptor in human mammary carcinoma: an assay based on isoelectric focusing in polyacrylamide gel. *Anal. Biochem. 85,* 461.
2. Silfverswärd, C., Gustafsson, J.-A., Gustafsson S.A. et al. (1980): Estrogen receptor analysis on fine needle aspirates and on histologic biopsies from human breast cancer. *Eur. J. Cancer 16,* 1351.

New assays: developments in assay procedures

P.M. Martin

We cannot obtain surgical samples from all patients with breast tumours; in some patients we can only perform drill biopsies and fine needle aspiration. For this reason it was necessary to develop a technique to use in the routine assay of micro samples. We have developed this technique with Dr Henri Magdelenat (Curie Fondation, Paris, France) and Dr Paul Kelly (C.M.V. Laval Quebec, Canada).

Until now we estimated the oestrogen or the progestin receptor content of small biopsy specimens of human breast tumours, down to 25 mg of tissue, using the dextran charcoal procedure, with R 2858, R 5020. We are now able to estimate both receptors on the same specimen.

Principle

Incubation of cytosol with ^{3}H-R 2858 ^{3}H-R 5020 and ^{3}H-R 1881 (in the presence of cortisol (F)) – adsorption and separation of hormone receptor complexes on hydroxylapatite (HPA) and/or incubation in glycerol/thioglycerol/EDTA/tris HcL buffer; (GTEM) pH 7.8.

- Alcohol or ether extraction of bound hormones (HPA) pellet or GTEM port DCC).
- Separation of ^{3}H hormones by high pressure liquid chromatography (HPLC) or by activated celite column or by LH20 column.

The number of hormone receptors that can be assayed simultaneously is unlimited, theoretically, provided HPLC, celite or LH20 separation of hormones can be achieved.

Methodology

Tissue sample 30–60 mg from drill or fine needle aspiration.

Homogenization (Potter) in 0.5 ml of tris (50 mM) phosphate 10 mM pH 7–8,

Table.

HPLC Conditions		Celite column				LH 20		
Column (25 cm)	Spherisorb 5 C18	Hyflow supercel (0.8 g)				LH 20 (0.5 g in Bz/Met (85/15)		
		Stationary phase: ethylene-glycol				Pre-equil phase: (ISO 8 BENZ/MET) 90 5 5		
Eluant	Methanol/water: (90/10)	Deposit	(Bz/ISO 8) 10 100	Volume 2 × 500 μl		(ISO 8/BENZ/MET) 90 5 5	Volume 2 × 100 μl	
Flow Injection	1 ml/mn 50 μl	Elution	(Bz/ISO 8) 10 100	4 ml	R 5020	(ISO 8/BENZ/MET) 90 5 5	6 ml	R 5020
Detection	UV: 283 nm		(EA/ISO 8) 30 100	3 ml	Discard	80 10 10	6 ml	R 1881
Retention time:			40 100	5 ml	R 1881	75 15 15	1 ml	Discard
R 2858	3.4 mn		60 100	6 ml	R 2858	50 20 30		R 2858
R 1881	5.2 mn							
R 5020	6.8 mn							

containing 10% glycerol and 0.4 Mkcl. Centrifugation for one hour at 105,000 g.

Incubation of 50 or 100 μl aliquots, 18 hourly at 4° C with ^{3}H-R 2858, ^{3}H-R 5020 and ^{3}H-R 1881.

1. 1 nM each
2. 1 nM each + 1,000 nM of unlabelled hormones
3. 5 nM each
4. 5 nM each + 1,000 nM of unlabelled hormones

A. Addition of 100 μl of HPA slurry (1/1) in buffer containing 20% glycerol, incubation for 30 min at 4° C with gentle agitation, addition of 300 ml of buffer (20% glycerol), centrifugation of HPA phase, at 1,500 g, 5 min at 4° C, and 2 washes with buffer (20% glycerol).

B. Partition using DCC technique.

Extraction (15 min) with 1 ml of methanol or with 4 ml of ether, twice, evaporation, recovery in 100 μl containing 3 (nM) of unlabelled hormones as carriers and internal standards for column.

Separation by chromatography (see Table)

When comparing the 3 techniques it was found that recovery varied from 89–98%, and that reproducibility was almost the same.

In fact the main difference was the cost of determination; the necessary material for the LH 20 column technique cost 10 French Francs and for HPLC the cost was 100,000 French Francs.

The difference between celite column and LH 20 remains that hyflow supercel needs to be activated at 500° C and that the procedure should be performed in dry atmosphere.

We used this technique for endometrial samples as shown in our presentation on endometrial carcinoma (see pages 333–349) and for the follow-up of many patients under therapy for breast carcinoma.

New assays: developments in assay procedures

J.A. Gustafsson

I would like to discuss some studies we have performed with an antiserum directed against the glucocorticoid receptor [1].

We have raised in rabbits polyclonal antibodies against the glucocorticoid receptor (Fig. 1). This is a typical glycerol density gradient centrifugation analysis of the glucocorticoid receptor. When the antiserum is added the peak is shifted to the bottom of the centrifuge tube. There are also other ways in which it can be shown that we actually have an antiserum against the glucocorticoid receptor.

We believe that the glucocorticoid receptor is a slightly cigarshaped molecule with a Stokes radius of 61 Å (6.1 nm) (Fig. 2). There is one site for the ligand, and another site for the DNA. We have also found that the antibody binding domain of the receptor seems to be at the far end of the receptor molecule. It is possible to separate these different domains using careful proteolytic digestion with various enzymes.

The Table summarizes the specificity of our antiserum. It reacts with the glucocorticoid receptor in rat liver, thymus and hippocampus. It also cross-reacts, although less so, with human glucocorticoid receptor derived from lymphocytes, hippocampus and leukaemia cells. It does not react with the proteolytic fragments that can be induced by trypsin, for instance. It does not cross-react with the androgen, oestrogen or progestin receptor, nor with transcortin or with the ligand itself. It seems, therefore, to be a reasonably specific antiserum.

Using this antiserum we have set up and indirect competitive enzyme-linked immunosorbent assay (ELISA). When there is an antigen present in the sample there is less colour reaction in the tube. We made analyses of the glucocorticoid receptor using a crude cytosol preparation. In these experiments we wanted to demonstrate whether the ELISA gave the same results as the radioactivity measurements. This is a Sephadex G-150 gel filtration of the [^{3}H]-triamcinolone acetonide-labelled glucocorticoid receptor. The glucocorticoid receptor is eluted at about 6.1 nm (Fig. 3). The ELISA method shows a

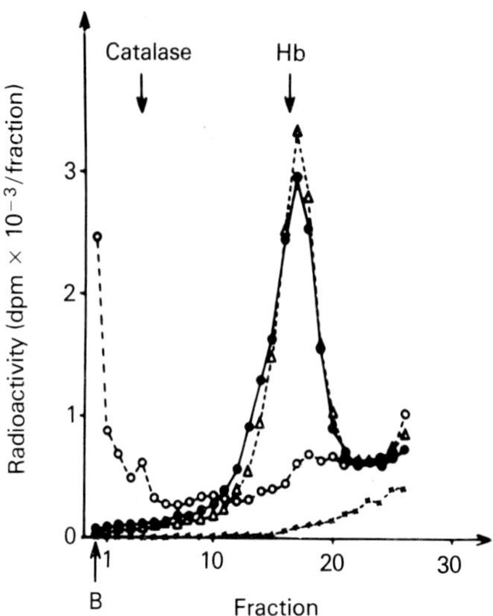

Fig. 1. Density gradient centrifugation of anti-gluco corticoid receptor-antiserum-treated gluco corticoid hormone-receptor complex from crude liver cytosol. Aliquots (0.15 ml) of cytosol containing 1.01 pmol [^{3}H]TA-GR complex were incubated with 50 μl of a solution of IgGi (5mg/ml) (○-----○), IgGn (5mg/ml) (•——•) or sodium phosphate buffer (50 nM, pH 7.4) (△-----△) for 2.5 h at 4° C in the presence of 0.15 M NaCl. A parallel incubation of cytosol with [^{3}H]TA in the presence of a 100-fold excess of unlabelled TA was also analysed by density gradient centrifugation (X-----X). The whole volumes of the incubation mixtures were layered on 4.5 ml 12–30% (w/v) glycerol gradients containing homogenizing buffer in the presence of 0.15 M KCl and centrifuged for 17 h in an SW 50.1 rotor in a Beckman Model L3–50 ultra-centrifuge at 200,000 X g. In the bottom of the centrifuge tube there was a layer of 0.4 ml 87% (w/v) of glycerol. Fresh human hemoglobin, 4.1 S, and bovine liver catalase, 11.3 S, were layered on parallel gradients for calculation of sedimentation coefficients. 'B' indicates the radioactivity adhered to the bottom of the tube after emptying of the gradient and gentle washing.

dip here in the colour reaction, where the radioactivity is eluted.

The same can be shown when using glycerol density gradient centrifugation. The radioactive peak occurs at the same place as the ELISA dip, so the immunoreactivity is identical to the radioactivity (Fig. 4).

Using isoelectric focusing in agarose gel, the radioactive peak focuses at pI 5.7, as does the ELISA dip (the immunoreactivity thus again being at the same place as the radioactivity) (Fig. 5).

We do have other methods that show the same results. In other words, we believe that we have at least a qualitative ELISA method with which the

Table. Specificity and cross-reactivity of IgG.

A. Cytosol GCR		
I. Rat:	liver ('61 Å' native receptor)	+
	thymus	+
	hippocampus	+
II. Human:	lymphocytes	+
	hippocampus	+
	chronic lymphatic leukaemia (lymphocytes)	+
III. Mouse:	liver	+
IV. Proteolytic fragments of the rat liver cytosol receptor:		
	'36 Å' fragment	–
	'19 Å' fragment	–
B. Nuclear GCR		
Rat liver:	'50–60 Å' receptor	+
	'30–36 Å' receptor	–
C. Other receptors		
Androgen receptor (rat prostate cytosol)		–
Oestrogen receptor (rat uterus cytosol)		–
Progestin receptor (rat uterus cytosol)		–
D. Other compounds		
Transcortin (rat serum)		–
Triamcinolone acetonide		–

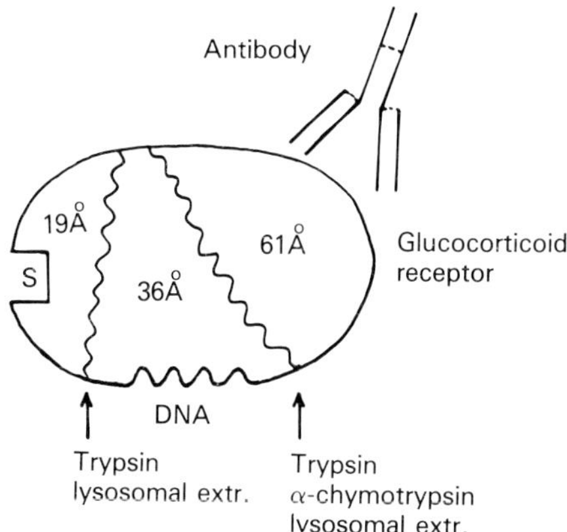

Fig. 2. Current concept of the structure of the glucocorticoid receptor.

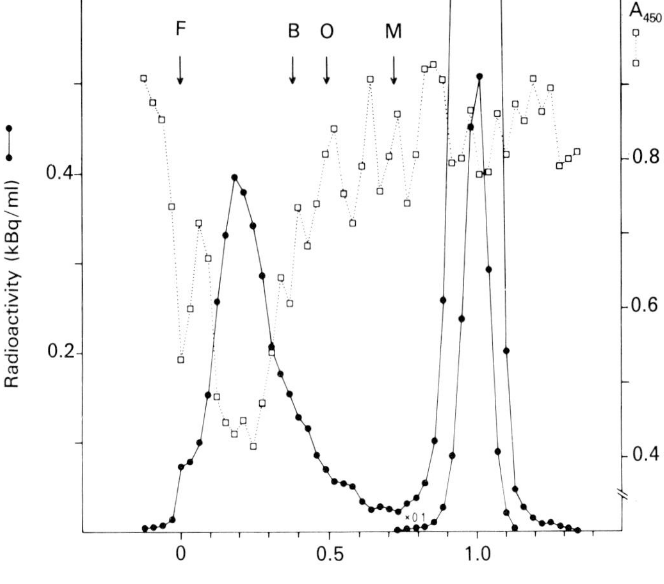
F
B
O
M
Radioactivity (kBq/ml)
A450
0.4
0.2
0.8
0.6
0.4
×0.1
0
0.5
1.0
Distribution coefficient

Fig. 3.

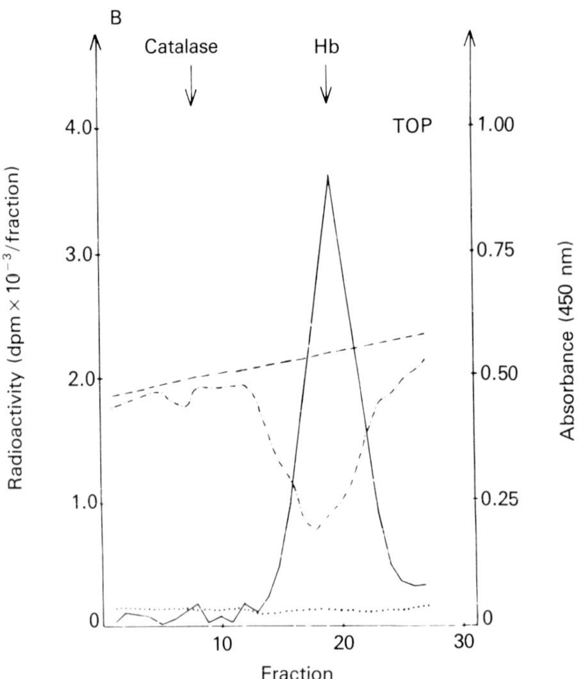
B
Catalase
Hb
TOP
Radioactivity (dpm × 10⁻³/fraction)
Absorbance (450 nm)
4.0
3.0
2.0
1.0
0
1.00
0.75
0.50
0.25
0
10
20
30
Fraction

Fig. 4.

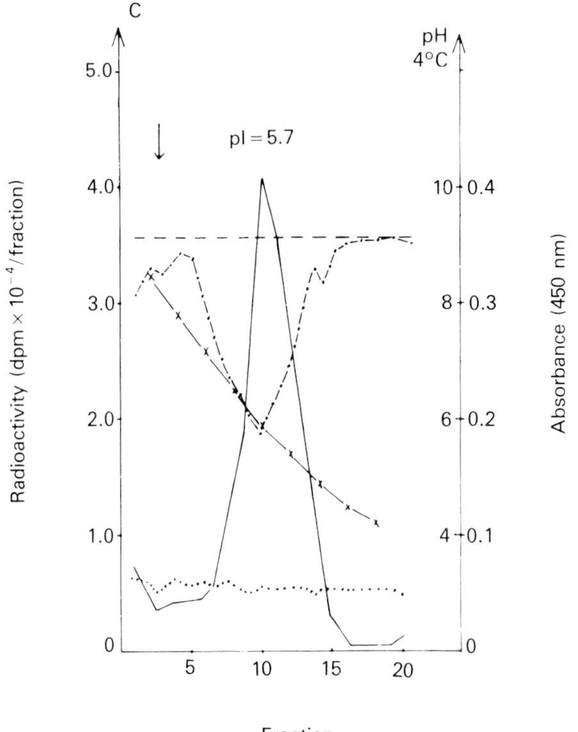

Fig. 5. Agarose isoelectric focusing of 8.8 pmol [³H]TA-GR complex/sample. After electrofocusing, the proteins were extracted from the gel. The extraction buffer was taken for analysis using ELISA or radioactivity measurement. pI, isoelectric point; X———X, pH-gradient. The arrow indicates the sample application point. For further details, see legend to Figure 3.

←

Fig. 3. Gel filtration of cytosol labelled with [³H]-triamcinolone acetonide on Agarose A-0.5m. After incubation with triamcinolone acetonide, the concentration of NaCl was adjusted to 0.15 M and the sample applied on the column which was eluted with EPG buffer containing 0.15 M NaCl and 0.02% NaN_3. After chromatography, the fractions were analyzed for radioactivity and for immunoactivity by ELISA (A_{450}). F = ferritin; B = bovine serum albumin; O = ovalbumin; M = myoglobin.

Fig. 4. Glycerol density gradient centrifugafraction of 1.77 pmol [³H]TA-GR complex. After centrifugation, the gradients were fractioned in 0.2 ml fractions. 50 μl of each fraction was assayed for radioactivity, while the rest (0.15 ml) was assayed using ELISA. Hemoglobin (4.1 S) and catalase (11.3 S) were used as standards. For further details, see legend of Figure 3.

glucocorticoid receptor can be detected. We are trying to develop a quantitative ELISA as well. We believe, however, that a monoclonal antibody may be better in this respect than polyclonal antibodies, and some effort is now being invested into raising such a monoclonal antibody.

If the glucocorticoid receptor is proteolysed with trypsin under very careful conditions, a smaller part of the receptor may be obtained (3.6 nm) – about half the native receptor (Fig. 6). The immunoreactivity now no longer coelutes with the radioactivity. There is one immunoreactive peak at 2.6 nm, and there is another immunoreactive peak at 1.4 nm. In fact, the 2.6 nm peak is converted into the 1.4 nm peak if the proteolysis is continued. It seems, therefore, that using this method we can detect other fragments of the receptor which are undetectable when using the conventional ligand-based method.

This can also be demonstrated using DNA-cellulose chromatography. In this case, the radioactivity elutes from the DNA-cellulose column as a sharp peak, as does the immunoreactivity (Fig. 7). If we treat with trypsin, now the

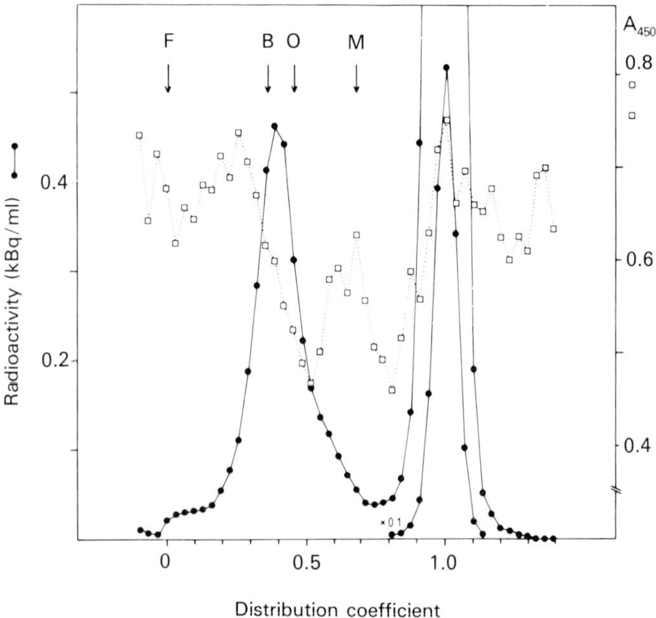

Fig. 6. Gel filtration of [³H]-triamcinolone acetonide-labelled cytosol treated with α-chymotrypsin. After incubation of the cytosol with triamcinolone acetonide, the labelled cytosol was incubated with α-chymotrypsin and the incubation was terminated by the addition of lima bean trypsin inhibitor. Chromatography on Agarose A-0.5m was performed as described in the legend to Figure 3.

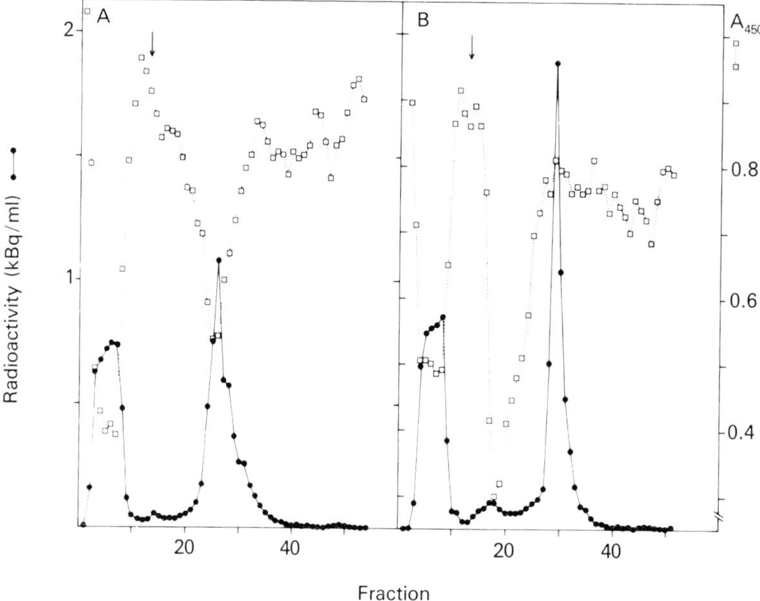

Fig. 7. DNA-cellulose chromatography of labelled cytosol treated (B) or not treated (A) with α-chymotrypsin. After application of the dextran-coated charcoal-treated samples, the columns were washed with EPG buffer and then eluted with a linear 0–0.5 M NaCl gradient. The arrow marks the start of the gradient.

smaller half of the receptor (the 3.6 nm peak) comes off slightly later from the DNA-cellulose column, indicating a higher DNA binding capacity of this receptor fragment (as we have shown previously). The interesting observation, however, is that the immunoreactivity does not co-elute with the radioactively-labelled receptor. We believe, therefore, that this immunoreactive fragment represents the immunoreactive domain which has been split off from the native receptor.

Our findings are summarized in Figure 8. We believe that the glucocorticoid receptor is made up of three domains: the A, B and C domains. The A domain binds the ligand, the B domain binds DNA and the C domain is the site to which the antibody binds.

I should add finally that these findings are of clinical interest because certain glucocorticoid-insensitive tumour cells have been demonstrated to contain a receptor fragment (A + B) which represents only part of the native receptor (A + B + C). In other words, we now have an antiserum against the

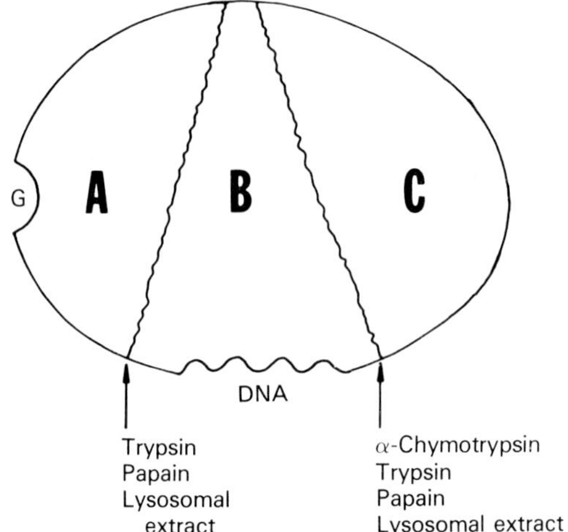

Fig. 8. Hypothetical model for the functional domains of the glucocorticoid receptor. Domain A contains the steroid binding site, domain B the DNA binding site and domain C the immunological determinant(s). The biological function of domain C is still unclear.

glucocorticoid receptor and we have an ELISA method, with which we can distinguish the native functional receptor from non-functional forms of the receptor which are still able to bind the ligand. Using such specific methods, perhaps it will be possible in the future to increase the predictiveness of steroid receptor-based tests.

Reference

1. Okret, S., Carlstedt-Duke, J., Wrange, Ö. et al. (1981): Characterization of an antiserum against the glucocorticoid receptor. *Biochim. Biophys. Acta 677,* 205.

New assays: developments in assay procedures. A new assay system for oestrogen and progesterone receptors: double labeling using (^{125}I)-oestradiol and (^{3}H)-R5020 as radioligands

K. Pollow

Determination of the level of oestrogen and progesterone receptors in breast tumour tissues has been shown to be of considerable value in the selection of breast cancer patients for endocrine therapies. The most widely used and generally accepted method for quantification of receptors is the dextran-coated charcoal assay. Analysis is run on a cytosol preparation from tumour tissue using ^{3}H-labeled oestradiol and R5020 for oestrogen or gestagen-receptor measurement, respectively.

Recently Thibodeau et al. published a new method for simultaneous determination of the concentrations of oestrogen and progesterone receptors in tumour cytosol [1]. The concentrations of these receptors are derived from separate Scatchard plot analyses of a single dextran-coated charcoal assay that incorporates both, radio-iodinated oestradiol and ^{3}H-R5020 as the labeled ligands. The 2 isotopes, radio-iodine and tritium, are easily discriminated with a liquid scintillation counter.

We would like to report first experiences with this new method for simultaneous determination of oestrogen and gestagen receptor concentrations using radio-iodinated oestradiol, that was characterized by Hochberg as a highly effective ligand for oestrogen-receptor measurement [2], and ^{3}H-R5020 for progesterone-receptor determination.

In Figure 1 the energy spectra of ^{3}H-R5020 (H-3) and radio-iodinated oestradiol (I-125) were determined in the presence of various quenching substances in a Beckman LS 7800 liquid scintillation counter. According to these spectra the energy windows were set. The quench curve was established using ^{3}H and radio-iodine reference sources with calibrated dpm-values. On channel I radio-iodinated oestradiol, on channel II ^{3}H-R5020 was measured and printed out as dpm. The β-energy of I-125 was automatically subtracted.

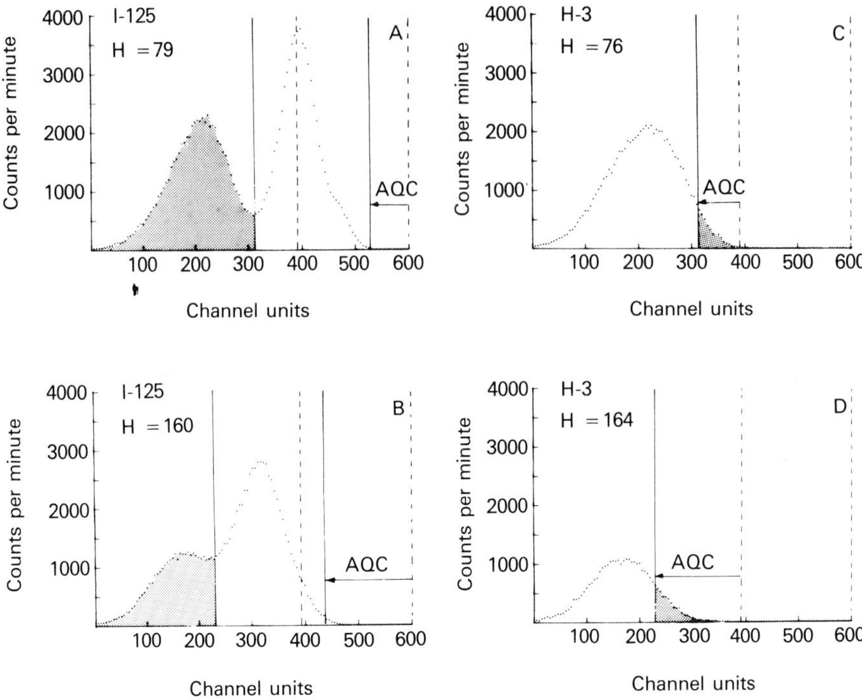

Fig. 1. Energy spectra of I-125 and H-3 in differently quenched samples. The energy spectra for I-125 and H-3 were determined on a Beckman LS 7800 liquid scintillation counter in order to adjust the counting channels for a double-labeling programme. The channels were adjusted as follows (dashed lines): I-125 on channel I (lower limit 390, upper limit 600 units); H-3 on channel II (lower limit 0, upper limit 390 units). The spill over (shaded areas) is automatically subtracted. By automatic quench compensation (AQC) the counter dynamically adjusts the channel settings according to the H-number, determined. Figures IA and C represent samples with low quench; B and D are highly quenched. The H-number is subtracted from the theoretical channel number (390 or 600), this provides individual and optimal channel setting for each sample. The H-number is determined by an external standard.

The maximal counting efficiency was 41% for radio-iodine and 45% for ^{3}H.

Figure 2 demonstrates that the newly available 16α-iodo-3,17β-oestradiol (^{125}I) binds with identical affinity to the oestradiol receptor compared to oestradiol.

Figure 3 shows the correlation of oestrogen receptor concentrations of 150 mammary tumours as determined by our standard assay and by the newly developed double-labeling assay. The correlation coefficient is r = 0.956.

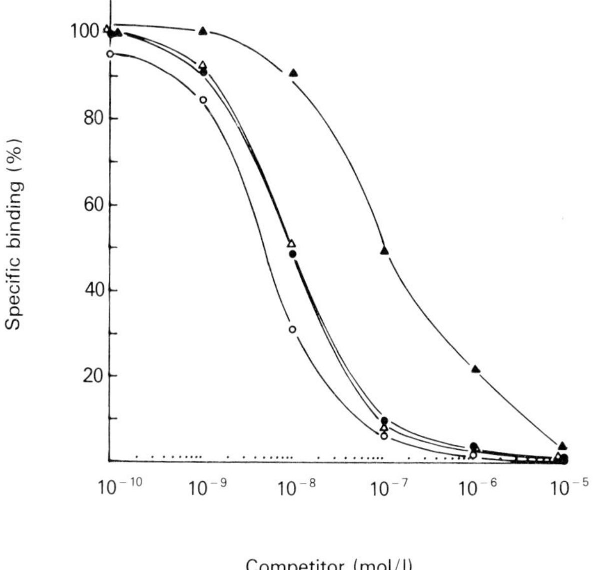

Fig. 2. Binding specificity of 16α-iodo-3,17β-oestradiol to the oestrogen receptor. Oestradiol (○), diethylstilboestrol (•), 16α-iodo-3,17β-oestradiol (△) and 16β-bromo-3,17β-oestradiol (▲) were investigated for their relative binding affinities (RBA) to human uterine oestrogen receptor. The tubes were prepared as follows: to each tube 50 μl of ^{3}H-oestradiol (in PENG-buffer) was pipetted to give a final concentration of 8 nmol/l. Then aliquots of 50-μl containing the various competitors (in PENG-buffer) at 6 different concentrations (10^{-10} – 10^{-5}mol/l) were added. Finally, to each tube 100 μl of human uterine cytosol were added and after gentle shaking the tubes were incubated overnight at 4 °C. The reactions were terminated by the addition of 0.5 ml of dextran-coated charcoal suspension. After 10 minutes of incubation under gentle shaking the tubes were centrifuged for 10 minutes at 1,500 g, 0.5 ml of the supernatant were transferred to scintillation vials and, after addition of 10-ml cocktail, counted for radioactivity. All determinations were carried out in triplicate.

The correlation of progesterone receptor concentrations are shown in Figure 4. A correlation coefficient of r = 0.989 was obtained.

This new assay offers several advantages. First, the amount of tissue necessary for a valid 5–6-point titration analysis can be reduced by half. This should be of interest for receptor determinations in needle biopsies, in lymphnodes or cell cultures. Secondly, time and costs for the assay can also be significantly reduced. We feel, that after careful further investigation, this double-labeling assay will replace the standard assay presently used.

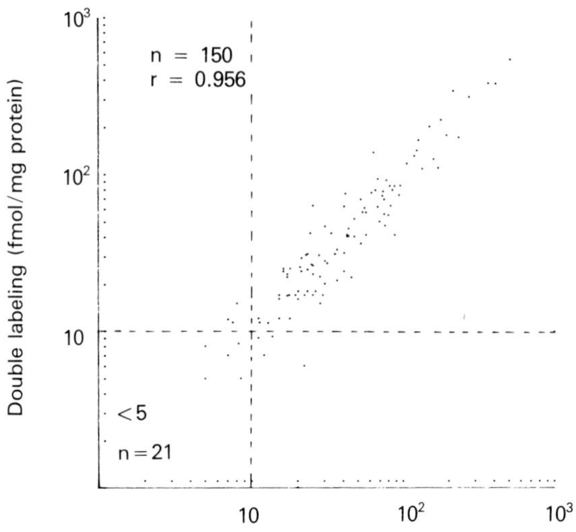

Fig. 3. Correlation of oestrogen receptor determinations as obtained by standard assay versus the double labeling assay (n = number of tissues investigated; r = coefficient of correlation; dashed line: clinical cut off level for being receptor positive). The double-labeling assay was performed as follows:

a. The tumour tissues were pulverized in a Micro Dismembrator (Braun Melsungen) and then suspended in PENGM-buffer (10 mmol/l KH_2PO_4, 10 mmol/l K_2HPO_4, 1.5 mmol/l EDTA, 3 mmol/l NaN_3, 10% glycerol, 5 mmol/l monothioglycerol, pH 7.5). The homogenates were centrifuged at 105,000 g for 30 minutes, the supernatant was taken as cytosol.

b. Five-point titration assay (double labeling): 50 μl of aqueous solutions of (^{125}I)-oestradiol and 50 μl of ^{3}H-R5020 – both in 5 concentrations – were pipetted into the same 75 × 9 mm glass tubes either alone (in duplicate, total binding) or in the presence of 200-fold excess diethylstilboestrol and R5020 (nonspecific binding). Then 100 μl of cytosol were added. The final concentrations of (^{125}I)-oestradiol were 0.5–8 nmol/l and of ^{3}H-R5020 were 1–16 nmol/l. The tubes were incubated overnight at 0–4°C. In a parallel experiment the routine assay using ^{3}H-oestradiol and ^{3}H-R5020 in separate tubes was performed. Dextran-coated charcoal (500 μl) were added to each tube and the tubes were incubated for 10 minutes. After centrifugation, 500 μl of the supernatant were withdrawn and counted for radioactivity. The data were all expressed as dpm either using the double-labeling programme or the regular ^{3}H-dpm programme. The receptor concentrations were calculated according to Scatchard [3] and expressed as fmoles receptor/mg of cytosol protein. Protein concentrations were determined according to Waddell [4].

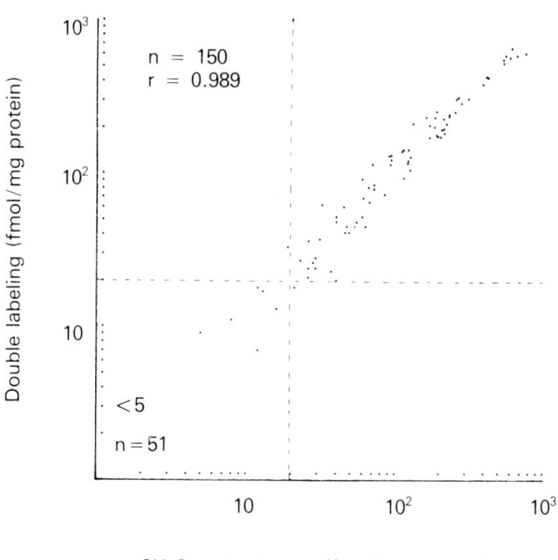

Fig. 4. Correlation of progesterone receptor determinations as obtained by standard assay versus the double-labeling assay.

References

1. Thibodeau, et al. (1981): *Clin. Chem. 27,* 687.
2. Hochberg, (1979): *Science 205,* 1138.
3. Scatchard, (1949): *Ann. N.Y. Acad. Sci. 51,* 660.
4. Waddell, (1956): *J. Lab. Clin. Med. 48,* 311.

W.L. McGuire: It is clear that the trend is to be able to develop more simple assays, or assays that can be used on much smaller specimens.

Discussion

W.L. McGuire: Professor Pollow, how much of this purified material, in μg, do you have at the present time?

K. Pollow: It has been possible to prepare between 200 and 400 μg of receptor protein.

E. Milgrom: Dr Weigel said that in her laboratory there is some evidence on the specific binding of the receptors to the ovalbumin gene. Could she say to which region of the ovalbumin gene the receptors are bound and also may we have some details about it?

N. Weigel: This work has just begun and the exact region of the ovalbumin gene has not yet been shown. It is known, though, that the receptors will also bind to a 5′-region of the Y gene, which is the analogue to the ovalbumin gene. However, when other eukaryotic genes are used, such as actin or the chicken globin gene, there is no binding. Receptor will bind in a simple assay, but in competition it will not bind very well. It much prefers the ovalbumin gene, which is I think similar to what has been observed with the glucocorticoid receptor. The exact site has not yet been localized.

E. Milgrom: Do you mean that the whole gene is used in this kind of assay?

N. Weigel: No, a piece of it – known as ovi–1.7, which is a small amount of the structural gene, most of which is the 5′-flanking region. That is what was used in the original assay. We are now in the process of cutting up that piece to see where the binding can be found and what feature of the DNA is being recognized, whether it is a specific sequence or, say, an AT-rich region. We know that it is not simply, for example, AT because plasmids with AT-linkers are not picked up.

A. Di Marco: If I understood correctly, Dr Weigel showed that the protein kinase which is cyclic-AMP-dependent has a regulatory function on the activity of the progesterone receptor ovalbumin gene. Is this regulatory function positive or negative? What is active, the dephosphorylated unit or the phosphorylated unit?

Secondly, is this regulatory effect on ovalbumin gene function a negative effect on oestradiol-induced proliferative activity?

N. Weigel: We do not know quite as much as that yet, but we know that if the receptor is dephosphorylated the second hormone binding site is lost. Presumably, therefore, the phosphorylated receptor would be the active receptor. I showed that the receptor displays as 3 spots, so there may well be 2 phosphorylation sites and 2 separate activities. So far, there has not been enough time to investigate what effect, for example, there is on specific DNA binding. It is known that the A protein used in the experiments that I described in which the specificity is seen is a mixture of the 3 forms – presumably looking very much like the preparation I showed which was predominantly dephosphorylated. We are currently developing methods to isolate those 3 forms in order to compare in various assays whether, for example, one form binds better to DNA. There has not been the opportunity yet to do those experiments.

P. Robel (Bicetre, France): Dr Weigel probably knows that progesterone receptor purified from French chicken is of the A type only, although it seems to bind nicely to DNA. Antibodies to that progesterone receptor can be obtained – which seems to be a reasonably purified molecule. Was an attempt made to get antibodies against the A and B forms of the progesterone receptor and then to see whether there is some immuno-cross-reactivity of both components?

N. Weigel: That is being done now. In fact, we have a collaborative project with Professor McGuire, and there are about 50 clones for me to assay on my return to our laboratory. When that has been done, we should be able to answer that question.

A. Fuchs (Freiburg, Federal Republic of Germany): With regard to clinical application, we can still remember the critical remarks made by Professor McGuire earlier in this symposium. What will be the new views about clinical application with regard to the work that has been going on about antibodies and other ways of purifying receptors? What do we as clinicians have to do so that in 4 years' time we can come back with results from different studies and withstand the critical views of the biochemists with regard to oestrogen receptor assays?

W.L. McGuire: Perhaps the question can be rephrased, asking each of the 5 speakers, Dr Weigel and Professors Milgrom, Di Marco, Gustafsson and Pollow, briefly to say what they hope to have accomplished, in 3–5 years, that might have some biological or clinical significance?

N. Weigel: As is known, we are attempting to obtain antibodies to our chicken progesterone receptor. These may or may not cross-react with human receptor. The project in which I am most involved that would have clinical relevance is the joint project in which we are currently involved with Upjohn attempting to determine the 3-dimensional structure of the progesterone hormone-binding site, with the idea that it would then be possible rationally to design various types of analogues of progesterone. We will be able then to do computer modelling and to look at the interaction in the hormone binding site to better develop various drugs that might be useful for people. My part of it will be to determine the amino acid sequence and to provide the hormone binding site for x-ray crystallography.

E. Milgrom: It is a very dangerous exercise because if we come back in 5 years' time probably what will have been accomplished will not be what we see now as likely to be accomplished, but other things which had not even been suggested. Obviously, even if our laboratory does not achieve it, some other laboratory or collaborative effort between laboratories will find immunological ways of measuring receptors. I am not sure that the use of receptors, for instance, in breast cancer, will continue to be of importance, but I am sure that it will become very easy to measure receptors – there will be kits sold by various firms, and everybody will be able to measure receptors without any difficulties.

The second thing that will probably have been achieved, as I said, is the use of markers of hormone action – which will I think be widespread and used to measure what the hormone is really doing, how much it is doing at any given moment.

These predictions will probably be false in 5 years' time, however.

J.A. Gustafsson: One might anticipate that within 3–5 years we will perhaps have monoclonal antibodies against the glucocorticoid, oestrogen and progesterone receptors, and that immunoassays based on these preparations are available. The problem will be the androgen receptor which so far has not been purified.

W.L. McQuire: Professor Di Marco, what would like to have accomplished in the next 3–5 years?

A. Di Marco: I have no programme on monoclonal antibodies.

K. Pollow: With the increasing success in producing highly-effective techniques of receptor purification perhaps it will become possible to establish a radioimmunoassay for such receptor proteins in the cytosolic fraction of target organs.

W.L. McGuire: I am disappointed to hear that everyone wants an immunological assay. With the recombinant DNA techniques, I would have hoped that someone would be talking about innovative ways of putting receptors into cells where they have not been previously, and so on. It is obvious that we cannot discuss that now.

Receptors in adjuvant disease

W.L. McGuire

I would like to present a follow-up on a study that has been going on for some time in Cleveland, Ohio, in which stage II breast-cancer patients were randomized to chemotherapy (CMF), chemotherapy plus tamoxifen, or chemotherapy, tamoxifen and BCG. They were all stage II, axillary node-positive patients, in all of whom the oestrogen receptor status was known (this was done in my laboratory) and, of course, their nodal status was also known. Almost 300 patients were entered into the study.

The new aspect that I want to mention is that the progesterone receptor was measured in all these patients as well as the oestrogen receptor.

The results can be summarized by saying that until 1981 in the oestrogen receptor-positive (ER-positive) group of patients there was an advantage of CMF plus tamoxifen over CMF alone.

Now, however, the *P* value is no longer significantly different between the 2 groups. We think that there are several reasons for this. First, that tamoxifen was stopped at 12 months. If we were to design a new adjuvant programme with tamoxifen, I think that we would continue tamoxifen well beyond 12 months. Nevertheless, this is the study that was originally designed, and these are the most up-to-date results for ER-positive patients by treatment. Let us now consider the most favourable group; let us pick ER-positive/progesterone receptor-positive (PgR-positive) patients. If there is ever a group that should respond to tamoxifen, *that* is the group. In fact, we have the same result; in other words, there is perhaps an early advantage with tamoxifen, but after a long time that positive effect disappears – again *perhaps* because the tamoxifen was given for only 12 months. That may explain the early positive effect.

What happens to disease-free survival in patients receiving tamoxifen if they are divided according to whether they are PgR-positive or PgR-negative? This question has been partially answered previously. There are suggestions (from France primarily) that irrespective of treatment, PgR-positive patients are more likely to have prolonged remission or delayed recurrence compared with PgR-negative patients. I think that this is an important findig, and something that I was trying to stress yesterday. If we are trying to compare treatments A and B, it is important to ensure that there is stratification of the factors affecting overall prognosis.

What about the amount of PgR? It is what might be anticipated. Greater than 50 fmol of PgR gives the best response. The intermediates, 5–19 fmol, or 20–50 fmol, are about the same. Less than 5 fmol is clearly inferior.

In summary, we have to start measuring things that have a known impact on recurrence and survival if we are to be able to evaluate the effects of our therapy.

Receptors in adjuvant disease

S. Saez

The results I shall present have been obtained in 2 different centres, one in Paris by the group working with Dr Milgrom and Marie-France Pichon, and the other series of patients comes from my own laboratory.

The results concern the prognostic value of oestrogen and progesterone receptors. A check was made to ensure that there had been no selection of patients in the group studied for this purpose. In fact, the same distribution of patients was found in the different categories of receptor status in this series, as in a larger unselected series of patients (Table).

Results are presented here only in relation to the determination of oestrogen receptors after a follow-up of 7 years (Fig. 1). Patients were entered into these series until 1978 and clinical data have been re-evaluated recently. We have reported previously that after 2.5 years the rate of recurrence was lower in oestrogen receptor (ER)-positive patients. However, after 7 years' follow-up the 2 curves are identical.

Figure 2 shows the results obtained by Marie-France Pichon concerning the progesterone receptors alone, and also the results obtained on the total

Table. Distribution of patients according to receptor status.

	Numbers of patients	ER+ (%)	ER− (%)	Numbers of patients	PGR+ (%)	PGR− (%)
Controls						
Total	621	69	36	621	35	65
Premenopause	155	58	42	185	39	61
Postmenopause	436	66	34	436	33	66
Present study						
Total	310	67	33	151	58	93
Premenopause	92	58	42	48	42	58
Postmenopause	195	72	28	90	37	63

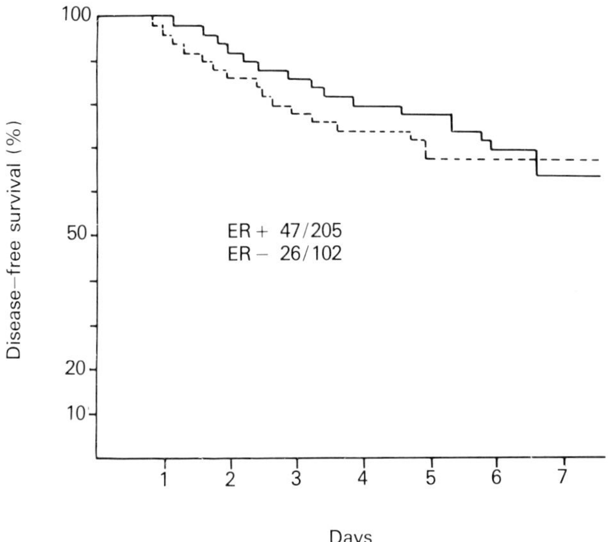

Fig. 1. Disease-free survival in ER-positive (——) and ER-negative (-----) patients. Follow-up was for 7 years.

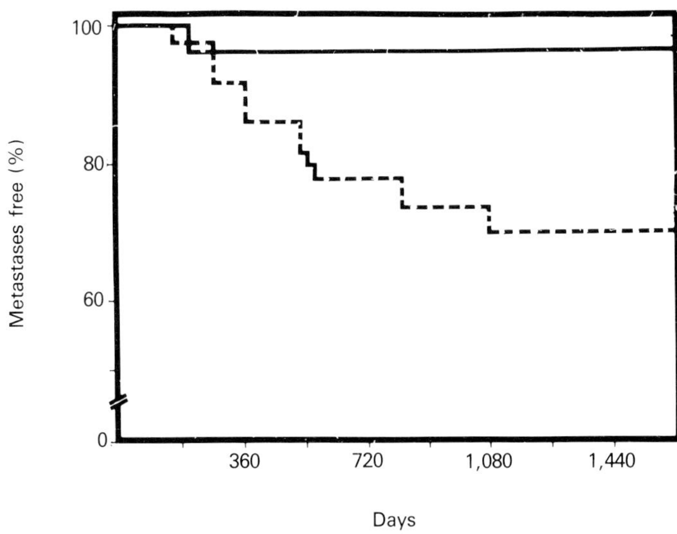

Fig. 2. Percentage of patients metastases free after almost 4 years, according to PgR status. PgR-positive (——) n = 44, PgR-negative (-----) n = 44; P = 0.02. Reproduced with permission of the Editor from Cancer Research 1980, 40 (3357–3360).

population after almost 4 years' follow-up. The percentage of patients without recurrence is lower in the patients with positive progesterone receptor (PgR), and it is very different from PgR-negative patients.

The patients shown in Figure 3 are a smaller group with poor prognosis because of their invaded nodes at the time of surgery. In this category of patients the difference is even more significant in relation to the presence or the absence of progesterone receptors. Even in these patients with poor prognosis there are very few cases of recurrence after 4 years in PgR-positive patients.

The results obtained in my laboratory (Fig. 4), show a similar significance to that of the series just shown. They relate to 150 patients followed for 5 years. There was the same difference between PgR-positive and -negative patients as observed in Pichon's work.

Figure 5 shows the results we obtained with a sub-population with poor prognosis because of their invaded nodes. We found a significant difference between the PgR-positive tumours and the PgR-negative tumours. The difference in favour of a longer disease-free interval in the PgR-positive cases is even more important at 5 years' follow-up. These data are very different from the results observed with oestradiol receptors alone – since the 2 curves of recurrences were similar after a longer follow-up.

I should add that in this series of patients adjuvant treatment has been ap-

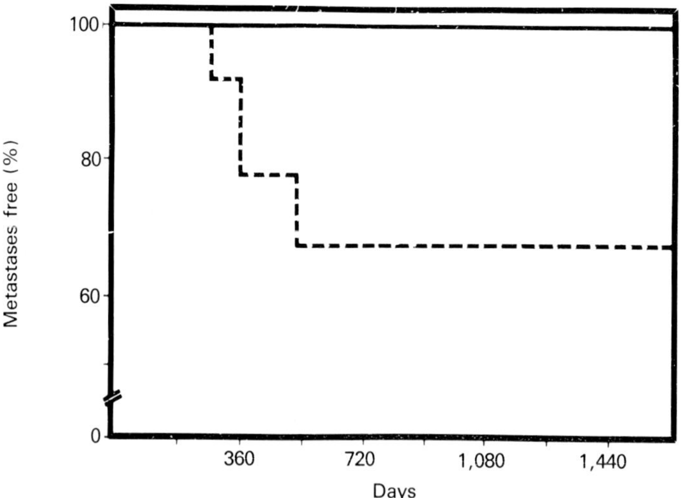

Fig. 3. Percentage of patients with poor prognosis who were metastasis free almost after 4 years, according to PgR status. PgR-positive (——) n = 25, PgR-negative (-----) n = 15; P = 0.005. Reproduced with permission of the Editor from Cancer Research 1980, 40 (3357–3360).

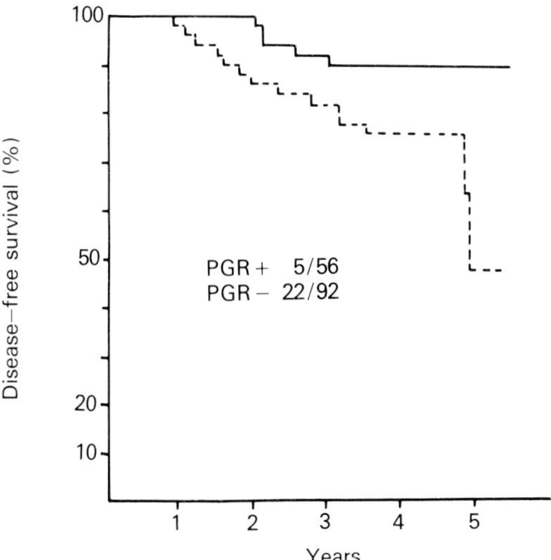

Fig. 4. Disease-free survival in 150 patients followed-up for 5 years according to PgR status. PgR-positive (——), PgR-negative (-----).

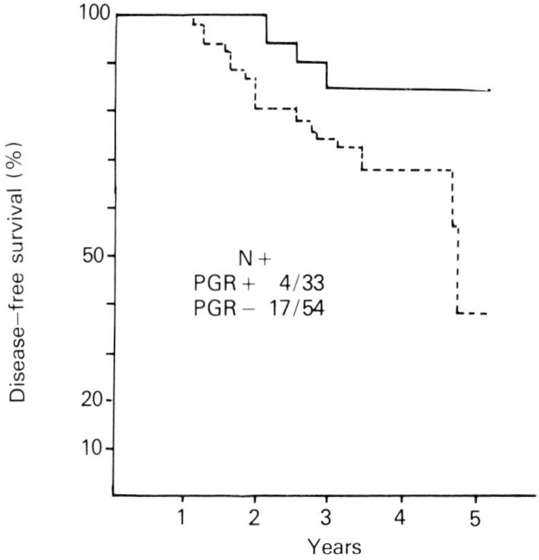

Fig. 5. Disease-free survival in a group of patients with poor prognosis. PgR-positive (——), PgR-negative (-----).

plied independently of the receptor status, so there has been no selection of patients by therapy between PgR-positive and PgR-negative status.

Receptors in adjuvant disease

Y. Nomura

First, I would like to present our data on the disease-free survival of the patients with operable breast cancer as a function of oestrogen receptors (ER). There were 202 ER-positive patients, 193 ER-negative patients and 85 with unknown ER status – that is, almost 500 patients in total. The patients were stage I, II and III, and there were no biases of the clinical factors among the groups. The median follow-up was 34 months. As can be seen from the Figure there are no differences among the groups in the disease-free curves of the patients. However, the metastatic site of the recurrence in ER-positive patients is mainly in the soft tissues. In 50% (18 out of 36) the metastatic site was in the soft tissues. In contrast, the patients with ER-negative tumours, visceral, particularly liver metastases are predominant – in 70% (19 out of 27). This may affect the survival rates of the patients in their future evaluation.

Since 1978 we have been carrying out a prospective randomized trial of adjuvant therapy in the operable breast cancer patients, based on the results of the determination of ER status and menopausal status of the patients. The adjuvant treatment for ER-positive premenopausal patients is divided into 3 categories:

1. tamoxifen following oöphorectomy;
2. chemotherapy with mitomycin C and long-term oral cyclophosphamide; and
3. tamoxifen plus the same chemotherapy.

Adjuvant treatment for ER-positive postmenopausal patients was:

1. tamoxifen alone;
2. chemotherapy alone; or
3. combination of tamoxifen and chemotherapy.

For ER-negative patients the treatment was:

1. chemotherapy; or
2. chemotherapy plus tamoxifen.

In all, 309 patients have been subjected to the adjuvant therapy and the median follow-up is 21 months after mastectomy.

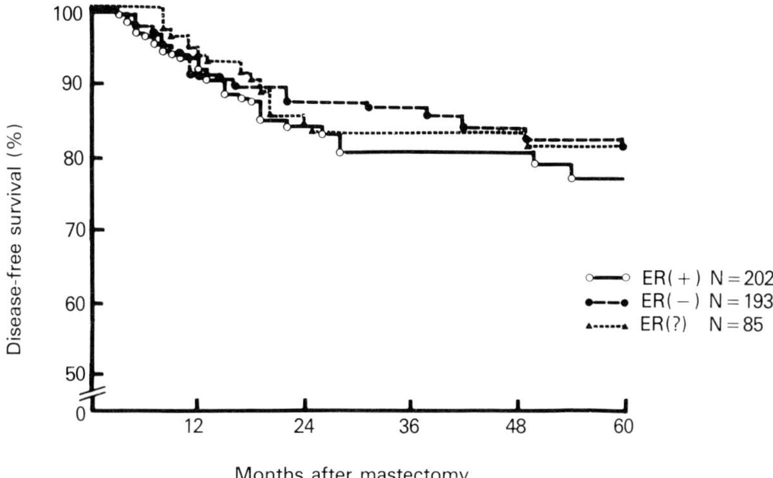

Figure. Disease-free survival in breast cancer patients according to ER. ER-positive (○——○) n = 202, ER-negative (•——•) n = 193, ER? (▲----▲) n = 85.

In ER-positive premenopausal patients oöphorectomy with tamoxifen treatment appeared to be as effective as chemotherapy alone – or perhaps more effective. This study is on-going, and more time and more patients are required before an evaluation can be made.

Discussion

W.L. McGuire: Let us not focus, in this discussion, so much on the results of treatment, but perhaps more on the role of receptors in the prognosis or in helping to select therapies in adjuvant disease.

W. Jonat (Bremen, Federal Republic of Germany): First, Professor McGuire showed that progesterone may be of prognostic value. On the other hand, although the patients in his group were divided into ER-positive, PgR-negative and so on (they were divided into different groups), as far as I understood all the patients were treated by CMF or by CMF plus tamoxifen.

Could the therapy influence the results obtained?

Secondly, with regard to Dr Hubay's CMF/tamoxifen versus CMF study, does he think that therapy may influence receptor content in the tumour so that after 6 years it makes no difference whether or not the patient is treated with tamoxifen because the tumour itself is entirely receptor-negative?

W.L. McGuire: In answer to the first question: since some of these patients were treated, what does it all mean? I should explain that this was a prospective, randomized trial with every patient receiving CMF. There were 2 other arms, in which the patients received CMF plus tamoxifen or CMF, tamoxifen and BCG. It turned out that in the latter 2 groups there was no difference in disease-free survival – so those 2 groups were combined for the purposes of this analysis. This means that we are talking about chemotherapy or chemotherapy plus tamoxifen. A multivariate analysis was done to see what was the most important factor, or factors, accounting for recurrence. First, we found that it was not treatment. The treatment effect was not significant in this study – so we can eliminate treatment.

The factor that came out first and foremost in predicting a short disease-free survival was the number of positive lymph nodes.

The second most important factor was progesterone receptor. If the progesterone receptor and lymph node status were known, there was no need to know anything else – oestrogen receptor or anything else. At the moment, that is all I can say. We are continuing to analyse the data into smaller subsets and so on. So far, those are unequivocal conclusions.

E. Milgrom: In the series shown by Dr Saez (and which we have published in *Cancer Research* in September 1980) there were 90 patients who received no treatment at all – and the prognostic effect of progesterone receptor was as shown, so this was completely independent of any treatment.

W.L. McGuire: It is as yet unpublished, but it may be recalled that in the NSABP protocol B09, chemotherapy plus or minus tamoxifen, based upon oestrogen receptor, they also measured progesterone receptor. Those data are now being analysed, and some very interesting results are being found. What I am saying is that until the French groups and our own group started to analyse progesterone receptor data something was being ignored. I think that there is something to be said for insisting upon the measurement of progesterone receptor.

E. Milgrom: In the group we studied there was a very significant difference between metastases and local recurrences. Progesterone receptor status predicted the occurrence of metastases very well, but did not predict the occurrence of local recurrence. Has Professor McGuire any experience of this; has he tried to study this point?

W.L. McGuire: That point has not yet been analysed.

F. Cavalli: I am perhaps going to make some trivial remarks, but I would not like to think that some people in the audience believe that there are already data in favour of using some kind of hormonal treatment in the adjuvant situation by the medical community. When we go for adjuvant treatment, we are bound to go for cure – nothing else matters. There are 3 large studies, each comprising between 1,500 and 2,000 patients (the NSABP trial, the ECOG trial and the Ludwig trial). There are, as yet, no meaningful data from these 3 trials, which are investigating the value of adding hormonal therapy to chemotherapy or of hormonal therapy alone. This is even considering the preliminary analysis published by Fisher, which, in my opinion, is not yet meaningful.

It must be stressed clearly, that for the time being there are no data. I would go one step further and say that we always hold the dogma that we go from the advanced situation to the adjuvant situation, taking the advanced situation as a model. When each of those groups started those trials 3, 4 or 5 years ago, everyone was much more enthusiastic than we are now about the value of combining chemotherapy and hormonal therapy in the advanced situation. Even on a theoretical basis, I think that today the ground for using hormonal therapy in the adjuvant situation is, at best, shaky.

W.L. McGuire: If we really want to pursue that point, what Dr Cavalli is saying is that endocrine therapy in advanced disease never cured anybody. How many patients in advanced breast cancer has chemotherapy cured? (*Several people said 'none'*).

F. Cavalli: I accept that there are good data in favour of the prognostic value of receptors in the patients who have been radically operated – that is all that is known today.

We have probably never cured even one patient with advanced disease with chemotherapy. I would go even further and say that probably even the data concerning the pure chemotherapy in the adjuvant situation are not yet sufficient to advocate a conventional use of chemotherapy in the adjuvant situation. To my mind, adjuvant chemotherapy is still a research tool. That is why in the latest trial of the group with which I co-operate we are now randomizing between peri-operative chemotherapy and the usual, conventional CMF chemotherapy. Even there, for the time being there are not sufficient data to tell the medical community that they should treat all the patients with chemotherapy.

W.L. McGuire: I think that we are in basic agreement – although it sounds like we are arguing – but the fact remains that we are dealing with a systemic disease at the time of surgery. At the moment, there are only 3 possible modalities of treatment: chemotherapy, endocrine therapy and 'immunotherapy'. That is all we have, and at the moment all of them are experimental, so we have to use them in single or some form of combination. That is what we are talking about: different protocols. To be dogmatic, and to say that we should not be trying endocrine therapy, or we should not be trying chemotherapy (I am not quoting Dr Cavalli here), is as wrong as saying that we should be doing all of them. We are in the stage of experimentation. But my point is that if 2 different therapies are going to be compared, a control versus an active agent or 2 active agents, we have to be sure that all the things known to affect prognosis have been measured. The purpose of randomization is not to take care of that. If something is known to affect prognosis, it must be measured. Randomization is only a hope that things that are not understood will be equalized.

My emphasis on receptors is not that receptors and hormones will cure cancer, but that at least we will be able to interpret the results of different treatment regimens.

F. Cavalli: I fully agree. I just wanted to make clear that it is not possible to base our treatment choice in the adjuvant situation today on the results of the receptors. But I agree – we have done that in our adjuvant trial comprising more than 1,600 patients and have measured the receptors in most of them.

W.L. McGuire: It sounds as though Dr Cavalli and I are arguing, but we are really not. If we all knew the answer, there would be no argument – but none of us knows the final answer. We have our biases, and that is what makes good competitive science.

F. von Eyben (Sweden): I work in the south of Sweden where we have an adjuvant study in which tamoxifen is being given for 12 months. I think it can be argued very well that much intellectual effort should be put into the stratification etc. and I think that there should be the same interest shown in the kind of treatment to be given. In my opinion it is treatment which has the potential for cure rather than a knowledge of the correct receptor status.

Therefore, I want to return to Professor McGuire's comment about how long to treat patients. He said that one of the things that could be done to change the design of the study would perhaps be to continue the hormone treatment for a period longer than 12 months. I think it could easily be argued that what is perhaps being done is that the fraction of the tumour cells which is positive and sensitive to this kind of treatment is being killed, and that what is left is a clone which is not sensitive to that treatment.

What kind of data does Professor McGuire have to support the suggestion that a longer period of some sort of hormonal treatment would be adequate in this situation?

W.L. McGuire: I have no facts to support the idea that 36 months' tamoxifen would be better than 12 months, but it is known clinically that patients who respond to tamoxifen and who then relapse can respond again to another endocrine therapy. By treating with tamoxifen we have not selected out a clone of ER-negative endocrine non-responsive cells – we know that is not true. I think that using long-term tamoxifen under those conditions is well justified.

If we are talking about chemotherapy, people are now talking about the old Nissen-Meyer data using peri-operative short-term therapy: his 20-year results show a 10% difference. There are very many ways of approaching the design and strategy of chemotherapy. I do not think that any of us here could produce the perfect plan because we all have our prejudices and biases.

G. Beretta: Firstly, a suggestion has been made in the literature that a difference in results may relate to the dosage level of the chemotherapy. Has Professor McGuire investigated to see whether the PgR-positive or PgR-negative receptor patients have received the same amount of chemotherapy?

Secondly, has the site of recurrence been investigated to find out whether the progesterone- or oestrogen-receptor content gives a different pattern of relapse?

W.L. McGuire: In Dr Hubay's study we have not looked at the pattern of relapse. Our San Antonio data have recently been analysed with regard to receptors and patterns of relapse, and it turns out that ER-positive patients tend to go much more frequently to bone metastases than ER-negative patients. The ER-negative patients go to visceral disease and, interestingly, to recurrence in local tissues. Most interesting of all is the lung because ER-positive premenopausal patients rarely have their primary, first recurrence in the lung as compared to postmenopausal patients who are also ER-positive. We are now in the process of writing this up. I present it now descriptively, not interpretatively.

In answer to the question about the dose level, in view of the Milan experience we are very interested in that – but I can only say that the doses chosen in this assay were low and would be homoeopathic by most standards.

G. Beretta: Thirdly, has any difference been observed in treatment with tamoxifen with or without BCG? The meaning of BCG in terms of receptors is not known.

W.L. McGuire: This study was designed in 1974 when BCG was popular. There is no difference in outcome in that arm.

Receptors in advanced disease

F. Cavalli

The Table shows the breakdown with regard to the receptors within our study. As I said in my presentation (see pp. 224–233), the receptors are known for 40 of the 150 evaluable patients. I want to stress that in almost every case the receptors are measured just before entering the study. Many of those patients had had their mastectomy many years previously, at which time the receptors were not measured.

In the group receiving high-dose MPA (Group A), which is about 650 mg daily, i.m. (whereas the low dose (Group B) is about 130 mg daily, i.m.) for 30 days, there was a response rate of 47% among the previous hormonal responders. In this low-dose group, however, the response rate among the previous hormonal responders was only 12%.

Looking at the results, ± indicates where the laboratory was only able to say qualitatively that the PgR was positive and could not give an exact figure.

Table. Receptor status in relation to response.

Receptor status	Treatment group A		Treatment group B	
	Number of patients in whom receptor status known	Number of patients showing response indicated	Number of patients in whom receptor status known	Number of patients showing response indicated
ER+, PgR+	7	5PR, 2NC	3	
ER+, PgR−	5	2PR, 1NC	5	1NC
ER−, PgR+	1	1PR	1	1NC
ER−, PgR−	7		6	1PR
ER+, PgR±	1	1NC	4	1PR
Totals	21		19	

ER = oestrogen receptor.
PgR = progesterone receptor.

With high-dose MPA, there is the usual pattern of response according to the receptors, whereas for the low-dose group, even based on this limited number, the usual pattern is not seen.

I do not like to draw conclusions from small numbers, so I am just presenting what we have found so far, but to me, it is striking that according to the breakdown as regards previous hormonal response and also according to those preliminary data on the receptors, there seems perhaps to be some dose-response relationship. For instance, it is known that Dr Tormek was able to show some dose-response relationship with tamoxifen. My very personal and philosophical conclusion for the time being is that this low dose is probably subtherapeutic and therefore this difference is observed.

Receptors in advanced disease

A. Pellegrini

Three years ago we decided to treat advanced breast-cancer patients, already unresponsive to any conventional treatment, with an alternating sequence of ethinyloestradiol (ETE) and medroxyprogesterone acetate (MPA). The rationale for this study was essentially based on 2 observations: 1. early experimental studies in DMBA-induced tumours in rats showed some response with a similar hormonal combination [1–4]; and 2. there have been recent advances in knowledge about hormone receptors and their reciprocal interactions with specific and aspecific hormones. We refer particularly to interactions between oestrogens and progesterone receptors, with the 'priming' activity of oestrogen itself. Therefore, we considered the possibility that a 'priming' with ETE, paving the target cells with progestin receptors, could re-induce or improve the response of the hormono-related breast-cancer cells to MPA. This was a pilot study that showed a response rate of about 30% with a partial response rate of 26% [5]. The study was successively enlarged and a follow-up of 30 months was reached with a response rate of 25% and a median response duration of 11 months (range 6–20 months). Modifications of the initial treatment sequence (essentially reducing MPA administration) markedly lowered the response rate.

More recently we have planned a multicentre study substituting tamoxifen (TAM) for ETE and its rationale was essentially based on the oestrogen-agonistic activity of the anti-oestrogen in 'priming' the target cell with progestin receptors. The main goal of these studies was to obtain better final results than with the single-agent treatment and, moreover, to reduce the high doses of MPA while keeping the same response though with fewer side-effects. A preliminary trial with a limited number of patients who were already resistant to any conventional treatment was highly suggestive of this.

The treatment schedule presents 3 different sequences: scheme A consists of 3 weeks' tamoxifen administration followed by oral MPA for another 3 weeks, then the 2 drugs are given in combination for 6 weeks; scheme B is based on an alternating schedule of 3 weeks' TAM and 3 weeks' MPA, followed by a 3-day interval – the cycle is then repeated; scheme C is an alternating sequential schedule of one week of TAM and one week of MPA, followed by a 3 days' interval, after which the cycle is repeated until progression of the disease. All patients in the trial will have been unresponsive to conventional treatment. They will be studied for oestrogen and progesterone receptor content of metastatic lesions (skin, soft tissues or breast etc.). The essential aim of reporting these preliminary data is to invite other workers to extend this trial. If our results are confirmed, further studies in receptors (selected populations and different schedules) may allow a more physiopathologic approach to the treatment of some hormone-related tumours.

References

1. Stollba (1967): Effect of Lyndiol, an oral contraceptive, on breast cancer. *Br. Med. J. 1*, 150.
2. (1967): Progestin therapy of breast cancer: comparison of agents. *Br. Med. J. 3*, 338.
3. Crowley, L.G. and MacDonald, I. (1965): Delalutin and estrogens for the treatment of advanced mammary carcinoma in the post-menopausal woman. *Cancer 18*, 436.
4. Laudau, R.L., Ehrich, E.N. and Huggins, C. (1962): Estradiol benzoate and progesterone in advanced human breast cancer. *J. Am. Med. Assoc. 182,* 136.
5. Pellegrini, A., Massidda, B., Mascia, V. et al. (1981): Ethinyl estradiol and medroxyprogesterone treatment in advanced breast cancer: A pilot study. *Cancer Treat. Rep. 65*, 1.

Receptors in advanced disease

Y. Nomura

Figure 1 shows the survival curves of 94 patients with oestrogen receptor (ER)-positive and ER-negative tumours after adreno-oöphorectomy as a function of response to therapy. The survival curves of the patients with ER-positive tumours not responsive to therapy (NC, PD) are very similar to those of the patients with ER-negative tumours.

In 58 of these 94 patients following major endocrine therapy the combination of oestrogen and progesterone receptor status was assayed. The survival curves of ER-positive/PgR-positive and ER-positive/PgR-negative cases are different from the survival curves of ER-negative/PgR-negative cases. However, there seems to be no difference between the survival curves of ER-positive/PgR-positive cases and ER-positive/PgR-negative cases (Fig. 2).

We have been carrying out a randomized trial with a combination of

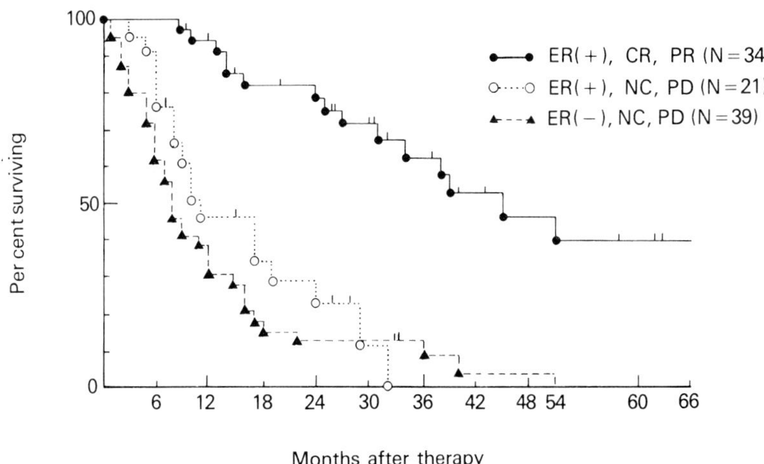

Fig. 1. Survival curves of patients with advanced breast cancer.

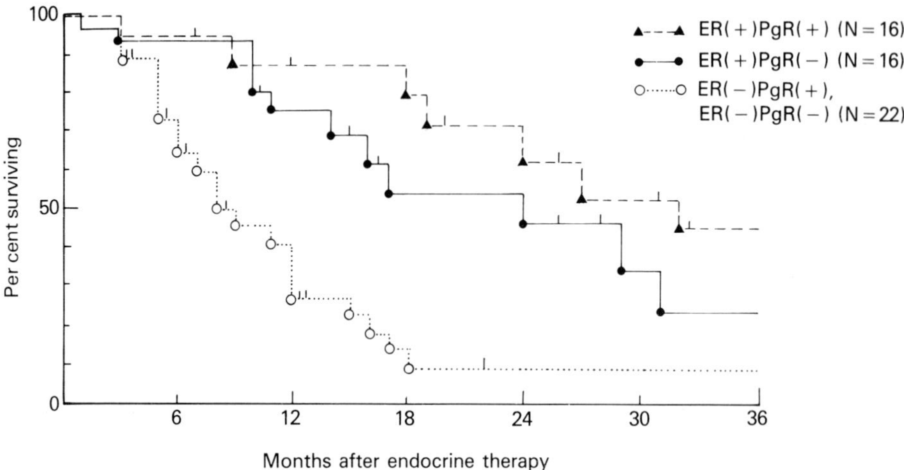

Fig. 2. Survival curves of advanced breast cancer after major endocrine therapy, according to oestrogen and progesterone receptors.

chemotherapy and endocrine therapy in advanced breast cancer patients. The trial has 4 aims:

1. adreno-oöphorectomy;
2. adreno-oöphorectomy plus FAC combination chemotherapy;
3. FAC combination chemotherapy alone; and
4. tamoxifen plus FAC combination chemotherapy.

Sixty-seven patients have been evaluated so far. There were about 60% showing complete or partial remission, except in the cases given endocrine therapy alone.

Oestrogen and progesterone receptors were assayed in these patients immediately before therapy, in the hope that it would be possible to select suitable patients for combined chemotherapy and endocrine therapy. The study is in very early stages and the number of cases entered is still small, but it seems that better responses are obtained in the ER-positive/PgR-positive cases regardless of the treatment given, including endocrine therapy alone. In ER-positive/PgR-negative cases, chemotherapy or chemotherapy plus endocrine therapy gave a better response. In ER-negative/PgR-negative cases the response rate was lower than in the patients with ER-positive tumours.

Receptors in advanced disease

E. Milgrom

I will present results, which are rather similar to those presented by Dr Cavalli, summarizing what has been found at the Centre René Huguenin, at St Cloud, using another progestogen, norethisterone acetate, in advanced breast cancer.

The results of this treatment were not good, because there were not many responsive patients. We wondered whether the response could be increased by selecting the patients on the basis of progesterone receptor measurement, and whether there could be a positive correlation between response and the presence of progesterone receptors. Results, however, were disappointing. There was a trend towards worse results in progesterone receptor-negative patients, but in this small series of 26 patients the predictive quality of the assay seemed very poor and is, therefore, probably not useful for individual patients. As has been said previously, progesterone receptors seem to be useful for predicting the outcome of breast cancer in its initial stages, but here, in advanced breast cancer, this assay has a poor predictive quality for progesterone therapy, at least in our series.

Discussion

W.L. McGuire: I am not sure that there is much merit in discussing the good and the bad points of studies with only 20 or 30 patients. Perhaps other questions might be asked of the Panel that might be of interest.

F. Cavalli: First, what does Professor McGuire think about the combination of tamoxifen and progesterone agents? I have been trying to repeat some published data on priming skin metastases with different periods of treatment with tamoxifen and have been unable to observe any clear-cut pattern of behaviour of the progesterone receptors after this priming with tamoxifen.

Secondly, and slightly more provocatively, I am sometimes afraid that as soon as people are able to measure something they stop thinking. With receptors we are able to spare some premenopausal women oöphorectomy, which is a main advantage that we have obtained with the receptors. I am wondering mainly about postmenopausal women where by means of a careful clinical evaluation we are, even before starting treatment, almost able to tell whether or not the patients will be hormonosensitive.

W.L. McGuire: The attitude can be taken that as more is learned about the biological basis of our treatments it should be possible to learn more about the type of patient who should respond to a therapy – and I do not mean just hormonal therapy. We might even talk along the lines of the clonogenic assay and so on. The approach can be taken that if all our single-agent chemotherapeutic agents give about 20% response rate, let us combine them all (let us use 4 or 5) and hopefully get a 60 or 70% response rate. That has been the traditional thinking with regard to combination chemotherapy. Someone who is used to that sort of thinking will have to come to grips with the rationale behind the clonogenic assay – *if* it becomes successful.

Let us turn to the receptor assays and tamoxifen. Let us say that tamoxifen is a benign drug (although it has a few side-effects); so should we give it to everybody and not worry about receptor assays? What happens if – by measuring progesterone receptors – there might be a group of patients who, if given chemotherapy and tamoxifen, would do worse than with chemotherapy alone. Would that be impressive? If I knew the progesterone receptor status of a group of patients, and I knew that tamoxifen added to chemotherapy might give inferior results than chemotherapy alone, would that be considered a reason for wanting to know the progesterone receptor level?

F. Cavalli: You are talking about very early data in the adjuvant premenopausal situation – and that is not my question.

W.L. McGuire: No – but the question is: how will those data be obtained unless the receptors are measured – unless the studies are done to find out exactly how valuable or useless the receptors are? I would hope that in 5 years' time we have some much better way to predict endocrine-dependence, chemotherapy-dependence and so on. But today, receptors are all we have – and they are by no means perfect. The studies of many of the Panelists have pinpointed the usefulness of receptors or their lack of usefulness. Now it is up to *you* – how do you practice medicine? What is your attitude? Do you feel that you know enough to be able to predict, with as good assurance, whether your patients will respond to an ablative or additive endocrine procedure, as with a receptor test? If you feel that way, by all means practice medicine that way. But if you are involved in group studies comparing treatments, then you must have all the prognostic information, so that the patients can be stratified. Receptors will have to be measured – it is that simple.

I do not know what the final outcome will be in 5 years' time, but the only way we shall know at the end of that time is by making all these measurements.

D. Razis: If the population of the cancerous tissue in breast cancer is not homogeneous (and this has been established), theoretically both treatments should be given, hormonal treatment and chemotherapeutic treatment. This may not be important in advanced disease, but perhaps it makes the difference between cure and non-cure in adjuvant disease. When we become fanatic about receptors, perhaps there will be good results in the short-term but not such good results in the long run.

W.L. McGuire: I agree. Tumours are very heterogeneous. If we focus on chemotherapy alone or on endocrine therapy alone, only part of the problem is being addressed. We are in a learning stage; we must use all the available information.

W. Jonat (Bremen, Federal Republic of Germany): With regard to the quantification of receptor content, it has just been shown that the quantitative value of oestrogen receptors may be of importance for prognosis, with regard to disease-free interval. It has also been shown that the quantitative value is important in the prediction of the outcome of endocrine therapy. On the other hand, Joe Allegra has shown that the quantitative value is not of importance with regard to survival of patients. Can Professor McGuire comment on that, and perhaps also Dr Nomura who has survival data?

W.L. McGuire: We are getting away from the topic of adjuvant studies. Like most things in medicine, there are data on both sides of the question. If we wanted to spend time examining both sides, that could be done. I suspect, though, that Dr Jonat and I, and people who are interested, should discuss this privately and not during the meeting. It is controversial and no conclusion or consensus will be reached.

W. Jonat: That is exactly what I want to hear – that the question of quantification is still open.

W.L. McGuire: Quantification is important. It has been shown to be important by too many people. Allegra's data was obtained in many patients who already had metastatic disease, which would bias the result. We can criticize every study, including our own – however, there is not enough time.

Changing receptor status

W.L. McGuire

Something that perhaps many people here do not know about, and which should be discussed briefly, is changing receptor status.

In our series in San Antonio, 238 patients could be analysed. Simultaneous assays were done in 76 patients – simultaneous meaning that within one week 2 separate biopsies were made. Sequential assays were done in 167 patients where we could follow them and have 2 biopsies.

I will summarize the results. First, if 2 biopsies are taken from the same patient, either at the same time or within one week, the discordance rate is 17%.

Secondly, with regard to sequential therapies, the overall discordance rate is 24%. It is higher going from positive to negative oestrogen receptors, and less (in fact, almost the same as the simultaneous rate) going from negative to positive oestrogen receptors. It was interesting that it really did not matter whether the biopsy was taken from a lymph node, liver or wherever – the site of the biopsy did not affect the discordance rate, nor did the time interval. That surprised me: I would have thought that, if there was a receptor-positive primary tumour, the longer the interval before measuring the metastatic site the more likely it would be to turn negative – but that is not true, time was not a factor.

An attempt was made to analyse the effect of intervening therapies. There were some patients who had received no therapy, some had received chemotherapy, others chemo-endocrine therapy or endocrine therapy alone. There was no clear-cut pattern of the effect of therapy, with the exception of tamoxifen. If a patient had received tamoxifen within 2 months, the oestrogen receptor value invariably changed from positive to negative, and that is known to correlate fairly well with the pharmacokinetics.

Changing receptor status

P.M. Martin

I agree with Professor McGuire about the variation of results when repetitive measurements are performed in the same patient, but this variation tends to both plus and minus directions. Without therapy our results are similar to Professor McGuire's results. Under therapy and when tumour regrowth is present, however, our results differ.

Figure 1 shows the determination of the oestrogen receptors in the primary and the metastatic sites without therapy at the time of determination. We now have a correlation for 100 patients. However, this correlation is not linear (plus or minus 15% for 85% of patients).

Figures 2 and 3 represent 5 years' work. For each patient the results were determined before therapy, and after chemo- and radiotherapy when the

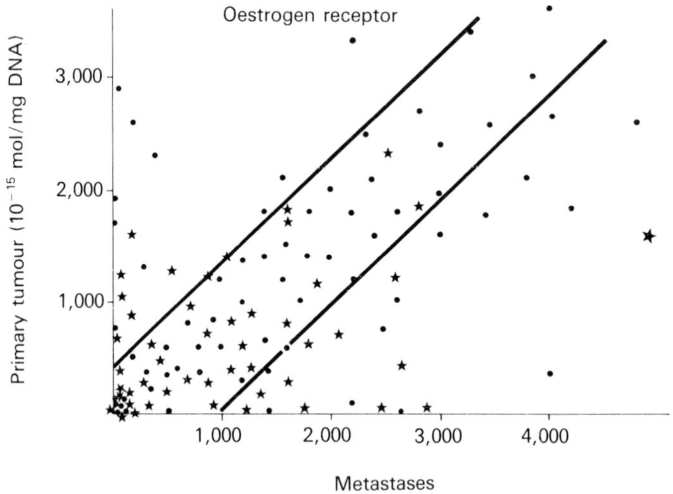

*Fig. 1. Correlation between primary tumours and metastatic sites without therapy; • = homogeneous cellular density; * = heterogeneous cellular density.*

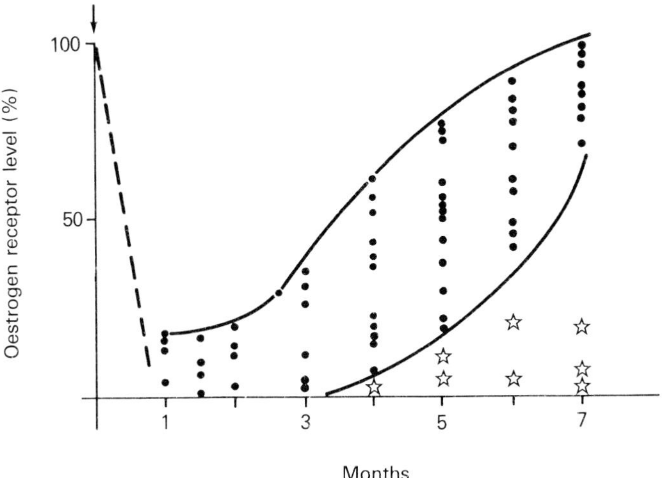

Fig. 2. Results obtained by comparison of the oestrogen receptor level in primary tumours (100%) with that in regrowing tumours (50%) after radiotherapy (in irradiated sites) from 1–7 months. (For symbol explanation, see Figure 1.)

tumour was regrowing (1–7 months). If the variation was only randomized, dispersion would have a variation (+ or −) for the second and third time, compared to the value of the first time (before therapy). In fact, after 2 months' chemo- or radiotherapy, the values we observed were always below those determined before therapy. It takes 4–6 months to get a correlation with the first determination. When the receptors are lower, short-time association of hormonotherapy with chemo- and/or radiotherapy is not performed under the most efficient conditions.

Figure 4 shows the receptor variation under hormonotherapy. At present, we have 28 patients treated with tamoxifen for progesterone receptor stimulation. Only one-third of these patients had a real stimulation of the progesterone receptors; we have never observed a zero stimulation. Every time we obtain a progesterone receptor stimulation, it appears that there was some progesterone receptor at a first determination if tamoxifen had been given for 2 weeks and a progesterone receptor had been analysed carefully.

Here is a good example of hormonotherapy screening of 2 patients who were given tamoxifen and MPA. What happened? First, there was a decrease of the oestrogen receptors under tamoxifen before MPA treatment and a rise of the progesterone receptors. The determination was made just before the MPA treatment and that gave an almost 2-fold increase of progesterone

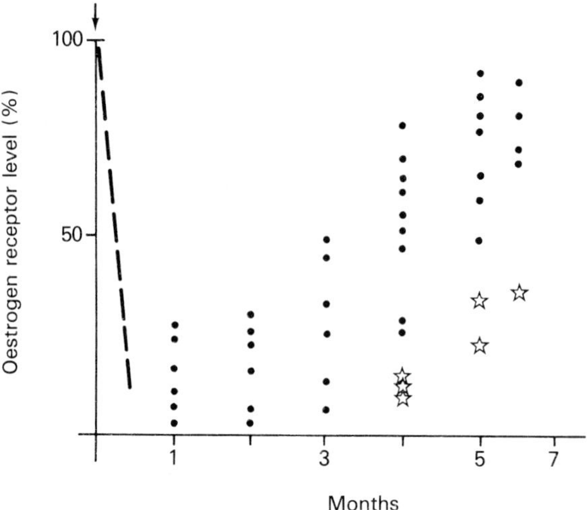

Fig. 3. Results obtained by comparison of the oestrogen receptor level in primary tumours (100%) with that in regrowing tumours (50%) after chemotherapy from 1–7 months. (For symbol explanation, see Figure 1.)

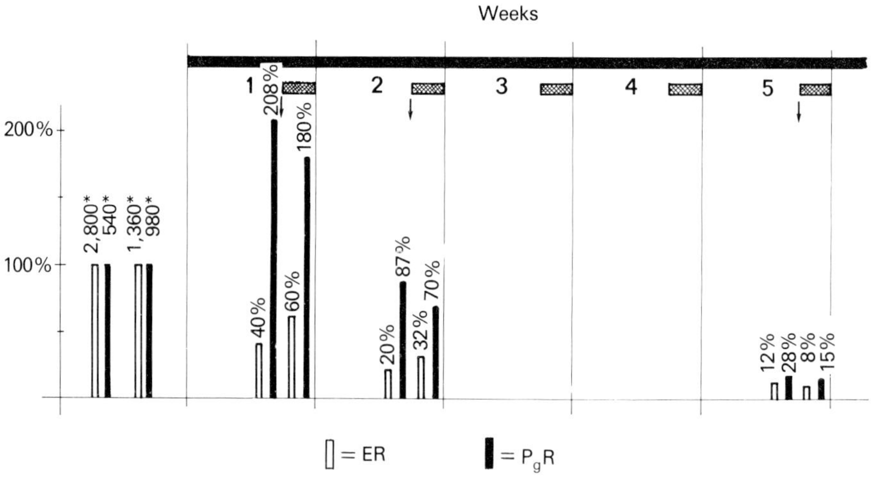

Fig. 4. Variation of the oestrogen and progesterone receptor (ER and PgR) levels under hormonotherapy; ▬ = continuously given tamoxifen; ▒ = discontinuously given MPA. The level determined before therapy is taken as 100% and the arrows indicate the timing for oestrogen receptor determination by micro-assay.

receptor. Under MPA treatment the progesterone receptor level decreased, but 4 and 5 months later under tamoxifen and MPA treatment, respectively, both the progesterone and oestrogen receptors decreased. These 2 patients no longer responded and the receptor assay at that time gave a very low value compared to the receptor status at the beginning. I think that timing is very important, and perhaps the second receptor determination helps to determine a good sequence of tamoxifen and MPA treatment for each patient. That is the reason we have developed a micro-assay for the oestrogen and progesterone receptors.

Changing receptor status

Y. Nomura

We have assayed oestrogen receptors (ER) in 940 breast cancer patients and progesterone receptors (PgR) in 773 patients.

The Figure shows the percentage of ER- and PgR-positive cancers in the malignancy stages – that is, primary tumours, first recurrence, second relapse and preterminal stages. The percentages of ER- and PgR-positive cancers in the metastatic regions at the time of the first recurrence are comparable to those of the primary tumours. However, after breast cancer had been treated with several kinds of therapy and malignancy progressed, the percentages of ER- and PgR-positive cancers clearly decreased. In the preterminal stages, only 20% of the cancers are ER-positive and only one of 29 tumours is PgR-positive. It may be that the hormone receptors in breast cancer tend to become negative, probably due to the treatment for or progression of the disease, but they remain positive in the first recurrence lesions in proportions similar to the primary tumours.

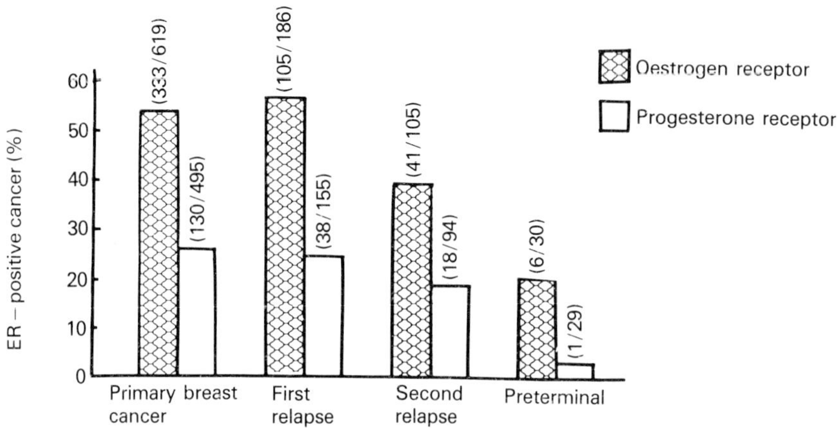

Figure. Proportion of ER-positive breast cancer during malignancy progression.

Sequential assays were carried out on primary and recurrence tumours in 42 patients. During the disease-free interval 63% (17/27) of ER-positive tumours remained positive, and all 15 ER-negative tumours remained negative, whereas 37% (10/27) of ER-positive tumours changed their status. The effects of adjuvant therapy seem to be inconclusive due to the limited number of patients. Changes in the combination of oestrogen and progesterone receptors indicate that changes from ER- and PgR-positive to ER- and PgR-negative or from ER-positive/PgR-negative to ER- and PgR-negative appear to be predominant – that is, progesterone receptor seems to be less stable.

Thirty-six patients were treated with adreno-oöphorectomy, anti-oestrogens, chemo-endocrine therapy or chemotherapy as a first-line therapy at the time of recurrence. When ER-positive tumours in the primary tumours remained positive in the recurrent tumours, endocrine therapy as well as chemotherapy was effective – except in cases given anti-oestrogens.

On the contrary, in patients whose tumours changed from ER-positive to ER-negative during a disease-free interval, neither endocrine nor chemo-endocrine therapy was effective.

The changes of oestrogen receptor content in advanced breast cancer during various kinds of treatment were investigated. In 38 patients there was an oestrogen receptor assay before the first-line treatment and also before the final therapy, after their having been subjected to more than 2 kinds of systemic treatment before the analysis. The time interval between the 2 oestrogen receptor assays varied from 2–82 months. Of 4 patients who had initially ER-positive assays, 19 (80%) lost their ER-positivity in the tumours after treatment. In only one of 14 ER-negative tumours did the oestrogen receptors became positive after therapy. Six of seven PgR-positive tumours

Table. Changes of oestrogen receptor contents in advanced breast cancer.

Treatment	Changes of oestrogen receptor			
	Positive → Positive	Positive → Negative	Negative → Positive	Negative → Negative
Anti-oestrogens	8 (53.3%)	7 (46.7%)	1 (16.7%)	5 (83.3%)
Adreno-oöphorectomy	7 (30.9%)	11 (61.1%)	0 (0%)	10 (100%)
Chemotherapy	5 (55.6%)	4 (44.4%)	3 (18.8%)	13 (81.2%)
Chemo-endocrine therapy	5 (33.3%)	10 (66.7%)	2 (20.0%)	8 (80.0%)
Between first and last treatment	5 (20.8%)	19 (79.2%)	1 (7.1%)	13 (92.9%)

became negative after therapy, and only one of 25 PgR-negative tumours became positive.

The Table shows the changes of oestrogen receptor content in 99 patients according to the type of treatment: anti-oestrogens, adreno-oöphorectomy, chemotherapy or chemo-endocrine therapy. Of these patients 56% (32/56) lost their ER-positivity during the treatment, whereas only 14% (6/42) of ER-negative tumours before therapy became positive after therapy. Thus, the apparent changes in ER-positivity are as follows: anti-oestrogens: 71–43%; adreno-oöphorectomy: 64–25%; chemotherapy: 36–32%; and chemo-endocrine therapy: 60–28%.

There was a most drastic change from ER-positive to -negative tumours by adreno-oöphorectomy or chemo-endocrine therapy, and by these treatments oestrogen receptor content also decreased significantly.

Discussion

W.L. McGuire: There is no doubt that receptors do change status.

A.T. van Oosterom (Leiden, The Netherlands): It is certain that the receptors in breast cancer change in about 20–25% of the patients. We heard earlier today (either in Dr Martin's or Dr Kauppila's presentation) that about 60% of the primary tumours in endometrial cancer are receptor-rich, but that in stage-III and stage-IV metastatic disease there are only about 10% receptor-rich tumours. Are there any data showing that in endometrial cancer the amount of receptor status change is higher than in breast cancer?

W.L. McGuire: Can anybody comment on endometrial carcinoma having very low or infrequent receptor content compared to the primary endometrial biopsy?

P.M. Martin: The problem is that in endometrium there is a lot of necrosis, and if we are not very careful in the determination many receptors are artificially lost.

A.T. van Oosterom: The response rate with MPA in endometrial cancer is 40%, so there is no good correlation between the receptor status and the response to this hormone treatment. If the receptor quality is so low in the tumour, I wonder whether an attempt might be made to raise it, for example, by pretreating metastatic endometrial cancer patients with tamoxifen, and giving them MPA afterwards.

W.L. McGuire: There is a fallacy with that, though. Who knows...?

A.T. van Oosterom: I do not know whether anybody is doing that, but it was suggested yesterday that the progesterone receptor can be increased by giving tamoxifen to the patients. When there is a tumour with a very poor receptor status, that procedure should be carried out to see whether it works.

W.L. McGuire: But does anyone know that the high-dose progestins (the low-dose may be another story) work through the progesterone receptor? Why is that assumption made?

A.T. van Oosterom: I hoped not to be asked that question!

W.L. McGuire: I do not think that there is any reason to assume that, when better responses are observed with very high MPA doses, the higher doses are necessarily working through the progesterone receptors.

F. von Eyben (Malmö, Sweden): What kind of biological impact does the change in receptor status have for those tumours in which such changes are observed, compared with those in which they are not?

W.L. McGuire: I do not think that anybody has analysed that yet – except that from Dr Nomura's slides it appeared that those patients who remained receptor positive had a better responsiveness to one or more of the endocrine therapies than those who changed. Is that correct, Dr Nomura?

Y. Nomura: Yes.

F. von Eyben: If I may return to what was discussed before about how long hormonal treatment should be given, Professor McGuire said that with tamoxifen there was a receptor change from positive to negative in 2 months. If I understood rightly, it was always seen...

W.L. McGuire: No, not always, but very frequently.

F. von Eyben: We, oncologists, mostly treat our patients until we see a relapse. That means that if we have an adjuvant trial we will stick to tamoxifen for one year and, if we listened to what Professor McGuire said, we might perhaps change the protocol to using it for 2 years. Then we get slightly confused, because the tumour receptor content has changed to negative.

W.L. McGuire: There are 3 ways to approach the receptors in a patient who has been on tamoxifen. The chances are that the receptor level in the cytoplasm will be low and unmeasurable – not always, but the chances are high. The progesterone receptor should be measured, because it may be elevated – that has been shown to be so enough times by enough people. If it is elevated, it should be used as we would use a high oestrogen receptor value. Alternatively, if there was a colleague working in an endocrine hormone research laboratory it would be possible to do a nuclear oestrogen receptor assay. Those are the only options.

A. Pellegrini: If I do not misunderstand you, you are saying that when high MPA doses are used they are certainly not working through receptors. Is that what you said, that the high MPA doses do not work through the progesterone receptors?

W.L. McGuire: For lack of any data showing that they do work through the progesterone receptors, I can give a number of theoretical reasons why they cannot.

A. Pellegrini: I agree completely. Do you think that oestrogen priming the progesterone receptors (as was mentioned earlier) can allow us to use lower doses, with less side-effects – perhaps with clinical improvement? This might be one of the reasons for the use of hormonal combination treatment.

W.L. McGuire: My bias is that the priming only identifies the patient who is likely to respond to MPA; in other words, it says that a patient is more likely to be an MPA-responder. I do not think that it increases the likelihood of response, but only identifies the patient; it is a marker.

F. von Eyben: Has an attempt been made to analyse another aspect – those patients who changed receptor status compared with those who did not? Was there anything different in how those patients were treated, so that in the future it would perhaps be possible to predict that if similar treatment was given to patients, those patients would be at a high risk of having receptor change compared with the other patients?

W.L. McGuire: That has been looked at and, as I said, we cannot find any patterns of response.

Receptors in non-classical tissues: analysis of oestrogen, gestagen and glucocorticoid receptors in human malignant melanoma

K. Pollow

Epidemiologic observations concerning possible hormonal influences on the survival of melanoma patients have been made (e.g., the differing prognosis favouring female patients' survival; the rarity of melanoma in prepubertal children; the improved prognosis for multiparous females; and the decline of prognosis in postmenopausal women). In addition, objective tumour regressions have occurred following additive and ablative hormonal manoeuvres.

Studies on the mechanism of action of steroid hormones have shown that cytoplasmic steroid receptors are a necessary, if not sufficient, requirement for steroid hormone responsiveness in target tissues. In the literature, at present only a few data are available about specific interaction between steroid hormones and receptor proteins in human melanomas [1–6]. Therefore, for further characterization we have analysed biopsy tumour specimens from patients with malignant melanoma for the presence of cytoplasmic receptors for oestradiol, progesterone and glucocorticoids.

For steroid hormone receptor quantification and characterization we used 2 techniques: first, a receptor assay based on a charcoal absorption procedure and Scatchard analysis of binding data; and secondly, a sucrose density gradient technique to further characterize the binding species for oestrogen. Sucrose density gradient analysis had to be performed because tyrosinase, present in most human melanomas, mimics oestrogen binding detected in melanoma cytosols. The binding of oestradiol to tyrosinase can be blocked by addition of an excess of L-dopa to the incubation mixture. Furthermore, sucrose density gradient analysis of ^{3}H-oestradiol binding to purified tyrosinase revealed binding with a sedimentation constant around 2.2 S, much lower than that of oestradiol receptor. We considered a negative receptor status to be lower than 5 fmol/mg of cytoplasmic protein. Separate oestrogen, progesterone and glucocorticoid binding activities were evaluated in a series of

32 patients with malignant melanoma (19 male, 13 female). Both primary and metastatic lesions from all sites were included in the study.

The Figure shows that 46% of females and only 26% of males had measurable oestrogen receptor activity. Progesterone receptor was detected in 30% of females but in 63% of males. Twenty-three out of 32 tumours showed ^{3}H-dexamethasone binding of less than 5 fmol/mg of protein.

The Table summarizes the mean values of binding capacity for oestradiol, R5020 and dexamethasone of the cytoplasmic fractions of various malignant

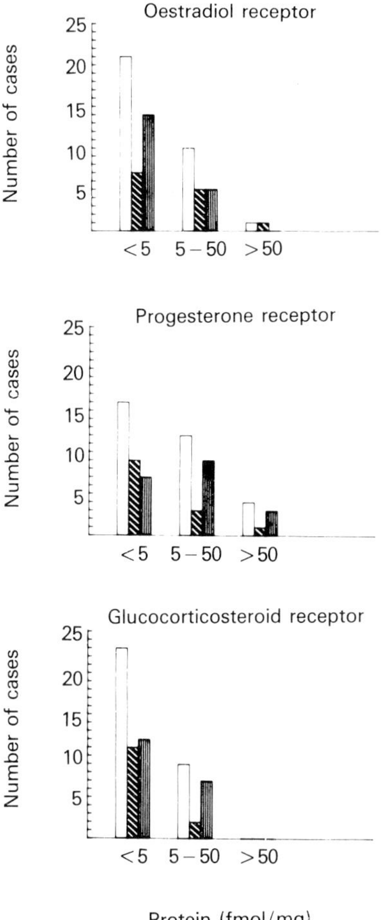

Figure. Distribution of oestrogen-, gestagen-, and glucocorticoid-receptor contents in human melanomas. □ = *total (n = 32);* ▧ = *female (n = 13);* ▥ = *male (n = 19).*

Table. Mean values of oestrogen, gestagen, and glucocorticoid receptors in human malignant melanomas.

	Oestradiol receptor	Progesterone receptor	Glucocorticoid receptor
Total	32	32	32
Arithmetic mean value			
(fmol/mg protein)	22.6	38.8	7.3
Range	0–107	0–362	0–43
Female	13	13	13
Arithmetic mean value			
(fmol/mg protein)	18.6	19.7	4.5
Range	0–107	0–194	0–39
Male	n = 19	n = 19	n = 19
Arithmetic mean value			
(fmol/mg protein)	4.5	52.3	9.1
Range	0–26.7	0–362	0–43

Human melanomas obtained from resections (tumour diagnosis was histologically verified) were directly brought to the laboratory and stored at −70° C until use. The tissues were minced, homogenized in PEM-buffer (10 mmol/l phosphate, 1.5 mmol/l EDTA, 5 mmol/l monothioglycerol, pH 7.5) using an all-glass homogenizer and centrifuged at 105,000 g to obtain cytosol. Due to the usually extremely small amounts of tissue, we decided to perform sucrose density gradient analysis together with a one-point receptor assay. Aliquots of cytosol were incubated in triplicates with: a. 8 nmol/l ^{3}H-estradiol alone (total binding) or together with a 200-fold excess of diethylstilboestrol (non-specific binding); b. 16 nmol/l ^{3}H-R5020 ± 200-fold R5020; and c. 16 nmol/l ^{3}H-dexamethasone ± 200-fold dexamethasone, respectively, for 6 h at 0–4° C. After adsorption of the unbound steroid with dextran-coated charcoal (DCC) and subsequent centrifugation, aliquots of the supernatants were removed and counted for radioactivity. When more than 200 mg of tissue were available, a 5-point titration assay with DCC separation and Scatchard plot analysis was performed [7]. In a similar setup aliquots for sucrose density gradient centrifugation were incubated and after DCC treatment 0.2 ml of each of the 6 fractions were layered onto a 5–20% sucrose gradient in the presence of L-dopa (2 μM/l). Centrifugation was performed in a swinging bucket rotor for 16 h at 50,000 rpm and 4° C. Protein concentrations were determined according to the method of Waddell using a Biorad protein standard [8].

melanomas tested in this study. The glucocorticoid receptor levels are low in all 32 tumour specimens.

Of particular note is the observation separating the results according to sex, in that in male tumour samples the mean value for oestrogen-binding activity is 4.5 compared to that of 18.6 in female samples. The values in male specimens ranged from 0–27, in females from 0–107. The mean value for progesterone receptors of melanomas deriving from females was 19.7, whereas the mean progesterone receptor concentration in male tumour samples investigated here was 52.3, which is surprisingly high. The values in male specimens ranged from 0–362, in females from 0–194.

Sucrose density gradient analysis of the oestradiol binding in the tumour cytosols confirmed the presence of saturable binding of this steroid hormone, which was observed by means of charcoal adsorption technique. In 8 of 11 oestrogen receptor-positive tissue samples, distinct 4 S peak could be detected in the sucrose gradient; whereas only 3 tumour samples were characterized by sedimenting of ^{3}H-oestradiol receptor complexes in the 4 S and 8 S region (data are not shown).

Finally we would like to say that studies in human breast cancer have shown that analysis of steroid hormone receptors in tumour specimens correlates significantly with the likelihood of an objective response following hormonal manipulation. Further studies will be necessary to determine whether a group of patients with malignant melanoma, who have a higher likelihood of response to endocrine manipulation, can be selected by steroid hormone receptor analysis.

References

1. Fisher, R.I., Neifeld, J.P. and Lippman, M.E. (1976): Oestrogen receptors in human malignant melanoma. *Lancet II*, 337.
2. Neifeld, J.P. and Lippman, M.E. (1980): Steroid hormone receptors and melanoma. *J. Invest. Dermatol. 74,* 379.
3. Karakousis, C.P., Lopez, R.E., Bhakoo, H.S. et al. (1980): Estrogen and progesterone receptors and tamoxifen in malignant melanoma. *Cancer Treat. Rep. 64,* 819.
4. Creagan, E.T., Ingle, J.N., Woods, J.E. et al. (1980): Estrogen receptors in patients with malignant melanoma. *Cancer 46,* 1785.
5. McCarty, K.S., Jr., Wortman, J., Stowers, S. et al. (1980): Sex steroid receptor analysis in human melanoma. *Cancer 46,* 1463.
6. Grill, H.J., Benes, P., Manz, B. et al. (1982): Steroid hormone receptors in human melanoma. *Arch. Dermatol. Res. 272,* 97.
7. Scatchard, D.G. (1949): The attraction of proteins for small molecules and ions. *Ann. N.Y. Acad. Sci. 51,* 660.
8. Waddell, W.J. (1956): A simple ultraviolet spectrophotometric method for the determination of proteins. *J. Lab. Clin. Med. 48,* 311.

Receptors in non-classical tissues

S. Saez

I want briefly to discuss the existence of steroid hormone receptors in 2 types of epithelia which are not usually considered as target tissues – but which really are target tissues.

The first site is the larynx mucosa and the second is the bladder mucosa. In the larynx specific binding was found for androgen in normal mucosa in both sexes, and there was the same kind of binding in tumours developed in this area (Figure).

Table I shows the amount of binding sites found in male and female larynx or pharynx normal mucosa and also in the epithelioma.

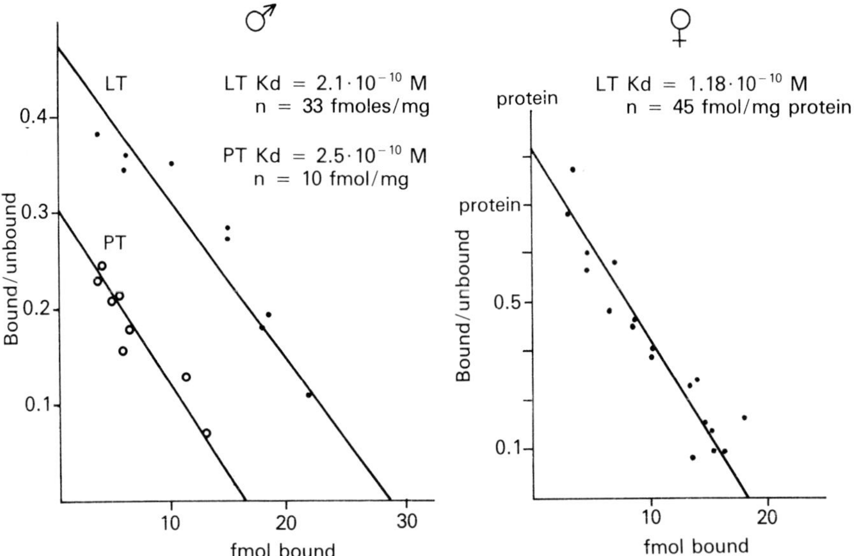

Figure. Scatchard plot of the binding of ^{3}H-DHT by the cytosol obtained from larynx (LT) and pharynx epithelioma (PT) in male and female. Reproduced with permission of the Editors from Steroid Receptors and the Management of Cancer Vol. I. CRC Press, 1979.

Table I. ^{3}H-DHT binding assay by larynx and pharynx epithelioma.

Epithelioma	Number of cases	Receptor content (fmol/mg protein)	Dissociation constant (10^{-10} M)
Male larynx	2	32–59	2.0 –2.1
Male pharynx	5	10–28	2.5 –2.7
Female larynx	2	33–45	1.18–2.1

The number of receptor sites and the dissociation constant have been calculated by the procedure of Scatchard. The numbers represent the range of values found. Reproduced with permission of the Editors from *Steroid Receptors and the Management of Cancer,* Vol. I. CRC Press, 1979.

Table II. Oestradiol and progesterone receptor data on bladder mucosa.

		Bound oestradiol (fmol/mg protein)	Sucrose gradient		Bound R5020 (fmol/mg protein)
Females					
Trigone area	Case 1	84	8S	Displaced	22
	Case 2	24	4S	ND	0
	Case 3	120	8S	Displaced	42
	Case 4	21	8S	Displaced	12
	Case 5	18	8S	Displaced	0
	Case 6	39	4S-8S	Displaced	12
	Case 7	20	8S	Displaced	0
	Case 8	12	4S	Displaced	0
	Case 9	0		0	0
	Case 10	0	8S	Displaced	0
Limit of the trigone	Case 11	0		ND	0
	Case 12	0		ND	0
Dome Males	10 Cases	0			0
	1 Case	30		8S	ND
Trigone area	7 Cases	0		ND	0
Dome	10 Cases	0			0
Tissue underlying the mucosa	10 Cases	0			0

ND = not displaced

Reproduced with permission of the editor from Saez, S. and Martin, P.R. (1981): Evidence of estrogen receptors in the trigone area of human urinary bladder. *Biochemistry 15,* 317.

Table II shows the binding data in one specific region of the bladder mucosa, the trigone, which is of the same embryonic origin as the vagina and which responds to hormones in the same way as does the vagina. Specific binding for oestradiol and progesterone was found in the majority of the females, but in fewer of the males. This specific binding was located only in the trigone, and was not found outside that region. The only link between these 2 kinds of data, on larynx and bladder, is that cancer may develop in these 2 areas which, in many cases, is determined by chemical carcinogenesis.

In the primary cancer of the larynx we found some effect of steroid hormones on the growth of the tumours, and some regulation of the tumour with anti-androgen treatment. However, in the bladder, there are no data on the effect of steroid hormones on the growth of these tumours. It is only in the experimental situation that some effect of the hormones on chemical carcinogenesis can be observed.

Receptors in non-classical tissues

D. Zava

I would like briefly to discuss the potential artifacts that can result when using the classic dextran-charcoal (DCC) assay system to assess the oestrogen receptor content in malignant melanoma. Let me first present a brief background on a unique biochemical property of the malignant melanocyte that is relevant to the measurement of the oestrogen receptor in malignant melanomas by the DCC assay. Both benign and malignant melanocytes often contain copious amounts of the enzyme tyrosinase which catalyzes the oxidative degradation of a wide spectrum of phenols to orthocatechols and then to the corresponding orthoquinones. The natural substrate for tyrosinase is tyrosine; however, many other phenols are oxidized by the same enzymatic pathway. In fact, tyrosinase has been shown to attack the phenolic A ring of oestradiol, hydroxylating it first to 2-hydroxyoestradiol and then oxidizing it to the corresponding orthoquinone of 2-hydroxyoestradiol (Figure). In the process of hydroxylation the 2-position hydrogen atom of the A ring of oestradiol is

Determination of oestrogen receptor by DCC assay system

	$(2,4,6,7-{}^3H)$ – oestradiol	$(6,7-{}^3H)$ – oestradiol
Breast tumour	196	225
Tyrosinase	973	38

Tyrosinase catalyzed hydroxylation and oxidation of $(2,4,6,7-{}^3H)$ – oestradiol liberated from the substrate in the form of water. One molecule of water is formed for each molecule of oestradiol hydroxylated. Since the 2-position hydrogen of (2,4,6,7–^{3}H)-oestradiol, but not (6,7–^{3}H)-oestradiol is tritium-substituted, the water liberated from the enzymatic attack of tyrosinase on the 4-labeled oestradiol is consequently tritium-labeled and thus will be resistant to DCC adsorption. We did a very simple experiment to illustrate this point, which was to incubate a breast tumour cytosol or purified tyrosinase with either (2,4,6,7–^{3}H)-oestradiol or (6,7–^{3}H)-oestradiol. After a specific time course of incubation, DCC was added to remove free (^{3}H)-oestradiol. The results demonstrate that near equimolar binding sites were present with the breast cytosols (196 vs. 225 fmol/100 μl cytosol), whereas in the presence of tyrosinase DCC-resistant binding was seen only in the presence of the 4-labeled oestradiol (973 vs. 38 fmol/100 μl cytosol). Since the 2- and 4-labeled oestradiols are identical in molecular structure and differ only in that the 2- and 4-position hydrogen atoms in the A ring of oestradiol are substituted by tritium, it may be inferred that the DCC-resistant radioactivity resulting from the interaction of tyrosinase with the 4-labeled oestradiol reflects the liberation of tritium from the 2-position A ring of 4-labeled oestradiol.

Discussion

W.L. McGuire: Professor Pollow, you did not use the 2,4,6,7-oestradiol, did you?

K. Pollow: Yes, we used 2,4,6,7-oestradiol as radioactive ligand for receptor measurement. It is clear that many malignant melanomas, producing melanin, are rich in tyrosinase, and that this enzyme is capable of binding [^{3}H]-oestradiol. But this binding is depressed by diethylstilboestrol and by L-dopa, respectively. Therefore, it is necessary to analyse oestradiol receptor in human malignant melanomas in the presence of L-dopa.

D. Zava: Here it should be emphasized that in previous studies on oestrogen receptor in malignant melanoma, the (2,4,6,7–^{3}H)-oestradiol was employed as the binding ligand. Thus the radio-activity resistant to DCC absorption after incubation of (2,4,6,7–^{3}H)-oestradiol with extracts of malignant melanoma containing tyrosinase may represent tritiated water rather than the tight binding of (^{3}H)-oestradiol to oestrogen receptor. We have done additional work with this system and have observed that the apparent binding present only with the 4-labeled oestradiol is abolished with diethylstilboestrol and with hydroxytamoxifen. In addition, we have found that the highly reactive orthoquinones of either the 2- or 4-labeled oestradiols are able to covalently complex with the nucleophilic groups of many different cellular molecules such as the sulphydryl groups of monothioglycerol, glutathione and bovine serum albumin. Each of these molecules was able to form covalent adducts with the quinones of either the 2-or 4-labeled oestradiols. In addition, these radioactive conjugates could be separated by sucrose gradients as 2S (glutathione) to 4S (BSA) components. Our conclusions are that if malignant melanoma does contain oestrogen receptor as described in breast cancer it will be extremely difficult to distinguish it from the products resulting from the interaction of tyrosinase with radio-labeled oestradiol. Furthermore, it is our belief that the oestradiol binding profiles previously reported by others in malignant melanoma more closely resembles the products resulting from the tyrosinase-catalyzed degradation of (^{3}H)-oestradiol to DCC-resistant radio-labeled products, [(^{3}H)-water and (^{3}H)-oestradiol-covalent adducts] rather than the binding of (^{3}H)-oestradiol to a true oestrogen receptor entity.

Concerning the use of L-dopa and the sucrose density gradient technique to assess the oestrogen receptor in malignant melanoma, several points should be emphasized. First, L-dopa stimulates the tyrosinase hydroxylation reaction in addition to acting as a competitive inhibitor of the same reaction at higher concentrations. Therefore, in the presence of excess L-dopa even minuscule amounts of (^{3}H)-oestradiol may be metabolized to (^{3}H)-water and covalent (^{3}H)-oestradiol adducts over a prolonged time course of incubation. Second, the covalent adducts of (^{3}H)-oestradiol that do form would be identified as a pseudo-oestradiol binding component by sucrose gradient analysis.

I have presented evidence to indicate that the apparent (^{3}H)-oestradiol binding component of extracts of malignant melanoma is not an authentic oestrogen receptor. Our data corroborates studies showing that the presence of this putative oestrogen receptor in malignant melanoma is not correlated to response of this disease to anti-oestrogen (tamoxifen) therapy. In breast cancer cells there is a true oestradiol binding protein, the oestradiol receptor, which mediates the biological effects of oestrogens and anti-oestrogens on these cells. In malignant melanoma, however, oestrogen receptor is probably not present. However, the oestradiol is a substrate for the enzyme tyrosinase, which is present in copious amounts within the malignant melanocyte. This enzyme system could potentially convert oestradiol or other hydroxy-compounds such as hydroxy-tamoxifen, into highly electrophilic compounds which could invoke cell damage or death selectively within the malignant melanocyte. Thus the antitumour effect seen with tamoxifen may be due to the tyrosinase-catalyzed oxidation of these otherwise innocuous drugs to harmful electrophiles.

G. Beretta: Has Dr Zava performed similar studies for progestin, androgen and glucocorticoid receptors? It is well-known, and has been published by the NCI group (Bethesda), that those types of receptors are present within melanoma cells.

D. Zava: No, we have not examined extracts of malignant melanoma for progestin, androgen or glucocorticoid receptors. However, I have found that neither progestins, androgens nor glucocorticoids are substrates for tyrosinase.

G. Beretta: I would like to take this opportunity to summarize the present data available in the literature, and my own experience carried out at the Medical Oncology Department of San Carlo Borromeo Hospital in Milan, concerning the results of hormonotherapy in malignant melanoma.

Data indicating a possible hormonoresponsiveness are: occasional reports on the influence of sex and pregnancy on the course of melanoma; the objective responses published after hormonal therapy (pregnane, diethylstilboestrol, i.m. medroxyprogesterone acetate (MPA), tamoxifen); and the evidence of oestrogen, progesterone and androgen receptors in both primary and metastatic melanoma.

In my group, we administered MPA at doses of 400–1,000 mg/day, continuously, to dacarbazine and/or nitrosourea-resistant patients. In 16 evaluable cases, we have obtained 2 partial responses of 2 and 5 months, and 4 stabilizations of 2 months, according to the WHO criteria. The median survival of all treated patients was 3 months, and of responders this was in excess of 5 months.

On the whole, considering also our previous experience with i.m. MPA after hormonotherapy in advanced metastatic melanoma, we have observed a 9.6% objective response in 31 evaluable patients. Partial responses were seen solely in females with soft tissue metastases, but NC was seen also in visceral metastases. There was no response, nor protection, as seen against brain localizations.

To conclude, MPA is active against malignant melanoma as 2nd- and 3rd-line treatments, and also is well tolerated, frequently with subjective benefits. The 10% response rate appears appreciable in this poorly responsive neoplasia, in which any 2nd-line chemotherapy usually induces objective responses in 5–8% of adequately treated patients. Further studies are necessary to elucidate: the activity of MPA as 1st-line therapy (eventually associated with dacarbazine and/or nitrosourea); the response rate after MPA in oestrogen and progesterone receptor-containing tumours; and the essence of mechanisms of action of this antitumour compound.

J.G.M. Klijn (Rotterdam, The Netherlands): There are some reports about a receptor for vitamin D in melanoma cells. Does Dr Zava know whether there is a relationship between the presence of a receptor for vitamin D and the presence of oestradiol and progesterone receptors?

D. Zava: I know of no correlation between vitamin D receptor and oestradiol and progesterone receptors in malignant melanoma.

W.L. McGuire: Vitamin D receptors are now being found in breast cancer and elsewhere.

Authors' index